Difficult Decisions in Digestive Diseases

Jamie S. Barkin, M.D., F.A.C.P., F.A.C.G.
Professor of Medicine
University of Miami School of Medicine
Chief, Division of Gastroenterology
Mount Sinai Medical Center
Miami, Florida

Arvey I. Rogers, M.D., F.A.C.P., F.A.C.G.
Professor of Medicine
University of Miami School of Medicine
Chief, Division of Gastroenterology
Veterans Administration Medical Center
Miami, Florida

YEAR BOOK MEDICAL PUBLISHERS, INC.
Chicago • London • Boca Raton

Copyright © 1989 by Year Book Medical Publishers, Inc. All rights reserved. No part of this publication may be reproduced, stored in a retrieval system, or transmitted, in any form or by any means—electronic, mechanical, photocopying, recording, or otherwise—without prior written permission from the publisher. Printed in the United States of America.

1 2 3 4 5 6 7 8 9 0 KE 93 92 91 90 89

Library of Congress Cataloging-in-Publication Data

Difficult decisions in digestive diseases.

   Includes bibliographies and index.
   1. Digestive organs—Diseases.   2. Gastroenterology—
Decision making.   I. Barkin, Jamie S.   II. Rogers,
Arvey, 1934–   . [DNLM: 1. Digestive System
Diseases—diagnosis.   2. Digestive System Diseases—
therapy.   WI 141 0569]
RC802.D52   1989   616.3   88-14239
ISBN 0-8151-0514-2

Sponsoring Editor: Richard H. Lampert
Assistant Director, Manuscript Services: Frances M. Perveiler
Project Manager: Carol A. Reynolds

$65.00

THE OTTO C. BRANTIGAN, M.D.
MEDICAL LIBRARY
SAINT JOSEPH HOSPITAL
7620 YORK ROAD
TOWSON, MD. 21204

RC
802
.D52
1989
89-121

Difficult Decisions
in Digestive Diseases

This book is dedicated to our colleagues, who over the years have taught us how and assisted us in making difficult decisions in digestive diseases; and to our students, who always ask the difficult questions.

Contributors

Ira Agatstein, M.D.
Senior GI Fellow
University of Miami School of Medicine
Mount Sinai Medical Center
Miami, Florida

Naurang M. Agrawal, M.D.
Professor, Tulane Medical School
New Orleans, Louisiana

Peter A. Banks, M.D.
Professor of Medicine
Tufts University School of Medicine
Harvard Medical School
Chief of Gastroenterology
St. Elizabeth's Hospital of Boston
Beth Israel Hospital
Boston, Massachusetts

Jamie S. Barkin, M.D.
Professor of Medicine
University of Miami School of Medicine
Chief, Division of Gastroenterology
Mount Sinai Medical Center
Miami, Florida

Stanley Bernard Benjamin, M.D.
Associate Professor of Medicine
Georgetown University
Chief, Gastroenterology
Georgetown University Hospital
Washington, D.C.

Leslie H. Bernstein, M.D.
Professor of Medicine
Director of G.I.
Albert Einstein College of Medicine
Program Director in Gastroenterology
Bronx Municipal Hospital Center
Montefiore Medical Center
Bronx, New York

John H. Bond, M.D.
Professor of Medicine
University of Minnesota
Chief, Gastroenterology Section
Minneapolis Veterans Administration
  Medical Center
Minneapolis, Minnesota

Lawrence J. Brandt, M.D.
Professor of Medicine
Albert Einstein College of Medicine
Director, Division of Gastroenterology
Montefiore Medical Center
Bronx, New York

Frank P. Brooks, M.D., Sc.D.(med)
Professor of Medicine and Physiology
University of Pennsylvania School of
  Medicine
Acting Chief, Gastrointestinal Section
Hospital of the University of
  Pennsylvania
Philadelphia, Pennsylvania

Lawrence B. Cohen, M.D., F.A.C.P.
Assistant Clinical Professor of Medicine
Mount Sinai School of Medicine of the
  City University of New York
Assistant Attending
Mount Sinai Hospital
New York City, New York

Sidney Cohen, M.D.
Professor of Medicine
Temple University School of Medicine
Chairman, Department of Medicine
Temple University Hospital
Philadelphia, Pennsylvania

Ghislain Devroede, M.D.
Professor of Surgery
Centre Hospitalier
Universitaire de Sherbrooke
Sherbrooke, Quebec, Canada

Harold O. Douglass Jr., M.D., F.A.C.S.
Associate Professor of Research Surgery
State University of New York at Buffalo
Associate Chief in Charge: Upper GI Oncology
Roswell Park Memorial Institute
Buffalo, New York

Murray Epstein, M.D.
Professor of Medicine
University of Miami School of Medicine
Associate Director
Nephrology Section
Veterans Administration Medical Center
Jackson Memorial Medical Center
Miami, Florida

Atilla Ertan, M.D.
Professor of Medicine and Physiology
Tulane University School of Medicine
Chief, Section of Gastroenterology
Tulane University Hospital
Veterans Administration Medical Center
New Orleans, Louisiana

Richard G. Farmer, M.D., M.S., F.A.C.P.
Chairman, Division of Medicine
Cleveland Clinic Foundation
Cleveland, Ohio

Michael J. Fisher, M.D.
Fellow, Division of Gastroenterology
University of Virginia School of Medicine
Charlottesville, Virginia

Robert S. Fisher, M.D.
Professor of Medicine
Temple University School of Medicine
Chief of Gastroenterology Section
Director, Functional Gastroenterology Tissues Section
Temple University Hospital
Philadelphia, Pennsylvania

Charles F. Frey, M.D.
Professor and Vice Chairman
University of California at Davis
Attending Surgeon
University of California at Davis Medical Center
Martinez Veterans Administration Hospital
Sacramento, California

Hans Fromm, M.D.
Professor of Medicine
Director, Division of Gastroenterology and Nutrition
George Washington University
George Washington University Medical Center
Washington, D.C.

John T. Galambos, M.D.
Professor of Medicine
Director, Division of Digestive Diseases
Emory University School of Medicine
Consultant, Emory University Hospital
Grady Memorial Hospital
Atlanta, Georgia

J.E. Geenen, M.D.
Clinical Professor of Medicine
Medical College of Wisconsin
Director, Digestive Disease Center
St. Luke's Hospital
Racine, Wisconsin
Froedtert Memorial Lutheran Hospital
Milwaukee, Wisconsin
Trinity Memorial Hospital
Cudahy, Wisconsin

Stephen G. Gerzof, M.D., F.A.C.R.
Professor of Radiology
Tufts University School of Medicine
Chief, Body CT
Boston Veterans Administration Medical Center
Boston, Massachusetts

Robert I. Goldberg, M.D., F.A.C.P.,
F.A.C.G.
Assistant Professor of Medicine
University of Miami School of Medicine
Associate, Division of Gastroenterology
Mount Sinai Medical Center
Miami, Florida

David Y. Graham, M.D.
Professor of Medicine
Professor of Virology
Baylor College of Medicine
Chief, Digestive Disease
Veterans Administration Medical Center
Houston, Texas

Norton J. Greenberger, M.D.
Professor and Chairman
Department of Medicine
University of Kansas College of Health
  Sciences and Hospital
Kancas City, Kansas

Steven E. Hahn, M.D.
Senior Fellow in Gastroenterology
University of Miami School of Medicine
Jackson Memorial Hospital
Miami Veterans Administration Hospital
University of Miami Hospital and Clinics
Miami, Florida

Lemuel Herrera, M.D., M.A., F.A.C.S.
Assistant Professor of Surgery
State University of New York at Buffalo
Cancer Research Surgeon
Roswell Park Memorial Institute
Buffalo, New York

Walter J. Hogan, M.D.
Professor of Medicine
Medical College of Wisconsin
Director, GI Diagnostic Lab
Froedtert Memorial Lutheran Hospital
Milwaukee County Medical Complex
Veterans Administration Hospital
Milwaukee, Wisconsin

Valerie J. C. Jagiella, M.D.
Fellow, Gastroenterology
Medical College of Georgia
Augusta, Georgia

Graham H. Jeffries, M.D., F.A.C.P.
University Professor of Medicine
Pennsylvania State University College of
  Medicine
University Hospital
Milton S. Hershey Medical Center
Hershey, Pennsylvania

Matin H. Kalser, M.D., Ph.D.
Professor of Medicine
Chief, Division of Gastroenterology
University of Miami School of Medicine
Director, University of Miami Hospital
  and Clinics
Miami, Florida

Keith A. Kelly, M.D.
Professor of Surgery
Department of Surgery
Mayo Medical School
Rochester, Minnesota

David Kelsen, M.D.
Associate Professor of Medicine
Cornell University Medical College
Associate Member
Memorial Sloan-Kettering Cancer Center
New York City, New York

Burton I. Korelitz, M.D.
Clinical Professor of Medicine
New York Medical College
Chief, Section of Gastroenterology
Department of Medicine
Lenox Hill Hospital
New York City, New York

Edwin N. Larkai, M.D.
Baylor College of Medicine
Veterans Administration Medical Center
Houston, Texas

Nicholas F. LaRusso, M.D.
Professor of Medicine
Associate Professor of Biochemistry and
  Molecular Biology
Mayo Medical School and Foundation
Rochester, Minnesota

Glen A. Lehman, M.D., F.A.C.P.
Professor of Medicine
Indiana University School of Medicine
Director of Clinical Gastroenterology
Indiana University Hospital
Indianapolis, Indiana

x / CONTRIBUTORS

Gary M. Levine, M.D.
Professor of Medicine
Temple University School of Medicine
Head, Division of Gastroenterology and Nutrition
Albert Einstein Medical Center
Philadelphia, Pennsylvania

Michael D. Levitt, M.D.
Professor of Medicine
University of Minnesota
Associate Chief of Staff for Research
Veterans Administration Medical Center
Minneapolis, Minnesota

Pedro P. Llaneza, M.D.
Diplomate, American Board of Internal Medicine
Diplomate, American Board of Gastroenterology
Attending, Baptist Hospital
Miami, Florida

Mauro Malavolti, M.D.
George Washington University School of Health Sciences
George Washington University Medical Center
Washington, D.C.

Richard M. McCallum, M.D., F.A.C.P., F.R.A.C.P. (Aust), F.A.C.G.
Professor of Medicine
Chief, Division of Gastroenterology
University of Virginia School of Medicine
Charlottesville, Virginia

Denis M. McCarthy, M.D., M.Sc., F.A.C.P.
Professor of Medicine
University of New Mexico
Chief of Gastroenterology
Veterans Administration Medical Center
Albuquerque, New Mexico

Thomas J. McGarrity, M.D.
Assistant Professor of Medicine
Pennsylvania State University
Assistant Professor of Medicine/ Gastroenterology
Milton S. Hershey Medical Center
Hershey, Pennsylvania

Angela Merlo, M.D., Ph.D.
Instructor, Temple University School of Medicine
Staff, Temple University Hospital
Philadelphia, Pennsylvania

Kevin P. Morrissey, M.D.
Clinical Associate Professor of Surgery
Cornell Medical College
Associate Attending Surgeon
The New York Hospital
New York City, New York

Nicholas J. Petrelli, M.D., F.A.C.S.
Assistant Professor of Surgery
State University of New York at Buffalo
Associate Chief, Colorectal Service
Roswell Park Memorial Institute
Buffalo, New York

John L. Petrini, Jr., M.D.
Associate Clinical Professor of Medicine
University of Southern California
Sansum Medical Clinic
Cottage Hospital
Santa Barbara, California

Richard S. Phillips, M.D., F.A.C.P., F.A.C.G.
Assistant Professor of Medicine
University of Miami School of Medicine
Associate, Division of GI
Mount Sinai Medical Center
Miami, Florida

Sigismund Stanley Pikul II, M.D.
Chief Resident of Surgery
Department of Surgery
University of California at Davis Medical Center
Sacramento, California

Jacques Poisson, M.D.
Professor of Surgery
University of Sherbrooke
Faculty of Medicine
Sherbrooke, Quebec, Canada

Daniel H. Present, M.D.
Associate Clinical Professor
Mount Sinai School of Medicine of the City University of New York
Associate Attending, Medicine
GI Division
Mount Sinai Hospital
New York City, New York

K. Rajender Reddy, M.D.
Assistant Professor of Medicine
University of Miami School of Medicine
Veterans Administration Medical Center
Miami, Florida

Joel E. Richter, M.D.
Associate Professor of Medicine/
　Gastroenterology
Bowman Gray School of Medicine at
　Wake Forest University
Staff Gastroenterologist
North Carolina Baptist Hospital
Winston-Salem, North Carolina

Robert H. Riddell, M.D., F.R.C.Path,
　F.R.C.P.(C)
Professor of Pathology
McMaster University
Chief of Service
Anatomical Pathology
Chedoke-McMaster Hospitals
Hamilton, Ontario, Canada

William Gardner Rowell, M.D.
Fellow, Department of Medicine
Division of Gastroenterology
University of Florida
Shands Hospital
Gainesville Veterans Administration
　Hospital
Gainesville, Florida

William B. Salt II, M.D.
Clinical Associate Professor of Medicine
Ohio State University
Director, Gastroenterology Laboratory
Director of Education in Gastroenterology
Mount Carmel Medical Center
Columbus, Ohio

Jean-Claude Schang, M.D.
Assistant Professor of Surgery
University of Sherbrooke
Faculty of Medicine
Sherbrooke, Quebec, Canada

Bernard M. Schuman, M.D.
Professor of Medicine
Medical College of Georgia
Professor of Medicine
Medical College of Georgia Hospital and
　Clinics
Augusta, Georgia

Sheila Sherlock, D.B.E., M.D.
Professor of Medicine
Royal Free Hospital School of Medicine
Consultant Physician
Royal Free Hospital
London, England

Jerome H. Siegel, M.D., F.A.C.P.,
　F.A.C.G.
Associate Clinical Professor of Medicine
Mount Sinai School of Medicine of the
　City University of New York
Chief, Gastroenterology
Doctors Hospital
New York City, New York

Stephen E. Silvis, M.D.
Professor of Medicine
University of Minnesota
Staff Physician in Gastroenterology
Veterans Administration Medical Center
Minneapolis, Minnesota

Michael V. Sivak, Jr., M.D.
Head, Section of Gastrointestinal
　Endoscopy
Department of Gastroenterology
Cleveland Clinic Foundation
Cleveland, Ohio

Stuart Jon Spechler, M.D.
Associate Professor of Medicine
Boston University School of Medicine
Associate Chief of Gastroenterology
Boston Veterans Administration Medical
　Center
Boston, Massachusetts

John E. Stone, M.D.
Assistant Professor of Medicine
Division of Gastroenterology
Medical College of Wisconsin
Staff Physician
Milwaukee County Regional Medical
　Center
Froedtert Memorial Lutheran Hospital
Milwaukee, Wisconsin

Francis J. Tedesco, M.D.
Professor of Medicine
Medical College of Georgia
Chief, Section of Gastroenterology
Medical College of Georgia Hospital and
　Clinics
Augusta, Georgia

W. Grant Thompson, M.D., F.R.C.P.(C)
Professor of Medicine
Assistant Dean, Clinical Affairs
University of Ottawa
Chief, Division of Gastroenterology
Ottawa Civic Hospital
Ottawa, Ontario, Canada

Phillip P. Toskes, M.D.
Professor of Medicine
University of Florida College of Medicine
Director, Division of Gastroenterology,
 Hepatology and Nutrition
Shands Hospital
Gainesville Veterans Administration
 Medical Center
Gainesville, Florida

David H. Van Thiel, M.D.
Professor of Medicine
Chief of Gastroenterology
University of Pittsburgh School of
 Medicine
Chief of Gastroenterology
Presbyterian University Hospital
Pittsburgh, Pennsylvania

Arnold Wald, M.D.
Associate Professor of Medicine
University of Pittsburgh School of
 Medicine
Head, Gastroenterology Division
Montefiore Hospital
Pittsburgh, Pennsylvania

Jerome D. Waye, M.D.
Clinical Professor of Medicine
Mount Sinai Medical Center
Attending Physician
Mt. Sinai Hospital
Lenox Hill Hospital
New York City, New York

Russell H. Wiesner, M.D.
Associate Professor of Medicine
Mayo Clinic and Mayo Foundation
Rochester, Minnesota

Bruce G. Wolff, M.D.
Assistant Professor of Surgery
Consultant in Colon, Rectal and General
 Surgery
Mayo Medical School
Consultant, Rochester Methodist
 Hospital and Saint Marys Hospital
Rochester, Minnesota

Preface

You would be justified in asking, "Why another textbook dealing with digestive diseases when there are so many already available?" The motivation to put forth the effort required to produce a textbook derives from any one or several sources and for as many reasons, both personal and professional. We would like to believe that our source was reliable and our reasons sound. We were the source. It was our perception that excellent texts already published did not fulfill an existing need in the study of digestive diseases: to provide expert "opinions" on specific issues that every day challenge professionals delivering health care. We all must make difficult management decisions. Each of us does so differently. It is comforting for many to know that we have colleagues with special expertise to whom we can look for guidance when necessary. Our patients, students, and colleagues frequently ask us, "What would you do in this situation?" Reaching a rational decision is not always easy. It is one thing to consult a textbook filled with useful facts written by experts, and yet still another to be able to apply those facts in the best way to resolve a difficult decision. It was our goal to make a textbook available that could provide immediate "consultation" or provide answers to questions most frequently asked in the management of patients with digestive disorders. In doing so, we felt we might facilitate the process of making *difficult decisions in digestive diseases*.

At the personal level, we thought it would be a challenge to tackle the task we envisioned, working together amicably and effectively in the process, and to interrelate with our many colleagues and friends across the country who would bring the idea to fruition.

We have not deluded ourselves into believing we have compiled a definitive list of difficult decisions. Rather, we would like to believe that we have included the majority of the more common management decisions we face. Nor have we included every expert as an author; this would have been impossible. We hope you will find *Difficult Decisions in Digestive Diseases* to be a reader-friendly consultant, a colleague in print who will provide comfort when you need it most.

The editors thank Ms Shirley Vance for her superb assistance in the completion of this book.

Jamie S. Barkin, M.D.
Arvey I. Rogers, M.D.

Contents

Preface

I
Esophagus 1

1
Chest Pain: Is the esophagus responsible? 3
JOEL E. RICHTER

2
Heartburn: What is an appropriate evaluation? 18
ANGELA MERLO, SIDNEY COHEN

3
Achalasia: What are the indications for medical or surgical approaches? ... 28
MICHAEL J. FISHER, RICHARD W. McCALLUM

4
Barrett's Esophagus: What should be done to reduce anxiety? 45
STUART JON SPECHLER

5
Esophageal Cancer: Who should be treated, and how? 55
DAVID KELSEN

II
Stomach and Duodenum 63

6
Gastroparesis: How should gastric emptying be assessed, and how should problems be managed? 65
ROBERT FISHER

7
Gastritis: Is it a distinct clinical entity? 74
THOMAS J. McGARRITY, GRAHAM H. JEFFRIES

8
Gastric Ulcers: Should all patients undergo endoscopy? What should be done with patients who heal "slowly"? 88
EDWIN N. LARKAI, DAVID Y. GRAHAM

9
Duodenal Ulcer: Is there a role for chronic prophylactic therapy? 95
DENIS M. McCARTHY

10
Gastric Volvulus: What is appropriate management? 108
PEDRO P. LLANEZA, WILLIAM B. SALT, II

11
Glandular Carcinoma of Gastric Origin 117
HAROLD O. DOUGLASS, JR.

III
Pancreas 131

12
Acute Pancreatitis: When should slow rsolution be cause for concern? 133
What is appropriate therapy for fulminant pancreatitis?
A. THE GASTROENTEROLOGIST'S VIEW: FRANK BROOKS 133
B. THE SURGEON'S VIEW: CHARLES F. FREY, SIGISMUND S. PIKUL, II 144

13
Common Duct Stones: Does a patient with intact gall bladder require surgery after endoscopic removal of common duct stones? 160
STEPHEN E. SILVIS

14
Pancreatic Pseudocyst and Abscess: Is percutaneous drainage
a reasonable option?... 181
   PETER A. BANKS, STEPHEN G. GERZOF

15
Pain of Chronic Pancreatitis: What are the management options?........... 192
   W. GARDNER ROWELL, PHILLIP P. TOSKES

16
Pancreas Divisum: Do the authorities now agree? 198
   GLEN A. LEHMAN

17
Pancreatic Cancer: What is a reasonable approach?........................... 207
   MARTIN H. KALSER

IV
Liver.. 215

18
Intractable Ascites: What should be done?....................................... 217
   JOHN T. GALAMBOS

19
Transplantation: Who? When? Where?.. 225
   DAVID H. VAN THIEL

20
Chronic Hepatitis: What are the newer approaches to management? 243
   SHEILA SHERLOCK

21
Hepatorenal Syndrome: What are the new concepts? 253
   MURRAY EPSTEIN

22
Hepatitis Immunization: Who? When? 264
   RICHARD S. PHILLIPS, K. RAJENDER REDDY

V
Biliary Tract 281

23
Gallstones: Dissolution? Fracture? Removal? 283
HANS FROMM, MAURO MALAVOLTI

24
Sclerosing Cholangitis: Treatment or transplant? 298
NICHOLAS F. LARUSSO, RUSSELL H. WIESNER

VI
Small Intestine 305

25
Chronic Diarrhea: How should we approach the diagnosis? 307
NORTON J. GREENBERGER

26
Work-up of the Patient with Recurrent Right Upper-Quadrant Pain 317
JOHN E. STONE, WALTER J. HOGAN, JOSEPH E. GEENEN

27
Small Intestinal Biopsy: Who? How? What are the findings? 326
ROBERT H. RIDDELL

28
Short Bowel Syndrome: How do we prolong life? 332
GARY M. LEVINE

29
Intestinal Gas: What do we offer the patient? 341
MICHAEL D. LEVITT

VII
Large Intestine 347

30
Fecal Incontinence: How should it be contained? 349
ARNOLD WALD

31
Ischemic Bowel: How often is it misdiagnosed? 359
LAWRENCE J. BRANDT

32
Ulcerative Proctitis: Tractable or intractable? 368
RICHARD G. FARMER

33
Colonic Crohn's Disease: What is a workable approach
to management? 380
BURTON I. KORELITZ

34
Intractable Perineal Fistulae in Crohn's Disease: Can life be made
worth living? 389
LESLIE H. BERNSTEIN

35
Toxic Megacolon: Is there a superior approach to management? 394
DANIEL H. PRESENT

36
Intestinal Surgery: How can we choose between pouches
and stomas? 402
KEITH A. KELLY, BRUCE G. WOLFF

37
Colon Cancer: Which therapeutic measures prolong life? 410
NICHOLAS J. PETRELLI, LEMUEL HERRERA

38
Heme-Positive Stool: What is the appropriate evaluation? 420
JOHN H. BOND

39
Massive Rectal Bleeding: What is a rational approach? 427
NAURANG M. AGRAWAL, ATILLA ERTAN

40
The Chronic Abdomen 433
W. GRANT THOMPSON

41
Infectious Colitis: What is an effective approach? 447
VALERIE JAGIELLA, BERNARD M. SCHUMAN, FRANCIS J. TEDESCO

42
Obstipation: What is the appropriate therapeutic approach? 458
GHISLAIN DEVROEDE, JACQUES POISSON, JEAN-CLAUDE SCHANG

VIII
Endoscopic Therapy 485

43
Bleeding in the Upper Gastrointestinal Tract: What is the rationale
for endoscopic intervention? 487
STEVEN E. HAHN, ROBERT I. GOLDBERG

44
Treatment of Bleeding Esophageal Varices 498
MICHAEL V. SIVAK, JR., JOHN L. PETRINI

45
Gastric Bubble Insertion: A rational approach to managing obesity? 523
STANLEY B. BENJAMIN

46
Colonoscopic Polypectomy of Polyps with Adenocarcinoma:
When is it curative? 528
LAWRENCE B. COHEN, JEROME D. WAYE

47
Nontoxic Megacolon: Is endoscopic therapy appropriate? 536
JAMIE S. BARKIN, IRA AGATSTEIN

48
Sigmoid Volvulus: Is it a difficult twist to manage?...........................543
KEVIN P. MORRISSEY

49
Endoscopic Sphincterotomy: When is it appropriate?........................551
JEROME H. SIEGEL

Index 559

I

Esophagus

1

Chest Pain:
Is the esophagus responsible?

JOEL E. RICHTER, M.D.

Coronary artery disease is a major cause of morbidity and mortality in the United States. Consequently, chest pain is taken seriously by both patient and physician, and frequently a complete cardiac work-up is undertaken. Up to 30% of patients with typical or atypical angina pain have normal coronary arteries on angiography.[1,2] With more than 500,000 coronary angiograms performed yearly,[3] more than 150,000 patients per year may be found to have noncardiac chest pain. These patients are primarily women with atypical chest pain unrelated to exertion. Some may have small vessel disease of the myocardium, coronary artery spasm, or misinterpreted angiograms. Nevertheless, their overall clinical prognosis is excellent. Since 1971, 12 studies have addressed the clinical outcome of over 2500 patients (60% female) with noncardiac chest pain.[4,5] With an average follow-up of approximately 3 years, myocardial infarctions (1.6%) and cardiac deaths (0.5%) are rare. However, these patients do suffer real disability if they are not given an alternative diagnosis for their complaints. They continue to have a limited life-style, frequently are unable to work, and often still believe they have heart disease.[6]

The heart and the esophagus have similar neural pathways for pain. Therefore, over the last 10 years, investigators have evaluated the importance of esophageal disease in patients with noncardiac chest pain. Incidence figures are quite variable and depend on the sophistication of study techniques used to identify esophageal diseases. In one study of patients discharged from a coronary care unit, esophageal disease was believed to be the cause of chest pain in 60% of patients.[7] In this series, detailed studies for gastroesophageal reflux disease (GERD), including 24-hour pH monitoring, found that 46% of these patients had chest pain secondary to acid reflux. Other studies, which employed barium esophagrams, endoscopy, esophageal manometry, and acid perfusion tests, have found that 18% to 58% of patients with normal coronary arteriograms may have their pain attributed to an esophageal cause.[8-13] Recently, ambulatory 24-hour esophageal pH and pressure monitoring have defined a clear association between chest pain and esophageal causes in about 35% of noncardiac chest pain patients.[14,15] In these studies, the esophageal diseases are generally evenly distributed between gastroesophageal reflux and motility abnormalities. If approximately 35% of the 150,000 chest pain patients with normal coronary angiograms have an esophageal cause for pain, then more than 50,000 new patients should be diagnosed yearly in the United States.

ORIGIN OF PAIN IN ESOPHAGEAL DISEASES

The specific mechanisms by which abnormalities of esophageal function may

3

produce chest pain are not clearly understood. The chest pain experienced by patients with esophageal motility disorders have occurred in association with esophageal contractions characterized by high amplitude, prolonged duration, and/or simultaneous onset. This pain might be explained by changes in esophageal wall tension stimulating mechanoreceptors. It is also possible that the pain of "esophageal spasm" is related to myoischemia, resulting from high intramural tension inhibiting blood flow for critical time periods. Although esophageal motility disorders may be evoked by acid perfusion,[16] dysmotility is not usually found during pain induction.[17,18] Therefore, acid-induced heartburn or pain is most likely related to stimulation of acid-sensitive receptors (chemoreceptors) in the esophageal mucosa. The issue of the origin of esophageal chest pain is further confounded by the possibilities that the patient may have a lower pain threshold than normal.[19] Thus, the patient may only perceive pain abnormally in response to physiologic events. Studies into the mechanisms of esophageal chest pain would be incomplete without an attempt to evaluate the individual patient's response to stress and/or possible estimate of pain perception.

ESOPHAGEAL ETIOLOGIES OF CHEST PAIN

Gastroesophageal Reflux Disease (GERD)

Although GERD is associated most often with substernal burning (heartburn) that occurs primarily after meals, in the recumbent position, or on bending and lifting heavy objects, some patients with reflux will experience exercise-induced pain or pain radiating into the arms or jaw. Up to 10% of reflux patients may have chest pain as their only symptom and will initially be diagnosed as having coronary artery disease. DeMeester et al. studies 50 consecutive patients initially believed to have heart disease, with documented normal coronary angiograms, and found 23 (46%) to have excessive acid reflux based on 24-hour pH monitoring.[7] Twelve patients had their typical chest pain reproduced during exercise stress testing, at which time the electrocardiograms (EKGs) were normal, but there was documented acid reflux. These patients had relief of chest pain with antireflux therapy. In six other studies, investigators found that 9% to 30% of patients with normal coronary arteriograms experience their typical chest pain after intraesophageal acid perfusion or when pH monitoring revealed acid reflux.[10,11,13,20–23]

It is extremely important to remember that GERD and coronary artery disease can coexist. In patients with both diseases, acid infusion can induce "typical angina pectoris" and also produce EKG changes indicative of myocardial ischemia and increased myocardial work load, as shown by an increase in the rate-pressure product.[23]

Esophageal Motility Disorders (EMDs)

EMDs in patients with angina-type chest pain have been reported since the 1930s. Early manometric studies describe these patients as having tertiary (repetitive, simultaneous, nonperistaltic) distal esophageal contractions, often with prolonged duration and increased amplitude. Usually they were given a diagnosis of diffuse esophageal spasm (DES). Over the years, this has become a generic term used by many to describe any type of painful EMD.

The development of low compliance infusion systems that permit accurate pressure recordings has brought studies of esophageal motility into the modern age. This new technology has allowed us to establish criteria for normal esophageal motility based on studies of large numbers of healthy adults and to better identify and characterize EMD.[24,25] Normal esophageal motility consists of the propagation of a progressive peristaltic wave down the esophagus. Manometrically, pressures are measured at approximately 3, 8, and 13 cm above the lower esophageal sphincter (LES).[24] Normal contraction amplitude after 5-ml water swallows ranges from 30 to 180 mm Hg, and the normal duration of contractions is 2 to 6 seconds. Contraction peaks are usually single, although double peaks may be seen in normal individuals.

It is now generally accepted that achalasia, DES, high-amplitude peristalsis (nutcracker esophagus), and hypertensive LES are primary disorders *associated* with chest pain. However, the degree of chest pain and/or dysphagia is a poor predictor of the type of motility abnormality.[26] In addition, there is a large group of patients with less dramatic contraction abnormalities who are given a diagnosis of nonspecific esophageal motility disorders (NEMDs). Criteria for defining EMDs are outlined in Table 1-1. It must be emphasized that these manometric criteria are not arbitrarily obtained but are based on extensive studies of 95 healthy volunteers with abnormality defined as outside two standard deviations.[24]

INITIAL EVALUATION

The patient evaluation for possible esophageal chest pain always should begin with careful exclusion of cardiac disease. This is particularly important because the prevalence of both diseases increases as the population grows older.[27] Therefore, the two problems may coexist in chest pain patients and may complicate their diagnostic evaluations.

The history and physical examination frequently may not be helpful in separating these two disease processes. Features that may distinquish esophageal from cardiac chest pain are outlined in Table 1-2. However, as many as 50% of patients with cardiac pain have some symptoms of esophageal pain; therefore, clinical features do not reliably discriminate the two groups.[28]

The extent of the cardiac work-up should be determined by the patient's age, family history, and cardiac risk factors. In general, cardiac disease in younger patients (less than 40 years old) usually can be excluded by a normal exercise stress test and echocardiogram. Older patients may require coronary angiography with possible ergonovine testing. After a negative evaluation, the patients can be reassured that the heart is normal and that the "noncardiac chest pains" will not lead to increased cardiac events or death.

The next step is to exclude musculoskeletal syndromes and evaluate the upper gastrointestinal (UGI) tract and gallbladder. The chest wall should be palpated for "trigger points" reproducing the patient's pain. A variety of syndromes, including costochondritis and Tietze's syndrome, are characterized by local tenderness and pain, often exacerbated by arm movements or breathing. Ten to 15% of patients may have a musculoskeletal cause for their chest pain. Structural lesions of the UGI tract should be excluded by barium studies or endoscopy. These studies may reveal an unusual cause of chest pain such as an esophageal or gastric ulcer. More commonly, reflux esophagitis is found, which strongly suggests an esophageal cause for chest pain. Most patients should also undergo a screening evaluation for gallstones.

ESOPHAGEAL TESTING

Esophageal testing for noncardiac chest pain is a primary indication for esophageal laboratory referrals. Over the last 3 years, my laboratory has evaluated 1250 patients for the following primary complaints: noncardiac chest pain (72%), dysphagia (20%), and miscellaneous (8%), i.e., prior to antireflux surgery and to exclude collagen vascular disease.[29] Routine esophageal testing should include esophageal manometry, acid perfusion test, edrophonium stimulation, and 24-hour ambulatory esophageal pH monitoring. More experimental studies may include esophageal balloon distention and ambulatory 24-hour pressure and pH monitoring.

TABLE 1–1.
Manometric Criteria for Primary Esophageal Motility Disorders

Motility Diagnosis	Required Criteria	Patient May Have:
Achalasia	Aperistalsis of esophageal body	Incomplete LES relaxation Elevated LES pressure (>45 mmHg) Elevated intraesophageal pressure
Diffuse esophageal spasm	Simultaneous contractions (>10% wet swallows) Intermittent normal peristalsis	Repetitive contractions (>2 peaks) Increased duration and/or amplitude Spontaneous contractions Incomplete LES relaxation Increased duration (>6 sec)
Nutcracker esophagus	Normal peristaltic contraction with increased distal amplitude (>180 mm Hg)	
Hypertensive lower esophageal sphincter (LES)	Elevated LES pressure (>45 mm Hg) Normal LES relaxation Normal peristalsis	
Nonspecific esophageal motility disorder	Any combination of criteria at right	Increased nontransmitted contractions (>20%) Prolonged duration contractions (>6 sec) Triple peaked contractions Retrograde contractions Low-amplitude peristalsis (<30 mm Hg) Absent peristalsis with normal LES

TABLE 1-2.
Esophageal versus Cardiac Chest Pain*

Features found more frequently in patients with esophageal pain:
1. Severe pain in onset which continues for several hours as a dull ache
2. Considerable variation in the degree of exercise that produces pain
3. Pain beginning as long as 10 min after exercise has stopped
4. Pain associated with swallowing, heartburn, or acid regurgitation
5. Pain provoked by stooping and recumbency
6. Pain awakening patient from sleep
7. Pain relieved by antacids

Features found more often in patients with cardiac pain:
1. Lateral radiation of central chest pain
2. Infrequent attacks of spontaneous chest pain

*Based on questionnaire results from 100 emergency admissions: 70 with anterior chest pain of cardiac (52) or esophageal (18) origin, and 30 with other sorts of chest pain. Alban Davies et al. J Clin Gastroenterol, 1985 (28)

Esophageal Manometry

Esophageal motility disorders may be found less frequently than commonly thought in noncardiac chest pain patients. Recently, I reviewed experience over 3 years with 910 patients referred for evaluation of noncardiac chest pain.[29] Only 255 patients (28%) had EMDs, compared to 132/251 patients (53%) referred for evaluation of dysphagia (Fig 1–1). In agreement with other series,[8, 25, 30-32] the nutcracker esophagus (48%) was the most common motility disorder in noncardiac chest pain patients, while classic DES (10%) was an infrequent finding. In contrast, achalasia (39%) was the most common motility diagnosis in dysphagia patients, while the nutcracker esophagus (10%) was an infrequent finding.

The documentation of an EMD *does not* conclusively prove it is the source of the patient's chest pain. In fact, when an EMD is observed the patient is usually pain free. Spontaneous chest pain with abnormal esophageal motility is a rare occurrence. Therefore, the presence of an EMD only suggests that the esophagus is a *probable* source of chest pain. Further provocative testing and/or ambulatory monitoring is required to identify the esophagus as a *definite* cause of chest pain.

Esophageal Provocative Testing

Because patients rarely experience their chest pain during manometry, provocative tests have been used to reproduce their pain. This is analogous to treadmill testing to elicit chest pain and EKG changes in patients with suspected an-

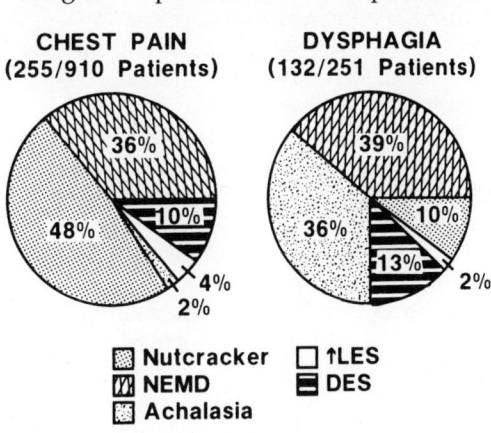

FIG 1–1.
Incidence of esophageal motility disorders in patients with noncardiac chest pain (left) and dysphagia (right). NEMD = nonspecific esophageal motility disorder; ↑LES = hypertensive lower esophageal sphincter; DES = diffuse esophageal spasm. (Reprinted with permission from Katz PO, Dalton CB, Richter JE, et al: Esophageal testing of patients with non-cardiac chest pain and/or dysphagia. Ann Intern Med 1987; 106:594)

gina. The ideal esophageal provocative test should be easily administered, highly sensitive and specific, and free from side-effects, and should not produce cardiac pain. Unfortunately, work has been hampered by the lack of a "gold standard" for diagnosing esophageal pain. Nevertheless, numerous approaches have been suggested based on the premise that increased esophageal contractile activity and acid reflux are potential causes of chest pain. Proposed provocative agents have included ice water swallows,[33] intraesophageal acid perfusion,[34] intraesophageal balloon distention,[35] and systemic injections of bethanechol,[36,37] edrophonium,[38,39] ergonovine,[40,41] and pentagastrin.[42] I have found intraesophageal acid perfusion and edrophonium to be the most reliable and safest provocative test for routine use in the clinical esophageal laboratory.

Acid Perfusion (Bernstein) Test

Since its introduction in 1958 by Bernstein and Baker, esophageal acid perfusion has been widely used as a clinical test for GERD.[34] When a positive test is defined as heartburn reproduction, it is an excellent screening study with a sensitivity and specificity approaching 80%.[43] It also may be a useful provocative test in reflux patients who present primarily with chest pain rather than heartburn. The largest series reported to date found that 61/910 patients (7%) with noncardiac chest pain had their pain reproduced by acid perfusion.[29]

The acid perfusion test is a simple procedure which may be performed in the office without manometric monitoring. The ideal method is to alternate saline with dilute acid (0.1 N HCl) to obtain a placebo control. These solutions are infused into the distal esophagus at a rate of 6 to 8 ml/minute. The saline should not cause chest pain; the acid must replicate the patient's chest pain to be called a positive test.

Edrophonium (Tensilon) Test

Edrophonium hydrochloride, a cholinesterase inhibitor, is a safe, specific test for esophageal chest pain. An intravenous dose of 80 µg/kg produces an increase in esophageal contraction amplitude and duration in *both* normal volunteers and chest pain patients[44] (Fig 1–2). This dose has provoked chest pain in 18% to 30% of patients, but not in over 150 asymptomatic volunteers.[38,44] Using a larger dose of edrophonium (10 mg bolus), other investigators have observed a positive response rate of 34%.[45] All studies report that baseline manometric abnormalities do not predict a positive pain response to edrophonium testing.[44,45]

Because edrophonium increases esophageal contractions, it was hoped that pressure changes might identify positive responders and clarify the relationship between chest pain and abnormal esophageal contractions. In our study,[44] edrophonium increased esophageal contraction amplitude and repetitive waves after wet swallows to a similar degree in age-matched controls and noncardiac chest pain patients, regardless of their pain response. The change in contraction duration was significantly greater in patients with edrophonium-induced chest pain. However, the overlap between individual patients with and without chest pain was considerable, thus preventing the establishment of a specific manometric criterion for a positive test. Other groups[46,47] also have failed to define specific contraction abnormalities after edrophonium provocation. Furthermore, Nasrallah and Hendrix found that the frequency of edrophonium-reproduced chest pain was similar in patients with EMDs or esophagitis.[46] This suggests that edrophonium-provoked pain is not specific for EMDs but rather highly sensitive for pain of esophageal origin. In contrast, Lee et al. found that edrophonium significantly increased amplitude, duration, and repetitive waves in positive responders.[45] The likely explanation for the discrepancy between this study and prior reports relates to the study design. The control group was not age-matched and manometric studies were performed following a series of dry swallows, a stimulus known to produce less predictable contraction pressures. Therefore, the key end point for a

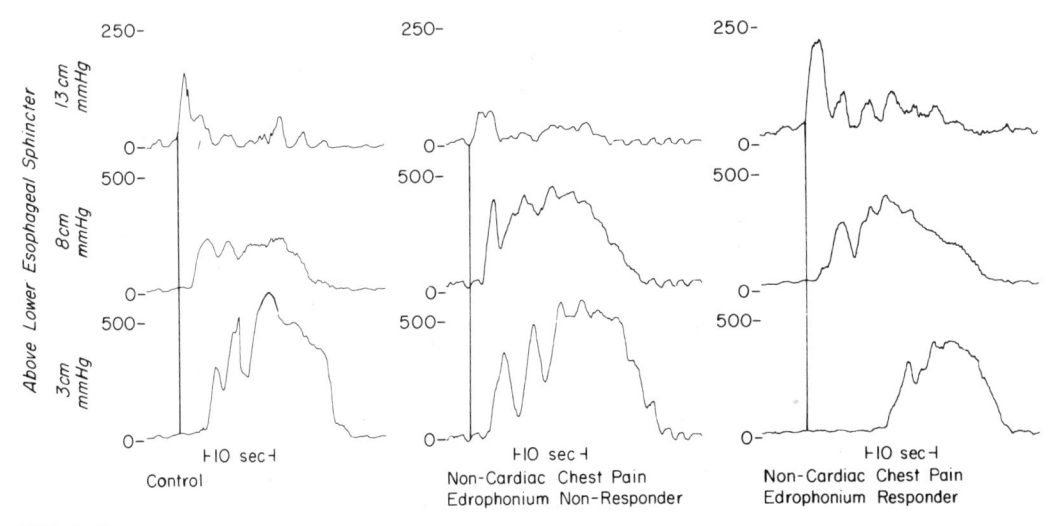

FIG 1–2.
Manometric response to edrophonium. After edrophonium (80 μg/kg intravenous bolus), esophageal contractions induced by wet swallows are peristaltic with waveforms characterized by increased amplitude, prolonged duration, and multiple peaks (repetitive contractions). Simultaneous contractions are not seen. Note, however, that esophageal contractile activity after edrophonium *does not* differentiate control subjects, patients with noncardiac chest pain who do not develop pain after edrophonium, and patients with noncardiac chest pain provoked by edrophonium. (Reprinted with permission from Richter JE, Hackshaw BT, Wu WC, et al: Edrophonium: A useful provocative test for esophageal chest pain. *Ann Intern Med* 1985; 103:16)

positive edrophonium test is *pain* rather than a specific change in esophageal motility.

In my laboratory, placebo (1 ml of 0.9% normal saline) and edrophonium (80 μg/kg) are consecutively administered intravenously in an order unknown to the patient, and each injection is followed by ten wet swallows. A positive test is the replication of the patient's chest pain within 5 minutes only after the edrophonium injection. In about 5% of patients, an uninterpretable test (pain after placebo or both placebo and edrophonium) may occur. Aside from occasional lightheadedness, nausea, and abdominal cramping, important side-effects are rare. Atropine may be used to reverse edrophonium side-effects, but I have not had to use this antidote in over 1500 patients. Unlike ergonovine, edrophonium does not promote myocardial ischemia by increasing heart rate or systolic blood pressure, nor does it reduce coronary blood flow by constricting epicardial vessels.[44]

Overall Usefulness of Provocative Testing

My laboratory's experience with 910 patients with noncardiac chest pain confirms the usefulness of the acid perfusion and edrophonium tests (Fig 1–3). Manometry was abnormal in 28% of patients, but this only suggested the esophagus was a *probable* cause of chest pain. Seven percent of patients had a positive Bernstein test, and 23% had a positive edrophonium test. If patients with both positive provocative tests are counted as a single positive, 27% of the patients had their chest pain reproduced in the laboratory and can be considered to have a *definite* esophageal source for their pain. A combination of patients with *definite* esophageal chest pain (27%) and *probable* esophageal chest pain (21%) gives an overall diagnostic yield of 48% for these simple esophageal studies.[29]

NON-CARDIAC CHEST PAIN
Esophageal Tests – 910 Patients

MANOMETRY ALONE

- Normal or Negative NOT Esophageal
- Abnormal Manometry Probable Esophageal
- + Bernstein ⎫
- + T+B   ⎬ Definite Esophageal
- + Tensilon ⎭

DIAGNOSIS
Not Esophageal – 655 (72%)
Probable Esophageal – 255 (28%)

MANOMETRY + PROVOCATIVE TESTS

DIAGNOSIS
Not Esophageal – 475 (52%)
Probable Esophageal – 192 (21%)
Definite Esophageal – 243 (27%)

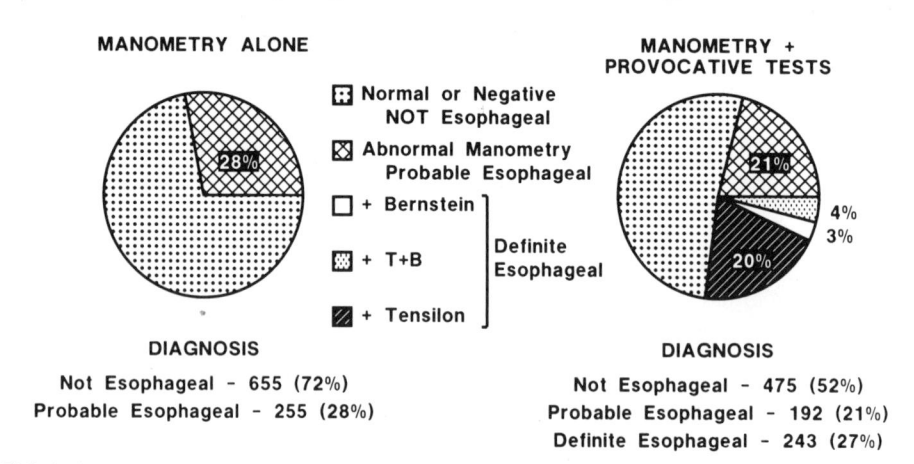

FIG 1–3.
Results of manometry and provocative tests in 910 patients with noncardiac chest pain. T + B = Tensilon and Bernstein tests.

AMBULATORY 24-HOUR ESOPHAGEAL pH MONITORING

The diagnosis of GERD and the specific relationship with symptoms may still be uncertain after the above tests. In this situation, prolonged monitoring of distal esophageal pH may be of value.[48, 49]

Briefly, a thin pH electrode is passed through the nose into the distal esophagus (5 cm above the LES). The patients alter their position, eat normal diets, and are told to record times of food ingestion, changes in position, and occurrence of symptoms. These studies are done on an outpatient basis in the home or work environment. Computer-analyzed programs

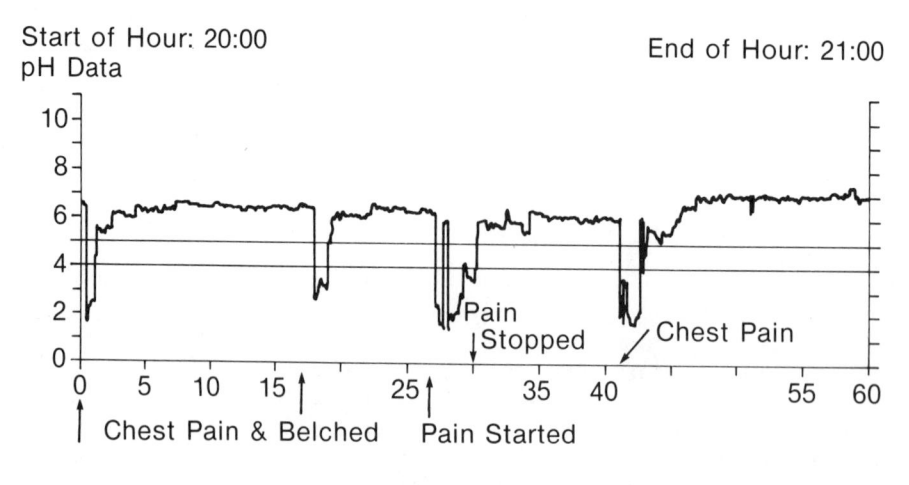

FIG 1–4.
Patient with noncardiac chest pain and frequent admissions to a coronary care unit. Prolonged esophageal pH monitoring showed good correlation between chest pain and acid reflux (pH < 4).

record the frequency and duration of reflux episodes in both the upright and supine position. More importantly, this study allows a direct comparison between symptoms and pH activity (Fig 1–4). This test may be particularly helpful in patients with suspected GER who hve normal endoscopy and negative Bernstein tests.

The algorithm shown in Fig 1–5 outlines my current approach to noncardiac chest pain patients. This schema takes into consideration that these patients are usually first evaluated by generalists, and certain esophageal tests, particularly manometry and pH monitoring, are not widely available. After excluding cardiac and musculoskeletal diseases, a UGI series should be done to rule out structural lesions of the esophagus, stomach, and duodenum. If unrevealing, acid perfusion and edrophonium testing with placebo controls can be done safely in the office without manometric monitoring. Patients with positive tests are diagnosed as having definite esophageal pain and are treated accordingly. Patients with negative tests should be referred to a gastroenterologist for further evaluation to include esophageal manometry and 24-hour pH studies.

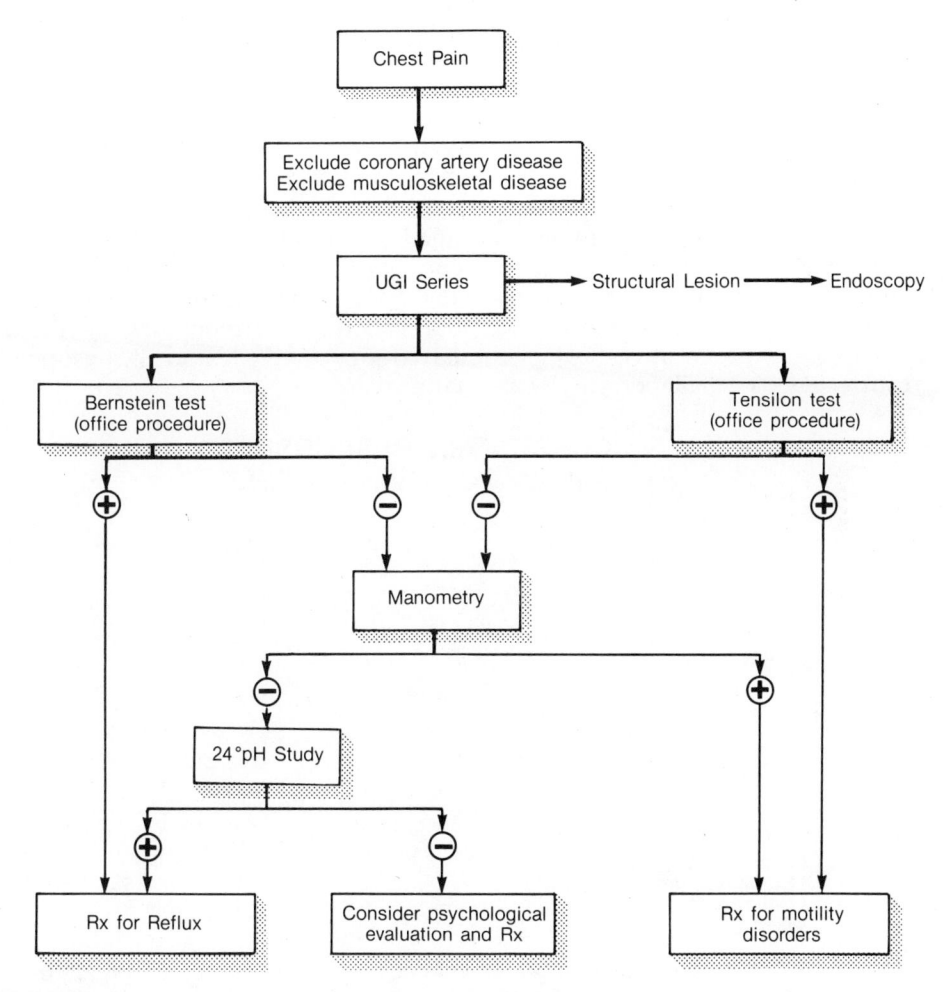

FIG 1–5.
Algorithm for the evaluation of noncardiac chest pain. This approach takes into consideration that these patients are usually first evaluated by generalists and certain esophageal tests, particularly manometry and pH monitoring, are not widely available.

NEW TESTS FOR ESOPHAGEAL CHEST PAIN

Current tests for esophageal chest pain have some limitations. The overall diagnostic yield is relatively low. Systemic drugs have potential side-effects and may provoke nonesophageal chest pain as the result of their generalized action. Furthermore, the provocative tests may simulate some of the natural events provoking esophageal chest pain but do not resolve the critical question of possible esophageal abnormalities responsible for *spontaneous* pain events. Several new exciting developments are on the horizon.

Esophageal Balloon Distention

Balloon distention of the esophagus, one of the earliest methods used to differentiate esophageal from cardiac chest pain, fell by the wayside with the development of the electrocardiogram. This nonpharmacologic provocative test has been resurrected. A small polyvinyl balloon is placed 10 cm above the LES and is inflated with 1-ml increments of air to a total volume of 10 ml. Pain occurred in 18/30 (60%) noncardiac chest pain patients and only 6/30 (20%) healthy volunteers.[19] Symptoms were unassociated with EKG changes and were resolved immediately with balloon decompression. Balloon pressures and esophageal contractions did not distinguish chest pain patients from control subjects. However, patients were observed to have lower pain thresholds for esophageal distention. This increased distention sensitivity is reminiscent of similar studies done with rectal balloons in patients with irritable bowel syndrome. Esophageal balloon distention subsequently was compared with acid perfusion and edrophonium in 50 noncardiac chest pain patients[35] (Fig 1–6). The conventional tests reproduced pain in 12 (24%) patients. Positive balloon studies occurred in 11 of these patients and identified an additional 13 patients, thus increasing the diagnostic yield from 24% to 48%. More patients need to be studied, but balloon distention may be the preferred provocative test to elicit esophageal chest pain.

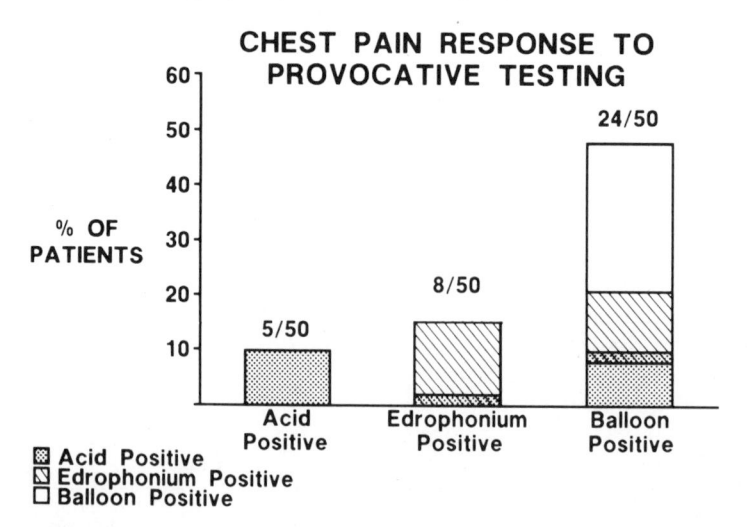

FIG 1–6.
Replication of noncardiac chest pain in 50 patients after acid perfusion, edrophonium injection, and intraesophageal balloon distention. A positive balloon study occurred in 11/12 patients with positive reponse to acid and/or edrophonium as well as identifying an additional 13 patients. Therefore, balloon distention increased the diagnostic yield of the provocative tests from 24% to 48%. (Reprinted with permission from Barish CF, Castell DO, Richter JE: Graded esophageal balloon distention: A new provocative test for non-cardiac chest pain. *Dig Dis Sci* 1986; 31:1296.)

Ambulatory 24-hour pH and Pressure Monitoring

As with prolonged pH studies, the ability to monitor esophageal pressures for 24 hours should help to clarify the complex relationship between chest pain and motility disorders. An ambulatory esophageal pH and pressure system has been developed and studies performed in 22 noncardiac chest pain patients.[14] A total of 92 spontaneous chest pain episodes were recorded—an average of nearly five episodes per patient. Thirty-three individual chest pain episodes (36%) correlated with abnormal motility (11 events), pH < 4, (18 events), or both (4 events), but 59 chest pain events (64%) were not associated with abnormal esophageal activity. Overall, 13/22 patients (59%) had at least one pain episode correlating with abnormal esophageal pH or motility. Patients could not distinguish chest pain episodes arising from motility or pH abnormalities from episodes not associated with abnormal esophageal activity. Using a comparable ambulatory system, a research group in Belgium has reported that a definite esophageal cause of chest pain could be identified in only 35% of their patients.[15]

NONCARDIAC CHEST PAIN—PART OF THE IRRITABLE BOWEL SYNDROME

The gastrointestinal tract is a sensitive organ of emotional expression. Although the stomach and colon have been the traditional sites for investigation of emotional influences on disordered intestinal motility, clinical experience and experimental observations indicate that esophageal motility is also affected by emotional stimuli. As early as 1892, Sir William Osler[50] wrote: "Esophagismus (esophageal spasm) is met with in hysterical patients and hypochondriacs. . . . The idiopathic form is found in females of a marked neurotic habit, but may also occur in elderly men." Subsequent studies have shown that startling noises and stressful interviews can trigger abnormal esophageal contractions. More recently, Clouse and Lustman[51] found that 21/25 patients (84%) with distal EMDs, compared to 4/13 patients (31%) with normal manometry, received a psychiatric diagnosis (primarily depression, anxiety, or somatization) during a structured psychiatric interview. Complementary results were obtained in a study of 20 patients with the nutcracker esophagus who were administered a psychologic inventory.[52] Patients differed significantly from controls but were comparable to irritable bowel patients on scales assessing somatic anxiety and the tendency to react to psychologic stress with an increase in gastrointestinal symptoms.

Many aspects of painful EMDs parallel the characteristic features of the irritable bowel syndrome. Both occur mostly in females and have similar associated psychiatric disturbances. Symptoms frequently overlap between groups. We have observed that 56% of patients referred to the laboratory for noncardiac chest pain have irritable bowel symptoms, compared with 26% of age-matched medical clinic patients ($p < 0.01$).[53] Noncardiac chest pain patients also have lower pain thresholds for esophageal balloon distention, an effect similar to rectal balloon studies in irritable bowel patients.[19, 54] Finally, both the esophageal and colonic disorders are manifested by abnormal contractions induced reflexly or by stress.[55, 56]

Therefore, it seems logical to suggest that painful EMDs may represent part of the spectrum of the irritable bowel syndrome, i.e., the "irritable esophagus." This phrase may serve to emphasize a point recently made by Marvin Schuster[57] that physicians need to begin to "look beyond the twitching of the esophagus to the feelings of the human beings." Until we better understand the complex interaction between emotional disorders, EMDs, and chest pain, therapeutic endeavors in this area will be fraught with frustrations.

THERAPY

Once a relationship between esophageal abnormalities and chest pain has

TABLE 1–3.
Therapy of Esophageal Motility Disorders

Treatment Modality	Dosage	Mode of Administration
Nitrates		
Nitroglycerin	0.4 mg sublingually	Before meals and prn
	10–20 mg P.O.	30 min. before meals
Anticholinergics		
Dicyclomine	10–20 mg P.O.	q.i.d.
Smooth muscle relaxant		
Hydralazine	25–50 mg P.O.	q.i.d.
Calcium channel blockers		
Nifedipine	10–30 mg sublingually or P.O.	q.i.d. or before meals
Diltiazem	90 mg P.O.	q.i.d.
Psychotropics		
Trazadone	50 mg P.O.	t.i.d.
Static dilatation	50 Fr	Repeat as needed
Pneumatic dilation	Progressive sizes	Repeat as needed
Esophagomyotomy		

been established, the critical question becomes the appropriate form of treatment. Unfortunately, over the years this has presented a major dilemma for the clinician. Because chest pain produced by GER may mimic EMDs, it is important to exclude the presence of acid reflux. This may require a trial of antireflux therapy for 4 to 8 weeks (see Chap. 2). The preferred treatment for primary EMDs, other than achalasia, and the irritable esophagus is not as easily identified. Many therapies have been proposed (Table 1–3), but most have not been examined in placebo-controlled trials. The following therapeutic suggestions are derived from clinical experiences and recently reported controlled trials.

Reassurance

Many patients will favorably respond to confident reassurance based on careful diagnostic studies. With the report that their symptoms are not due to cardiac disease and are caused by an esophageal problem, improvement may be noted. This supportive approach results in better patient acceptance of symptoms, less limitations in life-style, and frequently a diminution or resolution of chest pain.[58,59] Considering that other therapies are often less than satisfactory, simple reassurance during office visits and telephone conversations may be the simplest, safest, and most cost-effective approach.

Smooth Muscle Relaxants

Smooth muscle relaxants, including nitrates,[60] anticholinergics,[61] and hydralazine,[62] have been used with some success in patients with EMDs. Unfortunately, these drugs have not been effective in the majority of patients. Recently the calcium channel blockers, diltiazem[63] and nifedipine,[64,65] have been studied in patients with EMDs. The most dramatic effects have been reported with nifedipine with one study finding greater than 50% reduction in distal contraction amplitude after a single 30 mg oral dose.[65] In spite of these acute effects, two controlled studies have failed to show that nifedipine was better than placebo in relieving chest pain in patients with the nutcracker esophagus or diffuse esophageal spasm.[58,66] Conflicting reports on diltiazem therapy suggest a similar lack of efficacy.[67,68] These studies confirm that decreases in esophageal pressures alone may not improve chest pain. Smooth muscle relaxants may be useful in EMDs, but they need to be combined with other therapies or used when pain episodes show a clear relationship with simultaneously recorded abnormal esophageal contractions. Until these subsets can be easily defined, I recommend a trial of smooth muscle relaxants (particularly nifedipine or anticholinergics) in patients with more severe recurrent chest pains.

Psychotropic Drugs

Anectodal reports have suggested that psychotropic drugs can help patients with stress-related painful EMDs. In a recent placebo-controlled study, Clouse et al.[69] observed that low-dose trazodone (Desyrel, 100–150 mg/day) decreased the symptoms associated with abnormal esophageal contractions without changing esophageal pressures. Behavioral modification programs and biofeedback may also be beneficial. The contribution of emotional factors should be sought in all patients with noncardiac chest pain. A simple discussion of the relationship between stress and the patient's symptoms may be very helpful. More disturbed patients will require psychotropic drugs or referrals to psychiatrists or psychologists.

Dilatation and Surgery

Some physicians find that passage of a 50 French dilator will promote chest pain relief, but the response is likely a placebo effect.[70] Others suggest that patients with diffuse esophageal spasms (DES) may be treated with pneumatic dilatation.[71] This procedure should be reserved for patients with severe dysphagia and documented distal esophageal obstruction. A long surgical myotomy may help some patients with painful EMDs. However, surgical series are small with short follow-up periods. Failure of all medical regimens, including smooth muscle relaxants, psychotherapy, and reassurance, is quite unusual. Over the last 10 years, my colleagues and I have not needed to refer a single patient for surgical myotomy.[72] True intractibility must be quite rare!

References

1. Kemp HG, Vokonas PS, Cohn PF, et al: The anginal syndrome associated with normal coronary arteriograms: Report of a six year experience. Am J Med 1973; 54:735–742.
2. Proudfit WL, Shirey EK, Sones FM: Selective cine coronary arteriography; Correlation with clinical findings in 1,000 patients. Circulation 1966; 33:901–910.
3. Kennedy RH, Kennedy MA, Frye R, et al: Cardiac catheterization and cardiac surgical facilities. N Engl J Med 1982; 307:986–993.
4. Isner JM, Salem DN, Banas JS, et al: Long-term clinical course of patients with normal coronary arteriography: Follow-up study of 121 patients with normal or nearly normal coronary arteriograms. Am Heart J 1981; 102:645–653.
5. Wielgosz AT, Fletcher RH, McCants CB, et al: Unimproved chest pain in patients with minimal or no coronary disease: A behavioral phenomenon. Am Heart J 1984; 108:67–72.
6. Ockene IS, Shay MJ, Alpert JS, et al: Unexplained chest pain in patients with normal coronary arteriograms: A follow-up study of functional status. N Engl J Med 1980; 303:1249–1252.
7. DeMeester TR, O'Sullivan GC, Bermudez G, et al: Esophageal function in patients with angina-type chest pain and normal coronary angiograms. Ann Surg 1982; 196:488–498.
8. Brand DL, Martin D, Pope CE: Esophageal manometrics in patients with angina-like chest pain. Am J Dig Dis 1977; 22:300–305.
9. Henderson RD, Wigle ED, Sample K, et al: Atypical chest pain of cardiac and esophageal origin. Chest 1978; 73:24–27.
10. Kline M, Chesne R, Studevant RL, et al: Esophageal disease in patients with angina-like chest pain. Am J Gastroenterol 1981; 75:116–123.
11. Ferguson SC, Hodges K, Hersh T, et al: Esophageal manometry in patients with chest pain and normal coronary arteriograms. Am J Gastroenterol 1981; 75:124–127.
12. Areskog M, Tibbling L, Wranne B: Non-infraction coronary care unit patients: A three year follow-up with special reference to oesophageal dysfunction and ischemic heart disease as origin of chest pain. Acta Med Scand 1981; 209:51–57.
13. Alban-Davies H, Jones DB, Rhodes J: Esophageal angina as the cause of chest pain. JAMA 1982; 248:2274–2278.
14. Peters LJ, Maas LC, Petty D, et al: Spontaneous non-cardiac chest pain: Evaluation by 24 hour ambulatory esophageal motility and pH monitoring. Gastroenterology 1988; 94:878–86.
15. Janssens J, Vantrappen G, Ghillebert G: 24 hour recording of esophageal pressure and pH in patients with non-cardiac chest pain. Gastroenterology 1986; 90:1978–1984.
16. Siegel CI, Hendrix TR: Esophageal motor abnormalities induced by acid perfusion in patients with heartburn. J Clin Invest 1963; 42:686–695.
17. Richter JE, Johns DN, Wu WC, et al: Are esoph-

ageal motility abnormalities produced during the intraesophageal acid perfusion test? *JAMA* 1985; 253:1914–1917.
18. Burns TW, Venturatos SG: Esophageal motor function and response to acid perfusion in patients with symptomatic reflux esophagitis. *Dig Dis Sci* 1985; 30:529–535.
19. Richter JE, Barish CF, Castell DO: Abnormal sensory perception in patients with esophageal chest pain. *Gastroenterology* 1986; 91:845–852.
20. Brand DL, Ilves R, Pope CE: Evaluation of esophageal function in patients with central chest pain. *Acta Med Scan (Suppl)* 1981; 644:53–56.
21. Areskog M, Tibbling L, Wranne B: Oesophageal dysfunction in non-infarction coronary care unit patients. *Acta Med Scand* 1979; 205:279–282.
22. Chobanian SJ, Curtis DJ, Cattau EL, et al: Systematic esophageal evaluation of patients with non-cardiac chest pain. *Arch Intern Med* 1986; 146:1505–1508.
23. Mellow MH, Simpson AG, Watt L, et al: Esophageal acid perfusion in coronary artery disease: Induction of myocardial ischemia. *Gastroenterology* 1983; 83:306–312.
24. Richter JE, Wu WC, Johns DN, et al: Esophageal manometry in 95 healthy adult volunteers. *Dig Dis Sci* 1987; 32:583–592.
25. Clouse RE, Staiano A: Contraction abnormalities of the esophageal body in patients referred for manometry. *Dig Dis Sci* 1983; 28:784–791.
26. Riedel WL, Clouse RE: Variations in clinical presentation of patients with esophageal contraction abnormalities. *Dig Dis Sci* 1985; 30:1065–1071.
27. Svensson O, Stenport G, Tibbling L, et al: Oesophageal function and coronary angiogram in patients with disabling chest pain. *Acta Med Scand* 1978; 204:173–178.
28. Alban-Davies H, Jones DB, Rhodes J, et al: Angina-like esophageal pain: Differentiation from cardiac pain by history. *J Clin Gastroenterol* 1985; 7:477–481.
29. Katz PO, Dalton CB, Richter JE, et al: Esophageal testing of patients with non-cardiac chest pain and/or dysphagia. *Ann Intern Med* 1987; 106:593–597.
30. Benjamin SB, Gerhardt DC, Castrell DO: High amplitude, peristaltic esophageal contractions associated with chest pain and/or dysphagia. *Gastroenterology* 1979; 77:478–483.
31. Herrington JP, Burns TW, Balart LA: Chest pain and dysphagia in patients with prolonged peristaltic contractile duration of the esophagus. *Dig Dis Sci* 1984; 29:134–140.
32. Traube M, Abibi R, McCallum RW: High amplitude peristaltic esophageal contractions associated with chest pain. *JAMA* 1983; 250:2655–2659.
33. Meyer GW, Castell DO: Human esophageal response during chest pain induced by swallowing cold liquids. *JAMA* 1981; 246:2057–2059.
34. Bernstein LM, Baker LA. A clinical test for esophagitis. *Gastroenterology* 1958; 34:760–781.
35. Barish CF, Castell DO, Richter JE: Graded esophageal balloon distention: A new provocative test for non-cardiac chest pain. *Dig Dis Sci* 1986; 31:1292–1298.
36. Mellow M: Symptomatic diffuse esophageal spasm: Manometric follow-up and response to cholinergic stimulation and cholinesterace inhibition. *Gastroenterology* 197; 73:237–240.
37. Nostrant TT, Saves J, Haber T: Bethanechol increases the diagnostic yield in patients with esophageal chest pain. *Gastroenterology* 1986; 91:1131–1136.
38. Benjamin SB, Richter JE, Cordova CM, et al: Prospective manometric evaluation with pharmacologic provocation of patients with suspected esophageal motility dysfunction. *Gastroenterology* 1983; 84:893–901.
39. London RC, Ouyang A, Snape WJ, et al: Provocation of esophageal pain by ergonovine or edrophonium. *Gastroenterology* 1981; 81:10–14.
40. Alban-Davies H, Kaye MD, Rhodes J, et al: Diagnosis of oesophageal spasm by ergometrine provocation. *Gut* 1982; 23:89–97.
41. Eastwood GL, Weiner BH, Dickerson J, et al: Use of ergonovine to identify esophageal spasm in patients with chest pain. *Ann Intern Med* 1981; 94:768–771.
42. Orlando RC, Bozymski EM: The effects of pentagastrin in achalasia and diffuse esophageal spasm. *Gastroenterology* 1979; 77:472–477.
43. Richter JE, Castell DO: Gastroesophageal reflux: Pathogenesis, diagnosis and therapy. *Ann Intern Med* 1982; 97:93–103.
44. Richter JE, Hackshaw BT, Wu WC, et al: Edrophonium: A useful provocative test for esophageal chest pain. *Ann Intern Med* 1985; 103:14–21.
45. Lee CA, Reynolds JC, Ouyang A, et al: Esophageal chest pain: Value of high dose provocative testing with edrophonium chloride in patients with normal esophageal manometries. *Dig Dis Sci* 1987; 32:682–688.
46. Nasrallah SM, Hendrix EA: Comparison of hypertonic glucose to other provocative tests in patients with non-cardiac chest pain. *Am J Gastroenterol* 1987; 82:406–409.
47. Freiden N, Mittal R, McCallum RW: Is esophageal manometric recording during Tensilon test useful in non-cardiac chest pain? *Gastroenterology* 1987; 92:1395.
48. Johnson LF, DeMeester TR: Twenty-four hour pH monitoring of the distal esophagus: A quantitative measure of gastroesophageal reflux. *Am J Gastroenterol* 1974; 62:325–332.
49. Ward BW, Wu WC, Richter JE, et al: Ambulatory 24-hour esophageal pH monitoring. *J Clin Gastroenterol* 1986; 8(suppl I):59–67.
50. Osler W: *The Principles and Practice of Medicine*, ed 1. New York, Appleton, 1892.
51. Clouse RE, Lustman PJ: Psychiatric illnesses and contraction abnormalities of the esophagus. *N Engl J Med* 1982; 309:1337–1342.
52. Richter JE, Obrecht WF, Bradley LA, et al: Psychological similarities between patients with the nutcracker esophagus and irritable bowel syndrome. *Dig Dis Sci* 1986; 31:131–138.
53. McMahon TP, Richter JE: Non-cardiac chest pain and irritable bowel syndrome: Part of a continuum? *Gastroenterology* 1986; 90:1546.

54. Whitehead WE, Engel BT, Schuster MM: Irritable bowel syndrome: Physiological and psychological differences between diarrhea-predominant and constipation-predominant patients. *Dig Dis Sci* 1980; 25:404–413.
55. Stacker G, Schmeierer C, Kandgraf M: Tertiary esophageal contractions evoked by acoustic stimuli. *Gastroenterology* 1979; 44:49–54.
56. Anderson KO, Dalton CB, Bradley LA, et al: Stress: A modulator of esophageal pressure in healthy volunteers and esophageal chest pain patients. *Dig Dis Sci* (in press).
57. Schuster M: Esophageal spasm and psychiatric disorders. *N Engl J Med* 1983; 309:1382–1383.
58. Richter JE, Dalton CB, Bradley LA, et al: Oral nifedipine in the treatment of non-cardiac chest pain in patients with the nutcracker esophagus. *Gastroenterology* 1987; 93:21–28.
59. Ward WB, Wu WC, Richter JE, et al: Long-term follow-up of symptomatic status of patients with non-cardiac chest pain: Is diagnosis of esophageal etiology helpful? *Am J Gastroenterol* 1987; 82:215–218.
60. Kikendall JW, Mellow MH. Effect of sublingual nitroglycerin and long-acting nitrate preparation on esophageal motility. *Gastroenterology* 1980; 79:703–706.
61. Hongo M, Traube M, McCallum RW: Comparison of effects of nifedipine, probantheline bromide, and the combination of esophageal motor function in normal volunteers. *Dig Dis Sci* 1984; 29:300–304.
62. Mellow MH: Effect of isosorbide and hydralazine in painful esophageal motility disorders. *Gastroenterology* 1982; 83:364–370.
63. Richter JE, Spurling TJ, Cordova CM, et al: Effects of oral calcium blocker, diltiazem, on esophageal contractions. *Dig Dis Sci* 1984; 29:649–656.
64. Hongo M, Traube M, McAllister RG, McCallum RW: Effects of nifedipine on esophageal motor function in humans: Correlation with plasma nifedipine concentration. *Gastroenterology* 1984; 86:8–12.
65. Richter JE, Dalton CB, Buice RG, et al: Nifedipine: A potent inhibitor of contractions in the body of the human esophagus. *Gastroenterology* 1985; 89:549–554.
66. Alban-Davies H, Lewis MJ, Rhodes J, et al: Trial of nifedipine for prevention of oesophageal spasm. *Digestion* 1987; 36:81–83.
67. Frachtman RL, Botoman VA, Pope CE: A double-blind crossover trial of diltiazem shows no benefit in patients wtih dysphagia and/or chest pain of esophageal origin. *Gastroenterology* 1986; 90:14–20.
68. Spurling TJ, Cattau EL, Hirszel R, et al: A double blind crossover study of the efficacy of diltiazem on patients with esophageal motility dysfunction. *Gastroenterology* 1985; 88:1596.
69. Clouse RE, Lustman PJ, Eckert TC, et al: Low-dose trazodone for symptomatic patients with esophageal contraction abnormalities: A double-blind, placebo-controlled trial. *Gastroenterology* 1987; 92:1027–1036.
70. Winters C, Artnak EJ, Benjamin SB, et al: Esophageal bougienage in symptomatic patients with the nutcracker esophagus. *JAMA* 1984; 252:363–366.
71. Ebert EC, Ouyang A, Wright SH, et al: Pneumatic dilatation in patients with symptomatic diffuse esophageal spasms and lower esophageal sphincter dysfunction. *Dig Dis Sci* 1983; 28:481–485.
72. Richter JE, Castell DO: Surgical myotomy for nutcracker esophagus. To be or not to be? *Dig Dis Sci* 1987; 32:95–96.

2

Heartburn:
What is an appropriate evaluation?

ANGELA MERLO, M.D., PH.D.
SIDNEY COHEN, M.D.

Heartburn is a specific symptom of GERD. Esophagitis, esophageal ulceration, stricture, and Barrett's metaplasia are the sequelae of reflux. Heartburn is the most common esophageal disorder encountered in clinical practice. Asymptomatic reflux also occurs. It is important to recognize the clinical situations in which gastroesophageal reflux may occur, develop an appreciation for the proper use of diagnostic procedures, and embark on appropriate management.

PATHOGENESIS

Gastroesophageal reflux occurs when intragastric pressure overcomes the barrier of LES pressure. The LES is specialized circular smooth muscle measuring 3 to 5 cm in length in humans, with unique myogenic properties that enable it to generate a pressure of 12 to 30 mm Hg at rest. The LES relaxes normally in response to swallowing or proximal esophageal distension and is under complex neurohormonal regulation as shown in Table 2–1. LES pressure is increased by cholinergic and α-adrenergic agonists as well as a variety of hormones such as gastrin. LES pressure is decreased by β-adrenergic agonists, certain hormones, and xanthines such as coffee, chocolate, and theophylline. Neurohormonal stimuli or intrinsic alterations in myogenic properties may be the etiology of spontaneous fluctuations in LES pressure. The presence of a hiatal hernia does not alter LES function and is a poor predictor of GERD.[1] Symptoms of reflux are aggravated under conditions of increased intra-abdominal pressure such as occur with physical activity, after meals, when lying supine or wearing tight clothing. However, the clinical manifestations of gastroesophageal reflux and its sequelae are most common and severe when there is an esophageal motility disorder (EMD) in addition to a markedly incompetent LES.[2] This relation exists because peristalsis is the mechanism for clearing the esophagus of refluxed material. The clinical situations in which GERD occurs are listed in Table 2–2.

Although LES incompetence is the major determinant of GER, static measurements of LES pressure are not uniformly predictive of reflux. There is usually a statistical difference in mean LES pressures when large groups of patients with reflux symptoms are compared with asymptomatic subjects.[1, 3] However, there is overlap. The discrepancy may be due to technical difficulties in recording as pressure varies within the sphincter, or to the use of different methods of recording that do not yield identical measurements.[4] Some investigators have proposed that inappropriate relaxation of the LES is a more important determinant of reflux than basal LES pressure. Prolonged continuous monitoring of LES pressure using a Dent sleeve catheter system has demonstrated

TABLE 2–1.
Neurohumoral Agents Affecting Lower
Esophageal Sphincter (LES) Pressure

Increases LES	Decreases LES
Acetylcholine	β-adrenergic agonists
α-adrenergic agonists	Cholecystokinin
Bombesin	Dopamine
Cisapride	Glucagon
Met-Enkephalin	Histamine (H$_2$-receptor)
Gastrin	Nicotine
Metoclopromide	Nifedipine
Motilin	Progesterone
Pancreatic polypeptide	Secretin
Substance P	Vasoactive intestinal peptide
	Xanthines

TABLE 2–2.
Clinical Situations
Involving GERD

1. Idiopathic LES incompetence
2. Pregnancy
3. Chalasia of infancy
4. Scleroderma
5. Iatrogenic
   a. Medical
   b. Surgical
6. Hypothyroidism

that episodes of reflux correlate closely with transient sphincter relaxation unassociated with swallowing.[5]

Idiopathic LES Incompetence

Idiopathic GER, the most common category of LES incompetence, is considered to be a primary sphincter abnormality. The abnormalities in LES function are (1) basal LES incompetence, (2) diminished LES responsiveness to increases in intra-abdominal pressure, and (3) decreased LES pressure changes during feeding. Basal LES incompetence has been attributed to an abnormality in the mechanical properties of the smooth muscle comprising the LES. LES pressure in response to stretch is reduced in patients with LES incompetence.[6] This finding is consistent with the hypothesis that basal LES pressure depends on intrinsic myogenic factors. LES incompetence can also arise from a decrease in excitatory stimuli or an increase in inhibitory stimuli acting on the LES. Decreased fasting serum gastrin levels have been reported in some patients with GER, but, in general, serum gastrin levels correlate poorly with basal LES pressure.[7,8] Regardless of pathogenesis, the incompetent LES fails to respond normally to increases in intra-abdominal pressure.[9,10] In healthy individuals, an increase in intra-abdominal pressure leads to a compensatory rise in LES pressure such that reflux does not occur.[11] In LES incompetence, the LES pressure response is too small to compensate for the increase in intra-abdominal pressure allowing reflux of gastric contents into the esophagus. Patients with LES incompetence also show a reduced LES response to meal stimulus.[7,8]

The LES is a dynamic muscular structure with unique intrinsic myogenic properties and responsiveness to neurohormonal stimuli. Fluctuations in LES pressure lead to intermittent periods of reflux after the ingestion of certain foods or following unexplained stresses. GERD is a dynamic disorder which must be viewed in relation to the specific physical and neurohormonal factors in each patient. Clinically, episodes of reflux are most common (1) in the basal state when the patient is recumbent, (2) during physical activity when increased intra-abdominal pressure overcomes a poorly functioning LES, and (3) after meals when there is release of inhibitory hormones and an increase in gastric volume without a compensatory rise in LES pressure. It is noteworthy that the incompetent LES retains the ability to respond to neurohormonal stimuli such that endogenous cholecystokinin released after a fatty meal or exogenously administered theophylline will further reduce LES pressure.

Pregnancy

The prevalence of heartburn among pregnant women is 30% to 50%, most commonly occurring in the third trimester. Heartburn in pregnancy is accompanied by a reduction in LES resting pressure which returns to normal after delivery. There is convincing evidence that this transient LES incompetence is hormonally mediated. Reductions in LES pressure correlate closely with estrogen and progesterone levels during pregnancy,[12] and oral contraceptives induce similar reductions in LES tone in women[13] and animals.[14] Estrogen and progesterone impair LES responsiveness to neurohormonal stimuli in vitro.[15] Moreover, women with normal basal LES pressure in the first trimester of pregnancy exhibit abnormal LES responsiveness to neurohormonal agents.[16] These data indicate that transient alterations in LES during pregnancy probably reflect a generalized effect of female hormones on smooth muscle and that changes are apparent as early as the first trimester.

Chalasia of Infancy

Infants can regurgitate easily and exhibit significant GER. LES pressures in infants with reflux are reduced in contrast to those of normal infants which fall within the normal range of adults. This reflux is believed to be developmental and diminishes with growth. It most commonly resolves without complication and without medical intervention. However, gastroesophageal reflux has been associated with severe respiratory complications including aspiration pneumonia,[17] apnea,[18] and bronchospasm[19] and has been implicated in some cases of sudden infant death syndrome.[20] Cholinergic agonists often provide sufficient temporary amelioration, although a substantial number of antireflux surgical procedures are performed during infancy for refractory patients.[17,21,22]

Scleroderma

Scleroderma involves the esophagus in 74% of patients in manometric[23,24] and autopsy[25] series. The characteristic manometric features are a reduction in resting pressure of the LES and a reduction in the force of contraction in the distal two-thirds of the esophagus. There is gradual progression to total loss of distal esophageal function and a markedly incompetent LES with pressures less than 5 mm Hg. The incompetent LES leads to severe GER; the inability of the distal esophagus to propel refluxed material into the stomach produces erosive esophagitis in up to 50% of patients. Delayed gastric emptying may be a contributing factor. GER in conjunction with impaired motility is the etiology of symptoms. The symptoms are heartburn, dysphagia, odynophagia, and bronchopulmonary complications from aspirated material. Sequelae develop in up to 40% of patients; these are esophageal ulceration, stricture, and Barrett's metaplasia with an increased risk for developing adenocarcinoma.[26]

The pathogenesis of esophageal dysfunction in scleroderma is not well understood. The prominent lesion at autopsy is patchy smooth muscle atrophy with fibrosis and normal myenteric plexus.[25,27] However, physiologic dysfunction is not well correlated with these pathologic changes.[28] Abnormal motor function can be demonstrated in areas of intact smooth muscle. Indeed, some patients with esophageal dysfunction have a preserved response to direct muscle stimulants but not to agents requiring an intact cholinergic innervation.[23] These findings suggest that there may be a primary neuronal defect early in the disease course which later progresses to muscle atrophy and fibrosis. The esophageal manometric changes may precede by several years the characteristic skin changes of systemic sclerosis.

Esophageal motility disturbances identical to those of scleroderma have been found in patients with mixed connective-tissue diseases.[29] The overlap may stem from a common etiology for the esophageal dysfunction or merely the criteria used to categorize patients. Raynaud's phenomenon is the clinical feature most closely correlated with esophageal dysfunction in scleroderma.[29] Patients with mixed connective-tissue disease who have esophageal dysfunction also have Raynaud's phenomenon.[29, 30] Idiopathic Raynaud's disease and systemic lupus erythematosis (SLE) are not associated with aperistalsis of the esophagus.[23]

Therapy is aimed at preventing the development of reflux esophagitis and its complications. Aggressive medical management is necessary. Once formed, a peptic stricture requires repeated bougienage. Surgical intervention with fundoplication produces grim results because the aperistaltic esophagus can no longer empty. Barrett's esophagus requires close surveillance for malignancy.

Miscellaneous Causes

GER occurs in association with several other clinical conditions. Pharmacologic agents that reduce LES pressure (see Table 2–1) may cause or worsen GER. Reflux is common postoperatively after esophagogastrectomy for malignancies or Heller myotomy for achalasia when a fundoplication is not also performed. Diminished LES pressure in hypothyroidism is due to direct effects on smooth muscle.

CLINICAL SEQUELAE OF GER

GER does not lead to serious sequelae in most individuals. However, in some patients, reflux is complicated by erosive esophagitis, hemorrhage, esophageal ulceration, stricture, or Barrett's metaplasia. It can be difficult to predict which patients will have only heartburn and which will develop sequelae. Factors associated with the severity of the complication are the duration of symptomatic disease, the presence of reflux in the upright as well as recumbent position, the duration of each reflux episode, and the ability of the esophagus to clear refluxed material by peristalsis. In general, patients with sequelae will have reflux in all positions and will maintain a low esophageal pH for prolonged periods because of inability to clear refluxed acid.

The initial histologic alterations associated with reflux are basal cell hyperplasia, thinning of the surface squamous epithelium, and pit elongation. The mucosa may be normal to visual inspection or may show spotty erythema. With disease progression there is inflammatory cell infiltration of the lamina propria and mucosal and submucosal edema. These changes are associated with mucosal necrosis, morphologic evidence of edema, and punctate ulceration. Radiologically, the mucosa appears finely granular with nodularity, erosions, and thickened folds. Progression to erosive esophagitis accounts for 3% to 5% of upper gastrointestinal hemorrhage.

Esophageal Ulceration

Some patients with reflux develop a single large esophageal ulcer. These ulcers are located typically in the distal esophagus and found in conjunction with other manifestations of advanced esophagitis. Peptic esophageal ulceration is to be distinguished from pill-induced inflammatory changes, which are typically more proximally located. Ulceration may also occur in Barrett's epithelium where it is surrounded by relatively normal appearing mucosa. Shallow esophageal ulcers may heal completely. Deep ulceration is usually associated with scarring or stricture formation and possibly retraction of the adjacent esophageal wall.

Peptic Stricture

Peptic stricture of the esophagus is a serious sequela of GER. Strictures are more frequent in patients with an underlying EMD.[2] The stricture is caused by fibrosis in the submucosa and lamina propria and will be asymmetric if the underlying inflammation was eccentrically located in the esophageal wall. Esophageal strictures may be annular, long, or short tubular. Annular strictures are frequently confused radiographically and endoscopically with congenital lower esophageal rings which occur independently of reflux. The classic clinical presentation of a benign peptic esophageal stricture is slowly progressive dysphagia following longstanding symptoms of GER. In all patients with a stricture, endoscopic biopsies and cytologic studies are necessary to exclude malignancy. A benign esophageal stricture can be managed with medical therapy and repeated dilatations; antireflux surgery is reserved for refractory lesions.

Barrett's Esophagus

In Barrett's esophagus columnar epithelium replaces the normal squamous mucosal lining of the distal or mid-esophagus following prolonged GER. There can be different types of columnar epithelium resembling gastric or intestinal mucosa in varying degrees of maturation with jagged borders between zones and islands of columnar cells.[31] In a recent prospective study,[32] Barrett's esophagus was detected in 12.4% of patients with symptomatic GER. The aberrant mucosa is important clinically because it can be the site of ulceration or stricture or the origin or adenocarcinoma. Patients with esophageal adenocarcinoma typically present with rapidly progressive dysphagia; a history of symptomatic GER is often absent.[33-35] The tumors are usually far advanced at time of presentation[36] and sometimes multifocal.[37] The treatment of esophageal adenocarcinoma is surgical resection with the addition of adjuvant chemotherapy or radiotherapy for metastatic disease. Medical therapy for benign Barrett's metaplasia is aimed at preventing the sequelae of GER with endoscopic surveillance for the detection of dysplasia and early malignancies.

DIAGNOSIS

Controversy and confusion surround the diagnosis of GERD. Many diagnostic tests are available for the direct and indirect evaluation of reflux. Their potential value must be assessed in terms of purpose. Tests are presented in Table 2–3 in terms of their specific indication.

Measurement of GER

Direct measurement of GER is done with pH monitoring, radioisotope scintigraphy, or barium swallow.

TABLE 2–3.
Diagnostic Tests to Assess GERD

Test	Sensitivity*
A. Measurement of reflux	
1. pH reflux	
a. Standard acid reflux	Excellent
b. 24-hour esophageal pH monitoring	Controversial
2. Radioisotope scintiscan	Excellent
3. Barium contrast radiography	Poor
4. Esophagoscopy	Poor
B. Assessment of LES competence	
1. Intraluminal manometry	Excellent
C. Evaluation of sequelae of reflux	
1. Barium contrast radiography	Very good
2. Esophagoscopy with biopsy	Excellent
D. Provocation	
1. Bernstein test	Very good

*Sensitivity is the ability to detect positively as determined by the number of false-negative findings.

The standard acid reflux test demonstrates reflux by monitoring esophageal pH at a defined distance above the LES. An esophageal pH less than 4.0 indicates reflux. When the study is performed under basal conditions, a positive result is obtained in less than 70% of symptomatic patients but with no false positives.[38] The sensitivity approaches 100% with 25% false positives when 300 ml of 0.1 N HCl are infused into the stomach during examination. The standard acid reflux test is reliable.[39]

A recent modification of the standard acid reflux test is prolonged ambulatory recording of esophageal pH. This technique enables quantification of esophageal acid exposure and identification of the times reflux occurs, and may help identify provoking factors. Its use has been facilitated by computer analysis and the availability of compact recorders which enable the patient to pursue routine activities. Controversy surrounds the appropriate application of this technique and the criteria for distinguishing pathologic from physiologic episodes of reflux. Establishment of criteria for normality is complicated by the prevalence of mild symptoms in the general population, their occurrence in the absence of demonstrable GERD, and the presence of reflux in asymptomatic patients. Several complex scoring systems have been proposed[40,41] to weigh the frequency of reflux episodes and the cumulative duration of periods of high esophageal acidity. In general, (1) there is considerable individual variation in patterns of reflux; (2) basal LES pressure exhibits considerable temporal variation; (3) physiologic reflux is more common during the day and after meals than at night; and (4) patients who reflux both when recumbent and upright usually also have impaired esophageal clearing and the most severe esophagitis. Whether nocturnal acid reflux is as important a determinant of GERD as originally proposed[42] has recently been disputed.[5,43] The future of prolonged esophageal pH monitoring may lie in its ability to assess improvement from treatment strategies rather than provide an indication for surgical intervention. It may have some value as an extension of the more standard tests in select patients with negative cardiac and gastroesophageal evaluations in whom reflux is being sought as an etiology for atypical chest pain.

Radioisotope scintigraphy is a noninvasive method that quantifies GER by measuring radioactivity in the esophagus after ingestion of a radioisotope. Subjects swallow 300 ml of water mixed with technetium 99m sulfur colloid, and reflux is provoked by inflating an abdominal binder to increase intra-abdominal pressure. Radioactivity detected proximal to the gastroesophageal junction indicates reflux. This test is safe and reliable[39] and has a sensitivity of 79% to 98% in patients with mildly to severely symptomatic GERD.[44] It has been used to detect GER in children in the evaluation of sleep apnea, recurrent pneumonia, regurgitation, and failure to thrive.[45]

Barium contrast radiography is a poor modality for assessing GER. It can demonstrate reflux in the recumbent position but with low sensitivity. Sensitivity may be improved with use of provocative maneuvers, but a high false-positive rate is then obtained.

Assessment of LES Competence

Intraluminal manometry is the only test currently available that directly measures the competence of the physiologic LES. During routine esophageal manometry, LES pressure is determined as the mean of the peak inspiratory and expiratory pressures recorded from three or four catheters pulled slowly across the gastroesophageal junction. Repeated determinations are necessary because pressure is not uniform throughout the sphincter. In general, sphincter measurements can serve to distinguish patients with reflux from those without reflux. Mean sphincter pressure in normal subjects is 15 to 30 mm Hg above intragastric pressure. LES pressure in the extremes has excellent predictive value. Thus, a basal LES pressure of less than 5 mm Hg is highly predictive of reflux,[2] whereas LES pressure greater than 20 mm Hg virtually excludes it. Intermittent values may be more difficult to assess. Reflux can occur with LES pressures between 10 and 15 mm Hg, but these patients may or may not be symptomatic.[45] A second important application of LES pressure determination has been in the postoperative evaluation of fundoplication surgery. Successful surgical fundoplication results in elevation of LES pressure; a fundoplication that is inadequate or slipped or wrapped too tightly may be detected by this method. Esophageal manometry is helpful for the prediction of complications of reflux in that sequelae are more frequent in the presence of a motility disorder.[2]

Evaluation of the Sequelae of Reflux

GER may lead to esophagitis, ulceration, stricture, or Barrett's metaplasia. Methods for evaluating mucosal integrity are barium swallow and endoscopy with histologic evaluation of biopsy specimens. A barium swallow is usually the initial study. A barium swallow is performed not to diagnose reflux but rather to diagnose its sequelae. Ulceration and stricture are particularly amenable to radiographic detection. Barrett's esophagus can be accurately diagnosed in some cases with double-contrast radiography.[47] If the barium swallow is normal and the patient responds to antireflux therapy (see Table 2–4), then no further tests are indicated. Structural or mucosal lesions require further evaluation with endoscopy. Esophagoscopy with biopsy and cytologic brushings has become the best method for assessing the mucosa for inflammation, infection, metaplasia, or malignancy. Assessments of esophageal motility or LES competence during esophagoscopy are inaccurate, insensitive, and not recommended.

Provocation

The major provocative test to assess GER is the Bernstein test in which patient's symptoms are evaluated during perfusion of the distal esophagus with 0.1 N HCl and normal saline in a blinded control. The production of pain with acid but not saline perfusion is a positive result; it occurs in 90% of patients with symptomatic reflux with 10% false positives. The Bernstein test is valuable in confirming the presence of GERD but is less valuable in evaluating atypical chest pain. Some patients with symptomatic diffuse esophageal spasm have a false-positive Bernstein test.

TABLE 2–4.
Therapeutic Interventions for GERD

Stage I: Simple therapeutic maneuvers
  Dietary modifications
  Cessation of alcohol and tobacco
  Discontinuation of drugs that reduce LES pressure
  Avoidance of tight clothing
  Position
  Antacids
Stage II: Pharmacologic maneuvers
  H_2-receptor antagonists
  Bethanecol and metoclopromide
Stage III: Antireflux surgery
  Nissen fundoplication
  Hill procedure

MANAGEMENT

The management of GERD should be individualized according to severity of symptoms, the presence of complications, and response to previous therapy.

Stage I involves simple therapeutic maneuvers that can provide significant amelioration of symptoms when applied alone or in conjunction with pharmacologic agents. Smoking and injestion of foods, such as chocolate or coffee, that reduce LES pressure should be avoided. Weight reduction and wearing loose garments will prevent unnecessary increases in intra-abdominal pressure. Elevation of the head of the bed is helpful in counteracting gravitational effects. Antacids improve symptoms in 70% of patients, but they are inconvenient because they must be administered frequently.

Stage II involves pharmacologic manipulations to increase LES pressure or inhibit acid secretion. Bethanecol and metoclopromide increase LES pressure without increasing pH and provide symptomatic improvement in 60% to 70% of patients with GERD.[48] Bethanecol may have additional therapeutic value in improving peristaltic clearing of the distal esophagus, and metoclopromide may improve gastric emptying. Cimetidine and ranitidine act by reducing the acidity of refluxed material. (Famotidine, the most recently approved H_2-receptor antagonist, has not yet been tested clinically in patients with GERD.) Both cimetidine and ranitidine have been shown to improve the symptoms of GERD in a large number of clinical trials.[49] Objective evidence of healing on endoscopic biopsies has also been demonstrated. Both cimetidine and ranitidine are superior to antacids in alleviating symptoms and promoting healing. However, results of comparisons between H_2-receptor antagonists are less obvious. Observed differences may be more related to dose than drug. Both H_2-receptor antagonists are well tolerated and less associated with side-effects than metoclopromide whose use is often limited by extrapyramidal manifestations. Cimetidine, 1200 mg/day, is usually administered four times daily, and ranitidine, 300 mg/day, is administered two times daily. However, less frequent dosing may be equally efficacious, and higher doses may be safely administered if required to suppress acid output. The combination of metoclopromide and H_2-receptor antagonist may be beneficial in patients refractory to either drug alone, owing to differences in their mechanism of action.[50]

The usual treatment strategy is to continue stage I therapy alone if successful and add an H_2-receptor antagonist as needed. Mildly symptomatic patients will respond uniformly and to a variety of drug regimens. If the patient fails to improve after 6 weeks, reflux should be evaluated with standard tests (see Table 2–3). Subsequent treatment strategies are (1) reassessment after an additional 6 weeks of the same therapy (2) use of an increased dose of H_2-receptor antagonist if required for suppression of acid output, or (3) addition of metoclopromide to the regimen. Severe esophagitis may require 12 weeks to heal on combination medical therapy. Future developments in medical therapy for GERD are domperidone, a dopamine antagonist similar to metoclopromide but without central side-effects, and cisapride, a prokinetic agent to improve smooth muscle contraction. These drugs may prove important in the treatment of severe GERD when used in combination with inhibitors of acid secretion.

Surgery (stage III) is indicated to control otherwise unmanageable complications of reflux. The most widely accepted procedure incorporates a fundoplication around the distal esophagus. The Nissen fundoplication, a full 360-degree wrap of gastric fundus around the distal esophagus, provides clinical improvement with the most consistency. The Hill procedure, a posterior gastroplexy, is less reliable. The Belsey-Mark IV procedure is performed transthoracically—the gastric fundus is wrapped two-thirds around the anterior portion of the distal esophagus. Fundoplication improves LES function by restoring mechanical properties and increasing basal LES pressure.[51-53] Clinical improvement correlates with increases in LES pressure. Objective improvement in mucosal disease can also occur with regression of esophagitis or stricture after successful surgical repair.[53] The success of fundoplication approaches 90% in reported series.[54,55] In practice, results are less impressive. Surgical expertise is essential for excellent results. Postoperative complications are (1) obstructive symptoms such as dysphagia or an inability to belch or vomit from a fundoplication wrapped too tightly around the distal esophagus or (2) persistent reflux from an inadequate fundoplication. Many initially successful surgical repairs lose their effectiveness over time. Antireflux operations can be assessed postoperatively with esophageal manometry and double-contrast barium radiographs. The radiologic detection of surgical failures includes total disruption or incomplete breakdown of the wrap, slippage of the distal esophagus through an intact wrap, or slippage of the fundoplication below the gastroesophageal junction.[56] Reoperation for failed antireflux surgical procedures is common.[57] Acid-reducing operations such as vagotomy or antrectomy have no role in the management of GERD.

References

1. Cohen S: The diagnosis and management of gastroesophageal reflux. Adv Intern Med 1976; 21:47–75.
2. Antaridis G, Snape WJ, Cohen S: Clinical and manometric findings in benign peptic strictures of the esophagus. Dig Dis Sci 1979; 24:858–861.
3. Scheurer U, Halter F: Lower esophageal sphincter in reflux esophagitis. Scand J Gastroenterol 1976; 11:629–634.
4. Welch RW, Drake ST: Normal lower esophageal sphincter pressure: A comparison of rapid versus slow pull-through techniques. Gastroenterology 1980; 78:1446–1451.
5. Dent J, Dodds WJ, Friedman RH, et al: Mechanism of esophageal reflux in recumbent asymptomatic human subjects. J Clin Invest 1980; 65:256–267.
6. Biancani P, Zabinski MP, Behar J: Pressure, tension and force of closure of the human lower esophageal sphincter and esophagus. J Clin Invest 1975; 56:467–483.
7. Lipshutz WH, Gaskins RD, Lukash WM, et al: Hypogastrinemia in patients with lower esophageal incompetence. Gastroenterology 1974; 67:423–427.
8. Farrell RL, Castell DO, McGuigan JE: Measurements and comparisons of lower esophageal sphincter pressures and serum gastrin levels in patients with gastroesophageal reflux. Gastroenterology 1974; 67:415–422.
9. Cohen S, Harris LD: The lower esophageal sphincter. Gastroenterology 1972; 63:1066–1073.
10. Dodds WJ, Hogan WJ, Miller WN: Reflux esophagitis. Am J Dig Dis 1976; 21:49–67.
11. Holloway RH, Hongo M, Berger K, et al.: Gastric distention: A mechanism for postprandial gastroesophageal reflux. Gastroenterology 1985; 89:799–784.
12. Van Thiel DH, Gavaler JS, Joshi SN, et al: Heartburn of pregnancy. Gastroenterology 1977; 72:666–668.
13. Van Thiel DH, Gavaler JS, Stremple J: Lower esophageal sphincter pressure in women using sequential oral contraceptives. Gastroenterology 1976; 71:232–234.
14. Schulze K, Christensen J: Lower sphincter of the opossum esophagus in pseudopregnancy. Gastroenterology 1977; 73:1082–1085.
15. Fisher RS, Roberts GS, Grabowski J, et al: Inhibition of lower esophageal sphincter circular muscle by female sex hormones. Am J Physiol 1978; 234:E243–E247.
16. Fisher RS, Roberts GS, Grabowski CJ, et al: Altered lower esophageal sphincter function during early pregnancy. Gastroenterology 1978; 74:1233–1237.
17. Johnson DG: Current thinking on the role of surgery in gastroesophageal reflux. Pediatr Clin North Am 1985; 32(5):1165–1179.
18. Spitzer AR, Boyle JT, Tuchman DN, et al: Awake apnea associated with gastroesophageal reflux: A specific clinical syndrome. J Pediatr 1984; 104:200–250.
19. Boyle JT, Tuchman DN, Altschuler SM, et al: Mechanisms for the association of gastroesophageal reflux and bronchospasm. Am Rev Respir Dis 1985; 131 suppl:S16–20.
20. Leape LL, Holder TM, Franklin JD, et al: Respiratory arrest in infants secondary to gastroesophageal reflux. Pediatrics 1977; 60:924–929.
21. Cyr JA, Ferrara TB, Thompson TR, et al: Nissen fundoplication for gastroesophageal reflux in infants. J Thorac Cardiovasc Surg 1986; 92:661–666.
22. Fonkalsnid EW, Berquist W, Vargas J, et al: Surgical treatment of the gastroesophageal reflux syndrome in infants and children. Am J Surg 1987; 154:11–18.
23. Cohen S, Fisher R, Lipshutz W, et al: The pathogenesis of esophageal dysfunction in scleroderma and Raynaud's disease. J Clin Invest 1972; 51:2663–2668.
24. Matarazzo S, Snape W, Cohen S: Esophageal dysfunction in scleroderma. Clin Res 1975; 23:482.
25. D'Angelo WA, Fries J, Masi AT, et al: Pathologic observations in systemic sclerosis (scleroderma). Am J Med 1969; 46:428–440.
26. Katzka DA, Reynolds J, Saul SH, et al: Barrett's metaplasia and adenocarcinoma of the esophagus in scleroderma. Am J Med 1987; 82:46–52.
27. Atkinson M, Summerling MD: Oesophageal changes in systemic sclerosis. Gut 1966; 7:402–409.
28. Treacy WL, Baggenstoss AH, Slocumb CH, et al: Scleroderma of the esophagus. A correlation of histologic and physiologic findings. Ann Intern Med 1963; 59:351–356.
29. Stevens MB, Hookman P, Siegal CI, et al: Aperistalsis of the esophagus in patients with connective tissue disorders and Raynaud's phenomenon. N Engl J Med 1964; 270:1218–1222.
30. Garrett JM, Winkelman RK, Schlegel JF, et al: Esophageal deterioration in scleroderma. Mayo Clin Proc 1971; 46:92–96.
31. Spechler ST, Goyal RJ: Barrett's esophagus. N Engl J Med 1986; 315:362–371.
32. Winters C, Spurling TJ, Chobanian SJ, et al: Barrett's esophagus: A prevalent, occult complication of gastroesophageal reflux disease. Gastroenterology 1987; 92:118–124.
33. Sjogren RW, Johnson LF: Barrett's esophagus: A review. Am J Med 1983; 74:313–321.
34. Levine MS, Caroline D, Thompson JJ, et al: Adenocarcinoma of the esophagus: Relationship to Barrett's mucosa. Radiology 1984; 150:305–309.
35. Sarr MG, Hamilton SR, Marrone GC, et al: Barrett's esophagus: Its prevalence and association with adenocarcinoma in patients with symptoms of gastroesophageal reflux. Am J Surg 1985; 145:187–193.
36. Fein R, Kelsen DP, Geller N, et al: Adenocarcinoma of the esophagus and gastroesophageal junction. Cancer 1985; 56:2512–2518.

37. Smith RR, Boitnott LK, Hamilton SR, et al: The spectrum of carcinoma arising in Barrett's esophagus: A clinicopathologic study of 26 patients. *Am J Surg Pathol* 1984; 8:563–573.
38. Kaul B, Petersen H, Grette K, et al: Scintigraphy, pH measurement and radiography in the evaluation of gastroesophageal reflux. *Scand J Gastroenterol* 1985; 20:289–294.
39. Kaul B, Petersen H, Grette K, et al: Reproducibility of the gastroesophageal reflux scintigraphy and the SART. *Scand J Gastroenterol* 1986; 21:795–798.
40. Schindlbeck NE, Heinrich C, Konig A, et al: Optimal thresholds, sensitivity, and specificity of long-term pH-metry for the detection of gastroesophageal reflux disease. *Gastroenterology* 1987; 93:85–90.
41. Schlesinger PK, Donahue PE, Schmid B, et al: Limitations of 24-hour intraesophageal pH monitoring in the hospital setting. *Gastroenterology* 1985; 89:797–804.
42. DeMeester TR, Johnson LF, Joseph GJ, et al: Patterns of gastroesophageal reflux in health and disease. *Ann Surg* 1976; 187:459–469.
43. de Caestecker JS, Blackwell JN, Pryde A, et al: Daytime gastroesophgeal reflux is important in esophagitis. *Gut* 1987; 28:519–526.
44. Kaul B, Halvorsen T, Petersen H, et al: Gastroesophageal reflux disease: Scintigraphy, endoscopic and histologic considerations. *Scand J Gastroenterol* 1986; 21:134–138.
45. Rudd TJ, Christie DL: Demonstration of gastroesophageal reflux in children by radionucleotide gastroesophagraphy. *Radiology* 1979; 131:483–486.
46. Dodds WJ, Hogan WJ, Miller WN: Reflux esophagitis: Progress report. *Dig Dis Sci* 1976; 21:39–47.
47. Levine MS, Kressel HY, Caroline DF, et al: Barrett's esophagus: Reticular pattern of the mucosa. *Radiology* 1983; 147:663–667.
48. McCallum RW, Kline MM, Curry N, et al: Comparative effects of metoclopromide and bethanecol on lower esophageal sphincter pressure in reflux patients. *Gastroenterology* 1975; 68:1114–1118.
49. Cohen S, Merlo A: Gastroesophageal reflux: Evaluation and current treatment. *Postgrad Med* 1987; 81:203–218.
50. Lieberman DA, Keeffe KB: Treatment of severe reflux esophagitis with cimetidine and metoclopromide. *Ann Intern Med* 1986; 104:21–26.
51. Lipshutz WH, Eckert RJ, Gaskins RD: Normal lower esophageal sphincter function after surgical treatment of gastroesophageal reflux. *N Engl J Med* 1974; 291:1107–1110.
52. Behar J, Sheahan D, Biancani P, et al: Medical and surgical treatment of reflux esophagitis: A 38-month report on a prospective clinical trial. *N Engl J Med* 1975; 293:263–268.
53. Snape WJ, Cohen S: Gastroesophageal reflux: Advances in medical and surgical treatment. *Prog Gastro* 1977; 3:695–715.
54. Ellis FH, Crozier RE: Reflux control by fundoplication: A clinical and manometric assessment of the Nissen operation. *Ann Thorac Surg* 1984; 38:387–392.
55. DeMeester TR, Bonavina L, Albertucci M: Nissen fundoplication for gastroesophageal reflux disease. Evaluation of primary repair in 100 consecutive patients. *Ann Surg* 1986; 204:9–20.
56. Hatfield M, Shapir J: The radiologic manifestations of failed antireflux operations. *AJR* 1985; 144:1209–1214.
57. Stirling MC, Orringer MB: Surgical treatment after the failed antireflux operation. *J Thorac Cardiovasc Surg* 1986; 92:667–672.

3

Achalasia:
What are the indications for medical or surgical approaches?

MICHAEL J. FISHER, M.D.
RICHARD W. McCALLUM, M.D.

Achalasia is characterized by aperistalsis in the esophageal body coupled with inadequate relaxation of the lower esophageal sphincter (LES). It was the first described of all motility disorders, being recognized by Thomas Willis in the late seventeenth century.[1] Two centuries later, it became known as "cardiospasm," to denote spasm of the cardia as the site of the obstruction and the cause of the dysphagia. Hurst later coined the term "achalasia" to stress the failure of the LES to relax.[2] In order to examine best approaches toward management for achalasia, we should first review pathophysiology and diagnostic considerations.

ETIOLOGY AND PATHOGENESIS

Most cases of achalasia seen in this country are of unknown etiology. There are reports of achalasia occurring in monozygotic twins[3] and siblings,[4] but environmental factors are presumed to play a role in the idiopathic form. This notion is supported by prevalence studies in Britain that showed concentrations of cases in certain areas, as well as increases in age-specific incidence.[5] Other rare associations exist with certain malignancies,[6-8] with ganglioneuromatosis of the gastrointestinal tract,[9] and with submucosal esophageal hematoma.[10]

In South America there are large numbers of patients with Chagas' disease from infection with *Trypanosoma cruzi* who suffer an identical motor abnormality. Studies of chagasic esophageal disease have aided our understanding of the pathophysiology of achalasia.[11] A destruction of ganglion cells occurs in this infectious form of achalasia, resulting first in a dilatation of the esophagus, followed by compensatory hypertrophy of the musculature. With time this hypertrophied muscle becomes atonic and atrophic, leading to tremendous dilatation. Numbers of ganglion cells remaining correlate with symptoms, although the esophagus can function without symptoms becoming evident until approximately 20% of its ganglia are destroyed.

Pathologic study of the idiopathic form of achalasia reveals similar findings. Grossly, there is muscular thickening, especially of the circular layer. Microscopically, one sees decreased ganglion cells, mononuclear cell infiltration and fibrosis in Auerbach's plexus, and wallerian degeneration in vagal fibers and loss of nerve cell bodies in the dorsal motor nucleus of the vagus.[12] The smooth muscle cells appear normal under light microscopy, but under electron microscopy detachment of microfilaments and cellular atrophy are seen.[13] It is unknown whether these changes are primary or secondary to denervation.

Neuropharmacologic evidence suggests that the incomplete relaxation, or tonic contraction, in achalasia is caused by the absence or functional impairment of noncholinergic inhibitory nerves.[14] There are reduced numbers of vasoactive intestinal polypeptide (VIP) fibers in the esophagus as well,[15] consistent with the hypothesis that VIP is the inhibitory neurotransmitter mediating LES relaxation. It appears that the denervation process is selective because it has been shown that cholinergic excitatory innervation to the LES is intact in achalasics.[16] An exaggerated response to methacholine was noted years ago,[17] and edrophonium significantly increases LES pressure in achalasics[16] compared with normals. This is thought to result from the loss of postganglionic inhibitory nerves to the LES causing unopposed excitation and thus tonic contraction via the excitatory nerves. Serotoninergic nerves, or their absence, may play a role in the pathogenesis of achalasia. In Hirschsprung's disease, enteric serotoninergic axons are absent in aganglionic segments of bowel, and there may be an analogy in achalasia.[18]

An unusual syndrome of achalasia, alacrima (lack of lacrimation) and glucocorticoid deficiency have been described.[19] A possible defect in overall parasympathetic function is theorized in this syndrome. Because achalasia does not appear to involve the parasympathetic system, the inhibitory nerves that usually supply the LES might accompany the parasympathetic nerves or act through a second messenger via the cholinergic system. Evidence to support this concept is seen in some patients with achalasia who have denervation of the stomach and pancreas, as assessed by sham feedings.[20]

Achalasia generally presents in early middle-age adults, although it has been reported in persons as young as age 2 and as old as age 90. Because of this large age range, it has been suggested, but not proven, that there may be a slow virus or autoimmune process causing selective neural degeneration in achalasia. These theories are also supported by epidemiologic clustering of cases.

CLINICAL DATA

Achalasia is uncommon, but not rare, with an incidence of about 1 in 100,000 population per year. Any age can be affected, as mentioned, but the majority of patients present between the ages of 40 and 60. Reports indicate either no sexual predominance, or a slight female dominance with ratios of 3 to 2.

The classic symptom is progressive dysphagia for both solids and liquids. Patients are generally very accurate in localizing the obstruction to the distal retrosternal areas. Dysphagia may vary in severity from day to day while the disease is in its early stages. With time, however, the dysphagia worsens until it is present with every meal and with every single swallow. Regurgitation of undigested food, sometimes eaten a day or so previously, becomes commonplace, especially with bending, stooping, or sleeping. Patients will note food on the pillow in the morning. This is a crucial part of the history and separates achalasia from other motility abnormalities such as diffuse spasm and benign strictures of the esophagus. Of course, this regurgitation may lead to pulmonary complaints of wheezing, coughing, and nocturnal dyspnea from repeated aspiration of contents from the dilated, obstructed esophagus. Pneumonia and lung abscess are not unusual with achalasics. Weight loss may be striking, and patients may appear to the clinician as though they have an occult malignancy.

Chest pain may be the route of presentation with some achalasics, although 75% to 80% have no chest pain. This subgroup of achalasics with chest pain is more likely to be labeled as having "vigorous achalasia." They have the usual manometric characteristics of achalasia, namely impaired LES relaxation, but their nonperistaltic esophageal body contractions may have relatively high amplitudes (greater than 50 mm Hg). These patients may represent a transition phase from pure diffuse esophageal spasm to classic achalasia.[21]

Although clinical information may point the physician toward a diagnosis of achalasia, complete assessment must include radiologic, endoscopic, and manometric testing. Other entities included in the achalasic syndromes (Fig 3–1) may mimic the condition, and based on their presence, treatment will be altered significantly.

Radiology

A plain chest film can occasionally show mediastinal widening, outline of the esophageal wall, or absence of the gastric air bubble (50%) to yield the diagnosis. A lateral chest film may show the tracheal air column pushed anteriorly. A barium swallow will show characteristic features—dilation of the esophagus with a symmetric, smoothly tapering distal end in the shape of a "bird-beak," representing the tonically closed LES (Fig 3–2). There can be an air-fluid level in the upper to midesophagus caused by the retention of retained secretions and food. Dilatation can extend to the level of the upper

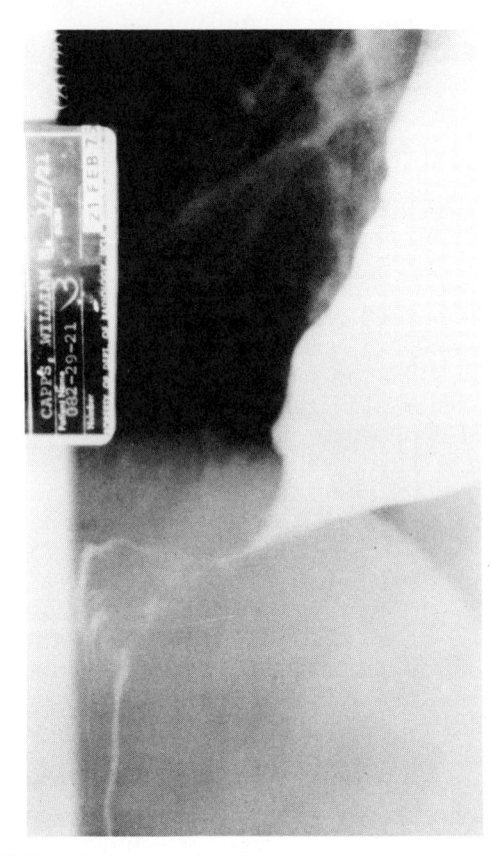

FIG 3–2.
Barium swallow demonstrating "bird-beak" of distal esophagus and LES.

esophagus where striated muscle begins, although typically the striated muscle is normal. Only small squirts of liquid barium from the esophageal column will pass into the stomach on fluoroscopy, or it will fail to pass at all. Peristalsis is absent, but sometimes nonperistaltic, "scalloped" (tertiary) contractions are seen. A severe form, called a "sigmoid" esophagus (Fig 3–3) because of its obvious resemblance, can be seen on some barium studies, as can epiphrenic diverticuli, and represents advanced disease.

THE ACHALASIC SYNDROMES

1. IDIOPATHIC ACHALASIA
    a) CLASSIC TYPE (LOW AMPLITUDE CONTRACTIONS IN ESOPHAGEAL BODY)
    b) "VIGOROUS" TYPE (CONTRACTION AMPLITUDES >50 mm Hg)
2. CHAGAS' DISEASE
3. ACHALASIA ASSOCIATED WITH MALIGNANCY
    - ADENOCARCINOMA OF GASTRIC FUNDUS
    - METASTATIC SITE
    - LYMPHOMA
4. GANGLIONEUROMATOSIS OF THE GASTROINTESTINAL TRACT (MEA, TYPE II,B.)
5. HYPERTENSIVE LOWER ESOPHAGEAL SPHINCTER SYNDROME (NORMALLY RELAXING LOWER ESOPHAGEAL SPHINCTER)

FIG 3–1.
The achalasic syndromes.

Radionuclide Studies

Esophageal emptying can be quantitated using a simple, noninvasive test—a radiolabeled meal.[22, 23] This test gives a

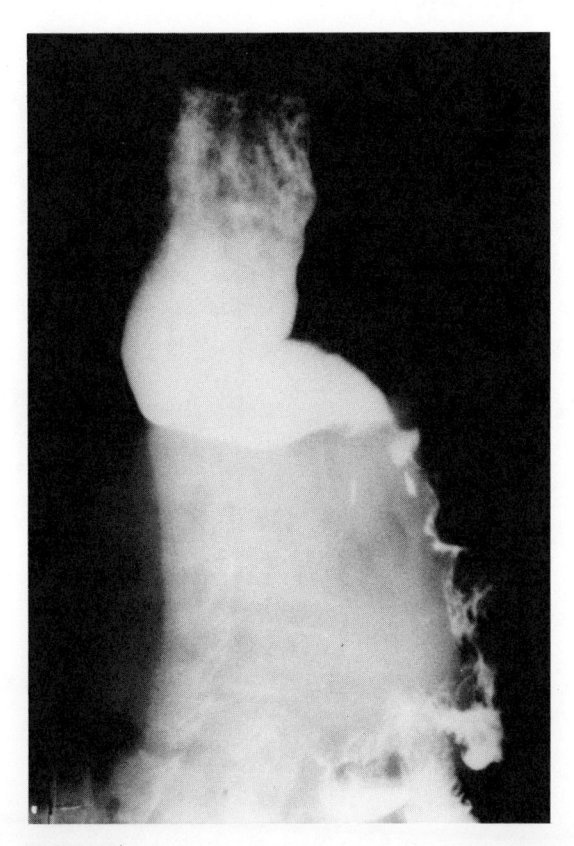

FIG 3–3.
Sigmoid esophagus.

significantly prolonged result when compared with normals and can be repeated posttreatment to assess the degree of improvement, which generally correlates with the changes in LES pressure (Fig 3–4 and 3–5). This technique can also be used as an objective parameter when new treatment options such as medical regimens are being considered. False-positives for achalasia using this technique, as well as barium radiography, have been seen in patients with the entity of isolated hypertensive LES.[24]

Endoscopy

Endoscopic examination is always required to exclude neoplastic processes at the location of the gastroesophageal junction. The only exceptions to endoscopy would be children and young adults under age 17. Although it may be necessary to lavage the esophagus to remove residual food debris prior to visualization, the endoscopic appearance of the mucosa is often normal. However, there may be changes of erythema, friability, or superficial ulceration consistent with stasis-induced esophagitis, and there may be overgrowth with bacteria or Candida. Generally, with gentle pressure the scope will traverse the LES, even if with slight difficulty. If the endoscopist cannot pass the scope into the stomach, one must seriously entertain the diagnosis of cancer causing pseudoachalasia. It is essential that a retroflexed view of the fundus and gastroesophageal junction is obtained at endoscopy. Biopsy is usually performed regardless of the mucosal appearance of the gastroesophageal junction and fundus because some tumors may lie just below a slightly abnormal mucosa.

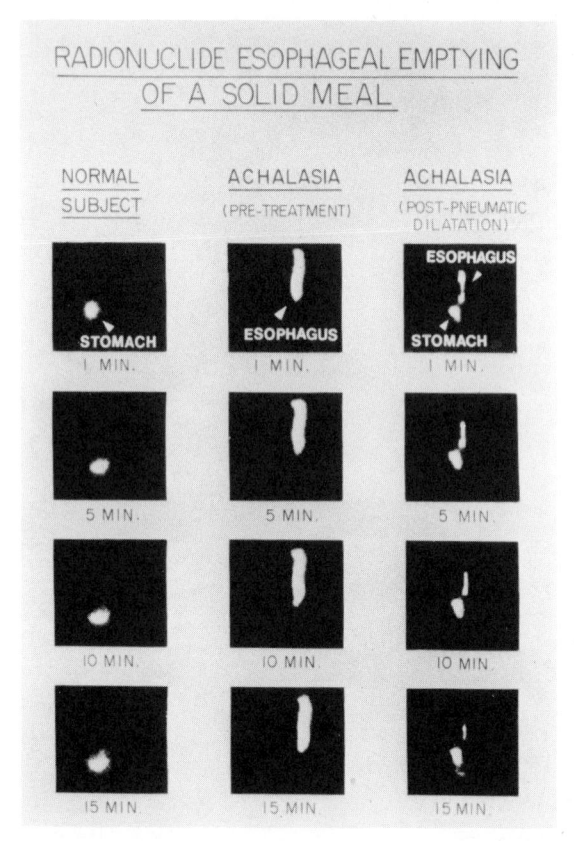

FIG 3–4.
Radionuclide esophageal emptying of a solid meal in a normal esophagus and in achalasia pre- and posttreatment. Note significant prolongation of tracer in achalasia pretreatment at 15 minutes. (From Holloway RH, Krosin G, Lange RC, et al: Radionuclide esophageal emptying of a solid meal to quantitate results of therapy in achalasia. Gastroenterology 1983; 84:771–776.)

pH Studies

Patients with achalasia before dilatation will have prolonged acid exposure times as a result of lactic acid production from decomposing retained food within the esophagus. This frustrates selection of patients who will have postdilatation or postsurgical reflux.[25] However, there would seem to be no justification for pursuing routine pH studies in this patient population.

Manometry

The diagnosis of achalasia should always be established by esophageal manometry[26, 27] (Figs 3–6 and 3–7). Features of significance include: (1) absent peristalsis in the esophageal body; (2) elevated resting intraesophageal pressure higher than intragastric pressure (reverse of normal); (3) LES resting pressure elevated (above 35 mm Hg) in approximately 60% of patients, sometimes to twice normal; and (4) incomplete (not absent) relaxation of the LES (less than 70% of the distance to gastric baseline pressure, range 10% to 70%) with wet swallows. Patients have also been subjected to more physiologic evaluation by measuring their esophageal pressures during eating[28] and have been shown to have lower contraction amplitudes but increased frequency of contractions when compared with normals. A sustained increase in esophageal body

LES relaxation despite other clinical criteria that point toward a diagnosis of achalasia.[29] This again is most likely related to the small size of the manometric catheter measuring the LES, which despite having a normal relaxation pressure, has a shortened duration of relaxation. This group represents a rare subset of patients with achalasia, who also have significantly less weight loss and dysphagia than more traditional achalasics. These findings lend credence to the hypothesis that there is a spectrum of motor disorders, with these patients being slightly different shades in that spectrum.

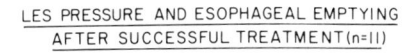

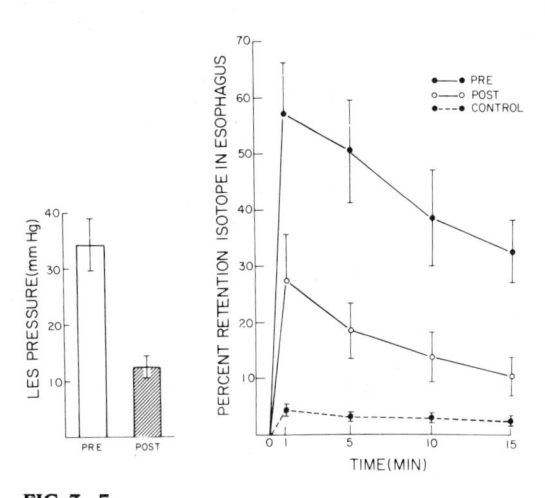

FIG 3–5.
LES pressure and esophageal emptying before and after successful treatment. (From Holloway RH, Krosin G, Lange RC, et al: Radionuclide esophageal emptying of a solid meal to quantitate results of therapy in achalasia. Gastroenterology 1983; 84:771–776.)

pressure is also seen in patients with achalasia during eating. This is most likely a catheter-induced artifact as the esophagus fills up with food. Other confusing manometric findings include apparent complete

PSEUDOACHALASIA

It is important, as previously mentioned, to exclude the presence of a malignancy at or near the gastric cardia giving manometric and radiographic features of achalasia. This is called pseudoachalasia or secondary achalasia. Most commonly these tumors are adenocarcinomas of the gastroesophageal junction, but reports exist of pancreatic, oat cell, squamous cell of the esophagus and lymphomas as causative neoplasms.[6, 8, 26, 30] The mechanisms is not clear, but in some cases infiltration of Auerbach's plexus has been

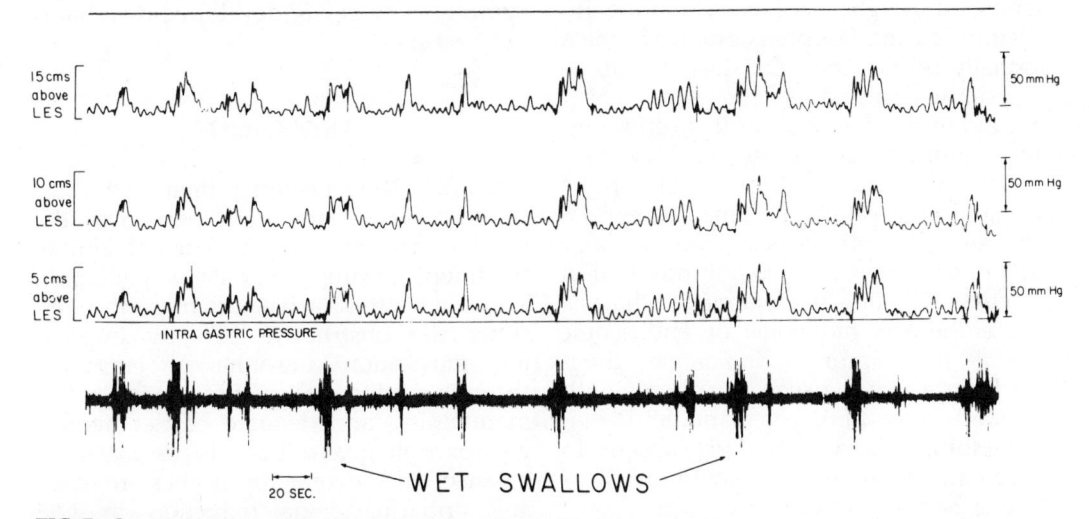

FIG 3–6.
Esophageal manometry of an achalasic patient, demonstrating absent peristalsis in the esophageal body.

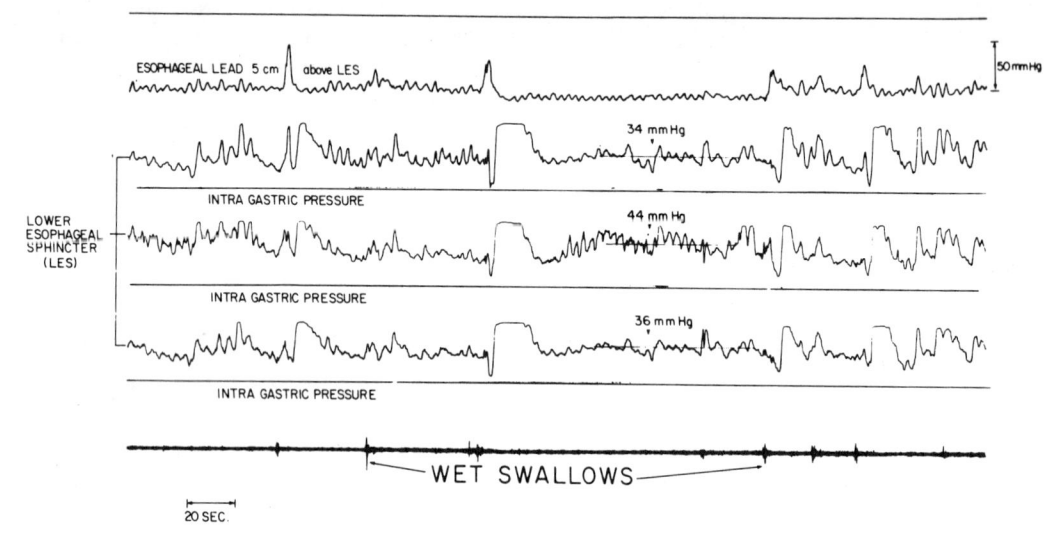

FIG 3–7.
Esophageal manometry showing increased "resting" LES pressure and incomplete relaxation of the LES.

noted. However, there are other reports of apparently non-neurogenic involvement by other tumors, such as bronchogenic carcinoma[31] and hepatoma[32] that cause achalasia from a distance, leading to suspicions of a paraneoplastic syndrome.

Patients with pseudoachalasia should be suspected in the proper clinical setting: patients in older age groups, shorter duration of symptoms (< 6 months), and significant weight loss. Amyl nitrate inhalation during esophagography, which normally relaxes the LES, does not do so in pseudoachalasia.[33] This test, which may aid in the diagnosis of this condition, should not replace endoscopy. However, even with endoscopy, tumors may not be seen and mucosal biopsies may be normal because of a submucosal process. Early exploratory laparotomy is not indicated in patients with newly diagnosed achalasia unless there is radiologic or endoscopic criteria for tumor.[34] Radiologic pseudoachalasia may be seen in patients with a hypertensive LES, yet manometric evidence for achalasia is otherwise absent. In these patients there is a delay in the clearance of barium from the esophagus.

There is some debate whether there is increased risk of carcinoma from longstanding achalasia. Late esophageal carcinoma with an incidence of 2% to 7% has been reported even after treatment of the achalasia.[35,36] However, a prospective follow-up of achalasics[37] could not substantiate this, and a retrospective review of cases of esophageal cancer over 10 years failed to produce a single case of associated achalasia. Thus, recommendations for routine follow-up endoscopy after treatment for achalasia appear unjustified and should be based on recurrence of symptoms or newly developed dysphagia or chest pain.

TREATMENT

Because the cause of primary achalasia is unknown, a cure must remain as the hope of the future. The current aim of treatment in this disorder is palliation. Those who treat achalasics hope to overcome the obstructive LES by improving gravitational esophageal emptying through reduction of LES tone, while maintaining an adequate barrier against gastroesophageal reflux. This is a delicate balance, and several approaches are available; pharmacologic reduction in LES pressure, forceful dilatation, and cardiomyotomy. Even after so-called successful dilatation or surgery, esophageal emptying never becomes normal because of the remaining aperistalsis (Fig 3–5). Patients can "normalize" but they will always have some limitation of the speed of eating.

Pharmacologic Treatment

This approach uses drugs active at the LES. In the past, it was found that nitroglycerin and anticholinergic drugs[38] had transient effects on the resting pressure of the LES, but clinically these drugs are of limited value. Anticholinergics can reduce LES pressure while promoting a reduction in salivation and hence in aspiration potential at night. Nitroglycerin may benefit those with achalasia and significant chest pain.

There has been, in recent years, success with isosorbide dinitrate[39] and nifedipine[40, 41] suggesting that the mechanism for this relaxation may be mediated by the inhibition of transmembrane calcium flux to the smooth muscle cell (Fig 3–8). Both of these drugs perform well clincially, improving symptoms of dysphagia in over 70% of patients with mild to moderate achalasia. Improvement is also demonstrated manometrically and by radionuclide esophageal emptying scan[42] (Fig 3–9). Dosages are begun at 5 mg for isosorbide dinitrate, sublingually, approximately 10 minutes before eating. Dosages can be increased if tolerated, but tachyphylaxis and headaches limit the drug's usefulness.

A double-blind randomized trial in this country showed that nifedipine administered sublingually was significantly better than placebo in relieving dysphagia.[43] Current recommendations for nifedipine as primary therapy in achalasia would be in the following settings: (1) elderly patients or those with significant medical problems such that if perforation accompanying forceful dilatation was to occur or if surgical intervention was required it would be accompanied by a high morbidity; (2) patients who refuse invasive forms

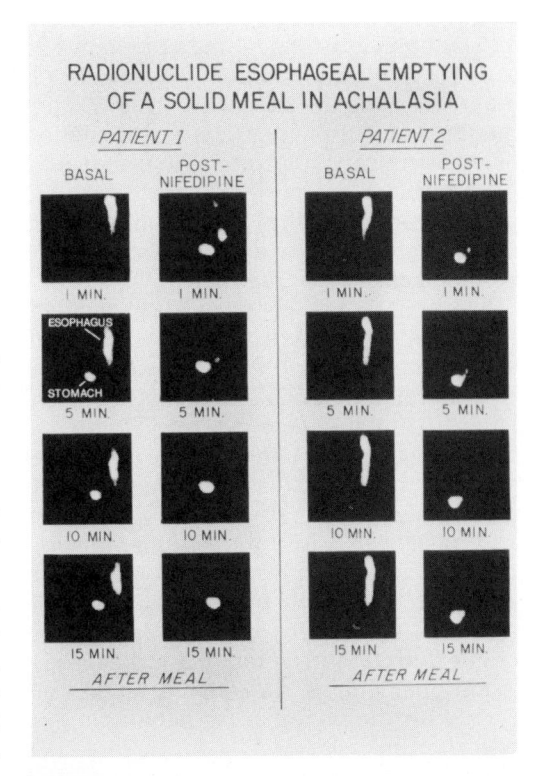

FIG 3–9.
Radionuclide esophageal emptying of a solid meal in two patients with achalasia. Nifedipine improves emptying of radionuclide from obstructed esophagus.

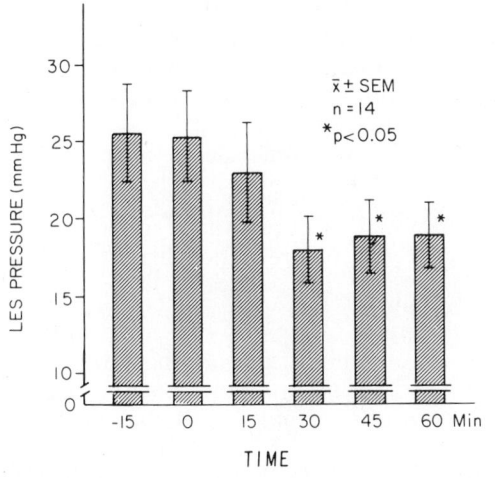

FIG 3–8.
Effect of sublingual nifedipine on LES pressure in patients with achalasia. There is a significant decrease in LES pressure 30 minutes after 20 mg sublingual nifedipine.

of treatment; and (3) patients whose mental state precludes adequate acceptance or cooperation for dilatation or surgery. It may also have an adjunctive role in augmenting or supplementing postdilatation or postsurgical symptoms. Finally, it may be used as a temporizing strategy while patients are deciding on definitive treatment or are trying to arrange for a time to be hospitalized for treatment.

Nifedipine has been used in adolescents[44] as a short-term relief of symptoms until more definitive long-term treatment is undertaken. It may be more effective when combined with anticholinergic drugs (Fig 3–10). Other calcium channel blocking drugs, diltiazem[45] and verapamil,[46] have been studied in achalasics and have been found to result in some reductions in LES pressure. Most experience has been with nifedepine, and one study found it to be more effective than either diltiazem or verapamil[47] (Fig 3–11). Additionally, it is the only drug in this class with the potential for sublingual administration.

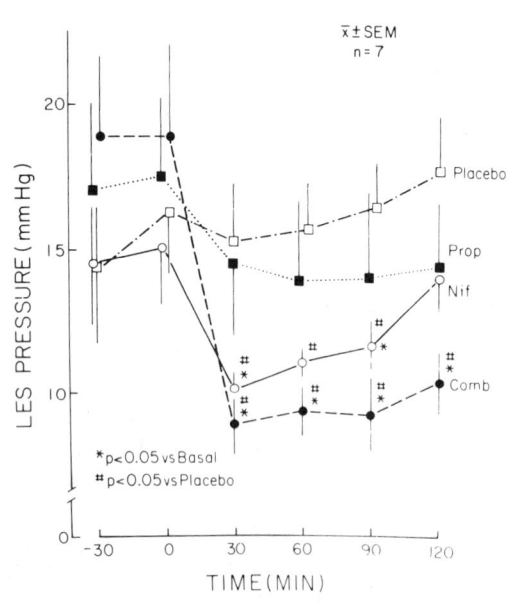

FIG 3–10.
Effect of nifedipine and propantheline on LES pressure. Note additive effect ("comb").

COMPARISON OF DILTIAZAM, VERAPAMIL, NIFEDIPINE, AND ANTICHOLINERGIC ON LES PRESSURE AND ESOPHAGEAL CONTRACTIONS

10 NORMAL ASYMPTOMATIC VOLUNTEERS HAD ESOPHAGEAL MANOMETRY ON 6 DIFFERENT OCCASIONS (ORR & ROBINSON ET AL GASTRO 84, ABSTRACT)

A. BASELINE   C. NIFEDIPINE   E. DILTIAZEM
B. VERAPAMIL D. HYOSCYAMINE F. NIFEDIPINE & HYOSCYAMINE

FINDINGS:

A. NIFEDIPINE ALONE PRODUCED A SIGNIFICANT DECREASE IN LESPRESSURE AND WAS SUPERIOR TO VERAPAMIL AND DILTIAZAM.
B. HYOSCYAMINE AND NIFEDIPINE PRODUCED SIGNIFICANT DECREASES IN AMPLITUDE.
C. HYOSCYAMINE ALONE WAS EQUIVALENT TO H + N.
D. NO AGENT HAD ANY SIGNIFICANT EFFECT ON ESOPHAGEAL TRANSIT.

FIG 3–11.
Comparison of diltiazem, verapamil, nifedipine, and hyoscyamine on LES pressure and esophageal contractions. (Data from Orr WC, Allen ML, Mellow M, et al: Differential effects of calcium channel blocking and anticholinergic agents on esophageal functioning (abstract). *Gastroenterology* 1984; 86:1202.)

Nifedipine can be administered in a dose of 10 mg sublingually (capsules are broken in the mouth) approximately 30 to 45 minutes before meals. The timing is important and plasma concentrations actually peak at 1 hour in achalasics rather than 30 to 40 minutes as in normals.[48] Increasing doses can lead to a higher incidence of side-effects including flushing, dizziness, headache, peripheral edema, and faintness. About 25% of the patients can tolerate a dose of 30 mg, three times a day. It is important to add a nocturnal dose of nifedipine to promote emptying of the esophagus overnight and to minimize regurgitation.

An oral β_2-adrenergic agonist, carbuterol, has been studied in achalasics[49] and a decrease in LES pressure was measured with minimal cardiovascular effects, but in more recent years attention has shifted to the calcium channel blockers.

Long-term treatment with medical therapy is generally disappointing. The drugs have short peak duration of action, tachyphylaxis often results, and the meal frequency is limited to the interval of drug administration. With increasing drug frequency, toxicity becomes the limiting factor and patients will opt for more permanent solutions to their problems. If long-acting and GI smooth muscle-specific relaxant drugs are developed, they may play a wider therapeutic role in achalasia.

Forceful Dilation

The major debate over the treatment of achalasia is between surgeons and dilators. There are patients in whom dilation is not the optimal therapy (Fig 3–12). In the elderly patient with significant and unstable medical disease, one who woud otherwise not be a surgical candidate, the decision to perform dilation, with its 2% to 7% perforation rate, should be reconsidered. A noncooperative or psychotic patient should not have dilation nor should the subset of patients who refuse the procedure.

Hydrostatic or pneumatic dilation depends on rapid distention of the LES with balloons that will disrupt muscle fibers at that zone. This is the reason why mercury-filled bougies (60F) will not provide adequate relief of symptoms even though they may provide short-term palliation. There are problems with control of the amount of forceful dilation required for effectiveness, because of differences in age, build, height, and tissue resistance. The success of the dilation may also correlate with the experience of the dilator. These variables make comparisons between methods and studies quite difficult. New dilation techniques have been developed in recent years to standardize the diameter of balloon dilation accomplished and attempt to bring more "science" and less "art" and "feel."

The most commonly used dilators consist of a single bag of fixed diameter, usually 3 to 4 cm, filled with air (Brown-McHardy, Mosher, Riser-Moeller) (Fig 3–13) or water (Plummer). Pressure is monitored with a gauge and the dilator is positioned under fluoroscopic guidance. The "waist" on the dumbbell-shaped dilator is placed at the manometrically located LES, and the bag is inflated to pressure. The "waist" is eliminated and kept in place for a variable amount of time, ranging from 15 seconds to 5 minutes (Fig 3–14). My personal approach (R.W. McCallum, M.D.) with the Brown-McHardy dilator is 30 seconds per dilation with two separate inflations (8 lb/in^2 and 10 lb/in^2) per session. The inflation should be rapid, over 5 to 10 seconds, and then 30 seconds of full pressure should be maintained. Difficulty with positioning of the dilator may be encountered in the tortuous or sigmoid-shaped esophagus of advanced achalasia.

All patients should be fasting at least 12 hours prior to the procedure, and all should be hospitalized for observation. Even after fasting for this long it may be necessary to pass a tube (large bore) to clean out the esophagus and minimize the chance of aspiration. In preparation for dilation, the patient is positioned in lateral position on a fluoroscopy table at a 60° angle. The pharynx is topically anesthetized, and an intravenous site is established. Atropine given at a dose of 0.6 mg IM 30 minutes before the procedure may minimize salivation and the potential for aspiration. Additionally, a small amount of benzodiazepine may be given to alleviate the patient's anxiety. More important, however, is that the physician fully explains the procedure and continually reassures the patient. The patient must be prepared to experience chest pain because

---

DISCUSSABLE CONTRAINDICATIONS TO PNEUMATIC DILATATION

1. A PHYSICIAN WHO HAS NOT RECEIVED ADEQUATE PRIOR TRAINING
2. INABILITY OF PATIENT TO COOPERATE - QUESTION OF RELATED PSYCHOSIS
3. CHILDREN AND UNDER AGE 17 - a) QUESTION OF COOPERATION; b) SHOULD DILATATION PRESSURES VARY?
4. UNABLE TO EXCLUDE AN ASSOCIATED CANCER OF GASTRIC FUNDUS MIMICKING ACHALASIA
5. A DISTAL EPIPHRENIC DIVERTICULUM - ? OF PERFORATION RISK
6. A SIGNIFICANT HIATAL HERNIA MAKES ACCURATE POSITIONING DIFFICULT - CAN OVERCOME WITH MANOMETRIC LES LOCATION
7. A SEVERELY TORTUOUS "SIGMOID" ESOPHAGUS AND PHYSICIAN NOT FAMILIAR WITH ALTERNATIVE TECHNIQUE
8. TWO OR MORE FAILED PNEUMATIC DILATATIONS

FIG 3–12.
Contraindications to pneumatic dilation in achalasia.

38 / ESOPHAGUS

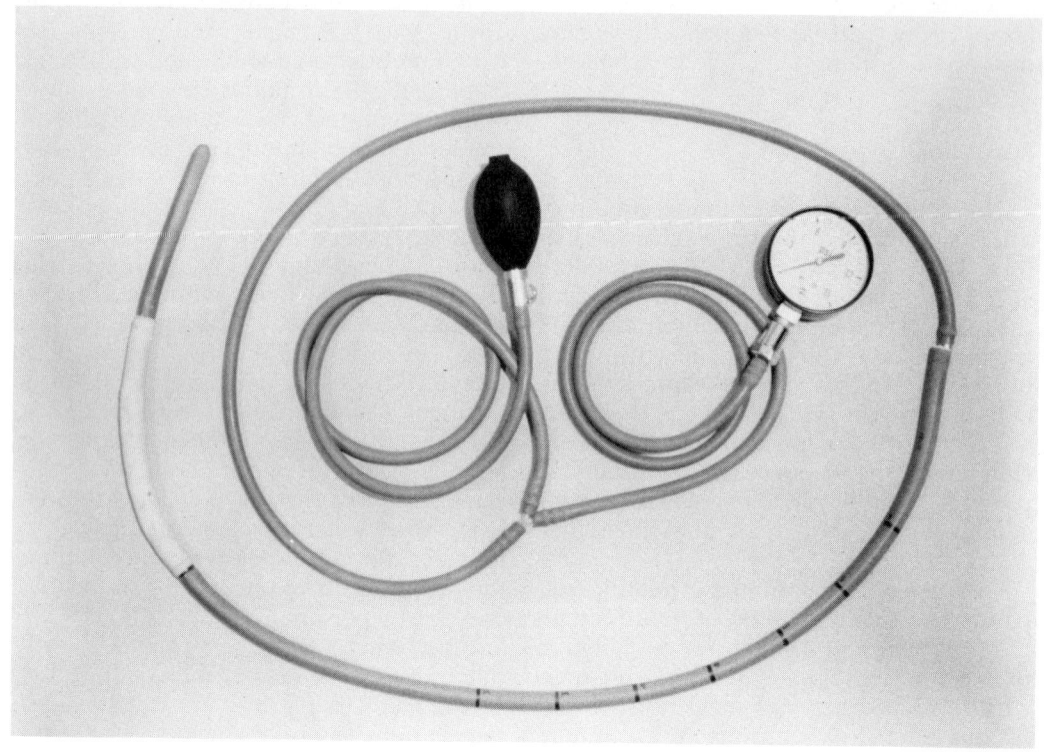

FIG 3–13.
Brown-McHardy bag dilator.

without it a successful muscle rupture cannot be achieved. After passing the dilator into the stomach, the patient is brought to a 90-degree upright angle for fluoroscopy and inflation.

To overcome problems with visualization and positioning in achalasia dilation, new dilators have been developed to fit over the endoscope[50] or over a guide wire.[51] These new dilators still require fluoroscopy to assist in the procedure, but they use modified polyethylene balloons which maintain a fixed shape and diameter when inflated (Fig 3–15). The use of excessive pressure will not enlarge the balloon but will only make it harder. If a rupture should occur, a safe longitudinal tear should theoretically occur rather than a transverse "blow-out" which could perforate the esophagus. A small amount of radiopaque contrast material injected inside the balloon prior to inflation can improve visibility but is unnecessary with the newer models with built-in radiopaque markers.

Blood on the surface of the dilator does not have any prognostic significance for complications but should be noted for completeness. After dilation, either a Gastrografin or thin barium esophagogram should be performed, and patients should be observed NPO (intravenous liquids) overnight for complications. A liquid-soft diet can be commenced the next day, and the patient may be discharged. Barium swallow or radionuclide tests to assess outcome are not indicated until 4 to 6 weeks after the procedure, to allow resolution of edema and mucosal disruption.

Successful dilations can be accomplished with a single procedure in 50% to 84% of patients.[52–54] In my hands (R.W. McCallum, M.D.) the figure is 50% for a single dilation when followed over 10 years. Sometimes repeat dilations are required with progressively larger diameter balloons, giving good to excellent results in 77% of patients.[55] Experience with two dilations (the second using two inflations of 10 and 12 lb/inch) gives a 70% success

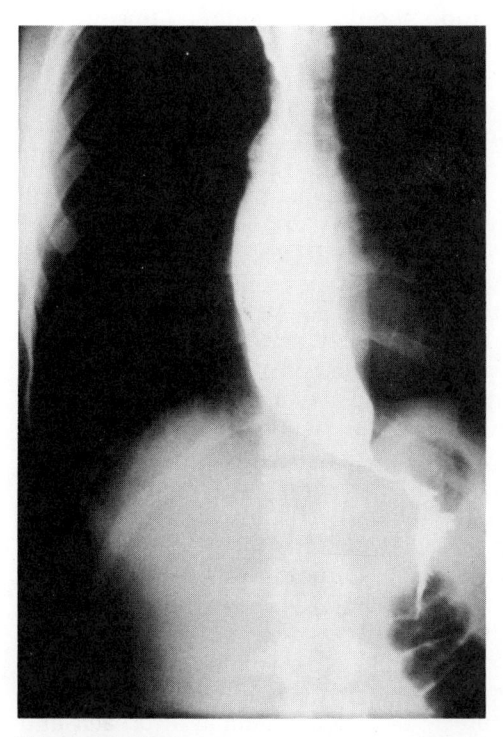

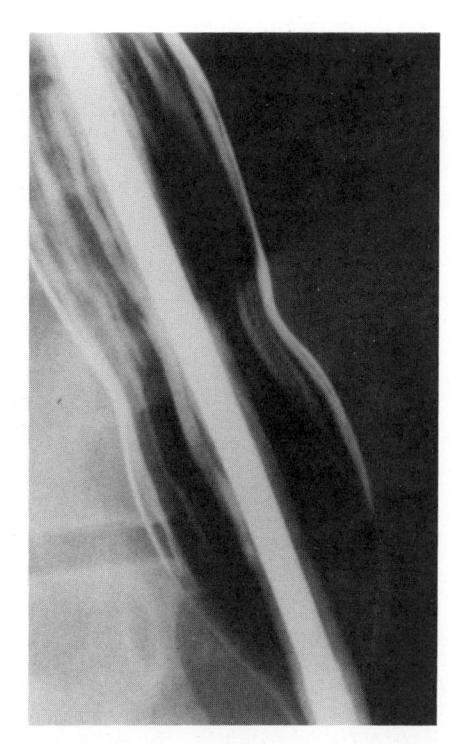

FIG 3–14.
A, typical barium esophagram in achalasia; **B,** Brown-McHardy bag in place at LES being inflated. Note "waist" on bag is being eliminated with inflation to pressure.

rate for patients followed over 10 years.[56]

Complications of forceful dilation are predominately in the form of perforations (Fig 3–16). The rate of perforation ranges from 2.2% in Vantrappen's series[57] to 7% in Nemir's study.[58] Only gastroenterologists who are fully trained and maintaining his or her skills should be performing dilations, with surgical back-up available in the event of a complication. Otherwise, dilations should only be performed at major referral centers. Dilation should be avoided for 1 week after biopsies of the gastroesophageal junction. Minimal, if any, sedation should be given during the procedure so that the patient can signal to the physican that disruption of the LES is occurring. The first symptom of perforation is thoracic pain. A perforation should be suspected if substernal pain persists postdilatation for more than 30 minutes, but especially if a new pain develops within the first 2 to 6 hours after the initial pain subsides. The new chest pain increases with respiration, refers to the back or lower thoracic region, and is usually accompanied by fever. A repeat esophagogram will demonstrate the disruption in most cases, and a chest x-ray may show a left pleural effusion, mediastinal air, or air under the diaphragm. Early laparotomy with closure of the laceration and cardiomyotomy is required in some cases,[59] but recently nonsurgical management has been advocated in this form of iatrogenic perforation, using parenteral alimentation, intravenous antibiotics, H_2 blockers and strict NPO.[57, 60] This conservative management is appropriate when signs of shock or massive hemorrhage are absent, of course. Despite the perforations, good long-term symptomatic relief from achalasia can still be obtained with nonsurgical treatment in these cases.

Since there is some residual LES pressure (usually 10 to 15 mm Hg), gastroesophageal reflux is rare after pneumatic dilation, occurring and continuing in fewer than 1% of patients. Patients have variable degrees of heartburn after return-

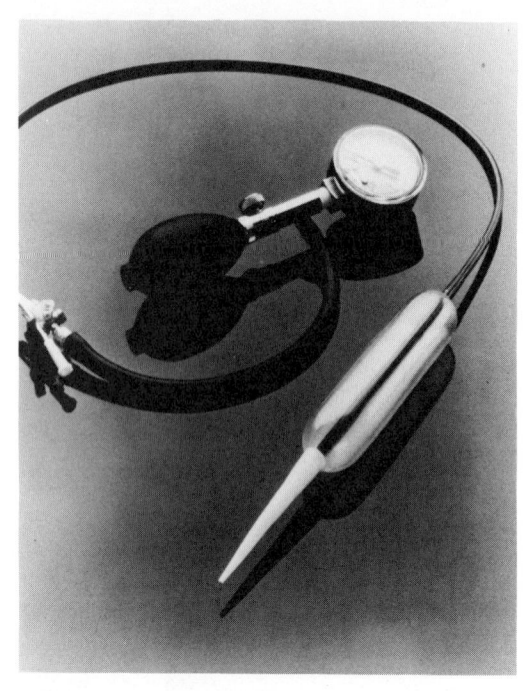

FIG 3–15.
New achalasia dilator. Strong polyethylene balloon inflates to set volume, reducing variable pressure effects during disruption of LES. (Courtesy of Microvasive, Inc. Milford, Mass.)

ing home, which last for as long as 4 to 8 weeks but which can be managed with antacids quite well. Barrett's esophagus has been reported in the postdilation achalasic esophagus,[61] with one case leading to adenocarcinoma within Barrett's epithelium.[62]

Successful outcomes have been achieved in children over age 9 with achalasia[63] although some authors[64] feel that repeat

```
          COMPLICATIONS OF PNEUMATIC DILATATION

1.  PERFORATION - GENERALLY REGARDED AS 2% BUT IN LITERATURE
    UP TO 7%.
    NEW CHEST PAIN, FEVER, (L) PLEURAL EFFUSION WITHIN 4-6
    HOURS OF PROCEDURE
    SURGICAL VS CONSERVATIVE (TPN) AND ANTIBIOTIC MANAGEMENT
2.  ASPIRATION PNEUMONIA
3.  BURNING CHEST PAIN REGARDED AS GE REFLUX RELATED TO
    CHANGE IN LES PRESSURE
```

FIG 3–16.
Complications of pneumatic dilation.

dilation should not be done after the failure of the initial dilatation.

Surgery

Indications for surgery are debated between surgeons and dilators. However, we feel that surgery should be undertaken when (1) there is a history of two failed dilations by experienced hands; (2) a knowledgeable and trained gastroenterologist is absent; (3) there is an experienced esophageal surgeon who performs this operation frequently; or (4) there is achalasia in children younger than 15 years old. Cardiomyotomy produces effective relief of achalasia symptoms in the majority of patients—85% to 90% in the large Mayo Clinic series.[65] Several different approaches are used, but the procedure with the widest acceptability is the modified Heller myotomy alone.[66] This procedure is performed by either a transthoracic or transabdominal approach and involves incising the circular and longitudinal muscles of the esophagus down to the mucosa. Modifications are based on length and how far to extend the myotomy onto the gastric musculature. In the vigorous achalasia subgroup, myotomy is often extended to the level of the aortic arch. There are trade-offs for the surgeon; to ensure that a full myotomy is made and no fibers remain that could allow dysphagia to persist the surgeon may extend the incision onto the gastric musculature, increasing the risk of reflux now that the main barrier for its prevention is obliterated. A major concern of the modified Heller operation is the roughly 10% incidence of reflux esophagitis that results.[57] Even though the dysphagia may be improved, a late peptic structure may become manifest. The incidence of reflux postoperatively appears to increase with time[67]—as much as 50% at 13 years.

This substantial incidence of postsurgical reflux esophagitis has led some surgeons to include an antireflux procedure during the initial esophageal myotomy.[68, 69] This proposal is still at issue with some surgeons who feel that in the achalasic, aperistaltic esophagus, a fundoplication can produce unpredictable obstruction.[63] Not only is there the question of whether to add an antireflux procedure, but once the decision is made to add it, another question arises as to which type of repair is best. Unfortunately, these questions have not been addressed by randomized trials. My personal recommendation (R.W. McCallum, M.D.) is the addition of a loose antireflux procedure—preferably a Belsey type done over a 60 French dilator. For the individual patient who undergoes operation for achalasia, the technique in which the surgeon has the most experience is the best for that patient, keeping in mind that GER may be asymptomatic in many patients and that if it presents, it can be approached medically.

A third procedure used to surgically treat achalasia is called a cardioplasty, a full-thickness incision through muscle and mucosa over which a gastric patch is sewn. The experience with this procedure is limited and is rarely done today.[70] For the patient with a "sigmoid" esophagus, the surgical approach involves pulling down and straightening the esophagus. Esophagojejunostomies or colonic interpositions should never be performed for classic achalasia. Patients with continued dysphagia after surgery may benefit from adjunctive nifedipine or anticholinergics. There is a role for forceful dilation in the postmyotomy setting, but this should only be attempted by experienced physicians.

Suggestions for Treatment

Before any treatment is instituted, it is assumed that a number of important criteria have been met. Organic strictures and achalasia secondary to carcinoma must be excluded by radiology and endoscopy. The degree of symptomatology will often dictate the direction of therapy after diagnostic studies have identified achalasia. Dietary modification is an important element of any treatment approach, and, in addition to a change in texture of food, eating in the evening should be limited to reduce nocturnal regurgitation. For the less severely symptomatic patient who is without nutritional impairment, a trial with nitrates or nifedipine is warranted as the initial therapy. Even as symptoms progress, maximization of the pharmacologic approach may abate symptoms and postpone more invasive means. However, in most patients the effect of smooth muscle relaxants is short-lived and the change in life-style that mandates their food intake to be linked to medication will be intolerable. Definitive therapy can then take either the surgical or dilatation route. Again it must be emphasized that to consider dilation is to consider surgery in view of the potential for complications. There may even be a rare patient who is best served with interval esophageal lavage with an Ewald tube in the physician's office and fluoroscopically guided mercury bougienage.

Pneumatic dilatation has the advantage of requiring only an overnight stay (with surgical stand-by for complications) in the hospital, compared to 10 to 14 days in the hospital for esophagomyotomy, added to intensive care unit if needed, chest tube, a 6-week recovery period, and loss of work for several months. In this era of DRGs, there is no comparison for the cost issue.

A general consensus favors dilation as the initial step in the management of achalasia. Unfortunately, the only randomized prospective study comparing pneumatic dilation and esophagomyotomy[71] was not only small but was biased against the dilated patients because of more pronounced dysphagia. In addition to this, the technique of dilation may have been insufficient. The conclusion favoring surgery over dilation in achalasia is thus debatable. Retrospective comparisons[52, 65, 72] of esophagomyotomy versus pneumatic/hydrostatic dilation identify higher initial success rates (90% versus 70%) and lower long-term recurrence rates (14% versus 59%) but as mentioned, a longer hospitalization and a higher incidence of complications related to this major operative procedure. Mortality for either procedure is less than 0.1%. Because there is no indication that forceful dilation predisposes to poor outcome from esophagomyotomy, we favor esophageal dilation as the initial step in long-term achalasia therapy. Greater than 50% of patients will have the expectation of a sustained successful outcome, and it may spare them from a major operation in approximately two-thirds of the time. Of those that relapse after initial dilation, 50% will do so within the first 12 months. A second dilation in this group of patients will have the same success rate as the initial dilation, as well as the same 2% risk of perforation. An overall success rate for both dilations will be approximately 70%. Those who fail to sustain the response from the second dilation should be offered esophagomyotomy by an experienced surgeon. A third dilation in this scenario is associated with an increase in the risk of perforation and we would counsel against further dilation. Inadequate myotomy or complications of surgery leading to persistent dysphagia may require reoperation. Remedial surgery for achalasia can correct the dysphagia in the majority of patients[73] although it is technically more demanding because of scar tissue distorting the anatomical relationships of the area.

Based on the above economic and statistical arguments alone it would seem logical to perform dilation as initial long-term therapy for achalasia. There has been in the past a regional factor to be reckoned with. Certain geographic areas may have experienced surgeons capable of esophagomyotomy but may not have adequately trained gastroenterologists who feel comfortable with a seldom-performed procedure such as dilation. The traditional techniques of pneumatic dilation involve variables that alter not only success rates but complications too. Recent additions to the therapeutic armamentarium are balloon dilators of fixed shapes and sizes which permit standardization of inflation pressures, widths, and times. These new tools should facilitate future prospective comparisons between surgery and dilation by removing some of these variables. They should also make the technique easier to learn and thus more widely available.

Acknowledgement

The authors wish to acknowledge the expert secretarial assistance of Joyce Dolan in preparing this manuscript.

References

1. Willis T: *Pharmaceutic Rationalis: Sive Diatriba De Medicamentorum; Operationibus in Humano Copore.* London, Hagae-Comitis, 1674.
2. Hurst AF, Rake GW: Achalasia of the cardia (so-called cardiospasm) *Q J Med* 1930; 23:491.
3. Stein DT, Knauer CM: Achalasia in Monozygotic twins. *Dig Dis Sci* 1982; 27:636–640.
4. Stoddard CJ, Johnson AG: Achalasia in siblings. *Br J Surg* 1982; 69:84–85.
5. Mayberry JF, Atkinson M: Variations in the prevalence of achalasia in Great Britain and Ireland: An epidemiological study based on hospital admissions. *Q J Med* 1987; 62:67–74.
6. Tucker HJ, Snape WJ Jr, Cohen S: Achalasis secondary to carcinoma: Manometric and clinical features. *Ann Intern Med* 1978; 89:315–318.
7. McCallum RW: Esophageal achalasia secondary to gastric carcinoma. Report of a case and review of the literature. *Am J Gastroenterol* 1979; 71:24–29.
8. Kline MM: Successful treatment of vigorous achalasia associated with gastric lymphoma. *Dig Dis Sci* 1980; 25:311–313.
9. Cuthbert JA, Gallagher ND, Turtle JR: Colonic and esophageal disturbance in a patient with multiple endocrine neoplasia, type 2b. *Aust NZ J Med* 1978; 8:518–520.
10. Hooper TL, Gholkar J, Smith SR: Recurrent submucosal dissection of the esophagus in association with achalasia. *Postgrad Med J* 1986; 62:955–956.
11. Koberle F: Pathogenesis of Chagas' disease. in *CIBA Foundation Symposium on Trypanosomiasis and Leishmaniasis, with special reference to Chagas' Disease.* Caracas, Venezuela, Feb. 13–15, 1973. Elsevier, Amsterdam, 1974, pp 137–158.
12. Vantrappen G, Hellemans J: *Diseases of the Esophagus.* Springer-Verlag, New York, 1974.
13. Casella RR, Ellis FH, Brown AL: Fine-structure changes in achalasia of the esophagus. *Am J Pathol* 1965; 46:279–288.
14. Dodds, WJ, Dent J, Hogan W: Paradoxical lower esophageal sphincter contraction induced by cholecystokinin-octapeptide in patients with achalasia. *Gastroenterology* 1981; 80:327–333.
15. Aggestrup S, Uddman R, Sundler F: Lack of vasoactive intestinal polypeptide nerves in esophageal achalasia. *Gastroenterology* 1983; 84:924–927.
16. Holloway RH, Dodds WJ, Helm J: Integrity of cholinergic innervation to the lower esophageal sphincter in achalasia. *Gastroenterology* 1986; 90:924–929.
17. Kramer P, Ingelfinger FJ: Esophageal sensitivity

to mecholyl in cardiospasm. *Gastroenterology* 1951; 19:242–254.
18. Gershon MD, Erde SM: The nervous system of the gut. *Gastroenterology* 1981; 80:1571–1594.
19. Pombo M, Devesa J, Taborda A: Glucocorticoid deficiency with achalasia of the cardia and lack of lacrimation. *Clin Endocrinol* 1985; 23:237–243.
20. Dooley CP, Taylor IL, Valenzuela JE: Impaired acid secretion and pancreatic polypeptide release in some patients with achalasia. *Gastroenterology* 1983; 84:809–813.
21. Minami H, McCallum RW: Chest pain: Differentiating esophageal disease from angina pectoris. *Compr Ther* 1982; 8:50–58.
22. Rozen P, Gelfond M, Zaltzman S: Dynamic, diagnostic, and pharmacologic radionuclide studies of the esophagus in achalasics. *Radiology* 1982; 144:587–590.
23. Holloway RH, Krosin G, Lange RC, et al: Radionuclide esophageal emptying of a solid meal to quantitate results of therapy in achalasia. *Gastroenterology* 1983; 84:771–776.
24. Traube M, Lagarde S, McCallum RW: Isolated hypertensive lower esophageal sphincter: Treatment of a resistant case by pneumatic dilatation. *J Clin Gastroenterol* 1984; 6:139–142.
25. Smart HL, Foster PN, Evans DF: Twenty-four hour oesophageal acidity in achalasia before and after pneumatic dilatation. *Gut* 1987; 28:883–887.
26. Fisher R, Cohen S: Disorders of the lower esophageal sphincter. *Annu Rev Med* 1975; 26:373–390.
27. Castell DO: Achalasia and diffuse esophageal spasm. *Arch Intern Med* 1976; 136:571–579.
28. Little AG, Skinner DB, Chen W: Physiologic evaluation of esophageal function in patients with achalasia and diffuse esophageal spasm. *Ann Surg* 1986; 203:500–504.
29. Katz PO, Richter JE, Cowan R: Apparent complete lower esophageal sphincter relaxation in achalasia. *Gastroenterol* 1986; 90:978–983.
30. Kahrilas PJ, Kishk SM, Helm J: Comparison of pseudoachalasia and achalasia. *Am J Med* 1987; 82:439–446.
31. Rock LA, Latham PS, Hankins JR: Achalasia associated with squamous-cell carcinoma of the esophagus: A case report. *Am J Gastroenterol* 1985; 80:526–528.
32. Feczko PJ, Halpert RD: Achalasia secondary to non-gastrointestinal malignancies. *Gastrointest Radiol* 1985; 10:273–276.
33. Dodds WJ, Stewart ET, Kishk SM: Radiologic amyl nitrite test for distinguishing pseudoachalasia from idiopathic achalasia. *AJR* 1986; 146: 21–23.
34. Sadler RS, Bozymski EM, Orlando RC: Failure of clinical criteria to distinguish between primary achalasia and achalasia secondary to tumor. *Dig Dis Sci* 1982; 27:209–213.
35. Just-Viera JO, Haight C: Achalasia and carcinoma of the esophagus. *Surg Gynecol Obstet* 1969; 128:1081–1095.
36. Heiss FW, Tarshis A, Ellis FH Jr: Carcinoma associated with achalasia. Occurrence 23 years after esophagomyotomy. *Dig Dis Sci* 1984; 29: 1066–1069.
37. Chuong JJH, DuBovic S, McCallum RW: Achalasia as a risk factor for esophageal carcinoma: A reappraisal. *Dig Dis Sci* 1984; 19:1105–1108.
38. Ona FV, Polintan LS: Vigorous achalasia. Manometric response to atropine and nitroglycerin. *Arch Intern Med* 1980; 140:1118–1120.
39. Gelfond M, Rozen P, Gilat T: Isosorbide dinitrate and nifedipine treatment of achalasia: A clinical, manometric and radionuclide evaluation. *Gastroenterology* 1982; 83:963–969.
40. Bortolotti M, Labo G: Clinical and manometric effects of nifedepine in patients with esophageal achalasia. *Gastroenterology* 1981; 80:39–44.
41. Berger K, McCallum RW: Nifedepine in the treatment of achalasia. *Ann Intern Med* 1982; 96:61–62.
42. Rozen P, Gelfond M, Solzman S: Radionuclide confirmation of the therapeutic value of isosorbide dinitrate in relieving the dysphagia in achalasia. *J Clin Gastroenterol* 1982; 4:17–22.
43. Traube M, DuBovik S, Magyar L, et al: Sublingual nifedipine in achalasia: A randomized, double-blind study. *Gastroenterology* 1986; 90:1670.
44. Maksimak M, Perlmutter DH, Winter HS: The use of nifedipine for the treatment of achalasia in children. *J Pediatr Gastroenterol Nutr* 1986; 5:883–886.
45. Silverstein BD, Kramer CA, Pope CE: Treatment of esophageal motor disorders with a calcium-blocker, diltiazem. *Gastroenterology* 1982; 81:1181.
46. Becker BS, Burakoff R: The effect of verapamil on the lower esophageal sphincter pressure in normal subjects and in achalasia. *Am J Gastroenterol* 1983; 78:773–775.
47. Orr WC, Allen ML, Mellow M, et al: Differential effects of calcium channel blocking and anticholinergic agents on esophageal functioning (abstract). *Gastroenterology* 1984; 86:1202.
48. Hongo M, Traube M, McAllister RG: Effect of nifedipine on esophageal motor function in humans: Correlation with plasma nifedipine concentration. *Gastroenterology* 1984; 86:8–12.
49. DiMarino AJ, Cohen S: Effect of an oral beta-2 adrenergic agonist on lower esophageal sphincter pressure in normals and in patients with achalasia. *Dig Dis Sci* 1982; 27:1063–1066.
50. McLeen TR, Bombeck CT, Nyhus LM: Endoscopic piggyback pneumatic dilation in the initial management of patients with achalasia. *Gastrointest Endosc* 1986; 32:290–292.
51. Cox J, Buckton GK, Bennett JR: Balloon dilator in achalasia: A new dilator. *Gut* 1986; 27:986–989.
52. Donahue PE, Samuelson S, Schlesinger PK: Achalasia of the esophagus. Treatment controversies and the method of choice. *Ann Surg* 1986; 203:505–511.
53. Dellipiani AW, Hewetson KA: Pneumatic dilation in the management of achalasia: Experience of 45 cases. *Q J Med* 1986; 58:253–258.
54. Fellows IW, Ogilvie AL, Atkinson M: Pneumatic dilation in achalasia. *Gut* 1983; 24:1020–1023.
55. Vantrappen G, Janssens J: To dilate or to oper-

ate? That is the question. *Gut* 1983; 24:1013–1019.
56. Hongo M, Baue AE, Rafelson S, et al: The long-term results of pneumatic dilatation and distal esophagomyotomy on symptoms and esophageal function in 109 patients with achalasia (unpublished data).
57. Vantrappen G, Hellemans J: Treatment of achalasia and related motility disorders. *Gastroenterology* 1980; 79:144–154.
58. Nemir P, Fallahnej MD, Bon B: A study of the causes of failure of esophagocardiomyotomy for achalasia. *Am J Surg* 1971; 121:143–149.
59. Slater G, Sicular AA: Esophageal perforations after forceful dilatation in achalasia. *Ann Surg* 1982; 195:186–188.
60. Swedland A, Traube M, Siskind BN: Non-surgical management of esophageal perforation from pneumatic dilatation in achalasia. *Dig Dis Sci* (in press).
61. Agha FP, Keren DF: Barrett's esophagus complicating achalasia after esophagomyotomy. A clinical, radiologic, and pathologic study of 70 patients with achalasia and related motor disorders. *J Clin Gastroenterol* 1987; 9:232–237.
62. Gallez JF, Berger F, Mouliner B: Esophageal adenocarcinoma following heller myotomy for achalasia. *Endoscopy* 1987; 19:76–78.
63. Boyle JT, Cohen S, Watkins JB: Successful treatment of achalasia in childhood by pneumatic dilation. *J Pediatr* 1981; 99:35–40.
64. Azizkhan RG, Tapper D, Eraklis A: Achalasia in childhood: A 20-year experience. *J Pediatr Surg* 1980; 15:452–456.
65. Okike N, Payne WS, Neufeld DN: Esophagomyotomy versus forceful dilation for achalasia of the esophagus: Results in 899 patients. *Ann Thorac Surg* 1979; 28:119–125.
66. Castrini G, Pappalardo G, Modarhan S: New approach to esophagocardiomyotomy: Report of 40 cases. *J Thorac Cardiovasc Surg* 1982; 84:575–578.
67. Jara FM, Toledo-Pereyra LH, Lewis JW: Long-term results of esophagomyotomy for achalasia of the esophagus. *Arch Surg* 1979; 114:935–936.
68. Black J, Vorbach AN, Collins JL: Results of Heller's operation for achalasia of the esophagus. The importance of hiatal repair. *Br J Surg* 1976; 63:949–953.
69. Bjorck S, Dernevik L, Gatzinsky P: Esophagocardiomyotomy and anti-reflux procedure. *Acta Chir Scand* 1982; 148:525–529.
70. Hirashima T, Sato H, Hara T: Results of esophagocardioplasty with gastric patch in treatment of esophageal achalasia. *Ann Surg* 1978; 188:38–42.
71. Csendes A, Velasco N, Braghetto I: A prospective randomized study comparing forceful dilatation and esophagomyotomy in patients with achalasia of the esophagus. *Gastroenterology* 1981; 80:789–795.
72. Mayberry JF, Smart HL, Atkinson M: Audit of surgical and pneumatic hydrostatic treatment of achalasia in a defined population. *J R Soc Med* 1986; 79:708–710.
73. Mercer CD, Hill LD: Reoperation after failed esophagomyotomy for achalasia. *Can J Surg* 1986; 29:177–180.

4

Barrett's Esophagus: What should be done to reduce anxiety?

STUART JON SPECHLER, M.D.

It is appropriate that patients with Barrett's esophagus have some anxiety regarding their condition. After all, they are predisposed to develop esophageal adenocarcinoma, an exceptionally virulent malignancy. Recent studies indicate that anxiety about cancer for patients with Barrett's esophagus need not be overriding, however. Their risk of esophageal cancer appears to be smaller than that suggested by earlier reports. Furthermore, regular endoscopic surveillance may provide the opportunity to detect tumors in Barrett's esophagus at an early, curable stage. Knowledge of the natural history of the disorder and the rationale for endoscopic surveillance should help to reduce anxiety for affected patients. These issues are discussed in this chapter.

BACKGROUND

Barrett's esophagus is the condition wherein the squamous mucosa of the distal esophagus is replaced by an abnormal columnar epithelium.[1] In most cases, the condition is acquired as a consequence of reflux esophagitis. The pathogenesis is judged to involve peptic ulceration of the esophagus; the ulcerated squamous mucosa may be re-epithelialized by immature cells which, in the presence of GER, differentiate into the columnar cells that comprise Barrett's mucosa.[2] Thus, Barrett's esophagus appears to be acquired through the process of metaplasia, the replacement of one adult cell type by another.

Barrett's mucosa is comprised of one or any combination of three types of epithelia.[3] The commonest type in adults is *specialized columnar epithelium* (often called intestinal, metaplastic, or distinctive epithelium). This epithelium resembles small intestinal mucosa with its villiform surface and crypts lined by columnar and goblet cells. The columnar cells of specialized columnar epithelium usually lack the well-defined brush borders that typify normal intestinal absorptive cells, however. The specialized columnar cells also contain glycoprotein secretory granules characteristic of gastric foveolar cells but not of intestinal absorptive cells. In addition to these columnar and goblet cells, the crypts of specialized columnar epithelium may contain Paneth's cells and enteroendocrine cells. *Junctional-type epithelium* resembles the mucosa of the normal gastric cardia with both its pitted surface and glands lined by mucus-secreting cells. *Gastric fundic-type epithelium* resembles that of the gastric fundus and body with its pitted surface lined by mucus-secreting cells and its glands that contain parietal cells and chief cells; compared to normal gastric mucosa, gastric fundic-type epithelium appears somewhat atrophic. Proof for the diagnosis of Barrett's esophagus requires the demonstration of at least one of these three epithelial types on an esophageal biopsy specimen obtained above the LES.

The average age at the time of diagnosis of Barrett's esophagus is approximately 55 years.[1] There is a male predominance, and the disorder is uncommon in blacks. Symptoms are primarily those of the associated GERD, including heartburn, regurgitation, and dysphagia. Ulceration and stricture of the esophagus complicate the majority of reported cases.

The most useful diagnostic techniques for Barrett's esophagus are radiography and esophagoscopy. A barium swallow revealing a benign-appearing stricture of the proximal esophagus strongly suggests Barrett's esophagus, but this finding is present in only the minority of cases.[4] For most patients, the radiographic changes are those of reflux esophagitis in general, and no radiographic finding is specific for Barrett's epithelium. Esophagoscopic examination characteristically reveals velvety, red Barrett's epithelium in the distal esophagus extending proximally as a circumferential sheet, or as irregular finger-like projections and islands that contrast sharply with the pale, glossy squamous epithelium.[5] These endoscopic features are not specific for Barrett's epithelium, however. Furthermore, Barrett's mucosa in children may be indistinguishable from squamous epithelium by endoscopic examination.[6] Therefore, the diagnosis always requires histologic confirmation.

In addition to an esophageal biopsy specimen revealing abnormal columnar epithelium, the diagnosis of Barrett's esophagus often requires some assurance that the specimen was obtained above the LES. Most authorities accept the diagnosis when endoscopic examination reveals velvety, red mucosa (biopsy specimens that show columnar epithelium) involving 3 cm or more of the distal tubular esophagus. For clinical purposes, any biopsy specimen obtained from the tubular esophagus that shows specialized columnar epithelium should be considered diagnostic, even when the extent of the columnar lining is not clear. With uncommon exceptions, specialized columnar epithelium is specific for Barrett's esophagus.[1]

ESTIMATION OF THE RISK OF ESOPHAGEAL CANCER

The presence of Barrett's mucosa per se causes no symptoms. In fact, some studies suggest that Barrett's epithelium may be less sensitive to painful stimuli than squamous mucosa.[7] Therefore, Barrett's esophagus would be merely a medical curiosity except for its association with esophageal adenocarcinoma. Because of that association, some authorities have recommended invasive therapies such as antireflux surgery to reduce the cancer risk.[8] Formulation of a rational management program for patients with Barrett's esophagus first requires a reasonable estimate of their risk for developing cancer, however. If that risk is high, invasive treatment programs may be warranted. Alternatively, a low risk of cancer might not justify the risks of invasive therapies.

Earlier estimates for the risk of cancer in this condition were based primarily on reports that described the frequency of esophageal adenocarcinoma in some series of patients with Barrett's esophagus.[9] These cancer prevalence rates ranged from 0% to 47%, with a mean of approximately 10%.[10] It is not appropriate to conclude on the basis of these data, however, that 10% of all patients with Barrett's esophagus will develop cancer. Very few of the patients with esophageal malignancies in those reports were known to have Barrett's epithelium prior to their initial presentations. Most of the cancer patients were seen initially because of their symptoms of esophageal cancer, and the Barrett's epithelium was discovered during their evaluations for cancer of the esophagus. In contrast, for the patients with benign Barrett's esophagus, the Barrett's epithelium was discovered during their evaluations for reflux esophagitis. Therefore, the reports described primarily the frequency with which adenocarcinoma was present at the time of the initial diagnosis of Barrett's esophagus, not the frequency with which cancer-free patients developed adenocarcinoma. Extrapolation of these data to estimate the risk of cancer development for patients with benign Barrett's epithelium would tend to exaggerate that risk.

Data on the incidence of adenocarcinoma in patients with Barrett's esophagus provide a better estimate for the risk of cancer development than do prevalence data. To obtain incidence data, one first identifies a group of cancer-free patients with Barrett's esophagus, and then follows them for the development of esophageal adenocarcinoma during a specified period.

The results of three studies on the incidence of esophageal cancer in patients with Barrett's esophagus are summarized in Table 4–1.[9, 11, 12] These data suggest that the incidence of esophageal cancer in Barrett's patients is approximately one case per 200 person-years, an incidence rate 30-fold to 40-fold higher than that of the general population. Pessimists might despair over this dramatic relative increase in the risk for esophageal cancer. Optimists might note that cancer of the esophagus is an uncommon tumor in the general population of the United States where it accounts for only 1% of all malignancies.[13] Even a 40-fold increase in the incidence of esophageal cancer represents a small risk for the *individual* patient. Clinicians must judge the importance of that risk and devise a management program for their patients with Barrett's esophagus.

IMPORTANCE OF THE CANCER RISK FOR PATIENTS WITH BARRETT'S ESOPHAGUS

One method for judging the clinical importance of the risk of cancer in Barrett's esophagus is to compare it to the risk of another common malignancy in the general population such as lung cancer. As previously noted, the incidence of adenocarcinoma in Barrett's esophagus is approximately one case per 200 person-years. Disease incidence rates are often reported as cases per 100,000 person-years. So expressed, the incidence of adenocarcinoma in Barrett's esophagus is 500:100,000 (1:200 = 500:100,000). Most series of patients with Barrett's esophagus are comprised of older white males.[1] As shown in Table 4–2, the incidence of esophageal cancer in patients with Barrett's esophagus is similar to the incidence of lung cancer in white men of the same age group in the general population.[13]

There are dramatic geographic variations in the incidence rates for esophageal cancer. The incidence is low in the United

TABLE 4–1.
Results of Studies on the Incidence of Cancer in Barrett's Esophagus*

	Study Center		
	Boston VA	Mayo Clinic	Lahey Clinic
Number of cancer-free patients followed	105	104	41
Mean length of follow-up	3.3 yr	8.5 yr	4.0 yr
Number of patients developing cancer during follow-up	2	2	2
Incidence of esophageal cancer (case/person-years)	1/175	1/441	1/81
Estimated increased risk above general population	40-fold	30-fold	NA

*Data from Spechler SJ, Robbins AH, Rubins HB, et al: Adenocarcinoma and Barrett's esophagus: An overrated risk? *Gastroenterology* 1984; 87:927–933; Cameron AJ, Ott BJ, Payne WS: The incidence of adenocarcinoma in columnar-lined (Barrett's) esophagus. *N Engl J Med* 1985; 313:957–959; and Sprung DJ, Ellis FH Jr, Gibb SP: Incidence of adenocarcinoma in Barrett's esophagus (abstract). *Am J Gastroenterol* 1984; 79:817.

TABLE 4–2.
Cancer Incidence Rates

Population	Cancer Type	Incidence (per 100,000)
Barrett's esophagus patients	Esophagus* (adenocarcinoma)	500
White men, ages 55–64	Lung†	227
White men, ages 65–74	Lung†	459
White men, ages 75+	Lung†	539
Chinese men in Linxian County	Esophagus‡ (squamous cell)	161

*Estimate based on data from Spechler SJ, Robbins AH, Rubins HB, et al: Adenocarcinoma and Barrett's esophagus: An overrated risk? *Gastroenterology* 1984; 87:927–933; Cameron AJ, Ott BJ, Payne WS: The incidence of adenocarcinoma in columnar-lined (Barrett's) esophagus. *N Engl J Med* 1985; 313:957–959; and Sprung DJ, Ellis FH Jr, Gibb SP: Incidence of adenocarcinoma in Barrett's esophagus (abstract). *Am J Gastroenterol* 1984; 79:817.
†1983 data from Sondik EJ, Yound JL, Horm JW, et al: *1985 Annual Cancer Statistics Review.* Bethesda, MD, National Cancer Advisory Board, 1985 (DHHS publication no. [NIH] 86-2789).
‡Data from Wu YK, Huang GJ, Shao LF, et al: Honored guest's address: Progress in the study and surgical treatment of cancer of the esophagus in China, 1940–1980. *J Thorac Cardiovasc Surg* 1982; 84:325–333.

States, while parts of China have such high rates that the government has sponsored mass esophageal cancer screening programs in those areas.[14] One such area is Linxian County of Henan Province, where the mortality rate from esophageal cancer in men (approximately equal to the incidence rate) is 161:100,000.[14] As summarized in Table 4-2, the incidence of cancer in Barrett's esophagus appears to be similar to that of lung cancer in the general population, and even greater than that for a high-risk area of China where mass esophageal cancer surveillance programs have been implemented. Based on these comparisons, the risk of cancer for patients with Barrett's esophagus appears formidable, albeit smaller than that suggested by earlier reports.

THE CASE FOR ENDOSCOPIC SURVEILLANCE

Rationale

A program of regular endoscopic and histologic surveillance to detect early, curable, malignancies has been proposed for patients with Barrett's esophagus.[1] While the efficacy of this program in reducing cancer mortality is not known, there is indirect evidence that supports the concept of endoscopic surveillance. One line of indirect evidence is the recent observation from China that esophageal cancers can grow for years before patients develop symptoms.[15] When a cancer of the esophagus has grown to the extent that it produces symptoms, the cure rate is dismal. Unfortunately, few esophageal cancers are discovered in an early, asymptomatic phase when cure may be possible. Endoscopic surveillance that resulted in the discovery and prompt treatment of an asymptomatic cancer of the esophagus presumably would improve the chance for cure.

More evidence supporting the concept of endoscopic surveillance emerges from studies suggesting that esophageal adenocarcinoma does not arise *de novo* in most cases, but rather evolves through a series of progressively severe dysplastic changes in the Barrett's epithelium.[10] The discovery of benign dysplasia on examination of esophageal biopsy specimens obtained during the endoscopic examination would provide opportunity for therapeutic intervention prior to the development of invasive cancer.

Dysplasia

Dysplasia in Barrett's epithelium is defined as an unequivocal neoplastic alteration of the esophageal columnar mucosa,[16] judged to be the precursor of invasive adenocarcinoma. Guidelines have been established to categorize dysplasia as high-grade or low-grade depending on abnormalities in the size, shape, staining characteristics, and position of the nuclei in the glandular cells; and on abnormalities of glandular architecture.[17, 18] Interpretation of these guidelines is a subjective skill, however. Disagreement among experienced pathologists in grading dysplasia is common, particularly in distinguishing low-grade dysplasia from regenerative changes in an injured epithelium.[19] Because the finding of dysplasia in Barrett's epithelium has such important clinical implications, it is prudent to have that finding confirmed by at least two expert pathologists.

Ironically, the contention that dysplasia is a premalignant lesion is based largely on the frequent association of dysplasia and Barrett's adenocarcinoma. Dysplasia has been found in the columnar epithelium surrounding Barrett's adenocarcinomas in 68% to 100% of cases,[1] and investigators have speculated that these cancers evolved from dysplastic changes that initially were benign. Dysplasia has been found in fewer than 10% of patients with Barrett's esophagus who have no apparent esophageal tumors.[16] The few reports available on the natural history of these cases suggest that patients found to have dysplasia in Barrett's epithelium frequently either will develop cancer or will already have an inapparent esophageal malignancy.[18, 20] It is important to recognize that perendoscopic biopsy specimens sample only a tiny fraction of the esophageal mucosa, and a small focus of invasive cancer can easily be missed because of biopsy sampling error. Problems with biopsy sampling error contribute to the uncertainty regarding the frequency of cancer development for patients with dysplasia in Barrett's esophagus. Despite these problems, the finding of dysplasia during an endoscopic surveillance examination might provide the opportunity to prevent cancer or to cure an asymptomatic esophageal malignancy.

Should We Do It?

When recommending procedures for a cancer-related health checkup, the American Cancer Society has identified four concerns: (1) that there be good evidence that the procedure is effective in reducing morbidity or mortality, (2) that the medical benefits outweigh the risks, (3) that the cost be reasonable compared to the expected benefits, and (4) that the recommended procedures be practical and feasible.[21] These concerns should be considered when recommending endoscopic surveillance for patients with Barrett's esophagus.

To address the first concern of the American Cancer Society, there is no direct evidence that endoscopic surveillance is effective in reducing the morbidity or mortality of esophageal cancer for patients with Barrett's esophagus. Unfortunately, such evidence is not likely to be available soon. Suppose one wants to design a controlled, randomized study to demonstrate that endoscopic surveillance decreases the mortality from esophageal cancer in Barrett's esophagus by 50%. Assuming an annual mortality rate from esophageal cancer for these patients of 500:100,000, such a study would require some 2,000 patients to be followed for approximately 10 years (power, 0.80; p value, 0.05).[22] Most reported series of patients with Barrett's esophagus are comprised of fewer than 50 cases. Furthermore, it has been estimated that programs for the early detection of lethal malignancies can reduce mortality rates by only about 10%, not 50%.[23] The number of patients and duration of follow-up necessary for a study to demonstrate a 10% decrement in mortality render the undertaking of such an investigation impractical.

The second concern proposed by the American Cancer Society can be answered easily. The risks of elective esophagoscopy are negligible.[24] Therefore, virtually any reduction in the mortality rate for esophageal cancer resulting from an endoscopic surveillance program would outweigh its risks.

The American Cancer Society's third concern, that the cost of endoscopic surveillance be reasonable compared to its expected benefits, cannot be answered in the absence of clear guidelines on what cost is reasonable. The cost of an endoscopic examination is substantial. The question is: How much is it worth to reduce the mortality from esophageal cancer? Stated differently, a conclusion on whether endoscopic surveillance is cost-effective requires that a financial value be placed on the lives saved.

Finally, upper gastrointestinal endoscopy is a widely available procedure. If reported series are representative, the number of patients with Barrett's esophagus is not so great that regular surveillance would overwhelm the endoscopic services of most institutions. Thus, in answer to the fourth concern voiced by the American Cancer Society, endoscopic surveillance of these patients seems both practical and feasible.

In summary, the rationale for endoscopic surveillance to detect curable esophageal neoplasms for patients with Barrett's esophagus is reasonable. It is improbable that proof for a beneficial effect of surveillance on mortality rates will be available in the near future given the large number of patients and long duration of follow-up required for a study to statistically confirm such an effect. Regular endoscopic surveillance is both safe and readily available. The major disadvantage is cost. Nevertheless, it seems inappropriate for the physician to withhold this potentially life-saving procedure from patients with Barrett's esophagus solely because of financial concerns.

THE CASE AGAINST ANTIREFLUX SURGERY FOR CANCER PROPHYLAXIS

Patients with Barrett's esophagus often require antireflux surgery to control severe manifestations of GERD such as persistent esophageal ulcerations and strictures, hemorrhage, pulmonary aspirations, and intractable symptoms of reflux esophagitis. In addition to these generally accepted indications, some authorities have recommended antireflux surgery for *all* patients with Barrett's esophagus, regardless of symptoms, specifically in an effort to reduce the risk of esophageal cancer.[8] Antireflux surgery is associated with substantial morbidity and mortality, however. Before recommending such a risky procedure, one should examine the evidence for efficacy.

Regression of Barrett's Epithelium

There is no direct evidence that antireflux surgery reduces the risk of cancer in Barrett's esophagus. Regression of Barrett's epithelium has been described after antireflux surgery,[25] and this regression has been proposed as an index for decreased risk of esophageal cancer. The assumption is that a therapy which is so successful as to result in regression of the aberrant epithelium must also decrease its propensity for malignancy. This seems reasonable, but one should recognize that it is a leap of faith to conclude that regression of Barrett's epithelium is tantamount to decreased risk of esophageal cancer.

Even if one accepts this tenuous premise that regression of Barrett's epithelium means less cancer risk, the frequency of such regression after antireflux surgery is unclear for at least two reasons:

1. Some investigators concluded that the Barrett's epithelium regressed after surgery on the basis of suction biopsy specimens of the esophagus.[25] Suction biopsy specimens are not usually obtained under direct vision. Rather, the biopsy tube is passed

through the mouth, and the specimen is obtained blindly when the biopsy port reaches a specified distance from the incisor teeth. In some studies, a postoperative biopsy specimen revealing squamous epithelium at the same level where a preoperative specimen showed columnar epithelium was interpreted as evidence of regression. Frequently, however, the Barrett's mucosa involves the esophagus eccentrically. As shown in Fig 4–1, a biopsy specimen taken at a level 35 cm from the incisor teeth could reveal either columnar or squamous epithelium, depending on which direction the biopsy port happened to face. The alleged epithelial regression in these reports could have been merely the result of sampling error.

2. The effects of antireflux surgery on esophageal mucosal architecture are not known. It is conceivable that what was interpreted as epithelial regression may only represent a mechanical effect of esophageal surgery which moves the squamocolumnar junction distally.

In summary, while it appears that regression of Barrett's epithelium can occur after antireflux surgery, conclusive evidence is not available, and the frequency of regression is not known.

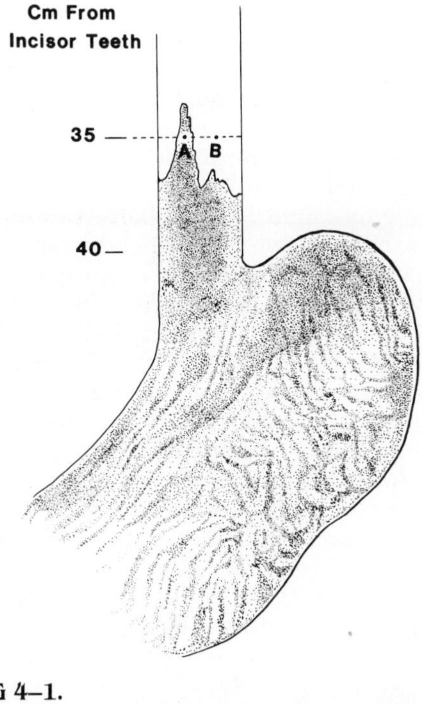

Antireflux Surgery and Dysplasia

If one accepts the concept that cancer in Barrett's esophagus evolves through progressive dysplastic changes, then the finding of dysplasia warrants therapeutic intervention. There are two basic approaches to therapeutic intervention for dysplasia. The direct approach is to resect the dysplastic epithelium. The indirect approach is to eliminate the factors driving the progression from dysplasia to cancer. It has been proposed (without proof) that GER promotes the development of benign epithelial dysplasia in the first place, and that continued reflux promotes the progression from benign dysplasia to invasive carcinoma. An extension of this argument suggests that elimination of reflux with antireflux surgery should cause dysplasia to regress and thus halt the development of cancer.

There are few data to support this hypothesis. One report described two patients who had apparent regression of dysplasia after antireflux surgery.[8] The authors concluded that successful antireflux surgery "leads to stabilization and possibly regression of the dysplasia in Barrett's epithelium." The same report described pre- and postoperative biopsy results for eight other patients; two of those patients had apparent *progression* of dysplastic changes. Overall in this study, antireflux surgery resulted in regression

FIG 4–1.
Diagram of esophagus and stomach illustrating eccentric involvement of esophagus by columnar epithelium. The stippled and unstippled areas represent columnar and squamous epithelium, respectively. A biopsy obtained at a level 35 cm from the incisor teeth could reveal either Barrett's epithelium, **A**, or squamous epithelium, **B**, depending on the orientation of the biopsy port.

of dysplasia for two patients, progression for another two, and no change for six others. These data are inconclusive, and it appears that the patients who had progression of dysplasia did not have successful control of their reflux by fundoplication. Nevertheless, these results do not provide overwhelming support for antireflux surgery alone as definitive treatment of dysplasia in Barrett's esophagus.

Cancer after Antireflux Surgery

There are some well-verified reports of patients who developed cancer in Barrett's esophagus after antireflux surgery. For example, in the series of cases from the Mayo Clinic discussed earlier in this report, both of the patients who developed esophageal cancer had previous fundoplications.[11] In most of the reports that describe cancers developing in Barrett's esophagus after antireflux surgery, it is not clear if the operation was successful in controlling GER. However, one particularly well-documented report from Johns Hopkins University described the development of adenocarcinoma in a patient for whom fundoplication was clearly successful in eliminating acid reflux as evidenced by extended postoperative esophageal pH monitoring.[26] Furthermore, antireflux surgery is not without risk in these cases. Of 209 Barrett's patients at the Mayo Clinic and at the Boston Veterans Administration (VA) Medical Center, followed from 1 month to 20 years, there were two deaths from esophageal cancer and five deaths from complications of antireflux surgery.[9, 11]

In summary, the case for antireflux surgery solely to prevent cancer in Barrett's esophagus is a house of cards comprised of unproved and largely untested hypotheses and questionable assumptions. The data do not support the practice of prophylactic antireflux surgery for the patient with uncomplicated Barrett's esophagus whose symptoms are easily controlled with conventional medications.

RECOMMENDATIONS FOR DISEASE MANAGEMENT

Barrett's esophagus is cause for concern, but not for panic. Education about the natural history of the disorder and the rationale for endoscopic surveillance should help to reduce anxiety for affected patients. As discussed, few data are available on the efficacy of therapy in reducing the cancer risk in this condition, and consequently there is much controversy regarding what constitutes proper patient management. A recommended approach is described below.[1]

Patients found to have Barrett's esophagus should have a careful endoscopic examination, and multiple esophageal biopsy specimens should be obtained to seek dysplasia or carcinoma. Patients who have signs or symptoms of reflux esophagitis should receive vigorous medical treatment. No specific medical or surgical treatment is recommended for patients who have no symptoms or objective signs of esophagitis. Antireflux surgery should be considered for patients found to have nonhealing esophageal ulcerations, progressive strictures, repeated pulmonary aspirations, or intractable symptoms of re-

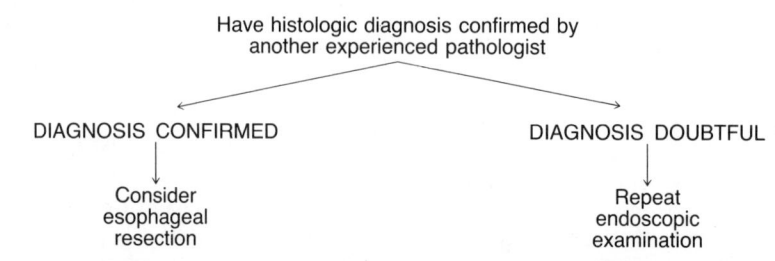

FIG 4–2.
Management recommendations for patients with high-grade dysplasia.

Have histologic diagnosis confirmed by another experienced pathologist

DIAGNOSIS CONFIRMED → Consider esophageal resection

DIAGNOSIS DOUBTFUL → Repeat endoscopic examination

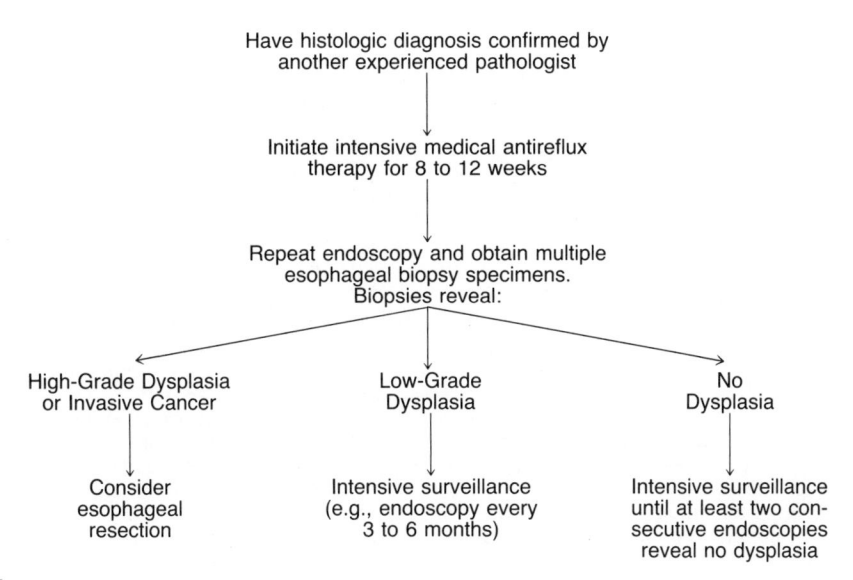

```
Have histologic diagnosis confirmed by
     another experienced pathologist
                    │
                    ▼
     Initiate intensive medical antireflux
        therapy for 8 to 12 weeks
                    │
                    ▼
     Repeat endoscopy and obtain multiple
       esophageal biopsy specimens.
              Biopsies reveal:
      ┌─────────────┼─────────────┐
      ▼             ▼             ▼
High-Grade Dysplasia  Low-Grade    No
or Invasive Cancer   Dysplasia  Dysplasia
      │             │             │
      ▼             ▼             ▼
   Consider    Intensive surveillance  Intensive surveillance
  esophageal   (e.g., endoscopy every  until at least two con-
   resection      3 to 6 months)       secutive endoscopies
                                       reveal no dysplasia
```

FIG 4–3.
Management recommendations for patients with low-grade dysplasia.

flux esophagitis after 8 to 12 weeks of vigorous medical therapy.

Patients with Barrett's esophagus, including those who have had antireflux surgery, should have careful routine endoscopic surveillance for dysplasia and early malignant disease. If dysplasia is detected, that finding should be confirmed by at least two expert pathologists. If any doubt remains, an endoscopic examination should be repeated as soon as possible to obtain more esophageal biopsy specimens for analysis. The diagnosis of high-grade dysplasia is sufficiently ominous to warrant immediate consideration of surgery to resect all of the esophagus that is lined by columnar epithelium. This approach is diagrammed in Fig 4–2. Management of low-grade dysplasia is particularly controversial. A recommended approach is diagrammed in Fig 4–3.

References

1. Spechler SJ, Goyal RK: Barrett's esophagus. *N Engl J Med* 1986; 315:362–371.
2. Hamilton SR: Pathogenesis of columnar cell-lined (Barrett's) esophagus, in Spechler SJ, Goyal RK (eds): *Barrett's Esophagus: Pathophysiology, Diagnosis, and Management*. New York, Elsevier Science Publishing Co., 1985, pp 29–37.
3. Trier JS: Morphology of the columnar cell-lined (Barrett's) esophagus, in Spechler SJ, Goyal RK (eds): *Barrett's Esophagus: Pathophysiology, Diagnosis, and Management*. New York, Elsevier Science Publishing Co., 1985, pp 19–28.
4. Agha FP: Radiologic diagnosis of Barrett's esophagus: Clinical analysis of 65 cases. *Gastrointest Radiol* 1986; 11:123–130.
5. Herlihy KJ, Orlando RC, Bryson JC, et al: Barrett's esophagus: Clinical, endoscopic, histologic, manometric and electrical potential difference characteristics. *Gastroenterology* 1984; 86:436–443.
6. Hassall E, Weinstein WM, Ament ME: Barrett's esophagus in childhood. *Gastroenterology* 1985; 89:1331–1337.
7. Johnson DA, Winter C, Spurling TJ, et al: Esophageal acid sensitivity in Barrett's esophagus. *J Clin Gastroenterol* 1987; 9:23–27.
8. Skinner DB, Walther BC, Riddell RH, et al: Barrett's esophagus: Comparison of benign and malignant cases. *Ann Surg* 1983; 198:554–565.
9. Spechler SJ, Robbins AH, Rubins HB, et al: Adenocarcinoma and Barrett's esophagus: An overrated risk? *Gastroenterology* 1984; 87:927–933.
10. Haggitt RC, Dean PJ: Adenocarcinoma in Barrett's epithelium, in Spechler SJ, Goyal RK (eds): *Barrett's Esophagus: Pathophysiology, Diagnosis, and Management*. New York, Elsevier Science Publishing Co., 1985, pp 153–166.
11. Cameron AJ, Ott BJ, Payne WS: The incidence of adenocarcinoma in columnar-lined (Barrett's) esophagus. *N Engl J Med* 1985; 313:857–859.
12. Sprung DJ, Ellis FH Jr, Gibb SP: Incidence of adenocarcinoma in Barrett's esophagus (abstract). *Am J Gastroenterol* 1984; 79:817.
13. Sondik EJ, Yound JL, Horm JW, et al: *1985 Annual Cancer Statistics Review*. Bethesda, MD, National Cancer Advisory Board, 1985 (DHHS publication no. [NIH] 86-2789).

14. Wu YK, Huang GJ, Shao LF, et al: Honored guest's address: Progress in the study and surgical treatment of cancer of the esophagus in China, 1940–1980. *J Thorac Cardiovasc Surg* 1982; 84:325–333.
15. Guanrei Y, He H, Sungliang Q, et al: Endoscopic diagnosis of 115 cases of early esophageal carcinoma. *Endoscopy* 1982; 14:157–161.
16. Schmidt HG, Riddell RH, Walther B, et al: Dysplasia in Barrett's esophagus. *J Cancer Res Clin Oncol* 1985; 110:145–152.
17. Riddell RH: Dysplasia and regression in Barrett's epithelium, in Spechler SJ, Goyal RK (eds): *Barrett's Esophagus: Pathophysiology, Diagnosis, and Management*. New York, Elsevier Science Publishing Co., 1985, pp 143–152.
18. Hamilton SR, Smith RRL: The relationship between columnar epithelial dysplasia and invasive adenocarcinoma arising in Barrett's esophagus. *Am J Clin Pathol* 1987; 87:310–312.
19. Reid BJ, Haggitt RC, Rubin CE, et al: Criteria for dysplasia in Barrett's esophagus: A cooperative consensus study (abstract). *Gastroenterology* 1985; 88:1552.
20. Lee RG: Dysplasia in Barrett's esophagus: A clinicopathologic study of six patients. *Am J Surg Pathol* 1985; 9:845–852.
21. American Cancer Society: Guidelines for the cancer-related check-up: Recommendations and rationale. *CA* 1980; 30:194–240.
22. Spechler SJ: Endoscopic surveillance for patients with Barrett esophagus: Does the cancer risk justify the practice? *Ann Intern Med* 1987; 106:902–904.
23. Eddy DM: The economics of cancer prevention and detection: Getting more for less. *Cancer* 1981; 47(suppl 5):1200–1209.
24. Goy JA, Herold E, Jenkins PJ, et al: "Open-access" endoscopy for general practitioners: Experience of a private gastrointestinal clinic. *Med J Aust* 1986; 144:71–74.
25. Brand DL, Ylvisaker JT, Gelfand M, et al: Regression of columnar esophageal (Barrett's) epithelium after anti-reflux surgery. *N Engl J Med* 1980; 302:844–848.
26. Hamilton SR, Hutcheon DG, Ravich WJ, et al: Adenocarcinoma in Barrett's esophagus after elimination of gastroesophageal reflux. *Gastroenterology* 1984; 86:356–360.

5

Esophageal Cancer:
Who should be treated, and how?

DAVID KELSEN, M.D.

Esophageal cancer, an uncommon but not rare tumor in the United States, causes substantial morbidity and mortality. In 1987 it is estimated that 9,700 new cases will be diagnosed; 95% of these patients will die. The treatment strategy for esophageal cancer remains controversial. This chapter will review current data regarding staging, conventional therapy, and the use of chemotherapy in the treatment of esophageal carcinomas both in palliation and in an adjuvant or neoadjuvant setting.

STAGING

The extent of disease evaluation, which determines the clinical stage of newly diagnosed patients, has shown little major change in the last 2 to 5 years. However, several new technical developments may improve our staging ability and help subdivide the local regional group into patients at high risk for relapse and those who are most likely to benefit from surgery alone or radiotherapy alone.

A detailed medical history and careful physical examination remain an important part of initial evaluation. The presence of supraclavicular nodes, hepatomegaly, or severe back pain still strongly suggests distant disease or direct extension to paravertebral tissues. Unfortunately a normal physical exam gives little help in the staging of most patients. A blood screening profile (SMA-12) is primarily aimed at evidence of liver or bone metastases, with the former being much more common. In the presence of a normal serum alkaline phosphatase, performance of a routine bone scan has a very low yield. A barium esophagogram and endoscopy both establish the diagnosis and aid in staging under earlier staging systems. All patients in whom the primary tumor is at the level of carina or higher (25–26 cm from the incisor teeth) should routinely undergo bronchoscopy. In approximately 5% to 15% of the patients with disease that otherwise appears to be limited, asymptomatic invasion into the trachea or mainstem bronchi is found. Tracheal invasion is an indicator of inoperability; it also has been repeatedly demonstrated that these patients are at extremely high risk for development of a tracheal esophageal fistula. Management of tracheal invasion or fistula is discussed below.

Computerized tomography (CT) scanning of the chest and abdomen has been studied extensively in esophageal tumors. A summary of several recent studies is shown in Table 5–1.[1] As can be seen, CT scanning is useful in determining the presence of liver metastases or adrenal metastases and is fairly accurate for determing impingement upon trachea, pericardium, or aorta. However, in the presence of normal-size lymph nodes, CT scanning is not a sensitive test. This is a critical point because the presence of lymph node metastases has a major impact on survival. The prognosis for these

TABLE 5–1.
Computerized Tomography (CT) Staging of Esophageal Cancer Predicting Invasion or Metastases—Results from Three Series*

Anatomical Area	Sensitivity† (T+/T+ +F−)	Specificity† (T−/T− +F+)	Accuracy† (T+ + T−/Total)
Aorta	88	92	92
Tracheobronchial	98	95	96
Pericardium	100	95	96
Periesophageal nodes	0	94	57
Liver	78	100	98
Adrenal	100	100	100
Abdominal nodes	76	93	87

*From Halvorsen R, Thompson W: Computed tomographic evaluation of esophageal cancer. *Semin Oncol* 1984; 11:101.
†Values expressed in percentages. F+ = False positive; F− = False negative; T+ = True positive; T− = True negative.

patients is only slightly better than that of those patients who present with distant metastases. Magnetic resonance imaging (MRI) is currently undergoing study in this area. MRI, especially using the sagittal view, can give a good estimate of the extent of disease and is probably, in this sense, superior to CT scanning. However, whether or not MRI is more useful than CT in determining the presence of regional lymphatic metastases is not yet known. Preliminary evidence suggests that it is not. Therefore, I consider MRI scanning to remain an investigational tool in this disease. CT scanning of the chest and abdomen should be performed in all patients prior to a decision involving surgery or radiotherapy.

A potentially useful new tool currently undergoing study in several centers (including Memorial Sloan Kettering Cancer Center—MSKCC) is endoscopic ultrasonography.[2] The esophagus is an ideal organ in which to use an endoscopic ultrasound. Although our preliminary impression is that this technique does demonstrate the presence of enlarged lymph nodes, it has not yet been determined whether it is superior (more accurate) to CT scanning or MRI. A prospective trial is currently underway at MSKCC comparing the three modalities, with confirmation at surgery. Until data are available, endoscopic ultrasonography should also be considered investigational.

The current staging system, developed by the American Joint Commission,[3] obviously has major drawbacks. Probably the biggest problem is the inability to distinguish among stage III patients (i.e., those who have tumor penetrating into periesophageal tissues alone (T3); or those patients who have lymph node metastases without distant metastases; or patients who have distant metastases). A new staging system, very similar to that used in gastric cancer, has been proposed. In the new schema, the depth of penetration through the esophageal wall determines the T stage (rather than the length of the lesion or the degree of obstruction as is currently used), and separate stages for lymph node metastases alone versus distant disease are employed. Because the aim of all staging systems is to aid in therapy, a new proposal must offer evidence that prognosis varies significantly with stage. New therapeutic modalities may be judged more accurately with more precise staging.

PROGNOSTIC VARIABLES

Many physicians hold the view that esophageal cancer is such a dismal disease that there is no use in separating out patient groups on the basis of prognostic variables. It is quite clear that cure for the vast majority of these patients is not possible with currently available techniques. Nonetheless, there are some prognostic variables between patient groups; these variables become crucial in the establishment of investigational protocols.

As mentioned above, *stage* is clearly of prognostic importance. Patients in pathologic stage I have a far better prognosis with surgical resection than do those in stage II or III (>80% 5-year survival versus 5%–15% 5-year survival, respectively).[4] Whether or not radiotherapy gives results for stage I tumors equal to surgery is not yet known with any certainty. Patients with stage III M1 disease or patients with regional lymph node metastases may not benefit from aggressive surgical approaches.

From the point of view of chemotherapeutic research trials, *performance status*, (i.e., the patient's general medical condition) also remains a critical prognostic factor. Patients with far-advanced disease who are bedridden (i.e., who have a Karnofsky Performance Status of less than 50) have much lower response rates to chemotherapy and are much more likely to suffer severe toxicity. Most research studies do not include patients with such poor general medical condition. I have rarely seen bedridden patients with esophageal cancer gain any significant benefit from any form of chemotherapy.

Several retrospective reviews identify *weight loss* as an important prognostic factor for patients with local regional disease.[5, 6] In general, patients who lose more than 10 lb appear statistically more likely to have a poor medium and long-term survival than do those without weight loss. This crude biologic end point is useful in assessing a preoperative population. An additional factor, which has been of some use in my experience (but which has not been studied prospectively), is the difference between the patient who has had weight loss because of mechanical obstruction and is still very hungry versus the patient who has had significant weight loss but has severe anorexia. Patients whose weight loss can be ascribed to mechanical obstruction will, following relief of obstruction, usually regain their lost weight rapidly. They are less likely to have distant metastases. Patients who have severe anorexia, even after they have had relief of obstruction, will continue to have weight loss; they are more likely to have distant metastatic disease. Why this happens is not clear, although one could speculate as to the role of substances such as cachexin.

THERAPY

Approximately 50% of patients will be found, after an evaluation as described above, to have disease limited to the local regional area (the esophagus and periesophageal tissues, clinical stage $T_1 = {}_2N_xM_o$). In spite of a large number of studies over the last 30 to 40 years, the optimum treatment for this group remains unclear. Conventional choices remain surgery alone or radiation therapy alone. A variety of investigational multimodality techniques are under study.

Surgery Alone

The data base of reports (almost all of which are retrospective) involving surgery as the major modality for the treatment of patients with esophageal cancer has been reviewed recently.[7, 8] It should be noted that it is almost impossible to determine from these reviews how many patients were treated with surgery alone and how many underwent surgery followed by postoperative radiation. Nonetheless, the end results of surgery has reported to date are as follows: Of 100 operable patients, approximately 70 will have resectable disease. The definition of resectable disease will vary tremendously from surgeon to surgeon. Some surgeons upon finding abdominal celiac nodal metastasis will deem the patient unresectable and will close. Others will resect celiac nodal disease and then proceed directly with esophagectomy. In many of these patients residual gross disease may be left in the mediastinum or small liver metastasis may be removed. Other surgeons will consider for resection only those patients who have no documented abdominal lymph nodes and who have a tumor which can be removed from the chest without any gross disease left behind. More recently, there are those who favor an extrathoracic esophagectomy, in which all surgery for esophageal cancer is deemed as primarily palliative and no attempt is made to dissect mediastinal lymph nodes.[9] Because these surgical approaches have not been compared head to head, it is difficult to say that a standard Ivor-Lewis procedure is superior to extrathoracic esophagectomy or to an extended radical esophagectomy as studied by Skinner et al. In the vast majority of surgical series, the operative mortality will be between 5% and 15%, and the median duration of survival will range from 12 to 18 months. Operative complications (morbidity) can be significant and include atelectasis and pneumonia, cardiac arrythmias, anastomotic leaks, and recurrent strictures at the anastomosis. If mechanical stapling devices are used to close the anastomosis, it is not uncommon for one-quarter to one-third of patients to require at least one and frequently repeated dilatations. Major changes in life-style are seen when a gastric pullup is used, although many surgeons think this is a simpler and safer technique than colon interpolation. Long-term survival remains poor with 5% to 10% of patients living for more than 2 to 3 years. Overall, there has been no significant improvement in survival outcome during the last 10 years with surgery alone.

Radiation Therapy

Radiation therapy is the conventional alternative of choice to surgery alone. The rationale for the use of radiotherapy lies in the lower mortality and lower morbidity during the treatment period. Results of radiotherapy have also been reviewed recently.[10] There are no reported prospective controlled trials comparing radiotherapy alone versus surgery alone for patients with similar clinical stage and general condition although several such studies are planned. The major problem with radiotherapy alone is the high local failure rate. This translates into recurrence of clinically significant dysphagia within a short time. The local failure rate (as first sign of tumor recurrence) is very hard to ferret out from the literature. Several studies have indicated that for patients who are receiving high (curative) doses (which is probably about 50% of the population referred for radiation), relief of dysphagia (suggesting local control) is achieved in about 80%. Unfortunately, the median duration of dysphagia relief is 2 to 4 months. By the end of 1 year, less than 20% of patients who are alive are able to swallow without significant difficulty. Thus, long-term palliation using standard techniques (including high-dose radiation with conventional fractionation) has been unsatisfactory because of local failure. This remains the major argument in favor of surgery.

Investigational Techniques

The most widely used multimodality techniques in the past have combined radiation and surgery. Two major choices are available: radiotherapy prior to surgery as a planned sequence, or radiotherapy after surgery. In the latter, radiotherapy is usually reserved for patients with lymph node metastasis or tumor through the wall of the esophagus. There have been a fair number of single arm phase II trials of preoperative radiation. The single arm trials in general proved that it was possible to give radiotherapy even in high dose with no increase in operative complications; treatment-related mortality rates appear to be similar to those seen with surgery alone. However, long-term survival for larger series with good follow-up remained extremely poor. The two prospective controlled randomized trials available for analysis[11, 12] have been criticized on the basis of unorthodox radiation therapy fractionation and scheduling. Lanouis and co-workers gave a total of 4,000 rads of radiation in an 8- to 12-day period, which is biologically the equivalent of a much higher dose. There was no difference in operability or resectability rates or in survival with an advantage to the surgery-only arm. Whether the poor long-term survival in the radiotherapy group may not be due to late complications of radiotherapy is unclear. In the second study by the European Organization for the Research and Treatment of Cancer (EORTC), a total of 3,300 rads of radiation was given in 8 to 10 days. Again, no differences in the key end points were noted. The conclusions of these investigators were that radiotherapy in a preoperative setting was not useful. Several other trials are investigating the use of radiotherapy in higher dose and more orthodox scheduling prior to surgery. Results are not yet available.

Data for postoperative radiation are far scantier than for preoperative radiation. There is, in fact, very little information available to indicate that giving radiation in a routine fashion following esophagectomy, even if regional lymph nodes were positive or tumor had penetrated through the esophageal wall, is effective in decreasing local recurrence rates. A randomized study organized by the European Organization for the Study of Esophageal Diseases (OESO) compares surgery followed by radiation to surgery alone. The third arm of the study involves neoadjuvant chemotherapy (see below). This trial and a proposed American trial may determine whether routine radiotherapy following surgical resection is useful. Thus, although postoperative radiation remains a commonly employed technique, there are no data to show that it is useful.

Therapy in Advanced Disease

For the 50% to 60% of patients in whom either distant metastases are documented or in whom the primary tumor is so extensive that there is no hope of cure, systemic chemotherapy has been employed in an attempt to improve palliation and survival.[13] Studies from the late 1960s to mid-1970s involved pooling data from a number of trials in which some patients with esophageal cancer were treated with a given agent as part of a larger study of that drug in many solid tumors. More recent phase II studies involve using a particular drug at a standard dose. Although the list of agents is still quite short, substantial progress has been made in the development of these trials. The most widely used drugs at the present time include cisplatin, vinca alkaloids such as vinblastine (a conventional analogue of the investigational drug vindesine), mitomycin C, fluorouracil, and bleomycin. As is the case in many solid tumors, the response rate to single agent therapy is low. Therefore, combinations have been investigated in an attempt to improve response rates and durations. The common denominator to almost all of these trials is cisplatin. There are few data to indicate that one cisplatin-containing combination is markedly superior to another. Toxicities are substantial but usually tolerable.

Patients with advanced metastatic esophageal cancer are candidates for chemotherapy if they are in reasonably good general medical condition (usually defined as a Karnofsky Performance Status of greater than 50), able to care for themselves in a home situation, and remain ambulatory. Bedridden patients with far advanced disease are highly unlikely to respond to these types of regimens but are much more likely to have severe toxicity. Using chemotherapy for palliation in the latter population is not recommended. Because there is no proof that one regimen is markedly superior to another, entrance into investigational studies is highly recommended. In the absence of an investigational trial, a cisplatin-based regimen (cisplatin-5FU or cisplatin-Velban) can be used, but my preference would be to avoid chemotherapy in a nonprotocol setting.

A special circumstance involves patients who have no evidence of distant metastatic disease but who have invasion into the tracheal-bronchial tree. They do not have resectable disease. Using radiation therapy has been difficult, because the induction of a tracheal-esophageal fistula (an almost inevitable natural consequence of this stage of disease) is the rule. An investigational approach has been used at MSKCC to induce response with chemotherapy followed by definitive radiation if the bronchus heals. Of a small group of 20 patients, four have had documented healing of the tracheal-bronchial tree on repeat bronchoscopy. All patients received radiation therapy following chemotherapy. Local control was achieved in several of these patients; however, no patient was cured, and the median duration of survival remained under 1 year.

Adjuvant chemotherapy has undergone fairly extensive study in esophageal cancer in the last 5 to 8 years. In almost all of these trials, chemotherapy has been given prior to surgery or radiotherapy or concurrently with radiotherapy if that is the primary treatment. The rationale for this neoadjuvant approach has both theoretical and practical considerations. Several in vivo tumor models have indicated that there is a therapeutic advantage to using chemotherapy prior to surgery. Because resection may play a major role in at least palliating patients with esophageal cancer, treatment that causes tumor regression may increase the resection rate. The use of chemotherapy alone enables one to assess whether or not these drugs in this patient or patient population are effective in causing tumor regression. A number of autopsy studies have demonstrated that in Western patients, esophageal cancer is widely disseminated even shortly after diagnosis. All of these points have led to the introduction of neoadjuvant chemotherapy, that is, giving chemotherapy prior to planned surgery or radiation.

The two major variations on this theme are the use of chemotherapy alone prior to surgery or the use of chemotherapy plus concurrent radiation prior to planned operation. Both approaches have been studied and a small number of published phase II trials address the technical feasibility of this approach.[14] In brief, use of chemotherapy alone prior to surgery is reasonably well tolerated and, if close attention is given to detail, then there appears to be no increase in operative morbidity or mortality. It should be emphasized that there are potential additive toxicities of this type of treatment plan. For example, bleomycin and mitomycin C are both potential pulmonary toxins when given prior to surgery, and an increased risk of severe postoperative pulmonary failure has been reported in several tumor types, including esophageal cancer. Careful attention to the amount of oxygen given during the operation (F_{IO_2}) is important. Studies from Memorial Hospital indicate that if the F_{IO_2} is kept below 30%, the risks of additional pulmonary toxicity appear to be minimal or no greater than that of surgery alone. When chemotherapy and radiation are given concurrently, the risk of pulmonary toxicity may be higher; it is not clear that controlling the F_{IO_2} fully removes this factor from consideration.

The key variables of either approach are the ability to control local disease, that is, the relapse pattern; and the impact on disease-free and overall survival. For the approach using chemotherapy plus concurrent radiation followed by surgery, a recent publication from the Southwest Oncology Group involving over 100 patients demonstrated that, unfortunately, the resection rate was not increased; only 48% of patients who entered the study, all of whom had operable disease at initiation, were able to undergo removal of the tumor.[15] The median survival was only 12 months which is no better than that seen with surgery alone. Although this was not a randomized trial, the results were disappointing enough so that future studies with the combination used in this program (cisplatin plus 5FU continuous infusion plus concurrent radiation followed by surgery) is not appealing.

Prospective randomized trials are now underway involving the use of preoperative chemotherapy alone followed by planned surgery. These trials include randomization against an arm of intensive pre-op radiation therapy (MSKCC) and a three-arm study being performed in Europe by the OESO, in which neoadjuvant chemotherapy with cisplatin, vindisine, and bleomycin is compared to surgery alone versus surgery followed by radiation. The results of all these trials will be forthcoming in the next several years and will be very useful in determining the role of this type of regimen in a neoadjuvant setting.

Because surgery has significant morbidity and mortality in its own right, a number of investigators have initiated studies using chemotherapy and radiation alone without a planned operative procedure. The technical factors in these trials vary as to whether radiation is given following chemotherapy or concurrently. The data to date are inconclusive. At the present time, phase II studies have demonstrated that it is technically possible to use this approach with tolerable side-effects. Whether or not there is a significant impact on disease-free overall survival is not yet known. Several randomized trials are underway. The preliminary results of one study from France comparing chemotherapy followed by radiation with radiation alone show no significant difference in disease-free overall or overall survival or in relapse pattern between the two arms. Cooperative groups in the United States have embarked on similar trials using *concurrent* radiation and chemotherapy. The approach of combining systemic chemotherapy with local control measures involving surgery and/or radiation is enticing, and is the focus of intense study at Memorial Hospital. However, it should not be considered a routine approach yet.[16] When chemotherapy is given carefully, toxicities are tolerable; still, they should not be underestimated. The optimal chemotherapy to use in these trials, the optimal timing of radiation, and the radiation dosage remain controversial. As is the case with the use of chemotherapy for patients with advanced disease, entrance of these patients into carefully designed clinical trials is highly recommended. However, if a research study is not available or the patient declines to enter research study, standard therapy at the present time, although still quite unsatisfactory, remains surgery alone or radiation alone.

References

1. Halvorsen R, Thompson W: Computed tomographic evaluation of esophageal cancer. *Semin Oncol* 1984; 11:101.
2. Fleischer D, Sivak M: Endoscopic Nd:YAG laser therapy as palliation for esophagogastric cancer. *Gastroenterology* 1985; 89:527–531.
3. Bearns O, Myers M (eds): *Manual for Staging of Cancer: Esophagus* Philadelphia, JB Lippincott, 1987, pp 61–66.
4. Yang CS: Research on esophageal cancer in China: A review. *Cancer Res* 1980; 40:2633.
5. Fein R, Kelsen D, Geller N, et al: Adenocarcinoma of the esophagus and gastroesophageal junction. Prognostic factors and results of therapy. *Cancer* 1985; 56:2512–2519.
6. Conti S, West DP, Fitzpatrick H: Mortality and morbidity after esophagogastrectomy for cancer of the cardia and esophagus. *Am Surg* 1977; 43:92–96.
7. Earlam R, Cunha-Menlo J: Oesophageal squamous cell carcinoma: A critical review of surgery. *Br J Surg* 1980; 67:381–390.
8. Skinner, B: Surgical treatment for esophageal cancer. *Semin Oncol* 1984; 11:136.
9. Orringer MB, Orringer JJ: Esophagectomy without thoracotomy: A dangerous operation? *J Thorac Cardiovasc Surg* 1987; 85:72–80.
10. Earlam R, Cunha-Menlo J: Oesophageal squamous cell carcinoma: A critical review of radiotherapy. *Br J Surg* 1980; 67:457–461.
11. Launois B, Delarue D, Compion J et al: Preoperative radiotherapy for carcinoma of the esophagus. *Surgery Gyn Obst* 1981; 153:690–693.
12. European Organization for the Research and Treatment of Cancer (EORTC): Pre-operative radiotherapy for carcinoma of the esophagus in DeMeestar T, Skinner D (eds): *Esophageal Disorders: Pathophysiology and Therapy.* 1986, pp 367–377.
13. Kelsen DP, Hilaris B, Martini N: Neoadjuvant chemotherapy and surgery of cancer of the esophagus. *Semin Surg Oncol* 1986; 2:170–176.
14. Kelsen DP: Chemotherapy of esophageal cancer. *Semin Oncol* 1984; 11:159–168.
15. Poplin E, et al: Combined therapies for squamous cell carcinoma of the esophagus, a Southwest Oncology Group study. *J Clin Oncol* 1987; 5:622.
16. Kelsen DP: Multimodality therapy of esophageal carcinoma: Still an experimental approach. *J Clin Oncol* 1987; 15:530–531.

II

Stomach and Duodenum

6

Gastroparesis:
How should gastric emptying be assessed, and how should problems be managed?

ROBERT FISHER, M.D.

To diagnose and treat gastroparesis effectively, an understanding of normal stomach physiology is most helpful. This chapter will review some of the highlights of normal gastric physiology and abnormal stomach emptying in patients with gastroparesis including clinical presentation, etiology, diagnosis, and treatment.

PHYSIOLOGY

The functions of the stomach are fivefold:
1. To act as a temporary storage receptacle for ingested food
2. To triturate the solid components of a meal to particles which are less than 1 or 2 mm in size so that they can be emptied into the duodenum through the pylorus
3. To initiate the early stages of digestion
4. To deliver nutrients into the duodenum and small intestine at a rate that will maximize digestion and absorption
5. To provide intrinsic factor for the absorption of vitamin B_{12}

Both the secretory and motor functions of the stomach are highly specialized activities, related to different anatomical regions of the stomach. For example, the fundus and body are rich in parietal and chief cells, which secrete acid and pepsinogen, respectively. The pyloric gland cells and other cells near the cardia secrete mucus. Similarly, the emptying of liquids and solids from the stomach is handled by different regional mechanisms. Emptying of liquids is controlled mostly by tonic motor activity in the cardia, fundus, and proximal body of the stomach. The distal body, antrum and pylorus act much as a conduit, carrying liquid from the proximal stomach into the duodenum. In contrast, emptying of solids is determined mostly by phasic motor activity in the distal body, antrum, and pylorus. The solid component of a meal empties rapidly from the proximal stomach, but is churned round and round in the distal two thirds until trituration is accomplished and emptying of chyme occurs.

Gastric motility is influenced by a number of factors. The volume of the meal may stimulate mechanoreceptors by distending the wall of the stomach. The chemical and physical composition of meals may interact with osmoreceptors, trigger a number of enterogastric neural reflexes, or stimulate the release of active peptides or chemicals from the small bowel mucosa. Some potentially important substances, in this regard, are gastrin, bombesin, cholecystokinin, motilin, serotonin, opiates, and prostaglandins.

Gastric motility is determined by myoelectrical activity within the longitudinal and circular muscle layers of the stomach (Fig 6–1). Although the proximal stomach is relatively quiescent, the myoelectrical activity of the distal two thirds of the stomach is characterized by slow waves (electrical control activity, pacesetter potentials) with superimposed spike potentials that correspond to muscle contractions. The frequency of the slow waves is variable in different anatomical locations throughout the stomach. The so-call pacemaker of the stomach is located high on the greater curvature in the body. Recordings of gastric myoelectrical activity (electrogastrogram) can now be obtained in human subjects using cutaneous electrodes. Their correlation with intragastric motor activity and their clinical relevance is currently being studied.

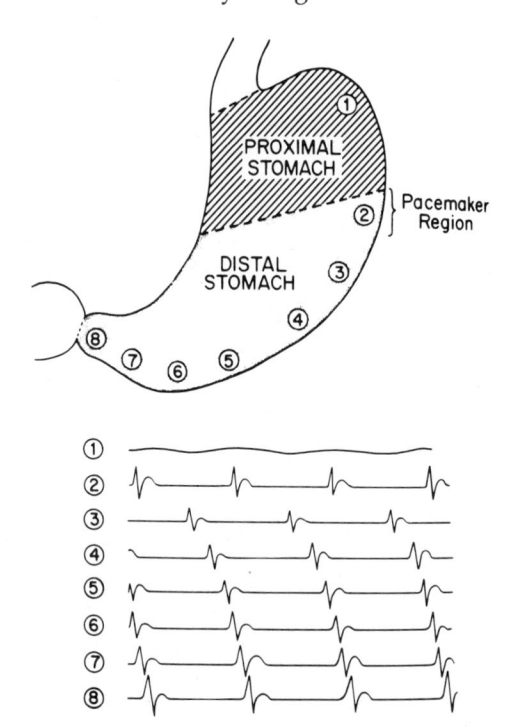

FIG 6–1.
Schematic of stomach showing pacemaker area and placement of serial myoelectric leads in different anatomical locations. Myoelectric tracings obtained from the different myoelectric leads are demonstrated.

SYMPTOMS AND ETIOLOGY OF GASTRIC EMPTYING DISORDERS

Abnormal gastric motility may be associated with rapid or delayed stomach emptying. Rapid emptying may produce a number of symptoms including lightheadedness, diaphoresis, palpitations, abdominal pain, and diarrhea. This constellation of symptoms has been referred to as the *dumping syndrome.* Some potential causes of the dumping syndrome are duodenal or jejunal overdistention, rapid intestinal transit, maldigestion, reactive hypoglycemia, and increased intestinal gas production. Symptoms may be mediated by the release of active agents, such as serotonin, prostaglandins, vasoactive intestinal polypeptides, insulin, opiates, and others. Clinically important rapid stomach emptying occurs rarely in patients with hyperthyroidism or gastrinoma. The full-blown dumping syndrome is usually a consequence of gastroduodenal surgery.

Delayed stomach emptying is much more common and can be subdivided into two major categories: delayed emptying due to increased gastroduodenal junction resistance, often referred to as *mechanical obstruction;* and delayed emptying due to failure of the stomach to generate an effective propulsive force (i.e., functional obstruction or gastroparesis). A variety of nonspecific symptoms may suggest that stomach emptying is prolonged. These include early satiety, postprandial abdominal distention or bloating, epigastric pain, nausea, vomiting, and weight loss. Vomiting of undigested food may occur immediately or hours after food has been ingested. An audible succussion splash over the abdomen may provide a clue to delayed emptying of the stomach.

A number of disorders may produce mechanical obstruction of the stomach (Table 6–1). Duodenal and pyloric channel ulcers, pyloric strictures, benign hypertrophic pyloric stenosis, and tumors of the stomach may all decrease the size of the lumen at the gastric outlet, thereby impeding gastric emptying. Both incomplete relaxation of the pylorus and gastroduodenopyloric dyskinesia are hypo-

TABLE 6–1.
Mechanical Obstruction of the Stomach

Duodenal ulcer
Pyloric channel ulcer
Pyloric stricture
Hypertrophic pyloric stenosis
Tumor of the distal stomach
Incomplete relaxation of the pylorus
Gastroduodenopyloric dyskinesia

TABLE 6–2.
Causes of Functional Obstruction of the Stomach (Gastroparesis)

Drugs
  Anticholinergic agents
  Beta-adrenergic agonists
  Calcium channel blockers
  Opiates
  Cytostatic drugs
  Dopamine agonists
Electrolyte imbalance
  Hypokalemia
  Hypocalcemia
  Hypomagnesemia
Metabolic disorders
  Diabetes mellitus
  Hypothyroidism
  Hypoparathyroidism
  Pregnancy
Vagotomy
Infiltrative gastropathy
  Amyloidosis
  Pernicious anemia
  Malignancy
Systemic diseases
  Scleroderma
  Dermatomyositis
Infections—nonbacterial (viral) gatroenteritis, Guillain-Barré syndrome, botulism
Crohn's disease
Psychiatric disorders
  Anorexia nervosa
  Psychogenic vomiting
Neuromuscular disorders
  Myotonic dystrophy
  Diabetes mellitus (autonomic neuropathy)
  Chronic idiopathic intestinal pseudo-obstruction
  Aberrant gastric pacemaker (i.e., tachygastria)
  Superior mesenteric artery syndrome(?)
  Familial megaduodenum syndrome
Idiopathic

thetical disorders that to date have not been clearly demonstrated. Incomplete relaxation of the pylorus might create a condition analogous to achalasia with its incomplete relaxation of the lower esophageal sphincter (LES). Gastroduodenopyloric dyskinesia might be associated with an ineffective gastroduodenal pressure gradient and/or poor timing between gastroduodenal contractions and pyloric relaxation. Clinical demonstration of these disorders will require an improvement in the techniques available for evaluating gastroduodenal motility.

There are many causes of gastroparesis, functional gastric outlet obstruction (Table 6–2). The subdivision is somewhat artificial, and there is certainly a great overlap between the groups. A comprehensive discussion of each of these disorders is clearly beyond the scope of this chapter. Nevertheless, the protean causes of gastroparesis must be considered in order to treat the problem effectively. A number of pharmacologic agents may alter the electromechanical events associated with normal gastric motility. In most cases these effects can be rapidly reversed when the agents are discontinued. Similarly, an imbalance of electrolytes may change gastric motility. Certain metabolic disorders may create electrolyte or abnormal neuromuscular reactivity by virtue of excessive or deficient release of hormones. Elevated blood glucose levels have been demonstrated in some cases to slow stomach emptying. Whether infiltrative gastropathies impedes gastric emptying by interfering with neural conduction or muscle contractility has not been determined. Certain systemic diseases have been associated with delayed stomach emptying.

Scleroderma and dermatomyositis may affect nerves or muscles directly or may disrupt gastric emptying by virtue of concomitant vasculitis. The mechanism by which Crohn's disease slows gastric emptying has not been elucidated. Infections with certain viruses such as the Norwalk agent have been identified as occasional causes of gastroparesis. Usually, these episodes are self-limiting and reversible over time. Recently, attention has been drawn to the occurrence of gastroparesis in certain psychiatric disorders such as anorexia nervosa and psychogenic vomiting. Positive responses to treatment with gastrokinetic agents have been reported.

Abnormal stomach emptying has been reported in a host of neuromuscular diseases. It could be argued that many of the causes of gastroparesis already listed also represent neuromuscular dysfunction, pointing out the difficulty with any classification of these disorders. Diabetic gastropathy has received the most attention and is probably a manifestation of the autonomic neuropathy often seen as a complication of longstanding diabetes mellitus. Chronic idiopathic intestinal pseudo-obstruction is a neuromuscular disorder which may involve any or all portions of the gastrointestinal tract. Abnormalities of the myenteric plexus have been shown in a number of patients. Several cases of an aberrant distal antral pacemaker, referred to as *tachygastria,* have been reported. Finally in our center, we are seeing an increasing number of patients with unexplained upper gastrointestinal tract symptoms due to gastroparesis. The majority of these patients are women. This experience is not unique to our center. One wonders whether gastroparesis may explain the symptoms in some patients previously labeled as having functional or nonulcer dyspepsia.

DIAGNOSIS AND TREATMENT

The first step in the treatment of delayed gastric emptying is diagnosis (Table 6–3). Symptoms such as nausea, vomiting, postprandial abdominal pain, bloating or abdominal distention, and early satiety should suggest the possibility of an abnormality in emptying of the stomach contents. The presence of a succussion splash on physical examination would corroborate this impression. A careful history and physical examination may provide important clues to the cause of gastric obstruction. A past history of peptic ulcer disease, pyloric stenosis of the newborn, pernicious anemia, scleroderma, thyroid disease, abdominal surgery, or psychiatric illness might be helpful. Similarly, findings of neuropathy or autonomic dysfunction might suggest certain etiologies. A common mistake in the evaluation of a patient for abnormal stomach emptying is to perform an upper gastrointestinal (UGI) tract barium roentgenogram followed by upper endoscopy as soon as the diagnosis is suspected. Usually, when these procedures are performed early, they do not succeed in including or excluding mechanical obstruction because of the presence of copious amounts of retained food in the stomach and marked gastric dilatation.

An acute emergency should be excluded by obtaining some routine laboratory tests, performing a roentgenographic obstructive series with erect and decubitus views, and ordering an ultrasonogram to examine the gallbladder, biliary tract,

TABLE 6–3.
Diagnosis of Gastroparesis

1. Suspicion
    History of physical examination
2. Exclude acute process
    Complete blood count (CBC), amylase
    Obstructive series (i.e., flat plate of abdomen)
3. Gastric lavage (Ewald tube) followed by nasogastric suction
    Peripheral or parenteral alimentation
4. Upper gastrointestinal endoscopy
5. Upper gastrointestinal roentgenography
6. Measurement of gastric emptying
    Intubation techniques
      Saline load test
      Residual volume measurement
      Nonabsorbable dyes
    Radionuclide gastric scintigraphy*
    Tomographic measurement of gastric impedance

*Method of choice.

and pancreas. An attempt should be made to remove retained food from the stomach using a large bore tube. Next, an indwelling nasogastric tube should be placed in the distal stomach and connected to intermittent suction in order to decompress the dilated stomach. Whether a patient has mechanical or functional gastric outlet obstruction, gastric decompression is an important early therapeutic step for restoring muscle tone to the walls of the stomach. For mechanical obstruction, the older literature suggests that decompression accompanied by intravenous fluid maintenance should be limited to 48 to 72 hours. Remember, however, that most of these reports were written before peripheral or parenteral alimentation was available to maintain or improve nutrition over extended periods. If there is a suspicion of peptic ulcer disease, intravenous H_2-receptor blockers should be administered empirically. I do not feel pressured to remove the nasogastric tube. Following serveral days of gastric decompression and nutritional support, endoscopic examination should be performed to detect benign or malignant lesions of the stomach and duodenum or a stricture of the gastric outlet. If endoscopy does not provide an answer, barium roentgenography should be considered. In most cases mechanical gastric outlet obstruction will be treated surgically.

If the endoscope passes easily through the gastroduodenal junction and no lesion is detected, this suggests that functional gastric obstruction, gastroparesis, may be the cause of the symptoms. The absence of a mechanical lesion may be confirmed roentgenographically with double contrast UGI. This impression can be documented by measuring gastric emptying using a test meal labeled with a gamma-emitting radionuclide. There are a number of patients with symptomatic gastroparesis in whom liquids empty normally from the stomach, but in whom solids are delayed. Therefore, a labeled solid test meal should be employed. Remember, however, administration of a solid test meal to a patient with mechanical gastric outlet obstruction would be a mistake. In those few cases in which functional and mechanical obstruction cannot be differentiated using endoscopic and roentgenographic techniques, a radionuclide solid test meal should be withheld until normal emptying of liquid is demonstrated by performing a saline load test and/or measuring the residual gastric volume after clamping the nasogastric tube overnight.

Over the years, several techniques have been used to measure gastric emptying. Barium roentgenographic studies are qualitative only and associated with high radiation burdens. Intubation techniques are inconvenient and uncomfortable, and they provide data only on emptying of liquids from the stomach. In 1966, Griffith and his colleagues introduced chromium-51-labeled porridge as a gamma-emitting radionuclide-labeled meal to quantitate gastric emptying. Over the years, simple gamma-counting probes positioned over the stomach were replaced by rectilinear scanners, which have now been supplanted by sophisticated gamma cameras on line to dedicated computers. Radionuclide scintigraphy, using solids alone or combined solid–liquid test meals, is the test of choice for making a diagnosis of gastroparesis. Labeled chicken liver or scrambled eggs are employed commonly as test meals. Gastric emptying can be observed by reviewing serial scintigrams obtained for either the solid or liquid component of a test meal (Fig 6–2) and using computerized data analysis. Emptying curves can be established for both components of the test meal (Fig 6–3).

Recently, a new technique using serial measurement of epigastric impedance as an index of gastric retention has been introduced. Already epigastric impedance measurements have been improved by using more cutaneous electrodes in a procedure called *applied impedance (potential) tomography*. The potential advantages of both of these techniques is that they are quantitative, noninvasive, radiation-free, and do not require an expensive gamma camera. Whether they can be performed for solid test meals has not been established.

Once a diagnosis of functional gastric outlet obstruction, gastroparesis, has been documented, an effort should be made to

70 / STOMACH AND DUODENUM

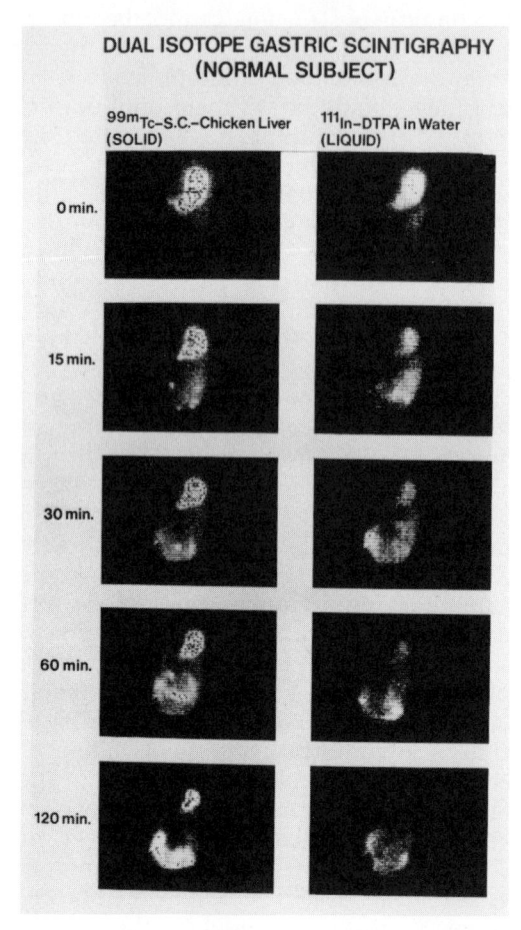

FIG 6–2.
Serial gastric scintigrams in a normal subject immediately and at 15, 30, 60, and 120 minutes after ingestion of a test meal. Emptying of both the solid component (technetium 99m chicken liver) and the liquid component (indium 111 water) is shown.

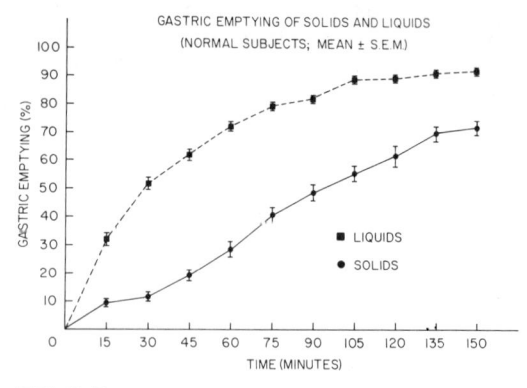

FIG 6–3.
Gastric emptying curves for both the liquid and solid components of the test meal in 10 normal subjects.

rule out correctable causes. For example, certain pharmacologic agents may be responsible. Also, certain reversible psychiatric or medical diseases may play a role. A comprehensive neurologic examination including computerized tomography of the head and evaluation of cranial and peripheral nerve function is essential. Medical disorders with specific treatments such as hypothyroidism, hypoparathyroidism, and Crohn's disease should be excluded. Esophageal and anal tonometry may provide clues to underlying systemic diseases.

Having made a diagnosis of gastroparesis, one must initiate specific therapy whenever possible and, if not, nonspecific therapy (Table 6–4). The efficacy of dietary alterations in the treatment of patients with gastroparesis has not been tested. After a period of gastric decompression using a nasogastric tube, it may be worthwhile to initially realiment a patient with low-volume, frequent liquid feedings. A number of patients tolerate liquids before the ability to handle solid food returns. It is probably best to limit

TABLE 6–4.
Treatment of Gastroparesis

1. Treat underlying medical illness
2. Eliminate causative drugs
3. Correct electrolyte imbalance
4. Dietary manipulation
   Small, frequent liquid meals
   Decrease lactose and/or fat in diet
   Enteral alimentation
   Home parenteral alimentation
5. Antiemetic agents
   Phenothiazines
   Antihistamines
   Anticholinergics (?)
6. Gastrokinetic agents
   Bethanechol
   Cisapride
   Metoclopramide
   Domperidone
   Serotonin antagonists (?)
   Opiate antagonists (?)
7. Behavior modification
8. Psychotherapy
9. Surgery

lactose and fat content during the initial stages of realimentation. In some patients it may be necessary to bypass the stomach for a time by instilling liquid supplements directly into the small intestine distal to the ligament of Treitz. This can be done with a jejunal feeding tube or by creating a feeding jejunostomy. Introduction of food into the stomach, duodenum, and small intestine may not be tolerated in a small group of patients. They may require home parenteral alimentation. In most cases the ability to tolerate oral feedings of relatively normal meals will return after a time.

For years the approach to pharmacologic treatment of gastroparesis was limited to treating its associated symptoms, nausea and vomiting. The phenothiazines, especially the halogenated forms such as prochlorperazine and thiethylperazine, are potent antiemetics by virtue of their action as dopamine receptor blockers at the chemoreceptor trigger zone. These agents are not usually effective against central types of vomiting and may be associated with side-effects such as sedation, hypotension, and extrapyramidal manifestations. On occasion, conventional antihistaminic agents (H_2 blockers) and antimuscarinic agents (anticholinergics) may be useful to treat or prevent vestibular-induced nausea and vomiting. However, these same agents may aggravate or exacerbate gastroparesis from other causes. Recently, marijuana (tetrahydrocannabinol) has been shown to be effective in treating severe nausea and vomiting due to cytostatic agents. A role for marijuana in treating symptomatic gastroparesis has not been established.

The most effective agents used to treat gastroparesis have been termed *prokinetic* (or, more specifically,) *gastrokinetic agents.* The prototypical gastrokinetic agents are the cholinomimetic agent, bethanechol, and the central and peripheral dopamine antagonist, metoclopramide.

Cholinomimetic agents reproduce totally or in part the effects of acetylcholine. They may be structural analogues, like bethanechol; they may inhibit acetylcholinesterase, like edrophonium; or they may release acetylcholine from nerve endings, like the new agent, cisapride. To date, bethanechol has received the most attention. Bethanechol has a selective muscarinic action with predominant effects not only on the bladder but also on the gastrointestinal tract. Increased amplitudes of esophageal, gastric, small intestine, colonic, and gallbladder contractions as well as elevated resting LES pressure have been reported. These effects would suggest that bethanechol might be potentially useful to treat patients with delayed esophageal transit, gastroesophageal reflux disease (GERD), gastroparesis, small intestinal motility disturbances and gallbladder stasis. Despite its multiple effects, there is little evidence that bethanechol is clinically effective in these conditions. Perhaps this is due in part to its potential side-effects, which include excessive salivation, blurred vision, headaches, abdominal cramps, nausea, vomiting, bladder spasm, flushing, and sweating. These side-effects limit the dose that can be administered. Cisapride has been employed in Europe and the United States to treat gastrointestinal motility disorders in a limited number of studies. To date, the results obtained in patients with idiopathic gastroparesis, reflux esophagitis, constipation, and idiopathic intestinal pseudo-obstruction have been encouraging. Furthermore, the side-effect profile has been very acceptable.

The other major category of gastrokinetic agent includes the dopamine antagonists. Metoclopramide, a drug chemically related to procainamide, exhibits dopamine receptor antagonism at both central and peripheral sites. Metoclopramide has a threefold mode of action: It may increase acetylcholine release from postganglionic cholinergic nerve terminals; it may sensitize muscarinic receptors to acetylcholine; and, most importantly, it antagonizes dopamine receptors. In addition to its prokinetic effects, metoclopramide has a central antiemetic action as well. Dopamine receptors are found throughout the body—not only in the gastrointestinal tract, but also in the central nervous system, the nigrostriatum, the emesis center, the chemoreceptor trigger zone, the medulla oblongata, the urinary bladder, the ureters, and in selected blood vessels. Blockade of dopamine receptors with metoclopramide has been reported to increase the amplitudes of esophageal, stomach, and small intestinal contractions. It may increase resting LES and pyloric pressures and may improve the coordination between antral and duodenal contractions and pyloric relaxation. Because of these effects, published data suggest that metoclopramide may be useful to treat patients with gastroparesis due to diabetes mellitus, vagotomy, GERD, anorexia nervosa, pregnancy, and unexplained causes. In addition, metoclopramide has been employed to empty the stomach before emergency anesthesia, endoscopy, or surgery.

Metoclopramide has been prescribed at doses ranging from 5 mg to 20 mg, 30 minutes before meals and at bedtime. An unfortunate aspect of metoclopramide use is the relatively high incidence, 20% to 30%, of side-effects which include agitation, irritability, drowsiness, akathesia, increased prolactin secretion, and extrapyramidal effects. Metoclopramide is available for both oral administration and intravenous use. A new prokinetic agent, under vigorous investigation in the United States and approved in many other countries throughout the world, is domperidone. Like metoclopramide, domperidone blocks dopamine receptors; but unlike metoclopramide, domperidone is predominantly a peripheral dopamine antagonist. Therefore, it has many fewer side-effects. Domperidone is being tested orally in doses ranging from 10 mg to 30 mg, administered 30 minutes before meals and at bedtime. Recent reports have suggested that certain serotonin and opiate antagonists may have gastrokinetic effects. These are only preliminary observations, however.

Other therapeutic modalities available to treat patients with gastroparesis include behavior modification, operant conditioning, hypnotherapy, and psychotherapy. Finally, surgical therapy may be employed in selected cases, but only after every effort is expended to assure normal esophageal, small intestinal, and colonic motility.

Bibliography

1. Cannon WB: The movements of the stomach studied by means of the Roentgen rays. *Am J Physiol* 1898; 1:359–382.
2. Cannon WB, Lieb CW: The receptive relaxation of the stomach. *Am J Physiol* 1911–12; 29:267–273.
3. Lind JF, Duthie HL, Schlegel JF, et al: Motility of the gastric fundus. *Am J Physiol* 1961; 201:197–202.
4. Kelly KA, Code CF, Elveback LR: Patterns of canine gastric electrical activity. *Am J Physiol* 1969; 217:461–470.
5. Hinder RA, Kelly KA: Human gastric pacesetter potential. *Am J Surg* 1977; 133:29–33.
6. Moore JG, Christian PE, Coleman RE: Gastric emptying of varying meal weight and composition in man. Evaluation by dual liquid- and solid-phase isotopic method. *Dig Dis Sci* 1981; 26:16–22.
7. Valenzuela, JE: Effect of intestinal hormones and peptides on intragastric pressure in dogs. *Gastroenterology* 1976; 71:766–769.
8. Kelly KA: Motility of the stomach and gastroduodenal junction, in Johnson LR (ed): *Physiology of the Gastrointestinal Tract* New York, Raven Press, 1981, pp 393–410.
9. Meyer JH, Ohashi H, Jehn D, et al: Size of liver particles emptied from the human stomach. *Gastroenterology* 1981; 80:1489–1496.
10. Rees WDW, Go VLW, Malagelada JR: Simultaneous measurement of antroduodenal motility, gastric emptying, and duodenogastric reflux in man. *Gut* 1979; 20:963–970.
11. Rees WDW, Go VLW, Malagelada JR: Antroduodenal motor response to solid-liquid and homogenized meals. *Gastroenterology* 1979; 76:1438–1442.
12. Fisher R, Cohen S: Physiological characteristics of the human pyloric sphincter. *Gastroenterology* 1973; 64:67–75.
13. Hinder RA, Kelly KA: Canine gastric emptying of solids and liquids. *Am J Physiol* 1977; 233:E335–E340.
14. Meyer JH, Thomson JB, Cohen MB, et al: Sieving of solid food by the canine stomach and sieving after gastric surgery. *Gastroenterology* 1979; 76:804–813.
15. Malagelada JR: Quantification of gastric solid–liquid discrimination during digestion of ordinary meals. *Gastroenterology* 1977; 72:1264–1267.
16. Meeroff JC, Go VLW, Phillips SF: Control of gastric emptying by osmolality of duodenal contents in man. *Gastroenterology* 1975; 68:1144–1151.
17. Chey WY, Hitanant S, Hendricks J, et al: Effect of secretin and cholecystokinin on gastric emptying and gastric secretion in man. *Gastroenterology* 1970; 58:820–827.
18. Malagelada JR: Physiologic basis and clinical significance of gastric emptying disorders. *Dig Dis Sci* 1979; 24:657–661.
19. Cooperman AM, Cook SA: Gastric emptying—

Physiology and measurements. *Surg Clin North Am* 1976; 56:1277–1287.
20. Goldstein H, Boyle JD: The saline load test—A bedside evaluation of gastric retention. *Gastroenterology* 1965; 49:375–380.
21. Malagelada JR, Longstreth GF, Summerskill WHJ, et al: Measurement of gastric functions during digestion of ordinary solid meals in man. *Gastroenterology* 1976; 70:203–210.
22. Meyer JH, MacGregor IL, Gueller R, et al: 99m-Tc-tagged chicken liver as a marker of solid food in the human stomach. *Am J Dig Dis* 1976; 21:296–304.
23. Heading RC, Tothill P, McLoughlin GP, et al: Gastric emptying rate measurement in man: A double-isotope scanning technique for simultaneous study of liquid and solid components of a meal. *Gastroenterology* 1976; 71:45–50.
24. Christian PE, Moore JG, Sorenson JA, et al: Effects of meal size and correction technique on gastric emptying time: Studies with two tracers and opposed detectors. *J Nucl Med* 1980; 21:883–885.
25. Holt S, McDicken WN, Anderson T, et al: Dynamic imaging of the stomach by real-time ultrasound—A method for the study of gastric motility. *Gut* 1980; 21:597–601.
26. Meeroff JC, Schreiber DS, Trier JS, et al: Abnormal gastric motor function in viral gastroenteritis. *Ann Intern Med* 1980; 92:370–373.
27. McCallum RW, Berkowitz DM, Lerner E: Gastric emptying in patients with gastroesophageal reflux. *Gastroenterology* 1981; 80:285–291.
28. Behar J, Ramsby G: Gastric emptying and antral motility in reflux esophagitis: Effect of oral metoclopramide. *Gastroenterology* 1978; 74:253–256.
29. Malagelada JR, Rees WDW, Mazzotta LJ, et al: Gastric motor abnormalities in diabetic and postvagotomy gastroparesis: Effect of metoclopramide and bethanechol. *Gastroenterology* 1980; 78:286–293.
30. Telander RL, Morgan KG, Kreulen DL, et al: Human gastric atony with tachygastria and gastric retention. *Gastroenterology* 1978; 75:497–501.
31. You CH, Lee KY, Chey WY, et al: Electrogastrographic study of patients with unexplained nausea, bloating, and vomiting. *Gastroenterology* 1980; 79:311–314.
32. Rees WDW, Miller LJ, Malagelada JR: Dyspepsia, antral motor dysfunction and gastric stasis of solids. *Gastroenterology* 1980; 78:360–365.
33. Perkel MS, Moore C, Hersh T, et al: Metoclopramide therapy in patients with delayed gastric emptying: A randomized, double-blind study. *Dig Dis Sci* 1979; 24:662–666.

7

Gastritis:
Is it a distinct clinical entity?

THOMAS J. McGARRITY, M.D.
GRAHAM H. JEFFRIES, M.D.

The clinical arena encompassing gastritis has been marked by confusion and semantic ambiguity. The histopathologic classification of gastritis based on the location and type of inflammatory cells in the mucosa bears little relationship to etiology, to clinical and endoscopic manifestations, or to the time course of the mucosal disease. The clinician encounters many patients with chronic dyspepsia who have no mucosal lesions; conversely, many patients with diffuse gastritis remain asymptomatic. In this review, gastritis is separated into erosive, nonerosive, and specific types[1] (Table 7–1).

EROSIVE GASTRITIS

The gastric mucosa is normally protected from the acid/peptic environment of the gastric lumen by multiple, interrelated events (Table 7–2). The layer of mucus on the mucosal surface provides a protective zone through which secreted bicarbonate establishes a gradient of pH values that approach neutrality at the epithelial surface. The surface epithelial cells are connected by tight junctions that limit the diffusion of electrolytes across the mucosa. Rapid replication and migration of surface mucous cells replaces damaged cells. Prostaglandins within the mucosa appear to play an important role in maintaining the blood flow that is necessary to support the epithelium as well as in regulating other protective events. A variety of exogenous agents and endogenous events may interfere with these normal protective mechanisms and cause mucosal erosions.

Stress-Related Acute Mucosal Injury (Stress Erosions)

Multiple superficial gastric erosions develop rapidly in morbidly ill patients under severe physiologic stress. These lesions have been termed *stress erosions* or *ulcers*, and *acute erosive or hemorrhagic gastritis*[2,3]; lesions in patients with extensive burns have been referred to as *Curling's ulcers*.[4] Ulcers that may complicate severe head trauma, neurosurgical procedures, or intracranial disease (Cushing's ulcers) may differ from other stress-related lesions; acid hypersecretion may play a major role in the pathogenesis of Cushing's lesions.[5–7]

Incidence

The best-studied group of patients with stress-related mucosal injury are burn patients.[4] Endoscopy documented gastric fundal lesions in 78% of patients with burns in excess of 35% of body surface area; these lesions occurred within 72 hours of injury.

The occurrence of stress gastritis in the critically ill medical or surgical patient is

TABLE 7–1.
Types of Gastritis

1. Erosive
   A. Stress gastritis
   B. Drug-induced gastritis
2. Nonerosive
   A. Chronic superficial
   B. Atrophic gastritis
      (1) Type A (autoimmune) atrophic gastritis
      (2) Type B atrophic gastritis
         a. Bile reflux gastritis
         b. *Campylobacter pylori* infection
3. Specific
   A. Menetrier's disease

proportional to the number and severity of risk factors present,[8,9] including sepsis; respiratory, hepatic or renal failure; hypotension; and coma. In Hastings' study of 100 critically ill patients, the incidence of overt or occult bleeding was 9% in patients with a single risk factor; this increased to 40% in patients with three to six risk factors.[10] This study, however, did not include endoscopy to define the presence of nonbleeding lesions.

Clinical Features

Bleeding is the most common and serious complication of stress-related mucosal injury. Prior to the routine use of prophylactic measures (antacids or H_2 blocking drugs), overt hemorrhage occurred in 11% to 22% of patients with severe burns (more than 35% of body surface area). Although occult bleeding was frequent in severely ill patients managed without antacid or H_2 blocker prophylaxis, clinically significant bleeding occurred in only 11% to 22% of patients.[3,4] Painless hematemesis is the most common manifestation of bleeding; melena alone is seen less often. In these critically ill patients, bleeding is associated with a high mortality (up to 50%).

Fewer than 10% of patients with stress erosions following thermal injury experience abdominal pain or dyspepsia. Stress-related mucosal lesions are usually superficial and thus do not lead to gastric perforation; ulcer perforation had been described in up to 12% of patients with severe burns.[11,12]

Pathology and Pathogenesis

Mucosal lesions have been detected within a few hours of the onset of injury. Foci of pallor and hyperemia are initial lesions seen almost exclusively in the fundus and body of the stomach (acid-secreting mucosa). Over 24 hours, these lesions evolve into multiple petechial hemorrhages and small (1–2 mm) red-based erosions. By 48 hours, the erosions are larger and may extend into the muscularis mucosa. With continued insult, lesions may extend to involve the antrum and proximal duodenum.[9,13] Microscopically, wedged-shaped mucosal hemorrhages and coagulation necrosis of the superficial mucosal cells are present. Inflammation, hemorrhage, and necrosis progressively extend to deeper layers of the mucosa, stomach, and duodenum.

Stress-related acute mucosal injury is the result of failure of gastric mucosal defense mechanisms (see Table 7–2) to resist acid/peptic autodigestion. Mucosal ischemia plays a major role in this injury.[14–16] Reduced mucosal blood flow due to circulatory collapse or microvascular injury may be a primary event that initiates mucosal damage by limiting oxidative metabolism,[17] by causing mucosal acidosis, or by decreasing surface cell replication. Back-diffusion of acid from the gastric lumen with loss of the mucosal barrier may accentuate ischemic injury by causing further damage to blood vessels in the mucosa.[18] Basal acid hypersecretion may increase the risk of mucosal injury and also the severity of mucosal lesions in patients with head injury, severe burns, and sepsis; acid hypersecretion does not appear

TABLE 7–2.
Components of the Gastric Mucosal Defense Mechanisms

Mucus
Bicarbonate secretion
Mucosal blood flow
Epithelial cell renewal
Prostaglandins

to be a significant factor in the pathogenesis of stress lesions in other patients.

Prophylaxis and Treatment

Because of the high mortality in patients with hemorrhage from stress-related acute mucosal injury, patients who are at high risk should be identified and managed prophylactically to prevent bleeding. The high-risk group of patients includes those with multiple organ failure (particularly in the presence of sepsis), extensive burns, and multiple trauma with head injury.

Antacid Prophylaxis. The administration of antacid hourly by nasogastric tube to maintain the gastric pH above 3.5 has been shown to be effective in preventing gastric mucosal bleeding. In Hastings' study of 100 critically ill patients who were randomly assigned to receive antacid prophylaxis or placebo, bleeding was detected in 2 of 51 patients receiving antacid versus 12 of 49 treated by nasogastric suction alone; in the majority of these patients, however, bleeding was detected only by tests for occult blood in gastric aspirates.[10] An analysis of 16 controlled trials comparing antacid prophylaxis, cimetidine prophylaxis, and placebo showed that overt bleeding occurred in 15% of patients treated without prophylaxis, and in only 3.3% of patients treated with antacid prophylaxis.[19]

Prophylaxis with H_2 antagonists. H_2 antagonists administered intravenously either by bolus injection of continuous infusion appear to be as effective as antacid prophylaxis in preventing stress-related bleeding. Prophylaxis with H_2 antagonists should be monitored by repeated measurements of gastric pH; in several studies it has been shown that bolus injections of H_2 antagonists even at high dosage may not effectively control gastric pH in critically ill patients.[20-22] Although early studies comparing cimetidine and antacid prophylaxis concluded that antacid prophylaxis was more effective than cimetidine in preventing bleeding,[23,24] this benefit appears to relate only to the frequency of occult bleeding. In an analysis of 16 controlled trials, Shuman and co-workers found that the frequency of overt bleeding was similar in patients receiving cimetidine (2.7%) or antacid (3.3%) prophylaxis.[19]

The potential for drug interactions with cimetidine,[25-27] and the problem of mental confusion with the use of this agent in elderly patients with hepatorenal failure[28,29] are relative contraindications for the use of this agent. Both ranitidine (50 mg every 6 hours IV) and famotidine (20 mg every 12 hours IV) are effective in maintaining the gastric pH above 4.[30] Other studies, however, are needed to document the safety and efficacy of these agents in preventing bleeding from stress lesions in critically ill patients.

Prophylaxis with Sucralfate. Controlled trials suggest that sucralfate (1 gm every 6 hours) may be as effective as antacid or cimetidine prophylaxis. In a study of 100 critically ill patients, bleeding occurred in 2 of 33 receiving cimetidine, in 2 of 33 receiving antacid, and in none of 34 receiving sucralfate[31]; patients who bled in the cimetidine and antacid prophylaxis groups did not have adequate control of gastric pH. Borrero[32] observed bleeding in 2 of 75 patients treated with antacids and in 3 of 80 patients receiving sucralfate.

The mechanism of sucralfate protection may relate to its antipeptic activity, or to mucosal protection via endogenous prostaglandin release rather than to an effect on gastric acidity. Protection without gastric neutralization has a potential advantage of decreasing intragastric bacterial overgrowth that could contribute to nosocomial pneumonia in ventilated patients.[33]

Prophylaxis with Prostaglandin Analogues. Theoretically, prostaglandins, which exert both an antisecretory and a mucosal protective action, would be ideal agents to prevent stress erosions and bleeding. In a single controlled study, prostaglandin E2 was compared with antacid prophylaxis. Bleeding was observed in 12 or 24 patients treated with prostaglandin and in only 3 of 22 patients receiving antacid ($p = 0.008$).[34]

Treatment of Patients with Stress-Related Mucosal Disease and Bleeding. The mainstay of treatment in patients with bleeding stress erosions is the correction of the underlying predisposing conditions. Careful monitoring of intravascular volume and treatment of acidosis and infection are mandatory. Coagulation abnormalities should be reversed with fresh frozen plasma. In the majority of critically ill patients, nasogastric aspiration of gastric content with installation of antacids to maintain gastric pH at 7.0 is associated with control of bleeding.[35,36] Peura and Johnson observed that cimetidine was of significant benefit in controlling blood loss (either observed endoscopically or determined by transfusion requirement) in patients admitted to a medical intensive care unit.[37] The use of intravenous or selective intra-arterial infusions of vasopressin (0.2 to 0.4 units per minute) may be of benefit, but the supporting data are limited[38,39]; the adverse cardiodynamic effect on vasopressin limits its use.

Although stress-related acute mucosal lesions are usually diffuse, endoscopy may identify bleeding sites; there has been limited clinical experience with the use of endoscopic therapy with electrocoagulation, thermal probes, and lasers, but these measures may be helpful in averting surgical therapy.[40]

Surgery to control stress bleeding is a measure of last resort; the operative mortality in patients who continued to bleed is in excess of 30%.[3,41] Vagotomy and pyloroplasty with oversewing of bleeding sites has been recommended for rapid control of bleeding,[41,42] but the rate of rebleeding is significant. A total gastrectomy may be the only other surgical alternative.

Drug-Induced Gastritis

It is now well documented that a variety of drugs, including aspirin, the nonsteroidal anti-inflammatory drugs (NSAID), and potassium chloride, may cause gastric mucosal damage. In most instances where a causal relationship between drug administration and gastric mucosal damage has been established, the possibility of gastric mucosal injury was first suspected because of dyspeptic symptoms following drug infection or because of bleeding. The relationship was then confirmed by studies in experimental animals and by controlled studies in patients or volunteers in which gastrointestinal blood loss was measured or serial endoscopic observations were performed.[43–46] It is likely that many other agents less commonly used than aspirin or NSAID also cause mucosal damage; in the absence of symptoms, they are less likely to be recognized as causing acute gastritis.

Incidence

The frequency and severity of mucosal injury following ingestion of aspirin or NSAID depends on the dose of drug, the amount of acid in the stomach following drug exposure, and on other undefined factors relating to patient resistance.

Aspirin. Serial endoscopic studies showed that the administration of 600 mg of aspirin with 10 mEq of hydrochloric acid caused petechial gastric hemorrhages in 50% of subjects, whereas similar lesions were found in only 17% of subjects given the aspirin alone.[47,48] Graham and Smith observed lesions in almost all patients who received a single 650-mg dose of aspirin; petechial mucosal and submucosal hemorrhages were evident 1 hour after drug ingestion and progressed to small erosions and ulcers within several hours.[49] In subjects receiving 2.6 gm of aspirin daily, focal erosions and submucosal hemorrhages were universally present within 24 hours but decreased in severity with continued daily drug administration over 7 days[50]; mucosal lesions resolved more rapidly following drug withdrawal in subjects who had received several days of drug exposure.

NSAID. Similar lesions are found on upper endoscopy following the acute administration of aspirin or NSAID.[44,48,51–53] The acute lesions following ingestion of NSAID are less severe than those caused by aspirin. In an endoscopic study of 60 volunteers given aspirin, sulindac, naproxen, or placebo, subjects receiving sulindac exhibited less mucosal damage than those receiving the other drugs[51]; it is possible that sulindac causes less acute gastric injury because it is converted to a prostaglandin inhibitor by hepatic metabolism.

Pathophysiology

The mechanisms for acute mucosal injury following aspirin exposure has been well defined in experimental studies. At an acid pH, aspirin is relatively lipid soluble and is able to penetrate the lipid surface membrane of the gastric epithelium. Epithelial cell damage is reflected by a disruption of the normal gastric mucosal barrier to the diffusion of ions and a loss of the normal transmucosal potential difference.[54-56] The back-diffusion of intraluminal acid through the damaged surface epithelium then causes disruption of surface cells with vascular injury and bleeding. As Davenport concluded from his experimental studies: "Salicylate opens the gates of the mucosal barrier, and acid pouring through the breeched defenses destroys capillaries and venules."[43]

The mechanism of mucosal injury following administration of NSAID is less well defined than that of aspirin injury. NSAID exposure does not lead to loss of the gastric mucosal barrier or transmucosal potential gradient[57]; prostaglandin inhibition with impairment of normal defense mechanisms is an attractive hypothetical mechanism.

There is a rapid adaptation of the gastric mucosa following injury. In this process of adaptation, termed *restitution*, the denuded surface epithelium is restored by the migration of cells from the underlying gastric pits. Epithelial restitution is not dependent on DNA or protein synthesis, cell proliferation, or endogenous prostaglandins; adequate calcium and actin microfilament function appears to be essential.[58] Mucosal healing with restoration of a normal population of surface epithelial cells depends on surface cell proliferation.

The relationship between acute mucosal lesions following drug exposure and the chronic gatric ulcers observed in patients who take aspirin and/or NSAID over long periods[59] has not been defined. The development of a chronic gastric ulcer in the setting of continued aspirin or NSAID treatment may reflect a failure of adaptive healing mechanisms.

Clinical Features

Multiple studies have shown that there is a poor correlation between symptoms and the presence of drug-induced gastric erosions or ulcerations.[44,51,52,59,60] An endoscopic study of 48 patients with rheumatoid arthritis treated with aspirin (at least 3.4 gm daily) revealed 19 patients (38%) with erosive gastritis, and 8 (16%) with gastric ulcers[59]; none had gastrointestinal symptoms.

Gastrointestinal hemorrhage is the major complication of acute and chronic drug-induced gastric mucosal lesions. In several epidemiologic studies it was found that aspirin ingestion was significantly more common in patients who suffered from acute upper gastrointestinal bleeding than in nonbleeding control patients. A national survey (ASGE) of patients with gastrointestinal bleeding showed that 27% of 3476 patients had ingested aspirin or NSAID before the bleeding event.[61] In another study of women over age 70 with acute upper gastrointestinal bleeding, 50% had NSAID-induced gastric ulcers.[62]

Prevention and Treatment of Drug-Induced Gastritis

Choice of Analgesic Agents. Acetaminophen, which causes no gastric mucosal damage, may be preferred as a temporary analgesic; in the absence of an anti-inflammatory action, however, this drug cannot replace aspirin or NSAID in patients with rheumatologic diseases. Commercially available buffered aspirin preparations (Bufferin, Ascriptin) do not contain sufficient alkali to protect the gastric mucosa from acid injury.[53] Enteric-coated aspirin, however, has been shown in endoscopic studies to produce significantly less gastric mucosal injury than buffered or plain aspirin.[53,59] Although sulindac (Clinoril) causes less acute mucosal injury than aspirin or naproxen,[51] it has not been established that this drug is less likely than other NSAID to produce chronic gastric ulcers.

Concurrent Use of Antiulcer Drugs. In experimental studies it has been shown that sucralfate, H_2 receptor antagonists, and synthetic prostaglandins protect against acute mucosal injury following aspirin or NSAID ingestion[63-66]; this protection may be due to decreased acid secretion or enhancement of the normal mucosal defense mechanisms. The concurrent use of antiulcer drugs and aspirin or NSAID would be both expensive and impractical; it has been estimated that 3% of the adult US population consume 15 or more aspirin tablets weekly.[49]

Management of Patients with Upper Gastrointestinal Bleeding and/or Gastric Ulcer due to Aspirin or NSAID. Aspirin and NSAID should be discontinued and subsequently avoided in patients without a strong indication for their continued use. Patients with documented gastric ulcer who require continued aspirin or NSAID heal their ulcers with conventional antiulcer therapy[67]; in these patients, maintenance therapy with sucralfate of H_2 antagonists should be used to prevent ulcer recurrence. Treatment with prostaglandin analogues has theoretical advantages in patients with aspirin or NSAID-induced ulcers. In a recent study, the prostaglandin analogue misoprostol was compared to placebo in the treatment of aspirin-induced gastric erosions and ulcers in 239 patients with rheumatoid arthritis. In spite of continued aspirin administration, there was healing of gastric erosions (77%) and ulcers (70%) after 8 weeks of misoprostol treatment; in placebo-treated patients the rate of healing was significantly less (39% and 29%, repectively).[68]

In patients who present with acute upper gastrointestinal bleeding following the use of aspirin or NSAID, these agents should be discontinued until gastric lesions have healed with appropriate antiulcer therapy. The value of sucralfate or H_2 receptor antagonists in preventing recurrent hemorrhage in patients who use aspirin or NSAID has not been established in long-term studies; theoretically, if gastric lesions can be prevented, recurrent bleeding should be less likely.

NONEROSIVE GASTRITIS

Nonerosive gastritis, also commonly called chronic gastritis, includes a variety of chronic lesions of differing and often poorly defined etiology. Infiltration of the lamina propria with acute and/or chronic inflammatory cells, variable atrophy of the specialized secretory cells in the gastric glands, and replacement of gastric epithelium by intestinal type epithelium characterize these lesions.

Chronic Superficial Gastritis

In chronic superficial gastritis, an increased number of lymphocytes and plasma cells infiltrate the lamina propria adjacent to the surface and gastric pits in the antrum and body of the stomach. An increased number of mitotic figures in the regeneration zone at the base of the gastric pits suggests that there is an increased loss and replacement of surface epithelial cells.[69]

The etiology and clinical significance of chronic superficial gastritis are unknown. Diffuse superficial gastritis is often associated with gastric ulcer in the body of the stomach and persists after ulcer healing.[70] Chronic colonization of the stomach with *Campylobacter pylori* may contribute to the development of chronic superficial gastritis; the frequency of both increase with age. The presence of superficial gastritis cannot be recognized clinically or endoscopically; it has not been proven that this lesion causes upper gastrointestinal symptoms, and the mucosa may appear normal on endoscopy.

Long-term follow-up of patients with biopsy-documented superficial gastritis suggests that this lesion may persist, improve, or progress to atrophic gastritis. Siurala and co-workers followed 50 patients over a 20-year period; 21 (42%) developed atrophic gastritis, 9 (18%) showed improvement, while 1 developed gastric carcinoma after 17 years.[71,72]

Atrophic Gastritis

Chronic atrophic gastritis is characterized pathologically by infiltration of the gastric mucosa with lymphocytes and plasma cells and atrophy of the gastric glands. The mucosal changes are diffuse and may be confined to the acid-secreting mucosa of the body and fundus with sparing of the antrum (type A) or may primarily involve the antrum (type B).[73] Both type A and type B atrophic gastritis increase in frequency with increasing age; this may relate to the increasing frequency of autoimmune disease with advancing age (type A) or to environmental factors (type B), rather than to the aging process alone.

Type A (Autoimmune) Atrophic Gastritis

In type A atrophic gastritis there is a selective atrophy of the gastric glands in the body and fundus of the stomach; this may be partial or complete. Normal surface mucous cells may be retained or may be partially or completely replaced by intestinal-type mucosa (intestinal metaplasia). The pyloric mucosa is unaffected and retains normal pyloric glands with hyperplastic endocrine cells. At endoscopy, the atrophic mucosa appears flat and pale with a prominent submucosal vessel pattern.[74] Functionally, the atrophy of gastric glands is associated with hypochlorhydria (partial atrophy) or achlorhydria due to a decreased parietal cell mass; there is a parallel decrease in intrinsic factor secretion from parietal cells.[75,76] The secretion of pepsinogen I (from chief cells) is decreased or lost. Antral mucosal function is preserved; high levels of serum gastrin result from G-cell hyperplasia and secretion in the absence of acid secretion.[77,78]

Pathogenesis. Both immunologic and experimental evidence supports the hypothesis that type A atrophic gastritis is an autoimmune disease.[79,80] The increased incidence in patients with other autoimmune diseases,[79] the presence of organ-specific parietal cell antibodies,[81–84] and the high frequency of atrophic gastritis and circulating antibodies in the relatives of patients with pernicious anemia[80] are consistent with an autoimmune etiology. The precise role of circulatory antibodies in the pathogenesis of atrophic gastritis remains uncertain. It is not established that circulating parietal cell antibody is responsible for the selective loss of parietal cells; parietal cell destruction may be cell mediated. In patients with pernicious anemia complicating autoimmune atrophic gastritis, the presence of intrinsic factor antibodies in serum and gastric juice may contribute to vitamin B_{12} malabsorption by inactivating small amounts of intrinsic factor that might otherwise be sufficient to maintain vitamin B_{12} absorption.

Clinical features. Type A atrophic gastritis is usually silent clinically. Intrinsic factor (IF) is normally secreted in considerable excess of the amount necessary for optimal vitamin B_{12} absorption[77,85]; thus, most patients with atrophic gastritis retain sufficient IF secretion to maintain normal vitamin absorption. A small fraction of these patients with advanced atrophic gastritis develop vitamin B_{12} malabsorption and present with manifestations of pernicious anemia when hepatic stores of this vitamin have been depleted.

Achlorhydria permits bacterial overgrowth both in the stomach and in the proximal small intestine. This bacterial overgrowth may be responsible for malabsorption (other than of vitamin B_{12}) in patients with treated pernicious anemia. Atrophic gastritis with achlorhydria may also contribute to bacterial overgrowth and malabsorption in patients with multiple jejunal diverticula.

Patients with atrophic gastritis (with or without pernicious anemia) are at increased risk for the development of multiple gastric carcinoid tumors and adenocarcinoma of the stomach. The development of carcinoid tumors may be related to a trophic action of sustained hypergastrinemia. An increased bacterial formation of nitrosamines in the achlorhydric stomach, and increased mucosal absorption of carcinogens may contribute to the late development of gastric carcinoma in these patients.[86,87]

Management. Patients who develop vitamin B_{12} deficiency require life-long parenteral replacement therapy (vitamin B_{12}, 1000 µg monthly). The benefit of endoscopic or radiographic screening programs for the earlier detection of gastric carcinoma in this group of elderly patients has not been established. An 18-fold increase in the risk of carcinoma in patients with pernicious anemia was calculated in an early study[88]; in a recent study, however, 152 patients with pernicious anemia were followed for 1550 patient-years, and carcinoma was documented in only 1 patient aged 96.[89]

Type B Atrophic Gastritis

Type B atrophic gastritis involves primarily the pyloric mucosa and extends proximally into the body of the stomach. The pyloric glands are thinned and infiltrated with mononuclear cells and variable numbers of polymorphonuclear cells which extend from the surface. Intestinal metaplasia may be patchy or diffuse. Type B atrophic gastritis is a nonspecific lesion that may result from bile reflux, chronic infection with *Campylobacter pylori*, or other undefined causes.

Bile Reflux Gastritis. Experimental studies have shown that exposure of the gastric mucosa to bile salts causes disruption of the surface epithelium with loss of the gastric mucosal barrier function, and back diffusion of acid.[18] Chronic exposure to bile salts may lead to degenerative changes and cellular infiltration of the deeper glandular zone to the gastric mucosa.[90,91] Bile reflux may be important in the pathogenesis of gastric ulcer and the associated antral gastritis. Following gastric surgery, particularly Billroth II operations, the reflux of bile into the gastric remnant in addition to a loss of the trophic effect of gastrin may be responsible for late fundic gland atrophy.[92-96]

The clinical significance of bile reflux gastritis (alkaline gastritis) is not well defined. It has been suggested that the clinical syndrome of postprandial dyspepsia, nausea, bilious vomiting, and weight loss following gastric surgery may be due to bile-induced gastritis. There is a poor correlation, however, between subjective symptoms and objective observations in these patients; the presence of a bile-stained hyperemic mucosa at endoscopy does not correlate with symptoms, with the severity of histologic changes on biopsy, or with quantitative measurements of bile reflux.[94,95,97-99] Medical treatment with antacids, sucralfate, or cholestyramine has not been successful in relieving symptoms.[100-102] Biliary diversion procedures with a Roux-en-Y reconstruction have been recommended for these patients; uncontrolled studies indicate a 50% to 95% success rate for remedial surgery. Unfortunately, preoperative evaluation cannot define those patients who would benefit from biliary diversion; thus surgery should be restricted to those patients with severe debilitating symptoms.[93-98]

An increased risk of gastric carcinoma has been suggested in patients 10 or more years after partial gastrectomy. Initial studies from Europe indicated that this risk was quite high,[103,104] but studies in the United States have not consistently confirmed this impression.[105-107] Schafer concluded in a study of 338 patients that the long-term risk of gastric cancer was not increased,[107] whereas Schuman reported adenocarcinoma in 4 and adenomatous polyps in 7 of 93 patients following operations for ulcer disease.[106] At the present time, there are limited and conflicting data supporting the use of surveillance gastroscopy in these patients; screening of young, asymptomatic patients 10 to 15 years after partial gastrectomy at intervals of 3 to 5 years appears to be a reasonable approach.

***Campylobacter pylori* infection.** There is increasing evidence that colonization of the stomach by *Campylobacter pylori* may cause both acute and chronic gastritis and may also relate to the pathogenesis of peptic ulcer disease.[108-112] This spirochete colonizes the surface mucous layer of the stomach, particularly in the antrum[113]; its attachment to surface epithelial cells may be responsible for the development of gastric mucosal lesions. Patients with *C. pylori* infection usually exhibit a chronic active antral gastritis characterized by mucosal infiltration with mononuclear and polymorphonuclear cells.

In 1979, 17 of 37 healthy volunteers participating in gastric secretory studies requiring repeated gastric intubation became acutely ill with epigastric pain; severe gastritis with hypochlorhydria or achlorhydria followed the acute illness[114]; a late follow-up of gastric biopsy specimens from these subjects revealed spiral organisms[108] and serologic studies suggested *C. pylori* infection.

A healthy person with histologically normal gastric mucosa ingested a culture of *C. pylori*; 7 days later he developed a mild acute illness that persisted for 7 days. Gastric biopsies showed gastritis with campylobacterlike organisms adherent to the epithelial cells.[115]

In multiple studies, it has been shown that there is a high frequency of *C. pylori* infection in patients with antral gastritis, gastric ulcer, and duodenal ulcer.[116] In both asymptomatic subjects and patients with ulcer disease, the frequency of *C. pylori* infection appears to increase with increasing age.[117]

The role of *C. pylori* in the pathogenesis of ulcer disease remains speculative. The presence of a bacterial protease that degrades gastric mucus suggests the possibility that the mucosal protective properties of surface mucus may be impaired.[118] The presence of campylobacterlike organisms in association with normal biopsies from the gastric body or antrum suggests that this organism may be part of the normal flora of the stomach. Further clinical, bacteriologic, and histologic studies correlating the presence of organisms with ulcer healing and recurrence may define the relationship between this organisms and ulcer disease.

Treatment. *C. pylori* is sensitive in vitro to tetracycline, erythromycin, penicillin, and cephalosporins and is susceptible to colloidal bismuth subcitrate.[119] Treatment of antral gastritis with bismuth compounds has resulted in temporary eradication of *C. pylori* with resolution of acute mucosal inflammation.[120–122] In a prospective, double-blind trial the organisms were cleared in 14 of 18 patients receiving bismuth, in 1 of 15 receiving erythromycin, and in none of 17 receiving placebo; patients with clearing of the organism were more likely to have relief of symptoms than those who did not.[121] Similarly, in duodenal ulcer patients with documented *C. pylori* infection, ulcer healing was increased and ulcer recurrence was decreased by eradication of the organism.[123]

PRIMARY HYPERTROPHIC GASTROPATHY

An increase in the thickness of gastric mucosal folds may result from infiltration with carcinoma or lymphoma or inflammatory cells, from hyperplasia associated with gastrin stimulation (Zollinger-Ellison syndrome), or from primary (idiopathic) hyperplasia of mucosal cells. Primary hyperplastic gastropathy has been classified pathologically into mucous cell hyperplasia (Menetrier's disease), glandular cell hyperplasia, and mixed mucous–glandular cell hyperplasia.[124] In Menetrier's disease there is hyperplasia of surface mucous and foveolar cells with tortuous or cystically dilated mucous-secreting glands. In the glandular cell type, there is hyperplasia of chief and parietal cells without hypergastrinemia.

Clinical Features

Hyperplastic gastropathy is most common in the fourth to sixth decades and has a 3:1 male predominance.[125,126] A transient, often benign form of Menetrier's disease has been described in children.[127] The common presenting symptoms are epigastric pain, vomiting, weight loss, and edema. Bleeding is an occasional complication. Edema and hypoproteinemia are due to an increased exudation of plasma proteins into the gastric lumen.[124,128,129] Radiographically, hypertrophic gastric folds are noted primarily in the body and fundus but may occasionally involve the entire stomach. Endoscopically, large, glistening, cerebriform mucosal folds are seen, often with overlying erosions. A full-thickness surgical or endoscopic snare biopsy is necessary to diagnosis and to exclude infiltrative disease.

Treatment

In adults with hypertrophic gastropathy, spontaneous remission is unusual.[126] Medical management may include a high-protein diet, diuretics, and antisecretory drugs. Anticholinergic drugs (atropine and propantheline bromide) have been helpful in decreasing protein loss[126,130-132]; cimetidine may also be of clinical value.[133-135] Protein loss, hypoproteinemia, and edema improved in one patient treated with prednisolone.[136] Surgery is usually reserved for bleeding, pyloric obstruction or unrelenting epigastric pain. If the disease is localized, partial or subtotal gastrectomy is effective. In Scharschmidt's series, 32 of 42 patients who underwent partial gastric resection had satisfactory results; there were seven postoperative deaths, however, of which five were from anastomotic leaks.[137]

REFERENCES

1. Weinstein WM: Gastritis, in Sleisenger MHN, Fortrand JS: Gastrointestinal Disease Pathophysiology Diagnosis Management. Philadelphia, W.B. Saunders, 1983, pp. 559–578.
2. Lucas CE: Stress ulceration: The clinical problem World J Surg 1981; 5:139–151.
3. Lucas CE, Sugawa C, Riddle J, et al: Natural history and surgical dilemma of "stress" gastric bleeding. Arch Surg 1971; 102:266–273.
4. Czaja MA, McAlhany JC, Pruit BA: Acute gastroduodenal disease after thermal injury. An endoscopic evaluation of incidence and natural history. N Engl J Med 1974; 291:925–929.
5. Bowen JC, Fleming W, Thompson JC: Increased gastrin release following penetrating central nervous system injury. Surgery 1974; 75:720–724.
6. Gordon MJ, Skillman JJ, Zervas NT, et al: Divergent nature of gastric permeability in gastric acid secretion in sick patients for general and neurological disease. Ann Surg 1973; 178:285–294.
7. Kamada T, Fusamoto H, Kawano S, et al: Gastrointestinal bleeding following head injury: Clinical study of 443 cases. J Trauma 1977; 17:44–47.
8. Schuster DP, Rowley H, Feinstein S, et al: Prospective evaluation of the risk of upper gastrointestinal bleeding after admission to a medical intensive care unit. Am J Med 1984; 76:623–630.
9. Onstead GR, Cass OW: Stress ulceration of the stomach. Practical Gastroenterology 1985; 9:6–11.
10. Hastings PR, Skillman JJ, Bushnell LS, et al: Antacid titration in the prevention of acute gastrointestinal bleeding. N Engl J Med 1978; 298:1041–1045.
11. Pruitt BA, Goodwin CW: Stress ulcer disease in the burned patient. World J Surg 1981; 5:209–222.
12. Bank S, Rahman N, Wise L: The incidence, distribution and evolution of stress ulcers in surgical intensive care patients (abstract). Am J Gastroenterol 1980; 74:76.
13. Marrone GC, Silen W: Pathogenesis diagnosis and treatment of acute gastric mucosal lesions. Clin Gastroenterol 1984; 13:635–650.
14. Ritchie WP: Pathogenesis of acute gastric mucosal injury. Viewpoints on Digestive Diseases 1983; 15:17–20.
15. Marrone GC, Silen W: Pathogenesis, diagnosis and treatment of acute gastric mucosal lesions. Clin Gastroenterol 1984; 13:635–650.
16. Kivilaakaso E: Pathogenic mechanisms and experimental gastric stress ulceration. Scand J Gastroenterol [Suppl] 1985; 20:57–62.
17. Menguy R: Role of gastric mucosal energy metabolism in the etiology of stress ulceration. World J Surg 1981; 5:175–180.
18. Ritchie WP: Role of bile acid reflux in acute hemorrhagic gastritis. World J Surg 1981; 5:189–198.
19. Shuman RB, Schuster DP, Zuckerman GR: Prophylactic therapy for stress ulcer bleeding: A reappraisal. Ann Intern Med 1987; 106:562–567.
20. More DJ, Raper RF, Monroe IA, et al: Randomized prospective trial of cimetidine and ranitidine for control of intragastric pH in the critically ill. Surgery 1985; 97:215–223.
21. Macci H, Fiasse R, Reynart M, et al: Effect of intravenous ranitidine on gastric acid secretion in severely ill patients admitted to an intensive care unit. The clinical use of Ranitidine. Medical Publishing Foundation Symposium Series 5, Oxford, 1982, pp. 269–274.
22. Walt RP, Male PJ, Rawlings J, et al: Comparison of the effects of ranitidine, cimetidine and placebo on the 24-hour intragastric acidity and nocturnal acid secretion in patients with a duodenal ulcer. Gut 1981; 22:49–54.
23. Priebe HJU, Skillman JJ, Bushnell LS, et al: Antacid vs cimetidine in preventing acute gastrointestinal bleeding. N Engl J Med 1980; 302:426–430.
24. Zinner MJ, Zuidema GD, Smith PL, et al: The prevention of upper gastrointestinal tract bleeding in patients in an intensive care unit. Surg Gynecol Obstet 1981; 153:214–220.
25. McGuigan JE: A consideration of the adverse

effects of cimetidine. *Gastroenterology* 1981; 80:181–192.
26. Sedman AJ: Cimetidine drug interactions. *Am J Med* 1984; 76:109–114.
27. Feely J, Wilkerson GR, Wood AJJ: Reduction of liver blood flow and propranolol metabolism by cimetidine. *N Engl J Med* 1981; 304:692–695.
28. Kimelblatt BJ, Cerra FB, Calleri G, et al: Dose and serum concentration relationships in cimetidine associated mental confusion. *Gastroenterology* 1980; 78:791–795.
29. Schentag JJ, Cerra FB, Calleri G, et al: Pharmacokinetic and clinical studies in patients with cimetidine associated mental confusion. *Lancet* 1979; 1:177–181.
30. Dammann HG, Burkhard F, Muller P, et al: Effect of intravenous fumotidine and ranitidine on intragastric pH and hormone levels in critical care patients (abstract). *Dig Dis Sci* 1985; 30:372.
31. Tryba N, Zeuvonou F, Torok M, et al: Prevention of acute stress bleeding with sucralfate, antacids or cimetidine: A controlled study with pirenzepine as a basic medication. *Am J Med* 1985; 79 (suppl):21–27.
32. Borrero BS, Margolis I, Schulman MD, et al: Comparison of antacid in sucralfate in the prevention of gastrointestinal bleeding in patients who are critically ill. *Am J Med* 1985; 79 (suppl): 28–34.
33. Craven DE, Driks MR: Nosocomial pneumonia in the intubated patient. *Seminars in Respiratory Infection* 1987; 2:20–33.
34. Skillman JJ, Lisbon A, Long PC, et al: 15(R)-15-methyl prostaglandin E_2 does not prevent gastric intestinal bleeding in seriously ill patients. *Am J Surg* 1984; 147:451–455.
35. Simonian SJ, Curtis LE: Treatment of hemorrhagic gastritis by antacid. *Ann Surg* 1976; 184:429–434.
36. McAlhany JC, Czaja AJ, Pruitt BA: Antacid control of complications from acute gastroduodenal disease after burns. *J Trauma* 1976; 16:645–649.
37. Peura DA, Johnson LF: Cimetidine for prevention and treatment of gastroduodenal mucosal lesions in patients in an intensive care unit. *Ann Intern Med* 1985; 103:173–177.
38. Athanasoulis CA, Baum S, Waltman AC, et al: Control of acute gastric mucosal hemorrhage. Intra-arterial infusion of posterior pituitary extract. *N Engl J Med* 1974; 290:597–603.
39. Fogel MR, Cnauer CM, Andres LL, et al: Continuous intravenous vasopressin in active upper gastrointestinal bleeding. *Ann Intern Med* 1982; 96:565–569.
40. Wara P: Endoscopic control of major stress ulcer bleeding. *World J Surg* 1981; 5:101–103.
41. Wilson WS, Gadacz T, Olcott C, et al: Superficial gastric erosions: Response to surgical treatment. *Am J Surg* 1973; 126:133–140.
42. Cody HS, Wichern WA: Choice of operation for acute gastric mucosal hemorrhage. Report of 36 cases and review of literature. *Am J Surg* 1977; 134:322–325.
43. Davenport HW: Salicylate damage to the gastric mucosal barrier. *N Engl J Med* 1967; 276:1307–1312.
44. Carruso I, Bianchi Porro G: Gastroscopic evaluation of anti-inflammatory agents. *Br J Med* 1980; 280:75–78.
45. Robert A, Nezamis JE, Lancaster C, et al: Cytoprotection by prostaglandins in rats. Prevention of gastric necrosis produced by alcohol, HCl, NAOH, hypertonic NACl, thermal injury. *Gastroenterology* 1979; 77:430–433.
46. Pierson RN, Holt PR, Watson RN, et al: Aspirin and gatrointestinal bleeding. Chromate 51 blood loss studies. *Am J Med* 1961; 31:259–265.
47. Thorsen WB, Western D, Tanaka Y, et al: Aspirin injury to the gastric mucosa. Gastrocamera observations of the effects of pH. *Arch Intern Med* 1968; 121:499–506.
48. Vickers NF: Mucosal effects of aspirin and acetaminophen: Report of a controlled gastroscopic study. *Gastrointest Endosc* 1967; 14:94–99.
49. Graham DY, Smith JL: Aspirin and the stomach. *Ann Intern Med* 1986; 104:390–398.
50. Graham DY, Smith JL, Dobbs SM: Gastric adaptation occurs with aspirin administration in man. *Dig Dis Sci* 1983; 28:1–6.
51. Lanza FL, Oryer GL, Nelson RS, et al: A comparative endoscopic evaluation of the damaging effects of nonsteroidal anti-inflammatory agents on the gastric and duodenal mucosa. *Am J Gastroenterol* 1981; 75:17–21.
52. Lanza FL, Royer GL, Nelson RS, et al: The effects of ibuprofen, indomethacin, aspirin, naproxen, and placebo on the gastric mucosa of normal volunteers. A gastroscopic and photographic study. *Dig Dis Sci* 1979; 24:823–828.
53. Lanza FL, Woyer GL, Nelson RS: Endoscopic evaluation of the effects of aspirin, buffered aspirin, and enteric-coated aspirin on gastric and duodenal mucosa. *N Engl J Med* 1980; 303:136–138.
54. Eastwood GL: Ultra structural effects of ulcerogens. *Dig Dis Sci* 1985; 30 (suppl):95S–104S.
55. Meyer RA, McGinley D, Posalaky Z: Effects of aspirin on tight junction structures of the canine gastric mucosa. *Gastroenterology* 1986; 91:351–359.
56. Baskin WN, Ivey KJ, Krause WJ, et al: Aspirin-induced ultrastructural changes in human gastric mucosa. Correlation with potential difference. *Ann Intern Med* 1976; 85:299–303.
57. Murray HS, Strottman MP, Cooke AR: Effect of several drugs on gastric potential difference in man. *Br Med J* 1974; 1:19–21.
58. Crithchlow J, Magee D, Ito S, et al: Requirements for restitution of the surface epithelium of frog stomach after mucosal injury. *Gastroenterology* 1985; 88:237–249.
59. Silvosa GR, Ivey JK, Butt JH, et al: Incidence of gastric lesions in patients with rheumatic disease on chronic aspirin therapy. *Ann Intern Med* 1979; 91:517–520.
60. Lanza FL, Nelson RS, Rack MF: A controlled endoscopic study comparing the toxic effects of sulindac, naproxen, aspirin and placebo on the gastric mucosa of healthy volunteers. *J Clin Pharmacol* 1984; 24:89–95.

61. Silverstein FE, Gilbert DA, Tedesco FJ, et al: National ASGE survey on upper gastrointestinal bleeding. Clinical prognostic factors. *Gastrointest Endosc* 1981; 27:80–93.
62. Jolobe OM, Montgomery RD: Changing clinical pattern of gastric ulcer: Are anti-inflammatory drugs involved? *Digestion* 1984; 29:164–170.
63. Kontorek SJ, Kwiecien N, Tolopeiwz W, et al: Double blind control study on the effect of sucralfate on gastric prostaglandin formation and micro-bleeding in normal and aspirin treated man. *Gut* 1986; 27:1450–1456.
64. Cohen MM, McCready DR, Clark L, et al: Protection against aspirin-induced antral and duodenal damage with enprostil. A double-blind endoscopic study. *Gastroenterology* 1985; 88:382–386.
65. Lanza FL, Aspinal RL, Suab EA, et al: A double blind placebo controlled endoscopic comparison of the cytoprotective effects of misoprostol and cimetidine on tolmetin induced gastric mucosal injury (abstract). *Gastroenterology* 1987; 92:1491.
66. Konturek SJ, Piastucki I, Brzozowski T, et al: Role of prostaglandins in the formation of aspirin-induced gastric ulcers. *Gastroenterology* 1981; 80:4–9.
67. Gerber LH, Rooney PJ, McCarthy DM: Healing of peptic ulcers during continuing anti-inflammatory drug therapy in rheumatoid arthritis. *J Clin Gastroenterol* 1981; 3:7–11.
68. Agrawal N, Roth S, Montoya H, et al: Misoprostol co-administration heals aspirin-induced lesions in rheumatiod arthritis patients (abstract). *Gastroenterology* 1987; 92:1290.
69. Whitehead R, Truelove SC, Gear MW: The histological diagnosis of chronic gastritis in fibreoptic gastriscope biopsy specimens. *J Clin Pathol* 1972; 25:1–11.
70. Gear WL, Truelove SC, Whitehead R: Gastric ulcer and gastritis. *Gut* 1971; 12:639–645.
71. Siurala M, Salmi HJ: Long-term follow-up of subjects with superficial gastritis or a normal gastric mucosa. *Scand J Gastroenterol* 1971; 6:459–463.
72. Ihamaki T, Saukkonen M, Siurala M: Long-term observation of subjects with normal mucosa and with superficial gastritis: Results of 23–27 years with follow-up examinations. *Scand J Gastroenterol* 1978; 13:771–775.
73. Strickland RG, Mackay IR: A reappraisal of the nature and significance of chronic and atrophic gastritis. *Am J Dig Dis* 1973; 18:426–440.
74. Meshkinpour H, Orlando RA, Arguello JF, et al: Significance of endoscopically visible blood vessels as an index of atrophic gastritis. *Am J Gastroenterol* 1979; 71:376–379.
75. Stockbrugger R, Angervall L, Lundqvist G: Serum gastrin and atrophic gastritis in achlorhydric patients with and without pernicious anemia. *Scand J Gastroenterol* 1976; 11:7–13.
76. Stockbrugger R, Larsson LI, Lundqvist G, et al: Antral gastrin cells and serum gastrin in achlorhydria. *Scand J Gastroenterol* 1977; 12:209–213.
77. Lewin KJ, Dowling F, Wright JP, et al: Gastric morphology and serum gastrin levels in pernicious anemia. *Gut* 1976; 17:551–560.
78. McGuigan JE, Trudeau WL: Serum gastrin concentrations in pernicious anemia. *N Engl J Med* 1970; 282:358–361.
79. Doniach D, Roitt IM, Taylor KB: Autoimmune phenomena in pernicious anemia. Serologic overlap with thyroiditis, thyrotoxicosis and systemic lupus erythematosus. *Br Med J* 1963; 1:1374–1379.
80. Varis K, Ihamaki T, Harkonen M, et al: Gastric morphology, function and immunology in first degree relatives of probands with pernicious anemia and controls. *Scand J Gastroenterol* 1979; 14:129–139.
81. teVelde K, Abels J, Anders GJ, et al: A family study of pernicious aenmia by an immunologic method. *J Lab Clin Med* 1964; 64:177–187.
82. Hennes AR, Sevelius H, Lewellyn T, et al: Atrophic gastritis in dogs. *Arch Pathol* 1962; 72:33–39.
83. Krohn K: Experimental gastritis in the dog, production of atrophic gastritis and antibodies to parietal cells. *Annual Medical Exp Fenn* 1968; 46:249–258.
84. Jeffries GH, Sleisenger MH: Studies of parietal cell antibodies in pernicous anemia. *J Clin Invest* 1965; 44:2021–2028.
85. Jeffries GH: Gastritis, in Sleisenger MH, Fortran JS (eds): *Gastrointestinal Disease*. Philadelphia. WB Saunders, 1973; pp 560–571.
86. Siurala M, Varis K, Wiljasalo M: Studies of patients with atrophic gastritis: A 10–15-year follow-up. *Scand J Gastroenterol* 1966; 1:40–48.
87. Siurala M, Vuorinen Y, Seppela K: Follow-up studies of patients with atrophic gastritis. *Acta Med Scand* 1961; 170:151.
88. Hitchcock CR, Sullivan WA, Wangensteen OH: The value of achlorhydria as a screening test for gastric cancer: A ten-year report. *Gastroenterology* 1955; 29:621–628.
89. Schafer LW, Larsen DE, Melton LJ, et al: Risk of development of gastric carcinoma in patients with pernicious anemia: A population based study in Rochester, MN. *Mayo Clin Proc* 1985; 60:444–448.
90. Cheng J, Ritchie WP, Delaney JP: Atrophic gastritis: An experimental model. *Fed Proc* 1969; 28:513.
91. Broadie TA, Sosin H, et al: Reflux gastritis: The consequences of intestinal juice in the stomach. *Am J Surg* 1976; 131:23–29.
92. Fischer AB, Graem N, Christiansen LA: Causes and clinical significance of gastritis following Billroth II resection for duodenal ulcer. *Br J Surg* 1983; 70:322–325.
93. Mosimann F, Sorgi M, Wolverson RL, et al: Bile reflux after duodenal ulcer surgery: A study of 114 asymptomatic and symptomatic patients. *Scand J Gastroenterol* 1984; 19(suppl 92):224–226.
94. Ritchie WP: Alkaline reflux gastritis: A critical reappraisal. *Gut* 1984; 25:975–987.
95. Boren CH, Way LW: Alkaline reflux gastritis: A re-evaluation. *Am J Surg* 1980; 140:40–46.
96. Van Heerden JA, Phillips SF, Adson MA, et al:

Postoperative reflux gastritis. *Am J Surg* 1975; 129:82–88.
97. Ludwig S, Ippoliti A: Objective evaluation of symptomatic alkaline reflux after antrectomy. *Dig Dis Sci* 1984; 29:824–828.
98. Sivelli R, Farinon AM, Sianesi M, et al: Technetium-99m HIDA hepatobiliary scanning and evaluation of afferent loop syndrome. *Am J Surg* 1984; 148:262–265.
99. Goldner FH, Boyce HW: Relationship of bile in the stomach to gastritis. *Gastrointest Endosc* 1976; 22:197–199.
100. Nicolai JJ, Speelman P, Tytgat GN, et al: Comparison of the combination of cholestyramine/alginates with placebo in the treatment of postgastrectomy biliary reflux gastritis. *Eur J Clin Pharmacol* 1981; 21:189–194.
101. Meshkinpour H, Elashoff J, Stewart H, et al: Effect of cholestyramine on the symptoms of reflux gastritis: A randomized, double blind, cross-over study. *Gastroenterology* 1977; 73:441–443.
102. Buch KL, Tedesco FJ, Weinstein MW: Sucralfate therapy in patients with symptoms of alkaline reflux gastritis: A randomized double blind study. *Am J Med* 1985; 79:49–54.
103. Stalsberg H, Taksdal S: Stomach cancer following gastric surgery for benign condition. *Lancet* 1971; 2:1175–1177.
104. Logan RF, Langman MJ: Screening for gastric cancer after gastric surgery. *Lancet* 1983; 2:667–670.
105. Ritchie MT, Kurtz RC: Gastric stump cancer. Selected summary. *Gastroenterology* 1984; 86:993–994.
106. Schuman BM, Waldbaum JR, Hiltz SW, et al: Carcinoma of the gastric remnant in the U.S. population. *Gastrointest Endosc* 1984; 30:71–73.
107. Schafer LW, Larson DE, Melton J, et al: The risk of gastric carcinoma after surgical treatment for benign ulcer disease. A population-based study in Olmstead County, MN. *N Engl J Med* 1983; 309:1210–1213.
108. Marshall BJ: *Campylobacter pyloridis* and gastritis. *J Infect Dis* 1986; 153:650–657.
109. Marshall BJ, Warren JR: Unidentified curved bacilli in the stomach of patients with gastritis and peptic ulceration. *Lancet* 1984; 1:1311–1315.
110. Marshall BJ, Warren JR: Unidentified curved bacilli on gastric epithelium in active chronic gastritis. *Lancet* 1983; 1:1273–1275.
111. Goodwin CS, Armstrong JA, Marshall BJ: *Campylobacter pyloridis*, gastritis and peptic ulceration. *J Clin Pathol* 1986; 39:353–365.
112. Price AB, Levi J, Dolby JM, et al: *Campylobacter pyloridis* in peptic ulcer disease: Microbiology, pathology and scanning electron microscopy. *Gut* 1985; 26:1183–1188.
113. Hazell SL, Lee A, Brady L, et al: *Campylobacter pyloridis* and gastritis: Association with intercellular space and adaptation to an environment of mucus as important factors in colonization of the gastric epithelium. *J Infect Dis* 1986; 153:658–663.
114. Ramsey EJ, Carey KV, Peterson WL, et al: Epidemic gastritis with hypochlorhydria. *Gastroenterology* 1979; 76:1449–1457.
115. Marshall BJ, Armstrong JA, McGechie DB, et al: Attempt to fulfill Koch's postulates for pyloric *Campylobacter*. *Med J Aust* 1985; 142:436–439.
116. Piper DW: Bacteria, gastritis, acid hyposecretion and peptic ulcer. *Med J Aust* 1985; 142:431.
117. Graham DY, Kline PD: *Campylobacter pyloridis* gastritis: The past, the present, and speculations about the future. *Am J Gastroenterol* 1987; 82:283–286.
118. Slomiany BL, Bilshi J, Murty VLN, et al: *Campylobacter pyloridis* degrades mucin and undermines gastric mucosal integrity (abstract). *Gastroenterology* 1987; 92:1645.
119. Marshall BJ, McGechie DB, Rogers PA, et al: Pyloric *Campylobacter* infection and gastroduodenal disease. *Med J Aust* 1985; 142:439–444.
120. McNulty CA, Gearty JC, Crump B, et al: *Campylobacter pyloridis* and associated gastritis: Investigator blind placebo controlled trial of bismuth salicylate and erythromycin ethylsuccinate. *Br Med J* 1986; 293:645–649.
121. Lambert JR, Borromeo M, Kormann MG, et al: The role of *Campylobacter pyloridis* in non-ulcer dyspepsia—A randomized control trial. *Gastroenterology* 1987; 92:1488.
122. Borody T, Hennessey W, Daskalopoulos G, et al: Double blind trial of De-Nol in non-ulcer dyspepsia associated with *Campylobacter pyloridis* gastritis (abstract). *Gastroenterology* 1987; 92:1324.
123. Marshall BJ, Goodwin CS, Warren JR, et al: Long term healing of gastritis and low duodenal ulcer relapse after erradication of *Campylobacter pyloridis:* A prospective double-blind study (abstract). *Gastroenterology* 1987; 92:1518.
124. Ming SC: *Tumors of the Esophagus and Stomach.* Washington, Armed Forces Institute of Pathology, 1972; pp 115-9, 153-4.
125. Simson JNL: Hyperplastic gastropathy. *Br Med J* 1985; 291:1298–1299.
126. Fieber SS, Richert RR: Hyperplastic gastropathy. *Am J Gastroenterol* 1981; 76:321–329.
127. Chouragui JP, Roy CC, Brocha P, et al: Menetrier's disease in children. *Gastroenterology* 1981; 80:1042–1047.
128. Raotma H, Angervall L, Dahl I, et al: Clinical and morphological studies of grant hypertrophic gastritis (Menetrier's disease). *Acta Med Scand* 1974; 195:247–252.
129. Weintraub G, Gelb AM: Exudative gastropathy due to giant hypertrophy of gastric mucosa. *Am J Dig Dis* 1961; 6:526–533.
130. Gordon MN, Schaefer EJ, Finkel M: Treatment of protein-losing gastropathy with atropine. *Am J Gastroenterol* 1976; 66:535–539.
131. Overholt BJ, Jeffries GH: Hypertrophic hypersecreting protein-losing gastropathy. *Gastroenterology* 1970; 58:80–87.
132. Kelly DG, Miller LJ, Molagelada JR, et al: Giant hypertrophic gastropathy: Pharmacologic effects on protein leakage and mucosal ultrastructure. *Gastroenterology* 1982; 83:581–589.
133. Florent C, Vidon N, Flourie B, et al: Gastric

clearance of alpha-1-antitrypsin under cimetidine perfusion. New test to detect protein-losing gastropathy? *Dig Dis Sci* 1986; 131:12–15.
134. Krag E, Fredericksen HJ, Olsen N, et al: Cimetidine treatment of protein-losing gastropathy. *Scand J Gastroenterol* 1978; 13:635–639.
135. Vendelboe M, Jespersen J: Hypertrophic protein-losing gastritis treated with cimetidine. *Acta Med Scand* 1981; 209:125–127.
136. Winney RJ, Gilmour HM, Matthews JD: Prednisolone in great hypertrophic gastritis (Menetrier's disease). *Dig Dis Sci* 1976; 12:337–338.
137. Scharschmidt BF: The natural history of hypertrophic gastropathy. *Am J Med* 1977; 63:644–652.

8

Gastric Ulcers:
Should all patients undergo endoscopy? What should be done with patients who heal "slowly"?

EDWIN N. LARKAI, M.D.
DAVID Y. GRAHAM, M.D.

Gastric ulcer is a common diagnosis. The true incidence of gastric ulcer is unknown, but clinical studies have suggested the frequency of new cases is about 1 per 2000 adults per year; the frequency in men and women is approximately equal. The prevalence of patients with gastric ulcer is higher because once ulcer disease begins ulcers tend to recur for many years. Studies in which "controls" have undergone endoscopy have shown that, on average, 1% of adults had a gastric ulcer at any one time.[1-3] The point prevalence of gastric ulcer in patients taking daily nonsteroidal anti-inflammatory drugs (NSAID) is about 10 times higher than those not taking NSAID (i.e., over 10%).[4]

The typical gastric ulcer is located on the lesser curvature of the stomach near the angulus incisura. It occurs as a symmetrical mucosal defect, between 1 and 2 cm in diameter with smooth, slightly overhanging edges and a white base.

The most common cause for presentation of patients with gastric ulcer is abdominal pain. Gastric ulcer pain is usually epigastric in location and relieved by the ingestion of food or antacids. The second most common presentation is upper gastrointestinal bleeding. The symptoms of gastric ulcer and duodenal ulcer cannot be reliably distinguished; location, periodicity, and episodic nature tend to be similar. Some patients with gastric ulcer complain of pain immediately after eating (possibly related to distention of the gastric wall and thus of the ulcer). Although this symptom suggests gastric ulcer, it is not completely reliable because it may be related by patients with duodenal ulcer. Patients with gastric ulcer who suffer pain with eating often lose weight, and the clinical diagnosis of gastric or pancreatic carcinoma may be erroneously considered, especially in elderly patients. There are no specific physical findings of gastric ulcer, although mild, nonspecific, epigastric tenderness is often present. Presence of an epigastric mass suggests gastric carcinoma instead of benign ulcer.

PATHOGENESIS

The pathogenesis of gastric ulcer remains unclear and, in all likelihood, is multifactorial. The presence of a chronic ulcer implies failure of the normal mucosal reparative processes. The pivotal factors that initiate a gastric ulcer and those that encourage spontaneous healing remain unclear. It is best to think of the pathogenesis of ulcer as a balance between potentially aggressive factors (such as acid and pepsin) and protective factors that serve to maintain the mucosal integrity despite the presence of high luminal acid concentrations and the ingestion of a variety of caustic substances (e.g., aspirin and jalapeno peppers) (Fig 8–1). Recently, a bacterium, *Campylobacter pylori*, has been associated with peptic ulcer. This bacterium causes a form of superficial gastritis; gastritis must interfere with normal mucosal function. Whether *C. pylori* plays an active or a contributory role in gastric ulcer remains to be shown, but it is clearly not the *cause* of gastric ulcer because most patients with *C. pylori* infection are asymptomatic and do not have peptic ulcer disease. *C. pylori* may be an important predisposing factor in gastric ulcer because it seems to be responsible for the gastritis so commonly associated with gastric ulcers. It has long been known that gastric ulcers occur most often in mucosa involved with gastritis with the ulcer having a predilection for the junction of normal mucosa and an area involved by gastritis.

DIAGNOSIS

Patients with gastric ulcer fall into two major categories: those with dyspepsia and those with upper gastrointestinal bleeding. The two modalities most commonly used to diagnose gastric ulcers are barium-contrast upper gastrointestinal (UGI) series and endoscopy. Endoscopy has greater diagnostic accuracy (>95%) than an UGI series, but it costs more. Many physicians still rely on the UGI series as their initial diagnostic test, so for many patients the presence of a gastric ulcer is first confirmed by UGI series. Following x-ray diagnosis, the patient is usually referred to a gastroenterologist for endoscopy to determine whether the ulcer is benign or is a gastric malignancy simulating a benign ulcer. This distinction is important because histologic examination of biopsies from the ulcer margins and base will identify that between 1% and 5% of radiographically benign-appearing gastric ulcers are malignant. The benign-appearing ulcerated gastric malignancy is often an "early gastric cancer," a lesion with a much better prognosis than typical advanced gastric cancer, so its identification is more than academic.

Gastric ulcers should be examined endoscopically. This "rule" is not meant to imply that every patient with a gastric ulcer should undergo endoscopy immediately after the diagnosis is made. A prudent approach would be to carefully examine the UGI series for signs that the

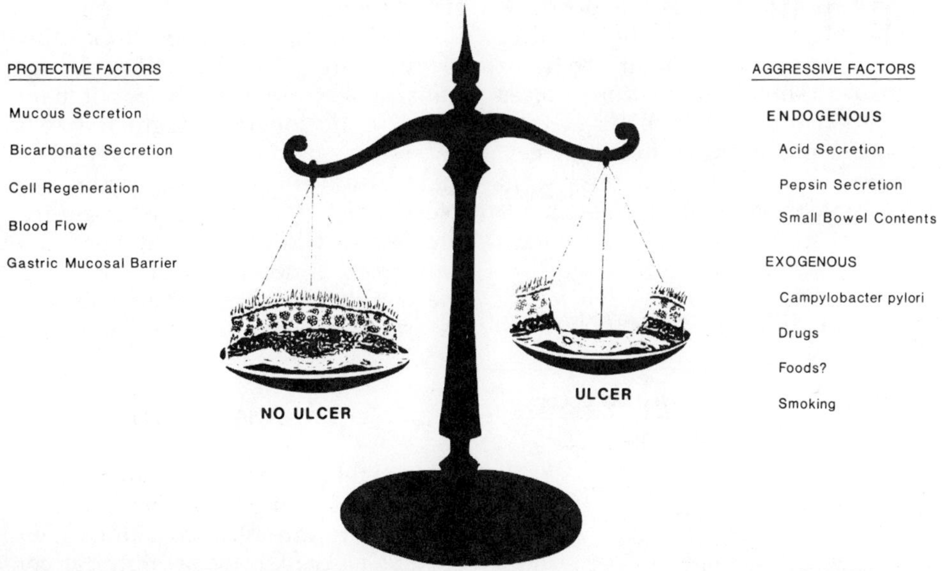

FIG 8–1.
The pathogenesis of peptic ulcer is depicted as a balance between aggressive and protective factors.

ulcer is benign. If the radiologist is certain that the ulcer is benign, endoscopy can be safely delayed until the first follow-up visit (i.e., 8 weeks). If the radiologist is uncertain (about 40% of cases in our experience), endoscopy should be performed. The strongest radiographic criteria for the benign nature of an ulcer are the presence of radiating folds, regular shape, a smooth ulcer crater, and location of the ulcer base on or outside the projection of the stomach wall. The most significant radiographic criteria of malignancy are the presence of an adjacent mass, gastric wall rigidity, and failure of the apex of the ulcer to project outside the stomach contour.

Clinical features that should prompt early endoscopy are anemia, presence of a mass, major weight loss, or signs and symptoms suggesting gastric outlet obstruction (Table 8–1). Endoscopic features that suggest gastric carcinoma include a stepwise depression of the ulcer edge; small extensions of the ulcer that may blur a portion of the wall; bleeding from the edge of the crater; a necrotic, dirty appearance of the ulcer crater; the presence of abnormal folds (clubbing or fusion of the tips); disruption of the mucosal folds before they reach the crater; and an irregular or moth-eaten appearance of the surroundings. Although these endoscopic features help one decide whether an ulcer is benign, biopsy is the final arbitrator and endoscopy should not be done unless one is prepared to obtain biopsies. We recommend a minimum of four biopsies, one from each quadrant of the ulcer's rim and one biopsy from the ulcer base, in addition to taking a specimen for cytology.[5] We advise taking an additional two to four biopsies if no cytologic examination is performed. Generally biopsies beyond the ulcer have a low yield.[6] We occasionally find that what appears endoscopically as a benign ulcer is really a gastric cancer, and this is consistent with the experience of others.[5, 7, 8]

When biopsies and cytologic specimens are negative, and the ulcer endoscopically has features that suggest, but are not diagnostic of, malignancy, we schedule a second endoscopic evaluation with biopsy. If the patient's condition does not otherwise suggest malignancy is present, this examination is scheduled after 2 to 4 weeks of therapy. This allows the ulcer to show significant healing and makes the determination easier. If the ulcer has not shown evidence of healing (at least a 30% reduction in size) and endoscopically still has features suggesting malignancy, the patient is referred for surgery.

Although early gastric cancers have been observed to heal,[9, 10] complete healing of the ulcer is a good criterion for the benign nature of the ulcer. Our concern for a possible gastric malignancy is also heightened whenever an apparently benign ulcer rapidly recurs at the same site.

The evaluation of patients with dyspepsia is changing (i.e., endoscopy is taking the place of the UGI series). Gastroenterologists rarely use the UGI series for the initial investigation of dyspeptic patients, and it is no longer thought that x-ray is necessary before endoscopy.[11, 12] The main disadvantage of endoscopy is cost. We predict that in the near future the problem of when to refer the gastric ulcer patient for endoscopy will be resolved by the fact that the initial diagnosis is made by endoscopy.

MANAGEMENT

Management of the patient with a gastric ulcer requires cooperation between the primary care physician and the endoscopist/gastroenterologist. Surgical consultation is also indicated for a small proportion of patients. The management of

TABLE 8–1.
Features Prompting Early or Delayed Endoscopy

Early Endoscopy	Delayed Endoscopy
Advanced age	Young patient
Long history	Short history
Weight loss	No weight change
Anorexia	Normal appetite
UGI bleeding/anemia	Normal blood count
Significant vomiting	Minor vomiting
No ulcerogenic drugs	NSAID therapy
Equivocal UGI series	Unequivocal benign ulcer

gastric ulcer can be broadly divided into three overlapping phases. The first phase is diagnosis, the second is dealing with any complications, and the third is healing the ulcer.

In general, the therapy of a gastric ulcer is the same as for duodenal ulcer (i.e., the same drugs are effective), only the duration of treatment is longer. Effective agents (currently available in the United States) for the treatment of benign gastric ulcers include antacids, H_2-receptor antagonists (cimetidine, ranitidine, or famotidine), and sucralfate. The relatively specific antimuscarinic anticholinergic, pirenzipine; several synthetic prostaglandins; and the substituted benzimidazole, omeprazole, are in clinical trial. Bismuth subcitrate and carbenoxolone sodium are effective but not available in the United States.

Antacids

Antacids accelerate healing of gastric ulcers. Antacids are best prescribed as liquid antacids to be taken seven times daily (1 and 3 hours after meals and at bedtime). Such therapy will achieve rates of healing identical to that achieved with H_2-receptor antagonists. Despite the effectiveness of antacids, they are inconvenient to use, and we generally prescribe antacids only as supplementary therapy. Antacids are especially useful for the first few days of treatment during which time the patients may still have pain. The addition of antacids to other therapies will neither accelerate the rate of healing nor produce symptomatic relief beyond that obtained with H_2-receptor antagonists alone.

H_2-Receptor Antagonists

The available H_2-receptor antagonists are all effective in accelerating healing of gastric ulcers.[13–16] Recent studies[16–18] have shown that a single nocturnal dose of an H_2-receptor antagonist is as effective as multiple-dose schedules. We now recommend that H_2-receptor antagonists be prescribed in single-dose therapy, with the drug being taken between 6 pm and 8 pm. The choice of agent should be based on the local cost. The dosages are cimetidine 300 mg qid (which is usually the cheapest program), ranitidine 300 mg in the evening, or famotidine 40 mg in the evening. The evening dose of cimetidine is 800 mg, although it may be less expensive to prescribe three 300-mg tablets instead.

Sucralfate

Sucralfate is a basic aluminum salt of sucrose octasulphate that promotes ulcer healing by forming a protective coating on the ulcer base to prevent access of noxious acid, pepsin, and bile salts. Although a cytoprotective mechanism was once suggested for sucralfate, this is no longer thought to be the case. More recent studies with synthetic prostaglandins have shown that the concept of "cytoprotectin," does not explain a response to therapy because doses of prostaglandins that are only cytoprotective were not effective in either healing ulcers or preventing their recurrence. The dosage of sucralfate is 1 gm qid, and it is as effective as H_2-receptor antagonists in accelerating healing of benign gastric ulcers.[19, 20]

General Measures

We advise patients who smoke to quit. Neither hospitalization nor bed rest is advised as specific therapy because neither accelerates ulcer healing. We do not prescribe a specific diet but advise the patient to avoid foods they have discovered will exacerbate their distress. Patients are also cautioned to avoid bedtime snacks because this will increase the acid secretion during the night.

What to Expect

Most patients obtain symptomatic relief within a few days of starting therapy (despite the persistence of the ulcer crater).

Gastric ulcers, on average, are larger than duodenal ulcers and thus require more time to heal. There is no apparent correlation between the status of ulcer healing and the presence of dyspepsia[21]; thus, an objective test must be done to ensure that ulcer healing has occurred. We use endoscopy to follow our patients. Follow-up endoscopy should be done at a markedly reduced charge, and the first follow-up for the uncomplicated ulcer is scheduled after 8 weeks of therapy. By this time approximately 85% of gastric ulcers will have healed.[14] The rate of healing of ulcers is a function of the initial size of the ulcer, and, thus, large ulcers may take longer. Ulcers in the elderly patient may also heal at a slower rate.[22, 23] If after 8 weeks of therapy, the ulcer is healing but is not yet fully healed, a third examination should be scheduled after an additional 8 weeks of treatment (Fig 8–2).

Surgery is recommended for patients whose ulcers remain unhealed after 16 weeks of adequate treatment. Surgical intervention should also be considered earlier in those that show no change in ulcer size after 8 weeks of treatment.

RECURRENCE OF GASTRIC ULCERS

The natural history of gastric ulcers is similar to that of duodenal ulcers (i.e., they heal and then recur). Rates of relapse within 1 year of healing as high as 70% have been recorded,[24] and a large proportion of gastric ulcer recurrences are asymptomatic.[21] The recurrent ulcer usually occurs near the site of the original ulcer. The most important fact predictive of early ulcer recurrence is slow healing of the index ulcer. The state of healing attained by the index ulcer may also be important (i.e., less frequent recurrence was noted when the state of "white scar" was attained compared to when healing only achieved "red scarring").[25] There does not seem to be a good correlation between ulcer size or location and the likelihood of recurrence.[26]

Prevention of Ulcer Recurrence

The rate of ulcer recurrence can be reduced by providing continued therapy with H_2-receptor antagonists or sucralfate.[2-29] Maintenance (preventive) therapy with H_2-receptor antagonists implies daily therapy at a lower dose than used to accelerate healing (e.g., 400 mg cimetidine, 150 mg ranitidine, or 20 mg of famotidine each taken in the evening). The maintenance dose of sucralfate is unclear; 1 gm qid may be required although 1 gm bid may also be effective. The problems with maintenance therapy include cost, the possibility of side-effects from the medications, drug interaction wtih other medications,[9] and the generally low symptomatic recurrence rate (most that receive maintenance therapy don't need it). We reserve maintenance therapy for those patients who have "slow-to-heal" ulcers, and those who have experienced a major complication such as bleeding but who are not surgical candidates. Patients with gastric ulcer who require continued nonsteroidal anti-inflammatory drug therapy may also be good candidates for maintenance therapy.

SPECIAL PROBLEMS

Benign giant gastric ulcers are arbitrarily defined as gastric ulcers with a diameter greater than 3 cm; 2% to 3% of gastric

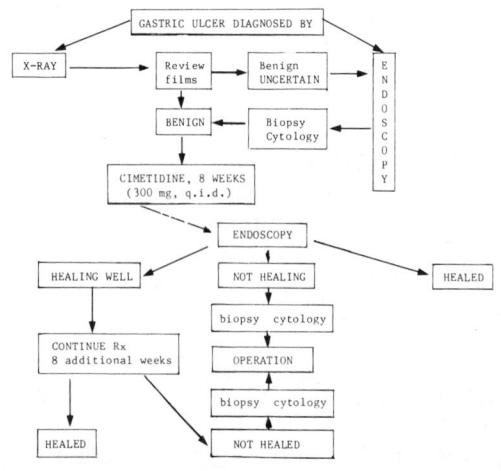

FIG 8–2.
Flow diaphragm for the evaluation and treatment of a patient with gastric ulcer.

ulcers qualify as giant ulcers. In the past, many physicians were inclined to treat giant gastric ulcers surgically based on (1) the anticipated, although unsubstantiated, high frequency of complication; (2) a belief that they are more likely to recur; and (3) a supposedly very high frequency of gastric cancer. None of these suppositions has been confirmed, and we believe that a reasonable attempt at medical therapy should precede surgical consideration of giant gastric ulcers. As noted earlier, 16 weeks of therapy may be needed for complete healing of these large ulcers.

Occasionally biopsies obtained from a benign gastric ulcer reveal the presence of hyphae of *Candida*. This is of no clinical significance. The addition of antifungal therapy will neither accelerate the rate of healing of these ulcers nor reduce the rate of recurrence.[30]

Gastric ulcers are very frequent in rheumatic patients taking aspirin and the other NSAID. Although the association has been most convincingly demonstrated with regular use of large doses of aspirin,[31] it appears that all NSAID agents can be responsible for gastric ulcers and that there is no major difference between them. We found a 10.7% point prevalence of gastric ulcers among arthritic patients receiving NSAID.[4] Endoscopically, NSAID-induced ulcers appear no different from any other chronic gastric ulcer, although often other changes of drug injury are evident (i.e., multiple small erosions and mucosal hemorrhages). NSAID-induced ulcers are usually silent unless a complication such as bleeding or perforation occurs. The NSAID-associated ulcer responds well to the standard therapy for gastric ulcer, and good results are to be expected even if the NSAID is continued. If possible, the NSAID should be discontinued. It is usually not possible to discontinue NSAID therapy in rheumatic patients; for those patients we recommend a change to another form or different NSAID. For example, if the patient is taking aspirin, an enteric-coated aspirin preparation or a different NSAID can be substituted. There is no evidence that there is any difference among NSAID in their propensity to cause ulcer. Thus, the notion that changing to a different NSAID might be helpful is based on the untested hypothesis that individual patients vary in their susceptibility to ulcer formation with different NSAID. Patients who do not need NSAID (both aspirin and the newer NSAID) should be advised to avoid them and use acetaminophen for pain relief, not only during the healing of the ulcer but "forever."

References

1. Akdamar K, Ertan A, Agrawal NM, et al: Upper gastrointestinal endoscopy in normal asymptomatic volunteers. *Gastrointest Endosc* 1986; 32:78–80.
2. Ihamaki T, Varis K, Siurala M: Morphological, functional and immunological state of the gastric mucosa in gastric carcinoma families: Comparison with a computer-matched family sample. *Scand J Gastroenterol* 1979; 14:801–812.
3. Lanza FL, Davis RE: Asymptomatic ulcers and erosions occur in normal volunteer populations. *Am J Gastroenterol* 1984; 79:820.
4. Larkai EN, Smith JL, Lidsky MD, et al: Gastroduodenal mucosa and dyspeptic symptoms in arthritic patients during chronic nonsteroidal anti-inflammatory drug use. *Am J Gastroenterol*, 1987; 82:1153–1158.
5. Graham DY, Schwartz JT, Cain GD, et al: Prospective evaluation of biopsy number in the diagnosis of esophageal and gastric carcinoma. *Gastroenterology* 1982; 82:228–231.
6. Hatfield ARW, Slavin G, Segal AW, et al: Importance of the site of endoscopic gastric biopsy in ulcerating lesions of the stomach. *Gut* 1975; 16:884–886.
7. Gugler R: Current diagnosis and selection of patients for treatment of peptic ulcer disease. *Dig Dis Sci* 1985; 30(suppl):30–35.
8. Isenberg JI, Peterson WL, Elashoff JD, et al: Healing of benign gastric ulcer with low-dose antacid or cimetidine: A double-blind, randomized, placebo-controlled trial. *N Engl J Med* 1983; 308:1319–1324.
9. Taylor RH, Menzies-Gow N, Lovell D, et al: Misleading response of malignant gastric ulcers to cimetidine. *Lancet* 1978; 1:686–688.
10. Sakita T, Oguro Y, Takasu S, et al: Observations on the healing of ulcerations in early gastric cancer. *Gastroenterology* 1971; 60:835–844.
11. Tedesco FJ, Griffin JW, Crisp WI, et al: "Skinny" upper gastrointestinal endoscopy—The initial diagnostic tool: A prospective comparison of upper gastrointestinal endoscopy and radiology. *J Clin Gastroenterol* 1980; 2:27–30.
12. Martin TR, Vennes JA, Silvis SE, et al: A comparison of upper gastrointestinal endoscopy and radiography. *J Clin Gastroenterol* 1980; 2:21–25.
13. Freston JW: Cimetidine in the treatment of gastric ulcer. *Gastroenterology* 1978; 74:426–430.
14. Graham DY, Akdamar K, Dyck WP, et al: Healing of benign gastric ulcer: Comparison of cime-

tidine and placebo in the United States. *Ann Intern Med* 1985; 102:573–576.
15. Hirschowitz BI, DeLuca V, Graham D, et al: Treatment of benign chronic gastric ulcer with ranitidine: A randomized, double-blind, and placebo-controlled six week trial. *J Clin Gastroenterol* 1986; 8:371–376.
16. Dammann HG, Walter TA, Hentschel E, et al: Famotidine: Nocturnal administration for gastric ulcer healing: Results of multicenter trials in Austria and Germany. *Digestion* 1985; 32(suppl):45–50.
17. Farley A, Levesque D, Pare P, et al: A comparative trial of ranitidine 300 mg at night with ranitidine 150 mg twice daily in the treatment of duodenal and gastric ulcer. *Am J Gastroenterol* 1985; 80:665–668.
18. Ryan FP, Jorde R, Ehsanullah RSB, et al: A single night time dose of ranitidine in the acute treatment of gastric ulcer: A European multicentre trial. *Gut* 1986; 27:784–788.
19. Marks IN, Lucke W, Wright JP, et al: Ulcer healing and relapse rates after initial treatment with cimetidine or sucralfate. *J Clin Gastroenterol* 1981; 3(suppl):163–165.
20. Martin F, Farley A, Gagnon M, et al: Short-term treatment with sucralfate or cimetidine in gastric ulcer: Preliminary results of a controlled randomized trial. *Scand J Gastroenterol* 1983; 18(suppl):37–41.
21. Jorde R, Bostad L, Burhol PG: Asymptomatic gastric ulcer: A follow-up study in patients with previous gastric ulcer disease. *Lancet* 1986; 1:119–121.
22. Okada M, Yao T, Fuchigami T, et al: Factors influencing the healing rate of gastric ulcer in hospitalized subjects. *Gut* 1984; 25:881–885.
23. Piper DW, Hunt J, Heap TR: The healing rate of chronic gastric ulcer in patients admitted to hospital. *Scand J Gastroenterol* 1980; 15:113–117.
24. Alstead EM, Ryan FP, Holdsworth CD, et al: Ranitidine in the prevention of gastric and duodenal ulcer relapse. *Gut* 1983; 24:418–420.
25 Miyake T, Ariyoshi J, Suzaki T, et al: Endoscopic evaluation of the effect of sucralfate therapy and other clinical parameters on the recurrence rate of gastric ulcers. *Dig Dis Sci* 1980; 25:1–7.
26. Hanscom DH, Buchman E: The follow-up period. *Gastroenterology* 1971; 61:585–597.
27. Marks IN, Wright JP, Girdwood AH, et al: Maintenance therapy with sucralfate reduces rate of gastric ulcer recurrence. *Am J Med* 1985; 79(suppl):32–35.
28. Jensen KB, Mollmann KM, Rahbek I, et al: Prophylactic effect of cimetidine in gastric ulcer patients. *Scand J Gastroenterol* 1979; 14:175–176.
29. Robinson M: Review of peptic ulcer maintenance trials. *Am J Med* 1984; 77(suppl):23–29.
30. Gotlieb-Jensen K, Andersen J: Occurrence of candida in gastric ulcers: Significance for the healing process. *Gastroenterology* 1983; 85:535–537.
31. Graham DY, Smith JL: Aspirin and the stomach. *Ann Intern Med* 1986; 104:390–398.

9

Duodenal Ulcer:
Is there a role for chronic prophylactic therapy?

DENIS M. MCCARTHY, M.D., M.Sc., F.A.C.P.

Duodenal ulcer is a term embodying two separate concepts: the "ulcer," a local defect in the mucosal surface of the duodenum, deep enough to reach or penetrate the muscularis mucosa; and "duodenal ulcer disease," the condition that leads to mucosal injury, pain, and ulceration. This problem has been discussed at length by Sprio,[1] who has pointed out the difficulties that arise when we build our concepts of duodenal ulcer around the crater as the cause of the problem, rather than trying to visualize the crater as a consequence of the disease—a chronic disturbance of gastroduodenal function, lasting throughout most of a patient's life, characterized by periodic pain and dyspepsia of variable severity, and interspersed with symptom-free periods.

Endoscopy has revealed that at times the periodic pain is accompanied by the presence of an ulcer and at times not, but that there is no predicatable relationship between the presence of an ulcer and the presence of pain. Certain risks of the disease (e.g., hemorrhage, perforation, penetration, or scarring) relate directly to the presence of an ulcer crater and do not occur in its absence. However, from the patient's point of view, overall management of the disease centers around the relief of pain and the restoration of a normal, risk-free life-style. Any strategy for managing duodenal ulcer disease must, on the one hand, include healing of ulcers and abolishing the risks that attend their presence, and on the other hand, dealing with their long-term impact on the patient's life, including the relief of pain, the avoidance or proper selection of surgical treatment, the lessening of the socioeconomic impact of the disease, and the avoidance of adverse consequences of treatment. Achievement of these objectives demands considerable knowledge of the natural history of the disease, more than we possess at the present time.

NATURAL HISTORY

Although modern studies have yielded much information helpful to formulating long-term policies, the data apply only to selected populations of duodenal ulcer patients. Some have more severe disease than average, necessitating their referral to academic centers where trials are performed; in others the opposite applies, that is entry criteria have excluded from the trials many of the more difficult kinds of patients seen in practice (e.g., those with very large, multiple, or complicated ulcers, those continuing to take aspirin and other anti-inflammatory drugs, those over age 60 to 65 years, or those with serious concurrent disease). A third problem is that clinical trials select from the ulcer disease population only those patients who have a crater present at the time of endoscopy. Various estimates suggest that this group constitutes only a minority

(3%–20%) of those with chronic duodenal ulcer disease.[2-4] Nevertheless, some valuable conclusions can be drawn and applied to the development of strategies for long-term management of duodenal ulcer.

Duodenal ulcer disease, a disease of this century, has from the outset been recognized by experienced physicians as a chronic disorder. In Moynihan's classic description,[5] he wrote: "It is not uncommon for a man, in answer to the question as to how long he has suffered, to reply 'all my life'." From an exhaustive contemporary review of the nature of ulcer disease,[6] certain generalizations can be made. Despite healing, almost all ulcers recur, although the frequency with which they do so, the severity of symptoms, the risk of complications, the response to treatment, and the ease with which their recurrence can be prevented, all vary markedly from person to person. In careful studies[6-9] the tendency to recurrence persists into late life, and the disease shows no tendency to "burn out" before age 75, with about 80% of patients ultimately having disease classified as "serious," if followed for long enough.[9] When first seen, over 50% of patients have had symptoms for at least 2 years. In the past decade, analysis of patients admitted to clinical trials of H_2-antagonist drugs showed that only one in ten duodenal ulcer patients was admitted for treatment of a first symptomatic episode[10]; most were recurrences.

Recurrences are thus an integral part of the disease itself and are not to be seen as failures of any particular kind of therapy. At present the cause of the disease is unknown and it cannot be cured, although a variety of medical and surgical interventions can alter its course (i.e., reduce symptoms, the frequency and severity of recurrence, the incidence of complications, the mortality and morbidity, and the socioeconomic impact of the disease). Despite a decade in which great advances have been made in our ability to employ new diagnostic modalities, new drugs, and new surgical operations to heal ulcer craters, our current view of duodenal ulcer disease is not unlike that advanced by Moynihan in 1910.[5] However, this view now rests on a much firmer foundation of data gleaned from large, well designed, blind, clinical trials, using prospective endoscopy as the "gold standard" for healing and recurrence of the ulcer crater. Despite differences among trials and observers as to what constitutes an "ulcer" at endoscopy, and what constitutes "healing," these studies have lent strong support to the notion of "once an ulcer, always an ulcer," and have shifted the focus of attention from the immediate to the long-term management problem (i.e., the prevention and treatment of the chronic disease).

INITIAL THERAPY

From a large body of information it can be reasonably stated that many forms of therapy effectively heal most ulcers and do so all at about the same rate. Thus, cimetidine, ranitidine, famotidine, and nizatidine—all H_2-receptor antagonists, antacids, antimuscarinic anticholinergic drugs (e.g., pirenzepine), various tricyclic antidepressants, antisecretory doses of several prostaglandin derivatives, and other mucosal protective agents such as sucralfate, colloidal bismuth, and various derivatives of licorice, all lead to healing of about 70% to 75%, 85% to 90%, and 95% of duodenal ulcers, with courses of therapy lasting 4, 8, and 12 weeks, respectively. With any of these drugs about 5% to 15% of ulcers fail to heal with 12 weeks of full-dose therapy and are deemed "refractory" or "resistant." Most of these latter can be healed by (1) doubling the dose of drug (e.g., cimetidine 800 mg hs increased to cimetidine 800 mg bid), or (2) by switching to another class of drug (e.g., from therapy with an H_2-antagonist to therapy with a mucosal protective agent—colloidal bismuth or sucralfate), or (3) by adding a nighttime dose of an anticholinergic drug (e.g., 10–20 mg isopropamide, to the regular nighttime dose of H_2-antagonist such as cimetidine 800 mg, ranitidine 300 mg, or famotidine 40 mg). Most refractory ulcers are encountered in males who are heavy smokers and/or who have high basal/nocturnal acid secretion. Refractory ulcers do not constitute a major problem in clinical practice.

The only drug to date which has achieved faster rates of ulcer healing is an experimental drug, the proton-pump inhibitor omeprazole, but only when given in doses of 60 mg/day or more. At this dose 100% of duodenal ulcers healed in 2 weeks.[11] However, because drug treatment is followed by rapid recurrence of ulcers, it is not clear that more rapid healing constitutes an advantage. When omeprazole is given in a dose of 20 mg/day or less, the dose now in most U.S. clinical trials of duodenal ulcer, healing occurs at about the same rate as that seen with the other drugs listed above. So far, ulcers "refractory" to omeprazole have not been reported.[12]

From the widespread availability of many drugs that heal most ulcers very effectively with 8 to 12 weeks of therapy, one might reasonably assume that duodenal ulcer should be disappearing rapidly. Unfortunately this is not the case. In most patients the initial course of therapy has healed the crater, but not eliminated or cured the underlying predisposition to relapse once full-dose therapy has ceased. In most studies, irrespective of the drug used to heal the ulcer, after therapy is discontinued most craters are seen to recur within 2 years when prospective endoscopic follow-up is performed whether or not the patient has symptoms. Only about half of the recurrences are symptomatic.[2, 6, 13, 14] In earlier studies of the natural history of ulcer disease,[9] only symptomatic recurrences were detected; consequently about 50% lower recurrence rates were reported.[6, 9] In some subgroups of patients (e.g., smokers), the rate of recurrence following medical therapy may be much more rapid. For example, in patients smoking more than 30 cigarettes per day, 100% had recurrences within 3 months of stopping drug therapy.[15] Until recently, prospective endoscopic studies have never been used to evaluate the total risk of ulcer recurrence (i.e., silent plus symptomatic) following surgical procedures, or the effect of smoking on this risk. But neither has it been shown that altering life-style (e.g., stopping smoking, changing diet, avoiding aspirin, reducing stress) reduces the risk of ulcer recurrence, following either medial or surgical therapy.

SYMPTOM–ULCER CRATER DISPARITY

In addition to the discovery that symptomless peptic ulcers were common, we have also learned that the presence of symptoms and the presence of ulcers are not clearly related. While there is a general tendency for healing of the crater to be accompanied by disappearance of or reduction in the patient's symptoms, the rate of relief of symptoms and the rate of healing are poorly correlated. Symptom relief is generally obtained in 1 to 2 weeks, but ulcer healing is much slower, taking 1 to 2 months in most cases. Analysis of the results of clinical trials indicates that while some patients with unhealed ulcers continue to have symptoms, most unhealed ulcers are asymptomatic, and furthermore most patients with persistent symptoms have healed ulcers.[16–18] For these reasons we are forced to conclude that relief of symptoms cannot be used as evidence that a crater has healed, nor can it serve as a basis for determining the required duration of treatment.[19, 20] In the same way we are frequently obliged to recognize that symptoms may be present at times when the crater is absent; the absence of a crater should not lead the doctor to withhold treatment with antiulcer drugs known to relieve the patient's pain when the ulcer crater is present.

DUODENITIS AND NONULCER DYSPEPSIA

Related to this issue, there is a growing realization that many people with classic ulcer symptoms do not have ulcer craters on endoscopy when first seen. Most of these "nonulcer dyspepsia" patients, with classic ulcer symptoms and relief by milk, antacids, and H_2-antagonists ("Moynihan's disease"), have duodenitis on endoscopy. Duodenitis has been closely linked to the risk of ulceration and recurrence, and it has been suggested that ulcer healing be redefined to include resolution of duodenitis as well as disappearance of the crater.[21] In an important long-term study of 219 patients with chronic erosive duodenitis,[22] Sircus has shown that while ulcer craters tend to occur seasonally, duodenitis is present uniformly throughout the year. He has also shown that during follow-up of patients with duodenitis, over 80% developed ulcer craters within 3 to 36 months. Such patients should not be confused with another subgroup of nonulcer dyspepsia patients, those with "flatulent dyspepsia," who generally do not have periodic pain or symptom relief from anatacids or H_2-anatagonists, in whom "gaseous distension" and "early satiety" are prominent, and who generally respond to prokinetic drugs (e.g., bethanecol or metoclopramide). What contribution, if any, chronic antral (type B) gastritis due to *Campylobacter pylori* infection (see below) makes to causing duodenal ulcer or flatulent dyspepsia cannot be assessed at the time of writing.[23]

From all of these considerations the conclusions that emerge are that duodenal ulcer disease is chronic, that ulcer craters are present only intermittently although related duodenitis may be present for longer periods, that only a minority of those with the long-term disease have ulcer craters at any particular time, that the presence of the ulcer does not correlate with symptoms or vice versa, and that when large populations are studied by radiographic screening,[24] endoscopy,[6] or autopsy,[25] about 50% of ulcer craters are found in asymptomatic subjects. The true prevalance of duodenal ulcer disease is underestimated considerably by studies requiring the presence of a crater on initial endoscopy. Many of these patients, with the "Moynihan's disease" variant of nonulcer dyspepsia, will probably turn out in time to have duodenal ulcer disease.

MAINTENANCE THERAPY

The most important recent change in our perspective of the disease derives from our renewed awareness of the high frequency of recurrences—60% to 100% during 2 years of follow-up. This has to be balanced against the fact that about half of the recurrences are symptomless and would not be detected clinically unless a complication developed. Initiation of maintenance therapy (following verified complete healing of the ulcer) with cimetidine 400 mg hs, ranitidine 150 mg hs, or famotidine 20 mg hs, lowers the recurrence rate considerably. Based on an analysis of 23 controlled trials the average duodenal ulcer relapse rate at 1 year was 27% for cimetidine and 25% for ranitidine. Based on much smaller numbers, the relapse rate on maintenance therapy with famotidine was 23.4%.[26] These rates are not significantly different from each other or from the relapse rates seen with maintenance sucralfate 1 gm bid. The average relapse rate on placebo for all these studies was 70% at 1 year. These figures include both symptomatic and asymptomatic recurrences.

In an excellent 2-year study of maintenance therapy, Bardhan[14] showed that when patients relapsed while on maintenance therapy, about half the relapses were silent and half were symptomatic. Among both silent and symptomatic patients, about half of the relapses were characterized by ulcers with or without erosions, and about half by erosions alone. People with ulcer craters were equally likely to have silent or symptomatic ulcers, but those with erosions alone were four times more likely to have silent disease. In the same population, cumulative symptomatic relapse rates at 1 and 2 years were 73% and 82%, respectively, in placebo patients, compared to cumulative rates of 22% and 32% in cimetidine-treated patients. Silent relapses were uncommon (11%, 12%) with most being symptomatic in the placebo group, but were as common as symptomatic relapses (50%) in the maintenance group. Most of those who relapsed did so within the first 6 to 12 months of therapy. No patient on maintenance therapy developed a complication at any time. The study also showed that relapses on maintenance therapy healed readily with full-dose therapy, following which a second course of maintenance therapy was likely to be as effective as the first. A single uncomplicated relapse was not necessarily an indication for abandoning maintenance treatment. Overall the treatment appeared to prevent relapse for as long as treatment continued.

Recent studies have shown that asymptomatic ulcer relapses during maintenance therapy did not usually reheal rapidly but persisted as active ulcers for at least 6 or 9 months,[27, 28] unless the maintenance dose of ranitidine was doubled.[29] Another study showed that those with active prepyloric ulcers and a history of chronic ulcer disease, or those who required more than 6 weeks to heal initially, required maintenance doses of cimetidine 800 mg hs to maintain healing.[3] These data suggest that about one patient in five may require higher maintenance doses. With regular maintenance therapy prolonged for up to 4 years of treatment with cimetidine 400 mg hs, there was a tendency for fewer first recurrences in the second, third and fourth years.[31–33] Ulcers that did not relapse in the first year usually remained healed for as long as treatment continued. However, since there was a gradual elimination of the worst cases (rapid relapses) from these studies, it is likely that the individual tendency to relapse was relatively unchanged over time in most subjects. It is premature to conclude that "the natural history of the ulcer disease has been altered" for the individual patient, unless by this one means that the individual's risk of recurrence has been deferred for the duration of maintenance therapy. About 10% of ulcers do not appear to recur on prolonged follow-up. Repeated relapses on higher dose maintenance therapy should generally lead to surgery, but alone should not be used to justify surgery more radical than parietal cell vagotomy, the operation of choice in intractable cases.

Not all subjects are equally likely to relapse. During maintenance therapy with cimetidine in 261 patients, Bardhan[14] found that among the minority of patients initially refractory to therapy (not healed in 3 months) the number of relapses on maintenance, the speed at which they occurred, and the likelihood that the relapse would be symptomatic, were all about twice as high as in nonrefractory patients. Other clinical features associated with increased ulcer relapse rates are smoking,[15] a long ulcer history,[16, 34] incomplete ulcer healing,[35] a slow initial response to therapy,[14, 30] and juxtapyloric location of the ulcer.[30] While the presence of one or more of these factors may be used to support a case for maintenance therapy in an individual patient, their predictive value or their overall impact are not yet sufficiently well defined to warrant their use in the formulation of general policies. Unsettled at the present time are two additional factors which may affect the rate of recurrence of ulcer, namely the presence of chronic persistent antral (type B) gastritis due to *C. pylori* infection, and the specific drug initially used to heal the ulcer.

CAMPYLOBACTER PYLORI

In recent years increasing attention has been focused on gram-negative spiral bacteria attached to the gastric mucosa, now designated *Campylobacter pylori* (CP). Their presence can be detected in histologic sections stained with Warthin-Starry, Giemsa, Wright's, and other stains. Pioneering sudies by Marshall, who himself ingested the organism, defined the natural history (now confirmed by others[36]) of acute gastritis caused by CP. Since then there has been a worldwide plethora of reports linking the organism with disease, which may be summarized as follows. Ingestion of the organism is followed by abdominal pain, nausea, halitosis, a sensation of fullness, and irritability. By the fifth day antral biopsies show acute gastritis with normal fundic histology and acid secretion. By the eighth day fundic biopsies show acute gastritis, and achlorhydria develops with gastric pH > 7.0. Symptoms subside at 11 to 14 days and with the development of immunity some recovery occurs. Acid secretion recovers slowly over 3 to 12 months. CP has fulfilled Koch's postulates as a cause of gastritis. In some untreated cases (estimated 50%), the condition appears to progress to classic chronic active type B gastritis, to persist for long periods particularly in antral mucosa, to be very difficult to eradicate completely, and to predispose patients to various other GI disorders, which include duodenal ulcer, gastric ulcer, symptomatic chronic gastritis, and/or the nonulcer dyspepsia syndrome.[23]

These conditions are all known to be associated with type B gastritis, and most cases are associated with the presence of CP in antral biopsies. Recovery of the organism from a duodenal ulcer crater is rare and may be associated with ectopic or metaplastic gastric epithelium at the site. From a variety of studies, CP seems to be found in antral biopsies in more than 90% of duodenal ulcer patients.[23, 37] While many drugs are active against CP in vitro, true eradication has been difficult in vivo, often requiring 4 to 6 weeks of treatment with furazolidone,[38] bismuth subsalicylate,[39] a combination of bismuth subcitrate and tinidazole, or of bismuth subsalicylate (Peptobismol) 1.q.i.d and amoxicillin 250 mg every eight hours.[40, 41] The bismuth drugs are of special interest in that they are highly effective agents in the healing of duodenal ulcer, heal the associated gastritis in about 60% of cases, reduce CP positivity of antral biopsies, and appear in some studies to be followed by a lower rate of duodenal ulcer recurrence than that which attends therapy with H_2-antagonists or antacids.[42] This lowering of recurrence rate may not be due to eradication of CP, but may relate to other antiulcer properties of the drugs. H_2-antagonists are devoid of activity against CP in vitro, and in most clinical trials healing of duodenal ulcer or gastric ulcer with H_2-antagonists in CP-positive cases is not accompanied by eradication of the organism, healing of gastritis, or reduction in the risk of recurrence. Peptic ulcers in CP-negative cases seem mostly related to other defined risk factors (e.g., heavy smoking, NSAID use, Zollinger-Ellison syndrome). Thus CP is very commonly associated with antral gastritis in patients with duodenal ulcer, but its precise role in pathogenesis of duodenal ulcer remains to be established. It may cause the disease in some patients, but seems unlikely to be the sole cause. It could also interact with other common etiologic factors (e.g., smoking, NSAID use) to produce ulcers.

INITIAL DRUG THERAPY AND RECURRENCE

When all recurrences (symptomatic and silent) are included it appears that duodenal ulcer recurs within a year in 80% to 90% of patients treated initially with H_2-antagonists. Some evidence now exists that relapse rates may be lower after treatment with other ulcer-healing drugs.[3, 4] The strongest body of information pertains to six comparative studies that showed that ulcer recurrence rates following healing with tripotassium dicitratobismuthate (Denol) were significantly lower than those following healing with H_2-antagonists. Combining all the data, 85% of patients relapsed in 1 year following H_2-antagonists compared to 59% (range 43%–62%) following Denol.[4] Other reputable studies have failed to find such differences (see Reference 3, Table 1). However, independent analyses of the positive results by two separate centers[3, 4] suggest that healing with cimetidine is followed by a fractional recurrence rate of 17% per month, compared to 7% per month recurrence rate following Denol.[4] One study showed that the recurrence rate following Denol therapy was as low as the recurrence rate on maintenance therapy with cimetidine.[3] However, the data are not strong, are even weaker when H_2-antagonists are compared to other mucosal protective agents such as sucralfate and antacids,[3] and are liable to suffer from sampling errors due to small numbers of cases. Furthermore, the data in these trials are in conflict with rates calculated elsewhere. For instance, data on

772 patients from noncomparative trials, in 22 different centers, showed that the recurrence rates following cimetidine healing were remarkably constant at 8.5%/month in those off the drug, and 2.5%/month in those who continued on maintenance therapy.[43,44] If the 8.5%/month rate is correct, the difference from the Denol rate (7%/month) is not significant. The strongest case for the existence of differences in the relapse rates derives from the fact that when a significant difference in relapse rates exists between an H_2-antagonist and another drug not dependent for its action on acid-secretory inhibition, it is consistently in favor of the latter drug.[3] Adequate follow-up data on the Denol-treated patients are lacking, and how long the benefit (if any) persists is currently unknown.

Differences in relapse rates off drug are not important if maintenance therapy is being universally employed, a course advocated by many experts.[29,44] They feel that because a recurrence may present with a lethal complication, prevention of relapse is the only rational goal of therapy. However, if intermittent courses of therapy at the time of relapse are employed as advocated by others, differences in relapse rates could have a significant effect on the number of duodenal ulcer patients requiring therapy at any time.[3,4,45] Calculations suggest that with intermittent therapy at least twice as many subjects would be using cimetidine or ranitidine as would require DENOL or possibly sucralfate, at any one time.[3,4] Preliminary data indicate that bismuth subsalicylate (Pepto-Bismol) is also effective in duodenal ulcer healing,[39] and that therapy with it is followed by a low relapse rate. Advocates of the theory that C. pylori causes peptic ulcers believe that recurrent infections cause ulcer recurrences, while eradication of the organism at least temporarily allows ulcer healing. They propose that the alleged superior efficacy of the bismuth drugs derives from their activities against C. pylori. However, these drugs have many properties; other possible mechanisms of action or of maintaining action have not be tested. At the present time these issues are unsettled. Bismuth-containing antiulcer drugs are not yet marked for such use in the United States.

CHOICE OF STRATEGIES

Given the many uncertainties that surround long-term therapy with antacids, anticholinergics, antidepressants, sucralfate, and a host of experimental drugs not yet available to U.S. physicians, this section will deal principally with the long-term use of H_2-antagonists, which dominate practice.

Because of the high probability of relapse, but a 50% chance that the relapse will be asymptomatic, some additional questions need to be examined before dealing with the choice of treatment strategy. First, what percentage of the ulcer population have frequent symptomatic relapses, and second, what are the consequences of relapse, symptomatic or silent? On the other side of the coin, we must assess the benefit to the patient of preventing all relapses, what this would cost, and to what extent would benefits be offset by iatrogenic consequences of therapy. We will then examine intermittent therapy, the alternative to maintenance therapy, and try to define patient subgroups who clearly need maintenance therapy.

Frequency of Relapse

Two studies have prospectively examined the number of symptomatic relapses that required therapy each year.[46,47] In the first study from the United Kingdom during 1 year of follow-up 36% had no symptomatic attack, 37% had one, 20% had two attacks, and 7% had three or more major attacks. In the second study from Australia, 25% had no attack, 29% had one, 29% two, and 17% had three or more attacks. Therefore, over 80% of subjects in both studies had zero to two attacks/year. However, as pointed out by Walan and colleagues,[48] frequency of attacks may be less important than their severity when evaluating maintenance therapy; this issue has not been formally examined. In the two studies quoted, subjects were treated either with intermittent 6-week courses of cimetidine[47] or Cimetidine 1 gm/day to healing.[46] This achieved satisfactory control with intermittent therapy in 50% of patients, compared to control of about 75% with maintenance therapy. However, no way of predicting an individual's prognosis could be found, nor could "failures" be identified in advance of therapy. In a third study,[49] where less adequate therapy (4 weeks) was employed, 19 of 65 patients (29%) had three or more relapses per year.

In deciding between intermittent therapy that allows relapse before treatment and prophylactic maintenance therapy that aims at preventing relapses, it is important to assess how much hazard the patient faces from a relapse. Looking at the total life-time risk from duodenal ulcer disease, the risk of death is about 2%, of perforation 5% to 15%, of pyloric stenosis 10% to 20%, and of clinically significant hemorrhage 36% to 39%.[6] Thus far, maintenance therapy has not been shown to influence mortality or perforation, as these occurred infrequently in both treated and untreated groups. Maintenance therapy may be associated with a slight increase in the development of pyloric stenosis,[50,51] but this is not established. However, in the case of hemorrhage, during 1 year of follow-up ulcer recurrence was accompanied by bleeding in 0% to 2% of those in maintenance therapy, as compared with 10% to 30% with bleeding in untreated groups. Among untreated patients 3.5% (range 0%–13%) presented with hemorrhage and were otherwise asymptomatic. It is believed that "silent ulcers" account for up to 25% of bleeding ulcers, but it is not known whether they mainly represent new acute ulcers or the recurrences of chronic duodenal ulcer disease. Presentation of silent ulcers with a complication occurs in 2% of those on maintenance therapy, in 10% to 20% of those off therapy,[6] and in almost 60% of those off ulcer therapy but on NSAID.[52,53] Of those who present with bleeding, at least 30% will bleed again during 5 years, 48% during 10 years, and 86% during 30 years of follow-up.[6] For these reasons most authorities feel that intermittent therapy should not be used in those with a history of hemorrhage but that such patients should be offered maintenance therapy or surgery.[48] This is particularly important in those who must continue to use NSAID (see below).

Other potential hazards to patients arise from toxic and side-effects of drugs. Because many of the side-effects of H_2-antagonists are dose-related, as expected side-effects during low-dose maintenance therapy are less than those seen at high dosage; overall limiting side-effects were 2.1% for cimetidine and 1.7% for placebo-treated patients.[54] Long-term studies of cimetidine use have shown over a 4-year period a progressive fall in the incidence of all side-effects attributable to the drug.[33] The incidence of all alleged side-effects fell from 8% in the first year to 4% in the second and third years and 1% in the fourth year. The incidence of serious or life-threatening side-effects was negligible.[31-33] While ranitidine has been in use for a shorter time, its safety record to date is excellent, and there is no reason to suppose that it will prove less safe than cimetidine with prolonged use. In choosing between different therapeutic strategies, dangers or side-effects attending the use of either drug long-term in maintenance doses can be dismissed. Famotidine appears similar but has not yet been adequately evaluated.

Costs of Disease

Diseases give rise to both direct and indirect costs. The direct costs of preventing, diagnosing, and treating the disease are constantly analyzed from different perspectives, depending on who has to pay them (i.e., the patient, the third-party provider, the profit-oriented corporation, or the local or federal health authorities). Largely ignored are the indirect costs—loss of productivity and income due to sick-leave, long-term disability, and premature death. Various estimates suggest that in the Scandinavian countries direct costs amount to between 22% and 30% of the total costs.[48] Drug therapy, including maintenance therapy, in Scandinavian countries accounts for about 2% to 3% of total and 8% to 14% of direct costs. In the United States direct costs are 46% of total costs, and drugs (based on intermittent therapy) account for 3.9% of total and 8.4% of direct costs (see Table 9–1). In either type of society the cost of the drugs used in treating and preventing the disease is only a small fraction of the total costs.

If the state has to bear either the total costs or the direct costs of the disease, there is little doubt that long-term maintenance therapy for all patients is the most economical (Table 9–1) and the most effective way to provide care[44] (hence the enthusiasm for this in countries such as the United Kingdom). However, in the United States, the focus is much more on the costs to the individual, who wishes to spend the least possible amount to take care of his particular ulcer, regardless of statistics. One way or another in the United States the costs are borne by the patient in about 70% of cases, with for-profit organizations leading the drive to reduce costs if not charges. In this climate, maintenance therapy should probably be reserved for those who need it, or who can afford it and choose to have it.

Indications for Maintenance Therapy

The list of indications for maintenance therapy in Table 9–2 is by no means exhaustive and reflects the author's views at this time. Some would add other indications (e.g., heavy smoking or continuing abuse of alcohol). In my view the doctor's energy should first be directed toward changing the behavior that creates the risk. However, when behavior cannot be altered, maintenance therapy is probably preferable to surgery in such cases provided that compliance is satisfactory. In the same way, others would include refractory ulcer, defined variously as an ulcer taking longer than 6, 8, or 12 weeks to heal, and juxtapyloric ulcer, both known to have high rates of recurrence. I would prefer not to include these as invariable indications, but instead to select such patients on the basis of their proven risk of recurrence (see indication #3 in Table 9–2). Indication #8, "severe ulcer disease," is deliberately left vague to allow inclusion of patients in whom the frequency of relapse is not high enough to meet indication #3, but in whom relapses when they occur may be severe, as judged by intensity of pain or other symptoms, amount of time lost from work, loss of income; or may be hazard-

TABLE 9–1.
Estimated Annual U.S. Cost of Ulcer Disease (1978)*†

Estimated Annual Cost for Duodenal Ulcer (U.S.)		Projected Annual Savings through Cimetidine Therapy (U.S.)	
TOTAL COST =	$2.19 billion	TOTAL SAVINGS =	$644 million
Absenteeism	$455 million	Absenteeism	$148 million
Disability	476	Disability	181
Mortality	245	Mortality	44
Drug therapy	85	Drug therapy	−34
Physician charges	186	Physician charges	47
Hospital care	732	Hospital care	258
Miscellaneous	13	Miscellaneous	—

*From Robinson Associates Inc.: *The Impact of Cimetidine on the National Cost of Duodenal Ulcers*. Bryn Mawr, PA, 1978.
†Based on 1 year of intermittent therapy, corrected appropriately for predicted recurrences.

TABLE 9–2.
Indications for Maintenance Therapy* in Duodenal Ulcer

1. Age > 65
2. Previous complications, especially hemorrhage
3. Two recurrences in 6 months, or three in 1 year
4. Severe coexistent diseases (e.g., cardiac, renal, respiratory or hepatic failure)
5. Poor surgical risk
6. Recurrence after previous ulcer surgery
7. Known hypersecretor (BAO > 10 mM/hr, MAO > 60 mM/hr)
8. Severe ulcer disease
9. Patient's choice
10. Provider policy for population

*Maintenance therapy to continue indefinitely.

ous due to poor access to medical care (e.g., seafarers) or to dangerous occupations. Because maintenance therapy is clearly effective and safe, I see no reason to discourage patients from having it, if they choose to do so following informed consent and possess the means to pay for it.

Many others would add continuing use of NSAIDs as an indication. There is a growing body of evidence[52, 55, 56, 57] that NSAID use markedly increases the risk of complications and death in both duodenal and gastric ulcer patients. NSAIDs seem to exacerbate and complicate existing duodenal ulcer rather than cause it, especially in females and in those over 65 years of age. To date no data show that these hazards are abolished or reduced by low-dose maintenance therapy. Because of the high proportion of asymptomatic ulcers, and because asymptomatic ulcers are particularly common in NSAID users,[52, 53] I advocate giving such subjects 800 mg of cimetidine or 300 mg of ranitidine indefinitely, at which doses asymptomatic ulcers should be very uncommon and the risk of hemorrhage much reduced. Not all NSAID users merit this approach but in the absence of adequate data, those with a history of peptic ulcer disease, a previous complication such as hemorrhage or perforation, or gastric surgery; those who are over 65; or those who have persistent occult blood in their stool must be handled with considerable care. The advent of prostaglandin-derivative drugs, which can be taken prophylactically and may prevent the adverse effects of NSAIDs may soon offer some relief for this difficult problem.

Intermittent Therapy

Intermittent therapy can be attempted in over 80% of duodenal ulcer patients, as long as doctor and patient agree to accept the small risk that a recurrence will present with any of a number of complications, some of which will be serious and a small minority of which will be fatal. There have been no precise determinations, based on large prospective trials, of the magnitude of these risks. Nevertheless at present they seem acceptably low. The impact of asymptomatic recurrence relates to the risk that it will lead to a complication before detection. There are no prospective data available to indicate what percentage of complications present without any warning symptoms in patients on intermittent therapy. If this figure proves high it will be much harder to justify intermittent therapy as a safe option. Available data suggest that this risk is low.[14, 46–49] In the meantime intermittent therapy reduces the cost per patient, the number of patients requiring maintenance therapy, and possibly the risk of side-effects, although because dosage is higher with intermittent therapy, this latter point also needs prospective evaluation. Three variants of intermittent therapy have been proposed—"seasonal" therapy,[58] "on-demand" therapy,[44] and "symptomatic" therapy[59,60]—but at the present time the numbers treated in these ways are too small to allow evaluation of the strategies.

Implications

The average patient presenting for care with a symptomatic uncomplicated duodenal ulcer should be told to stop smoking and should be treated for 8 weeks; therapy should then be discontinued unless the patient belongs to one of the categories listed in Table 9–2. Those who are symptomatic at 8 weeks require detailed investigation. Those who are asymptomatic may be discharged and told to return if they develop symptoms or a complication. If the same symptoms recur they should be retreated without reinvestigation with full-dose therapy for 8 weeks, and therapy should be discontinued again. They should also be strongly readvised to stop smoking and put in formal contact with one of the many organizations or programs who offer help in this area. Failure to stop smoking is commonly associated with an adverse course of disease. In one study placebo patients who were nonsmokers did better than patients on maintenance cimetidine; the best results were seen in nonsmokers on maintenance therapy.[61]

If recurrences become frequent (two to three attacks in 1 year), maintenance therapy should be prescribed indefinitely. If one recurrence occurs during maintenance therapy, the patient should be retreated on full dose therapy for 8 weeks and returned to maintenance therapy. If there is a second recurrence on maintenance therapy, the dose should be increased to 800 mg cimetidine hs or 300 mg ranitidine hs, and continued long-term, provided that there are no side-effects.

If side-effects develop or there is further recurrence, surgery should be recommended. Before recommending surgery the physician should strongly advise patients to stop smoking; the benefits of this should be assessed for at least 6 months before proceeding to surgery. To recommend surgery for a patient who is reluctant to stop smoking constitutes poor medical advice, given the large number of health hazards associated with smoking, the increased risks of surgical mortality and morbidity in smokers, and the probability that smoking adversely affects the outcome of surgery. However, some will persist in smoking and demand an operation. For these and for the small percentage of patients, who for reasons of serious alcohol abuse, poor compliance, side-effects of drugs, or poor access to drugs and health care, surgery should be recommended early in the course of care. Many other factors concerning the decision for surgery are well reviewed elsewhere.[62,63] Postsurgical recurrences are now easily treated long-term with H_2-antagonists. For this reason the emphasis should be on choosing an operation with negligible mortality and morbidity such as parietal cell vagotomy.[61,62,63] For those with severe intractable disease a surgical solution is more cost-effective than 5 years or more of maintenance therapy, but costs vary greatly in different geographic regions. Maintenance therapy can be recommended with great confidence as safe and effective, for those who can afford it, but intermittent therapy appears to be a reasonable alternative in 80% of duodenal ulcer patients at this time.

References

1. Spiro HM: Moynihan's disease: The diagnosis of duodenal ulcer. N Engl J Med 1974; 291:567–569.
2. Pounder RE: Model of medical treatment for duodenal ulcer. Lancet 1981; 1:29–30.
3. McLean AJ, Harrison PM, Ioannides-Demos L, et al: The choice of ulcer healing agent influences duodenal ulcer relapse rate and long-term clinical outcome. Aust NZ J Med 1985; 15:367–374.
4. Miller JP, Faragher EB: Relapse of duodenal ulcer: Does it matter which drug is used in initial treatment. Br Med J 1986; 293(6555):1117–1118.
5. Moynihan BGA: Duodenal Ulcer. Saunders and Co., Philadelphia, 1910, p 379.
6. Boyd EJS, Wilson JA, Wormsley KE: Recurrent ulcer disease, in Misiewicz JJ, Wood JR (eds):

Ranitidine: Therapeutic Advances. Amsterdam, Excerpta Medica, 1984, pp 14–42.
7. Elashoff JD, Van DeVenter G, Reedy TJ, et al: Long-term follow-up of duodenal ulcer patients. *J Clin Gastroenterol* 1983; 5:509–515.
8. Grossman MI: *Peptic Ulcer, A Guide for the Practicing Physician.* Chicago, Year Book Medical Publishers, 1981, for the CURE Foundation, UCLA.
9. Krause U: Long-term results of medical and surgical treatment of peptic ulcer. *Acta Chir Scand* 1963; 125(suppl 310):1–15.
10. Boyd EJS, Wilson JA, Wormsley KG: Review of ulcer treatment; Role of ranitidine. *J Clin Gastroenterol* 1983; 5(suppl 1):133–142.
11. Gustavsson S, Loof L, Adami HO, et al: Rapid healing of duodenal ulcers with omeprazole: Double-blind dose-comparative trial. *Lancet* 1983; ii:124–125.
12. Friedmann G: Omeprazole. *Am J Gastroenterol* 1987; 32:188–191.
13. Gudmand-Hoyer E, Jensen KB, Krage E, et al: Prophylactic effect of cimetidine in duodenal ulcer disease. *Br Med J* 1978; 1:1095–1097.
14. Bardhan KD, Hinchcliffe RFC, Bose K: Low dose maintenance treatment with cimetidine in duodenal ulcer: Intermediate-term results. *Postgrad Med J* 1986; 62:347–351.
15. Korman JG, Hansky J, Eaves ER, et al: Influence of cigarette smoking on healing and relapse in duodenal ulcer disease. *Gastroenterology* 1983; 85:871–874.
16. Ippoliti AF: Prognostic factors in ulcer disease: Are they real, are they relevant? *J Clin Gastroenterol* 1985; 7(5):445–446.
17. Peterson WL, Sturdevant RAL, Frankl HD, et al: Healing of duodenal ulcer with an antacid regimen. *N Engl J Med* 1977; 297:341–345.
18. Ippoliti AF, Sturdevant RAL, Isenberg JI, et al: Cimetidine versus intensive antacid therapy for duodenal ulcer. *Gastroenterology* 1978; 74:393–395.
19. Flind AC, Beresford J: Controlled trial of cimetidine for symptomatic treatment of duodenal ulcers. *Br Med J* 1983; 286:1284–1285.
20. Cleur KA: Cimetidine for symptomatic treatment of duodenal ulcers. *Br Med J* 1983; 286:1358.
21. Prichard PJ, Kerr GD: Duodenitis and ulcer relapse. *Lancet* 1985; 2:102–103.22.
22. Sircus W: Duodenitis: A clinical, endoscopic and histopathologic study. *Q J Med* 1985; NS56 (221):593–600.
23. Graham DY, Klein PD: *Campylobacter pyloridis* gastritis: The past, the present and speculations about the future. *Am J Gastroenterol* 1987; 82:283–286.
24. Dunn JP, Eher LE: Inadequacy of the medical history in the diagnosis of peptic ulcer. *N Engl J Med* 1962; 266:68–72.
25. Gibbs JD: Study of 219 cases of peptic ulcer in a series of 2301 consecutive necropsies. *Quart Bull Northwestern Univ Med School* 1946; 20:328–338.
26. Texter EC, Navab F, Manteu G, et al: Maintenance therapy of duodenal ulcer with famotidine. A multicenter U.S. study. *Am J Med* 1986; 81(suppl 4B):20–23.
27. Boyd EJS, Wilson JA, Wormsley KG: The fate of asymptomatic recurrences of duodenal ulcer. *Scand J Gastroenterol* 1984; 19:808–812.
28. Bianchi-Porro G, Lazzaroni M, Petrillo M, et al: Natural history of silent duodenal ulcer. *Gut* 1985; 26:A1145.
29. Wormsley KG: Ulcer disease: Medical treatment. *Current Opinion in Gastroenterology* 1986; 2:855–868.
30. Strom M, Berstad A, Bodemar G, et al: Results of short- and long-term cimetidine treatment in patients with juxtapyloric ulcers, with special reference to gastric acid and pepsin secretion. *Scand J Gastroenterol* 1986; 21:521–530.
31. Rohner HG: Long-term cimetidine therapy for the prevention of recurring peptic ulcer: A multicenter study. *Z Gastroenterol* 1985; 23:403–411.
32. Anglo Irish Long-Term Cimetidine Study Group: Prophylaxis against duodenal ulcer and gastric ulcer recurrence using maintenance treatment with cimetidine: 4 year results. *Gastroenterology* 1985; 88:1307.
33. Walan A, Bianchi-Porro G, Hentschel E, et al: Maintenance treatment with cimetidine in peptic ulcer disease for up to 4 years. *Scand J Gastroenterol* 1987; 22:397–405.
34. Gough KR, Bardhan KD, Crowe JP, et al: Ranitidine and cimetidine in prevention of duodenal ulcer. *Lancet* 1984; ii:659–661.
35. Paoluzi P, Ricotta G, Ripoli F, et al: Incompletely and completely healed duodenal ulcers outcome in maintenance treatment: A double-blind controlled study. *Gut* 1985; 26:1080–1085.
36. Morris A, Nicholson G: Ingestion of *Campylobacter pyloridis* causes gastritis and raised fasting gastric pH. *Am J Gastroenterol* 1987; 82(3):192–199.
37. McKenna D, Humphrey's H, Dooley C, et al: *Campylobacter pyloridis* and histological gastritis in duodenal ulcer. *Gastroenterology* 1987; 92(5):1528.
38. Gilman R, Leon-Barua R, Ramirez-Ramos A, et al: Efficacy of nitrofurans in the treatment of antral gastritis associated with *C. pyloridis. Gastroenterology* 1987; 92(5):1405.
39. Eberhardt R, Kasper G, Dettmer A, et al: Effect of oral bismuth subsalicylate on *Campylobacter pyloridis* and duodenal ulcer. *Gastroenterology* 1987; 92(5):1379.
40. Marshall BJ, Armstrong JA, McGechie DB, et al: Attempt to fulfill Koch's postulates for pyloric *Campylobacter. Med J Aust* 1985; 142:436–439.
41. Marshall BJ, McGechie DB, Rogers PA, et al: Pyloric *Campylobacter* and gastroduodenal disease. *Med J Aust* 1985; 142:439–444.
42. Goodwin CS, Warren JR, Murray R, et al: Long-term healing of gastritis and low duodenal ulcer relapse after eradication of *Campylobacter pyloridis:* A prospective double-blind study. *Gastroenterology* 1987; 92(5):1518.
43. Burland WL, Hawkins BW, Beresford J: Cimetidine treatment for the prevention of recurrence of duodenal ulcer. *Postgrad Med J* 1980; 2:173–179.
44. Pounder RE: Approaches to the long-term treatment of duodenal ulcer, in Misiewicz JJ, Wood

JR (eds): *Ranitidine: Therapeutic Advances*. Amsterdam, Excerpta Medica, 1984, pp 1–13.
45. McLean AJ, Harrison PM, Byrne AJ, et al: Relapse rates are more important than healing rates in determining the long-term outcome of duodenal ulcer therapy. *Gastroenterology* 1985; 89:480–482.
46. Bardhan KD: Intermittent treatment of duodenal ulcer with cimetidine. *Br Med J* 1980; 281(6232): 20–22.
47. Hetzel DJ, Hecker R, Shearman DJC: Long-term treatment of duodenal ulcer with cimetidine. *Med J Aust* 1980; 2:612–614.
48. Walan A, Strom M: Prevention of ulcer recurrence—Medical vs. surgical treatment: A physician's view. *Scand J Gastroenterol* 1985; 20(suppl 110):83–88.
49. Rune SJ, Mollman KM, Rahbek I: Frequency of relapses in duodenal ulcer patients treated with cimetidine during symptomatic periods.
50. Gray ER, Smith IS, McWhinnie D, et al: Five-year study of cimetidine or surgery for severe duodenal ulcer dyspepsia. *Lancet* 1982; i:787–788.
51. Rohner HE, Blomer A, Echterhof, et al: Chirurgische Behandlung der Ulkuskrankheit 5 Jahre vor und nach EinFuhrung von cimetidin. *Z Gastroenterol* 1983; 21:585–592.
52. Armstrong CP, Blower AI: Non-steroidal anti-inflammatory drugs and life-threatening complications of peptic ulceration. *Gut* 1987; 28:527–532.
53. McLaurin BP, Richards DA: Indomethacin-associated peptic ulceration. *NZ Med J* 1978; 88:439–421.
54. Burland WL: Treatment of chronic duodenal ulcer with cimetidine, in Truelove SC, Hayworth MF (eds): *Topics in Gastroenterology, Vol. 6*. Oxford, Blackwell Scientific, pp 327–343.
55. Cockel R: NSAIDS—Should every prescription carry a government health warning. *Gut* 1987; 28:515–518.
56. Collier DSEJ, Pain JA: Non-steroidal anti-inflammatory drugs and peptic ulcer perforation. *GUT* 1985: 26; 359–363.
57. Sommerville K, Faulkner G, Langman M: Non-steroidal anti-inflammatory drugs and bleeding peptic ulcer. *Lancet* 1986; i:462–464.
58. Palmas F, Andriulli A, Verme G: Seasonal treatment with ranitidine. *Lancet* 1984; ii:698–699.
59. Lance P, Gazzard BG: Controlled trial of cimetidine for symptomatic treatment of duodenal ulcers. *Br Med J* 1983; 286:937–939.
60. Gustavsson S, Adami HO, Loof A, et al: Symptomatic cimetidine treatment of duodenal and prepyloric ulcers. *Dig Dis Sci* 1986; 31:2–6.
61. Sontag S, Graham DY, Belsito A, et al: Cimetidine, cigarette smoking and recurrence of duodenal ulcer. *N Engl J Med* 1984; 311:689–693.
62. Andersen D: Prevention of ulcer recurrence—Medical vs. surgical treatment—A surgeon's view. *Scand J Gastroenterol* 1985; 20(suppl 110): 89–92.
63. Mullholland MW, Debas HT: Recent advances in the treatment of duodenal ulcer disease. *West J Med* 1987; 147:301–308.

10

Gastric Volvulus
What is appropriate management?

PEDRO P. LLANEZA, M.D.
WILLIAM B. SALT, II, M.D.

Gastric volvulus is an uncommon acquired torsion of the stomach upon itself that results in gastric outlet obstruction. Males and females are equally affected with a peak incidence occurring during the fifth decade of life.[1] Although more common in adults, gastric volvulus can occur in infants and children.[2,3] In adults, the majority of cases occur in those with a portion or all of the stomach assuming an intrathoracic location through an acquired or traumatic diaphragmatic defect. Paraesophageal hernia is commonly present. In children, the most commonly associated conditions are a congenital hernia (e.g., Bochdalek's hernia) or eventration of the diaphragm. The clinical presentation can be acute, chronic, or intermittent. Presenting symptoms include severe epigastric or low anterior chest pain and retching without productive vomiting. Treatment is usually surgical.

HISTORY

The first report of gastric volvulus in the literature was provided by Berti in 1866; the lesion was found at the autopsy of a 60-year-old woman.[4] Berg was the first to report successful operative correction in 1897,[5] and Rosselet first described the radiologic findings in 1920.[6] Four large collective reviews of the literature on gastric volvulus have been published: Buchanan in 1930 (33 patients),[7] Dalgaard in 1952 (150 patients),[8] Wastell and Ellis in 1971 (206 patients),[1] and Cole and Dickinson in 1971 (44 children).[9] Over 300 patients with gastric volvulus have been described in the literature.[10]

DEFINITION

Some consider that the diagnosis and definition of gastric volvulus require an acute presentation and either the presence of complete closed-loop gastric obstruction or compromise of the gastric blood supply, or the surgical demonstration of abnormal rotation of the stomach within the abdominal cavity.[11,12] Gastric rotation of lesser severity is considered "torsion," large paraesophageal hernia, or incarcerated hernia.[9,13] Such terminology can be confusing and does not lend itself well to description of chronic, partial, and intermittent forms of gastric volvulus, which we and others believe may account for the majority of cases seen in clinical practice.[1,10] We consider the term *gastric volvulus* to mean a rotation of the stomach exceeding 180 degrees, causing partial or complete closed-loop obstruction.

CLASSIFICATION

The classification of gastric volvulus can be based on type, extent, direction, etiology, and severity. Table 10–1 presents the

TABLE 10–1.
Classification of Gastric Volvulus*

1. **Type** (based on axis of rotation)(a)
   - Organoaxial (b): rotation upward around the long (cardiopyloric) axis, an imaginary line drawn from the gastric cardia to the pylorus. This type of gastric volvulus is the upside-down stomach seen with the large paraesophageal hiatus hernia. It was the most common type (59%) in the series of Wastell and Ellis[1]
   - Mesenteroaxial (c): rotation around the long axis of the gastric mesenteries, a line approximately perpendicular to the cardiopyloric line. The twist usually occurs right to left, although occasionally it is left to right. This type accounted for 29% of cases in this series[1]
   - Combined or unclassified type: a combination of the organoaxial and mesenteroaxial types. It was the least common type (12%) in this series[1]

2. **Extent**
   - Total: entire stomach rotates, except for the part attached to the diaphragm
   - Partial: rotation is limited to one segment of the stomach, usually the pyloric portion

3. **Direction**
   - Anterior: rotating part passes anteriorly
   - Posterior: rotating part passes posteriorly

4. **Etiology**
   - Secondary: results from disease in the stomach or adjoining organs
   - Idiopathic: no specific cause-and-effect relationship established

5. **Severity**
   - Acute: acute abdominal symptoms: emergent surgical intervention is necessary
   - Chronic: symptoms (i.e., pyrosis, dyspepsia, upper abdominal pain, bloating, belching, nausea, and vomiting) are chronic

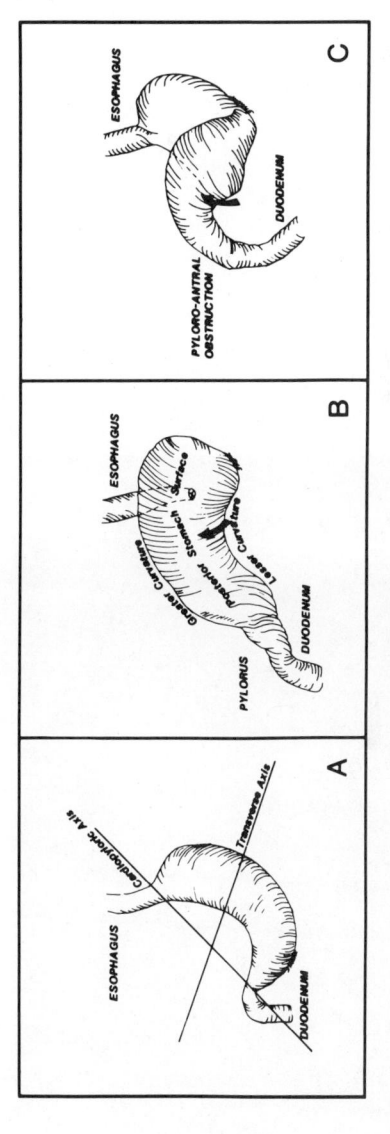

a. Anteroposterior view of stomach's imaginary cardiopyloric and transverse axes. b. Organoaxial volvulus, with rotation of stomach along cardiopyloric axis. c. Mesenteroaxial volvulus, with rotation of stomach along transverse axis and displacement of pyloroantral segment superiorly.

*From Llaneza PP, Salt WB: Gastric Volvulus: More common than previously thought? *Postgrad Med* 1986; 80:279–288. Copyright by McGraw-Hill, Inc.

topographic classification first described by von Haber in 1912[14] and later modified by Singleton in 1940.[15]

Rotation of the stomach of more than 180 degrees along its long axis, or cardiopyloric line, causes organoaxial gastric volvulus. This form of volvulus produces the "upside-down stomach" seen in association with large paraesophageal hernia. Rotation of the stomach along the long axis of the gastric mesenteries, an imaginary line from the middle of the lesser curvature to the middle of the greater curvature perpendicular to the cardiopyloric line, causes mesenteroaxial gastric volvulus. The twist occurs usually, although not invariably, left to right. A combined or unclassified type of gastric volvulus reflects the presence of both organoaxial and mesenteroaxial forms. Wastell and Ellis found the most common type of gastric volvulus to be organoaxial (59%), followed by mesenteroaxial (29%), and combined or mixed type (12%).[1]

PATHOGENESIS

Laxity of the ligaments that normally secure the stomach in the abdominal cavity is the most important factor that permits gastric volvulus to occur. The structures that fix the stomach include:

1. The gastrohepatic ligament, or omentum minus, attaching the lesser curvature to the liver
2. The gastrosplenic and gastrocolic ligaments attaching the greater curvature to the spleen and transverse colon, respectively
3. The esophagus and gastrophrenic ligaments anchoring the stomach cephalad
4. The relatively fixed retroperitoneal

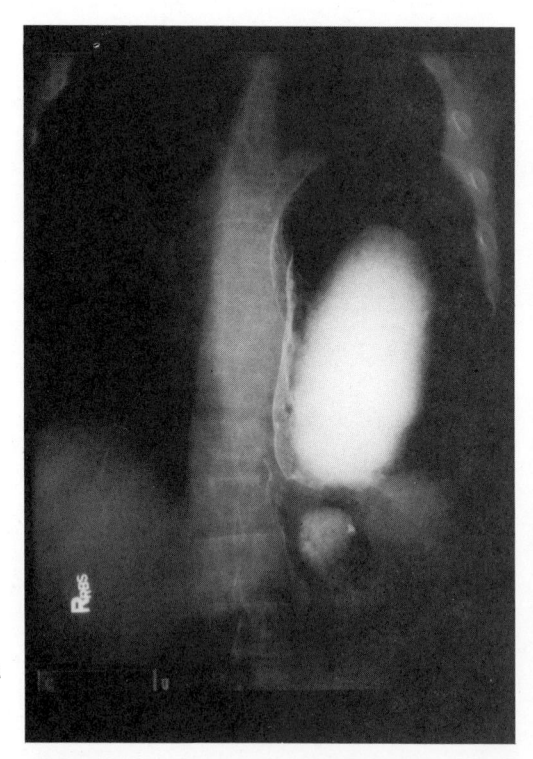

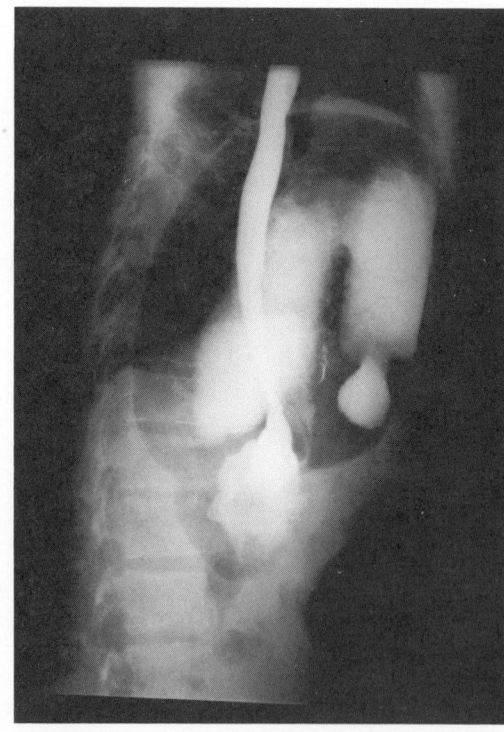

FIG 10–1.
Upper gastrointestinal radiographs of a mesenteroaxial volvulus. **A,** Anteroposterior view, showing massive gastric distention and complete obstruction of the pyloroantral outlet. **B,** Lateral view, showing esophagogastric junction inferior to its normal position. (From Llaneza PP, Salt WB: Gastric volvulus: More common than previously thought? *Postgrad Med* 1986; 80:279–288. Copyright by McGraw-Hill, Inc.)

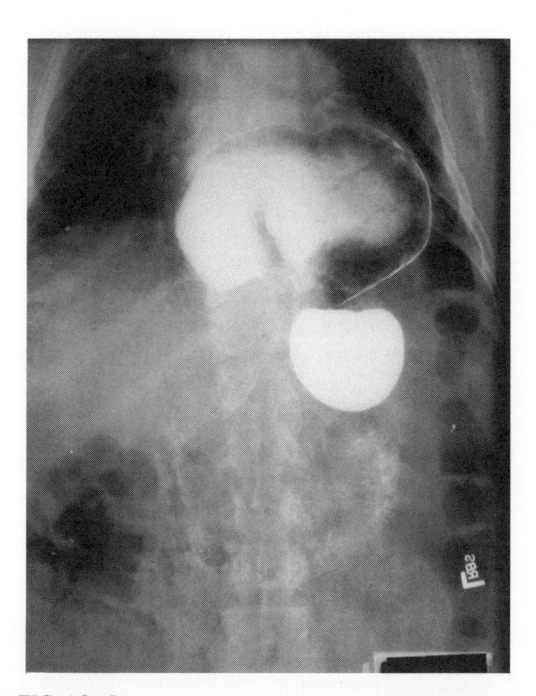

FIG 10–2.
Upper gastrointestinal radiograph, anterioposterior view, demonstrating an organoaxial volvulus. Note that the stomach is upside down and that the greater curvature lies superior to the lesser curvature. (From Llaneza PP, Salt WB: Gastric volvulus: More common than previously thought? *Postgrad Med* 1986; 80:279–288. Copyright by McGraw-Hill, Inc.)

second portion of the duodenum maintaining the gastric position caudad

Dalgaard used cadavers to show that the stomach could not be rotated 180 degrees unless either the gastrocolic or gastrosplenic ligament, or both, were severed.[8] Thus, in order for gastric volvulus to occur, abnormal relaxation of the ligamentous attachments of the stomach must be present sufficient to permit torsion of 180 degrees along or perpendicular to the cardiopyloric axis. Occasionally, one or more ligaments may be either congenitally absent or traumatically ruptured. Dalgaard also showed that an atonic and fluid-filled stomach could be twisted more easily than could an empty stomach.[8]

Once the integrity of the ligamentous support system of the stomach is compromised, movement of the greater curvature in a cephalad direction will result in an organoaxial gastric volvulus, or "upside-down stomach," while movement of the pylorus toward the cardia will produce a mesenteroaxial gastric volvulus (Figs 10.1 and 10.2).

Several conditions or disorders predispose those with gastric ligamentous laxity to the development of gastric volvulus. First and most important is the presence of an abnormal extension of the abdominal cavity that permits the stomach to enter the extension and twist. Such extensions include:

1. Paraesophageal hernia, in which the gastric volvulus is usually organoaxial
2. Eventration of the left hemidiaphragm related to phrenic nerve paralysis or resection of a portion or all of the left lung,[16, 17] in which the volvulus is usually mesenteroaxial
3. Traumatic injury of the diaphragm[18]
4. Large incisional ventral hernia

Second, normal gastric anatomy may be altered by extrinsic compression from adjacent organs or masses. Intrinsic gastric lesions, including ulcer and benign or malignant tumor, may also distort normal anatomy and allow the stomach to twist.

Third, gastric rotation in a susceptible individual can be precipitated by an overly distended or fluid-filled stomach, as can occur after a heavy meal. This is consistent with Dalgaard's observation that an atonic and fluid-filled stomach could be twisted more easily than could an empty stomach.[8]

Finally, rare conditions associated with gastric volvulus include congenital obstructive bands,[19] abdominal adhesions, pneumatosis cystoides intestinalis,[20] and long, redundant mesocolon.[21, 22]

CLINICAL FEATURES

The clinical presentation of gastric volvulus can be acute, chronic, or intermittent. Symptoms range from sudden, severe epigastric abdominal pain associated with retching in the acute process, to milder symptoms of epigastric discomfort, dyspepsia, and postprandial bloating, nausea, and discomfort in the chronic or intermittent form.

Acute Gastric Volvulus

Acute gastric volvulus is often dramatic and may be associated with shock. In 1904, Borchardt described a clinical triad that characterizes the acute presentation:
1. Violent retching with production of little or no vomitus
2. Sudden onset of severe and constant epigastric pain
3. Great difficulty in advancing a nasogastric tube into the stomach[23]

Clinical experience has confirmed these observations,[1] although the classic triad can be difficult to recognize in infants and children.[24] A history of trauma to the chest or abdomen can be important, because acute gastric volvulus can occur months to years later.[18] The upper abdomen can be very distended, while the lower abdomen remains relatively soft and flat.[12] Carter and colleagues reported 25 cases of acute gastric volvulus and emphasized that abdominal findings may be minimal if the stomach is located in the thorax.[25] Auscultation of the chest may yield bowel sounds,[26] or a succussion splash may be heard over either the chest or abdomen. The presentation of acute gastric volvulus can be confused with that of myocardial ischemia or infarction. Chest pain can be significant, and electrocardiographic changes mimicking myocardial infarction have been described.[27] Other authors contend that these changes actually reflect myocardial ischemia.[28]

Chronic Gastric Volvulus

Chronic gastric volvulus can be asymptomatic and remain undiagnosed for years. When symptoms occur they are usually vague and include dyspepsia, postprandial epigastric discomfort, singultus, belching, bloating, or nausea.[29, 30] Although symptomatic gastroesophageal reflux is uncommon, esophagitis was commonly found at endoscopy in one series.[31]

The pain of intermittent gastric volvulus may be similar to that seen in acute gastric volvulus, although less severe. Because of its constant character, it can be confused with pain of pancreatobiliary origin. Chronic and intermittent gastric volvulus should be considered in an individual with a paraesophageal hernia who has attacks of intermittent upper abdominal pain, particularly if vomiting or retching occurs.[32, 33]

COMPLICATIONS

The complications of gastric volvulus are listed in Table 10–2. By definition, some degree of gastric obstruction is present in gastric volvulus. The sites of obstruction vary with the type of volvulus. Organoaxial volvulus tends to obstruct both the gastric cardia and the pylorus. This closed-loop obstruction can result in rapid gastric distention and acute symptoms. By contrast, mesenteroaxial volvulus effects approximation of the pylorus and esophagogastric junction resulting in obstruction at one location, usually the mid-stomach or gastric outlet. Such obstruction is usually incomplete, and symptoms tend to be chronic. Because of the rich blood supply of the stomach, gastric gangrene is infrequent. Most reports estimate the occurrence of strangulation to be approximately 5%, however, Carter and his co-workers found strangulation in 28% of their series.[25]

DIAGNOSIS

Although inability to pass a nasogastric tube into the stomach in a patient with the acute onset of severe epigastric pain and retching without productive vomiting is characteristic of gastric volvulus,[23] the definitive diagnosis is based on radiographic assessment. Menuck described the classic findings of gastric volvulus on upright chest and abdominal radiographs:

TABLE 10–2.
Complications of Gastric Volvulus*

Complete gastric obstruction
Gastric infarction with gangrene
Gastric hemorrhage[34]
Perforation
Shock
Volume deficit
Electrolyte imbalance
Pulmonary complications (aspiration pneumonia, atelectasis)
Splenic rupture
Extrahepatic biliary tract obstruction[35]
Myocardial ischemia[28]

*From Llaneza PP, Salt WB: Gastric volvulus: More common than previously thought? *Postgrad Med* 1986; 80:279–288. Copyright by McGraw-Hill, Inc.

a double air–fluid level, one beneath the left hemidiaphragm representing the proximal stomach and the other in the retrocardiac mediastinum representing the distal stomach.[36] Pneumoperitoneum indicates gastric perforation, while air within the gastric wall suggests the presence of gangrene.

Barium contrast study of the upper gastrointestinal tract can be performed if gastric volvulus is suspected.[37-39] In the mesenteroaxial form, the esophagogastric junction is located below the level of the diaphragm in an abnormally low position while the distal stomach positioned cephalad (see Fig 10–1). With complete obstruction in the acute form, a "beak" may be noted at the level of the esophagogastric junction. In the organoaxial form of gastric volvulus, the stomach appears inverted, or "upside down," with the greater curvature superior to the lesser curvature and the cardia and pylorus pointing downward at the same level (see Fig 10–2). Gastric distention can occur with both types of volvulus. The angiographic appearance of the gastric volvulus has been described.[40]

Diagnosis can difficult in the chronic or intermittent form of gastric volvulus. Ideally, the upper gastrointestinal radiograph should be performed during acute symptoms. Demonstration of either eventration of the diaphragm or paraesophageal hernia in a patient with chronic or sporadic symptoms of upper abdominal pain and vomiting or retching should raise a consideration of the diagnosis of gastric volvulus.[10] If hiatal hernia is noted on the upper gastrointestinal series, it is important that the radiologist demonstrate the relationship of the esophagogastric junction to the diaphragm. In typical sliding hiatal hernia, the junction is located above the diaphragm. Failure to demonstrate that the junction is located below the diaphragm can result in failure to recognize the much less common paraesophageal hernia.

Upper gastrointestinal endoscopy offers little in establishing the abnormal anatomical configuration of the stomach in a gastric volvulus; however, difficulty in passing the instrument into the stomach argues for the diagnosis. Torsion may actually be reducing during the examination; thus, the diagnosis might not be recognized. Endoscopy is indicated if volvulus is suspected, because recognition of esophagitis, malignancy, or ulcer may have therapeutic implications as regards surgical management.

TREATMENT

Acute Gastric Volvulus

Acute gastric volvulus is managed surgically. Initial effort should be directed to correction of any volume deficit and electrolyte disorder. If vomiting, retching, succussion splash, or radiographic evidence of gastric distention is present, then nasogastric tube decompression of the stomach can be attempted. Because the esophagogastric junction is often obstructed by the torsion, passage of the nasogastric tube can be difficult or impossible. Because perforation of the esophagus or stomach with the nasogastric tube has been reported, particularly in children,[9] it is advisable to avoid the use of force if difficulty or resistance is encountered. If further effort is made to pass the nasogastric tube, it can be facilitated by the use of a radiopaque tube with fluoroscopic guidance. Needle decompression of a massively dilated stomach can be performed at the time of operation, if necessary.[41] Decompression of gastric volvulus as the only therapy has not been shown to prevent recurrence.[42]

Endoscopy is indicated to assess for endoscopic evidence of esophagitis, tumor, or ulcer. Direct aspiration of the stomach and decompression can provide symptomatic relief if a nasogastric tube cannot be passed. Endoscopic derotation of both acute[43] and chronic gastric volvulus[44] has been reported. Eckhauser and Ferron recently reported the successful treatment of intermittent chronic gastric volvulus by use of dual percutaneous endoscopic gastrostomy placed in both the body and antrum of the stomach.[45]

Once the patient has been stabilized, then emergency laparotomy is indicated. Operative objectives include gastric decompression, reduction of the gastric volvulus, fixation of the stomach, and correction or repair of any causative factors. The transabdominal approach is often used; however, the transthoracic approach may be preferred for reduction and repair of volvulus induced by traumatic injury of the diaphragm.[18] If gastric infarction is found, then subtotal gastrectomy or total gastric resection may be required, depending on the extent of gastric ischemic injury. Fixation of the stomach with an anterior gastropexy is generally recommended. Temporary gastrostomy after derotation may suffice to fix the stomach if the patient is a high surgical risk.[25] Precipitating disorders should be corrected or repaired, including diaphragmatic hernia or eventration, adhesions or bands, ulcer or malignancy. An antireflux procedure such as fundoplication can be included in the surgical repair if there is endoscopic evidence of esophagitis in patients with a paraesophageal hernia; however, its routine use is probably not advisable.

Chronic Gastric Volvulus

The selection of patients with chronic gastric volvulus for surgery can be difficult. Surgery is indicated to relieve troublesome chronic and recurrent symptoms, and to prevent acute gastric volvulus with its potential complications. If the entire stomach is located in the thorax, or paraesophageal hernia is present, surgery is probably advisable to prevent an acute event.[13] The association of iron deficiency anemia with large hiatal hernia has been recognized for many years.[46, 47] A recent report has suggested that the explanation for this association is linear gastric erosions caused by mechanical trauma as the hernia slides back and forth across the diaphragm.[48] The complication of iron deficiency anemia can provide a contributing indication for surgery.[49]

The clinician and patient must weigh the potential benefits of surgery against operative risk. If surgery is either not accepted by the patient or not recommended by the physician, then the patient should understand the risk of the possible future development of acute gastric volvulus and its complications.

Tanner has published a comprehensive review of surgical treatment of chronic or recurrent gastric volvulus.[19] He and others[50, 51] recommend reduction of the gastric torsion, gastropexy, and subphrenic transposition of the colon in those with gastric volvulus associated with eventration of the diaphragm. Those with organoaxial volvulus and an "upside-down" stomach associated with paraesophageal hernia require fixation of the stomach and diaphragmatic hiatal repair. Fundoplication is recommended if esophagitis is demonstrated endoscopically. In children with a foramen of Bochdalek's hernia, the abdominal approach is preferred with closure of the defect from below.[52]

Simple gastropexy or gastrostomy has been used with varying results. Antrectomy with or without vagotomy and gastroduodenostomy (Billroth I) may be necessary if an intrinsic lesion is identified.[19] If the duodenal stump is not suitable for anastomosis and a gastrojejunostomy (Billroth II) is necessary, colonic displacement with gastropexy may be advisable to prevent the potential development of a volvulus of the gastric remnant.[50]

References

1. Wastell C, Ellis H: Volvulus of the stomach. Br J Surg 1971; 58:557–562.
2. Campbell JB, Rappaport LN, Skerker LB: Acute mesentero-axial volvulus of the stomach. Radiology 1972; 103:153–156.
3. Idowu J, Aitken DR, Georgeson KE: Gastric volvulus in the newborn. Arch Surg 1980; 115:1046–1049.
4. Berti A: Sigolare attortiglamento dell'esofago col duodeno seqito da rapida morte. Gazz Med Ital Prov Ver 1866; 9:139.
5. Berg J: Qwei falle von axendrehung des magens; operation; heilung. Nord Med Ark 1897; 30:1.
6. Rosselet DJ: Contribution a l'etude du volvulus de l'estomac. J Radiol Electrol 1920; 4;341.
7. Buchanan J: Volvulus of the stomach. Br J Surg 1930; 18:99.
8. Dalgaard JB: Volvulus of the stomach. Acta Clin Scand 1952; 103:131–153.
9. Cole BC, Dickinson SJ: Acute volvulus of the stomach in infants and children. Surgery 1971; 70:707–717.
10. Llaneza PP, Salt WB: Gastric volvulus: More common than previously thought? Postgrad Med 1986; 80:279–288.
11. Haller JA, Bohrer SL: Gastric volvulus, gastric fistulas, and gastric trauma, in Scott HW, Sawyers JL (eds): Surgery of the Stomach, Duodenum, and Small Intestine. Boston, Blackwell Scientific Publications Inc, 1987, pp 489–498.
12. Camblos JF: Acute volvulus of the stomach. Am Surg 1969; 35:505–509.
13. Payne WS: Paraesophageal hiatal hernia, in Nyhus LM, Baker RJ (eds): Mastery of Surgery. Boston, Little, Brown & Co., 1984, pp 329–337.
14. von Haber H: Volvulus des magens vei carcinoma. Dtsch Z Chir 1912; 115:497.
15. Singleton AC: Chronic gastric volvulus. Radiology 1940; 34:53–61.
16. Creedon PJ, Burman JF: Volvulus of the stomach. Report of a case with complications. Am J Surg 1965; 110:964–966.
17. Carlisle BB, Hayes CW: Gastric volvulus. An unusual complication after pneumonectomy. Am J Surg 1967; 113:579–582.
18. Pillay SP, Argorn IB, Baker LW: Gastric volvulus unassociated with hiatal hernia. S Afr Med J 1977; 52:880–885.
19. Tanner NC: Chronic and recurrent volvulus of the stomach. Am J Surg 1968; 115:505–515.
20. Elidan J, Gimmon Z, Schwartz A: Pneumoperitoneum induced by pneumatosis cystoides intestinalis associated with volvulus of the stomach. Am J Gastroenterol 1980; 74:189–195.
21. Ascherman SW, Bednarz WW, Olix ML: Gastric volvulus. Arch Surg 1958; 76:621–629.
22. Jones WM, Jones CD: Volvulus of the transverse colon associated with organoaxial volvulus of the stomach. Am J Surg 1972; 124:404–406.
23. Borchardt M: Zur pathologie und therapie des magenvolvulus. Arch Klin Chir 1904; 74:243–260.
24. Campbell JB: Neonatal gastric volvulus. AJR 1979; 132:723–725.
25. Carter R, Brewer LA, Hinshaw DB: Acute gastric volvulus. A study of 25 cases. Am J Surg 1980; 140:99–106.
26. Smith RJ: Volvulus of the stomach. J Natl Med Assoc 1983; 75:393–397.
27. Farr C, Graver K, Curry RW, et al: Electrocardiographic changes with gastric volvulus. N Engl J Med 1984; 310:1747–1748.
28. Eagle KA, Yurchak PM: Transient myocardial ischemia resulting from gastric volvulus. N Engl J Med 1985; 312:121.
29. Bell JW: Chronically incarcerated hiatus hernia. Arch Surg 1972; 104:831–835.
30. Stremple JF: A new operation for the anatomic correction of chronic intermittent gastric volvulus. Am J Surg 1973; 125:360–363.
31. Pearson FG, Cooper JD, Ilves R, et al: Massive hiatal hernia with incarceration: A report of 53 cases. Ann Thorac Surg 1983; 35:45–51.
32. Babb RR, Peck OC, Jamplis RW: Gastric volvulus and obstruction in paraesophageal hiatus hernia. Dig Dis Sci 1972; 17:119–128.
33. Chessick KC, Hoye SJ: Paraesophageal hernia and gastric volvulus. J Fla Med Assoc 1975; 62:30–34.
34. Metcalfe-Gibson C: A case of haemorrhage from volvulus of the gastric fundus. Br J Surg 1975; 62:224–225.
35. Llaneza PP, Salt WB, E. Partyka: Extrahepatic biliary obstruction complicating a diaphragmatic hiatal hernia with intrathoracic gastric volvulus. Am J Gastroenterol 1986; 81:292–294.
36. Menuck L: Plain film findings of gastric volvulus herniating into the chest. Am J Roentgenol 1976; 126:1169–1174.
37. Ziprkowski MN, Teele RL: Gastric volvulus in childhood. AJR 1979; 132:921–925.
38. Kilcoyne RF, Babbitt DP, Sakaguchi S: Volvulus of the stomach. A case report. Radiology 1972; 103:157–158.
39. Eisenberg RL: Gastrointestinal Radiology—A Pattern Approach. Philadelphia, JB Lippincott, 1983, pp 286–290.
40. Fink DW: Gastric volvulus: The angiographic appearance. Am J Roentgenol 1972; 115:268–270.

41. Guernsey JM, Connolly JE: Acute, complete gastric volvulus. *Arch Surg* 1963; 86:423–429.
42. Gosin S, Gallinger WF: Recurrent volvulus of the stomach. Report of a case with recurrence after simple decompression. *Am J Surg* 1965; 109:642–646.
43. Haddad JK, Doherty C, Clark RE: Acute gastric volvulus-endoscopic derotation. *West J Med* 1977; 127:341–346.
44. Patel NM: Endoscopic correction of chronic gastric volvulus. *Gastrointest Endosc* 1983; 29:63.
45. Eckhauser ML, Ferron JP: The use of dual percutaneous endoscopic gastrostomy (DPEG) in the management of chronic intermittent gastric volvulus. *Gastrointest Endosc* 1985; 31:340–342.
46. Schwartz SO, Blumenthal SA: Diaphragmatic hiatus hernia with severe iron deficiency anemia. *Am J Med* 1949; 7:501–510.
47. Cameron AJ: Incidence of iron deficiency anemia in patients with large diaphragmatic hernia. A controlled study. *Mayo Clin Proc* 1976; 51:767–769.
48. Cameron AJ, Higgins JA: Linear gastric erosion. A lesion associated with large diaphragmatic hernia and chronic blood loss anemia. *Gastroenterology* 1986; 91:338–342.
49. Johns TNP, Clements EL: The relief of anemia by repair of hiatus hernia. *J Thorac Cardiovasc Surg* 1961; 41:737–747.
50. Schreiver H, Flickinger EG, Eichelberger MR, et al: Colonic displacement. Proposed treatment for gastric remnant volvulus due to eventration of the diaphragm. *Am J Surg* 1980 139:719–722.
51. Thorpe JA: Chronic gastric volvulus—aetiology and treatment. *Br J Clin Pract* 1981; 285:29–30.
52. Lilly JR, Haase GM, Karrer FM: Surgical treatment of pediatric digestive disease, in Moody FG, Carey LC, Jones RS, et al (eds): *Surgical Treatment of Digestive Disease*. Chicago, Year Book Medical Publishers, 1986, p 102.

11

Glandular Carcinoma of Gastric Origin

HAROLD O. DOUGLASS, JR., M.D., F.A.C.S.

If "Difficult Problems in Gastroenterology" are judged by our failure in early diagnosis and general lack of therapeutic success, then gastric adenocarcinoma certainly fits the picture. No more than 10% of patients in the United States in whom this diagnosis is eventually made will survive 5 years. In less than 1%, will the diagnosis be made sufficiently early to virtually ensure cure with proper treatment. The dozen or more different staging systems in use during the past two decades underline our continuing failure to fully understand this disease complex. Surgical procedures performed frequently fall short of ideal; however, the "optimal" operations for gastric cancers arising in various sites are still subject to argument. We have no proven adjuvant therapy and few candidate therapies for controlled trials. While our best treatments for advanced disease cause significant numbers of partial tumor regressions, complete regressions are few and their impact on overall survival often approaches zero.

Against this background, review of ten aspects of the complex of diseases lumped together under the diagnosis of gastric cancer will evaluate the facts at hand and how they can be applied to improve the management of patients with gastric neoplasia. The problems to be examined are:
1. Early diagnosis: Why gastric cancer is not diagnosed until late in its course.
2. Barrett's mucosa of the esophagus: How a better understanding of this metaplastic process can avoid its not-infrequent complications.
3. Staging: How resolution of the confusion can lead to better treatment planning.
4. The extent of surgery: Is more better?
5. The spleen: Its removal was once part of the standard radical gastrectomy.
6. Results of surgery: Identifying patients as candidates for surgical adjuvant trials.
7. Locally incurable disease: Proposal of a program that may improve survival.
8. Metastatic gastric cancer: Importance of the patterns of failure.
9. Surgical adjuvant therapy: Reasons for failure of previous trials and suggestions for success in the future.
10. Chemotherapy for advanced disease: Possible reasons for failure and the potential new approaches.

These discussions should lead to conclusions that only in-depth pathologic evaluation will clarify whether gastric cancer is one or several diseases, that modifications of the surgical approach may yield modest increases in long-term patient survival, and that with more explicit histopathologic evaluation, new therapeutic approaches may improve the survival of patients with advanced disease.

EARLY DIAGNOSIS

It has often been considered that the key to enhanced survival is an early diagnosis. Indeed, for patients with breast cancer, a patient with a 1-cm tumor has a better prognosis than the patient with a 2-cm tumor, and a far better prognosis than one with a 4-cm tumor. But where in the life cycle of that cancer, from the time of first neoplastic change until the patient's demise, is that 1-cm tumor? Because neoplastic cells behave as true parasites and, unless severely deprived, metabolize at a maximum rate, one can assume that the doubling time of a cancer is more or less constant during the earliest portions of its life history. A 1-cm tumor contains approximately 1 billion cells. To reach this volume, that first neoplastic cell and all of its daughter cells would have to have divided a total of 30 times. By the time of the 40th doubling, the tumor will weigh a kilogram, far more tumor than can be found in most patients. It takes three doubling times for that 1-cm tumor to become a 2-cm tumor, and three more to become a 4-cm tumor. Before four more doublings, the patient has usually died.

Although in large tumors, individual clones of cells may double in less than a day, for most solid tumors, the average doubling time appears to be in excess of 40 days. Some tumors double as quickly as every 18 days, while others may double no more than once every 120 days. Obviously, the more rapidly growing tumors take considerably less time to reach the 1-cm size. The average tumor probably has reached this size in approximately 3.25 years. The rapidly growing tumor may reach this size in 1.5 years. The slowly growing tumor may well have been present for 10 years.

Thus, that 1-cm tumor has parasitized the host for a considerable duration of time. Depending on the growth rate, once the cancer is diagnosed, the patient can be expected to survive between 6 months and 3 years, unless effective therapy is offered.

There is one further concern in this process of the basic cellular biology of cancer. It is estimated that for each million cells, there is a risk of a further mutation resulting in the formation of a new clone of tumor cells. This new clone may have a different (and generally more rapid) growth rate and different (usually increased) resistance to treatment. The significance of this will become apparent later.

What does all of this mean to the patient with a 1-cm tumor, be it in the breast, the esophagus, the stomach, or elsewhere? First, the diagnosis really isn't early. Second, there is certain heterogeneity already in the composition of the tumor. Third, the symptoms related to that tumor are not necessarily new. Chronic symptoms of months' or even years' duration may all be related to the growing cancer.

Nightly television commercials attest to the fact that we survive in a society where heartburn and vague epigastric distress are rampant. Were this not the case, there would not be so many antacids, anticholinergics, and assorted other medications available. In some parts of our society, it is most unfashionable not to at least have heartburn. Against this background, the physician must ask, "Why does the patient come for medical attention at this time? Are these new symptoms or has there been a change or progression of the symptomatology?" In the patient with cancer of gastric origin, the greatest difficulty is the confusion with the signs and symptoms of benign disease: heartburn, gas, pain, burning sensation, nighttime distress, postprandial pain, relief with milk or food, nausea, anemia, dysphagia, and so forth.

Symptoms severe enough to bring the patient to a physician are probably severe enough to warrant a diagnostic study. If the barium meal demonstrates a duodenal ulcer, the problem is solved. It's when the x-ray does not reveal an ulcer that the question remains. A classic gastric ulcer of typically benign appearance that heals at least partially after 3 to 4 weeks of treatment is no guarantee of the absence of cancer. The failure to demonstrate any pathology may even be more ominous. Perhaps the most treacherous finding is a hiatal hernia because one tends to accept it as the cause of many symptoms despite the fact that most people with hiatal hernias have no symptomatology whatsoever.

The solution is endoscopy. At the time of endoscopy, initial brushings of the mucosa may be far more revealing than any biopsy, particularly in the lower esophagus and at the diaphragmatic hiatus. Once a biopsy has been obtained, the inevitable trace of blood may make the cytologist's job impossible.

What if no pathology is found endoscopically? The pancreatobiliary tree and liver must then be studied, because it is "most likely" that the stomach is not the site of the symptoms. "Most likely" does not totally eliminate the stomach, which should be restudied if the symptoms persist without establishing a diagnosis for 3 months or more. Linitus plastica can masquerade in a normal stomach, with normal biopsies and cytology.

A greater problem is a cytologic report of atypical cells. Atypia mandates a promptly repeated gastroscopy and cytology, preferably with cytologic specimens obtained from several different parts of the stomach, carefully identified and labeled. Atypia does not necessarily indicate neoplasia nor will metaplastic cells necessarily appear atypical. Esophagitis, gastritis, and bile reflux may, on occasion, also lead to atypical appearances of mucosal cells.

If at the time of repeat endoscopy, atypical cells are no longer seen, gastroscopy should probably be repeated at a year, or sooner if symptoms persist. If the atypia is once again noted, a second repeat gastroscopy should be delayed for no longer than 3 months and then repeated again at 6 months and a year from the initial study. Cytopathologic consultation should be enlisted to determine if the atypia is becoming more or less severe.

If an area of ulceration or other pathology is identified, three to five biopsies, at a minimum, should be obtained. In an ulcerated lesion, the yield of malignant disease may be higher as a result of biopsing the side walls of the ulcer, rather than the base, which may be composed entirely of granulation tissue. Combining biopsies and brushings, the accuracy of diagnosis of cancer should exceed 95%.

Polyps of the stomach should be biopsied and excised endoscopically. As long as there is no evidence of malignant degeneration, new polyps can be excised repeatedly as needed. For many of these patients, the potential for endoscopic removal of polyps has eliminated the need for gastric resection.

GLANDULAR MUCOSA IN THE ESOPHAGUS (BARRETT'S ESOPHAGUS)

The incidence of heterotopic spread of gastric mucosa into the lower esophagus is unknown. Patients with Barrett's mucosa do demonstrate a loss of lower esophageal sphincter (LES) tone. Most likely, this phenomenon occurs as a result of resultant esophagitis with loss of the squamous mucosa and an ingrowth of the more rapidly growing columnar mucosa. Most patients with hiatal hernias are symptom free, as are many with esophagitis. Autopsy studies have not delineated the incidence of this metaplastic change, nor whether (as is the case with hiatal hernia) it is more common in overweight individuals. At least one report has suggested Barrett's dysplasia to be more common in white male smokers. The attention of the gastroenterologist is not drawn to all patients with metaplastic mucosa in the lower esophagus, but rather only to those whose esophagi are symptomatic. Thus, when metaplastic mucosa is found endoscopically, the question to be raised is why the patient is symptomatic now and not previously. The mere presence of this columnar mucosa indicates a chronic problem for which ingrowth of gastric mucosa has been a healing mechanism. In the absence of a mucosal lining, healing of esophagitis results in the formation of scar which, as it matures, contracts. The result is a narrowing of the esophageal lumen or a stricture. Metaplastic mucosa may be found well above levels of stricture, because this represents an old rather than recent injury to the esophageal lining.

Because gastroesophageal reflux (GER), by itself, is not sufficient to explain symptomatology in all patients, a search for another cause must be undertaken. In the absence of cancer, a Nissen fundoplication may halt progression of this disease.

Unfortunately, the risk of neoplasia in patients with Barrett's mucosa in the esophagus is unknown, largely because the actual incidence of Barrett's mucosa is unknown. Nevertheless, this mucosa must be considered premalignant. Endoscopic brushings and random biopsies should be performed every time dysplastic mucosa is identified.

In any operation in which the esophagus is being removed for a tumor arising in the Barrett's mucosa, all mucosa up to the level of the squamocolumnar junction must be removed. Residual mucosa left behind in the esophagus is a prime site for recurrence or further malignant degeneration. A frozen section at the site of an esophageal transection is necessary to ensure that circumferential squamous mucosa is present, in addition to ruling out proximal extension of the malignant process in the submucosa. Unless the upper limit of infiltration has been very carefully demarcated endoscopically, the surgeon must be prepared to resect the esophagus all the way up to the hypopharynx, if necessary. For this reason, we strongly recommend the classic lateral right thoracotomy as the most appropriate approach to the esophagus.

It is uncertain as to whether the mucosa, from which the heterotopic Barrett's cells arise, is from the fundus of the stomach or is antral. Both types of cells have been described in the esophagus, although fundic cells tend to be found closer to the cardioesophageal junction.

A number of different cell types make up the lining of the stomach. The major histologic differences are found between the cells of the body and fundus of the stomach compared to those of the antrum. While anatomically the antrum is considered to extend across from the incisura to the greater curvature, in reality the physiologic antrum extends far up the gastric wall along the lesser curvature, often to or above the esophageal inlet. Empirically, surgeons of the 1940s and 1950s found that peptic ulcer recurrence was reduced when the gastric resection extended high along the lesser curvature to the level of the esophagus. Studies showed that benign gastric ulcers tend to occur at the junction of antral and acid-bearing mucosa. That these ulcers can occur high on the lesser curvature and occasionally above the level of the esophageal inlet is well established. Unfortunately, there is insufficient information to establish the relative frequencies of gastric or antral mucosa in the distal esophagus. It is also unknown whether the histologic origin of this metaplastic mucosa in any way affects the nature of the neoplasia that occur. The hypothetical potential differences in the responsiveness of cancers of antral or fundic origin to act as major determinants of the outcome of antineoplastic therapy have yet to be considered clinically or experimentally.

STAGING

The past two decades have seen several different methods for staging gastric cancer in the United States and throughout the world. These alterations in the staging systems may have improved their predictive values. Comparison of published results becomes difficult if not impossible when those reported results are given by "stage." Staging systems used by the Japanese, by Americans, and by the World Health Organization (WHO) all differ. In addition, staging systems have evolved for specific protocols in an attempt to evaluate specific questions. The situation is further complicated by the tendency of many surgeons to appropriate the staging system designed for evaluating colorectal cancer, originally developed by Cuthbert Dukes and modified by several investigators over the past half century, and to adapt this system to describe gastric cancer. In many ways, this use of Dukes staging is as prognostically accurate as many of the various staging systems, and far easier for most surgeons to remember.

Weaknesses in the various staging systems reflect the spread of gastric cancer by four different routes. Liver metastases are not the most frequent cause of treatment failure. True liver metastases are a result of vascular (venous) invasion and metastases via the portal circulation. Far more common are lymph node metastases and the transperitoneal seeding of peritoneal surfaces (which includes the surface of the liver, the bowel, the abdominal wall, the omentum, the pelvis, and the ovaries). Direct invasion of contiguous organs such as the mesocolon, the liver, the pancreas and the spleen, usually do not eliminate the potential for curative surgical resection but do reduce the patient's chances for survival.

Any amount of ascitic fluid found in the peritoneal cavity at the time of gastric resection should be subjected to cytologic examination. In the absence of free fluid, washings of the stomach and upper abdomen should be performed. Positive cytology from these washings suggests peritoneal invasion that may not be clinically obvious. Negative washings in the face of apparent peritoneal invasion suggests that transperitoneal dissemination of the tumor may not yet have occurred and that a potential for curability by surgical resection is still present.

Japanese staging has long recognized the significance of peritoneal invasion. Their original staging system had considered transmural invasion of the serosa to carry a worse prognosis than lymph node metastases. The extent of invasion was considered important and was subdivided into microscopic invasion or gross invasion of the serosa.

Both the site at which the lymph node metastases are found (lymph node group) and the number of lymph nodes involved by the metastatic tumor process are important prognostic signs. No surgeon questions the prognostic difference when one or two nodes immediately adjacent to the tumor contain metastases, compared to a report of 26 out of 27 nodes on a specimen with metastatic cancer. Most recognized cancer lymphatics of the gastric wall at the site of surgical resection suggests a virtual 100% risk of recurrence (disease being left behind). Metatases into the first level of lymph nodes in the immediate vicinity of the tumor affect the patient's prognosis considerably less than do metastases in the next level of lymph nodes. However, the sites of primary and secondary levels of lymphatic drainage vary depending on the location of the cancer within the stomach and on its size.

Rigid definitions of levels of potential lymph node metastases become difficult to describe and even more difficult to remember. One staging system determined that the first level of lymph nodes were those within 3 cm of the tumor. While one would easily acknowledge that it is clearly possible to resect all lymph nodes 3 cm from a tumor at the incisura, for cancers at the cardioesophageal junction, the high left gastric, celiac and para-aortic lymph nodes are all within 3 cm of the primary tumor. Yet, involvement of the celiac lymph nodes should not deter their resection in continuity with the primary cancer, while involvement of periaortic lymph nodes is tantamount to surgical incurability. Under the Japanese staging system, celiac lymph nodes would be considered level 3, para-aortic nodes are considered level 4.

Staging criteria are further complicated by the realization that early gastric cancers, which are highly curable, can have metastases in the immediately adjacent nodes. Similarly, another malignancy that is highly curable (if a total gastrectomy is performed) is the superficial spreading cancer. Lymph node metastases also occur with this disease, yet do not seem to significantly alter prognosis if they are removed as part of the total gastrectomy.

Sites of lymph node metastases that do signify surgical incurability include those at the hilum of the liver, in the periaortic region particularly at the level of celiac axis, and those around the superior mesenteric artery at its takeoff from the aorta. This last site of involvement occurs more commonly than is generally realized.

Which groups of lymph nodes should we consider to be in the second echelon? Metastases in lymph nodes that do not lie between the primary tumor and the periaortic lymphatic drainage suggest the presence of proximal lymphatic obstruction and retrograde flow. For tumors on the lesser curvature of the stomach, lymph node metastases along the greater curvature are second level deposits, and vice versa. However, metastases in lymph nodes at the hilum of the spleen in the presence of an antral tumor could be considered part of the third level of lymph nodes, suggesting that the potential for curative surgery is lost unless the lymph nodes along the superior border of the pancreas and splenic artery are carefully dissected with the specimen. Lymph node metastases at the celiac axis represent the third echelon of lymph nodes, except when the gastric cancer is in the lower esophagus or at the cardioesophageal junction (for which they are only the second echelon of lymphatic defense). For lesser curvature cancers, lymph node metastases along the left gastric artery beyond the immediate vicinity of the tumor must also be considered in the second echelon.

Contiguous invasion of adjacent structures does not define nonresectability but the potential for cure falls significantly when the body and tail of the pancreas, the transverse colon, or the lateral segment of the left lobe of the liver must be removed with the specimen. Apparent contiguous spread often reflects earlier involvement of the peritoneal cavity: the lesser sac may have been penetrated when the tumor has invaded the pancreas; the peritoneal cavity must be crossed for the cancer to invade the left lobe of the liver. Invasion of the transverse mesocolon is almost uniformly associated with peritoneal invasion.

Tumor differentiation is another prognostic factor ignored by most staging systems. As is the case with most cancer patients, patients with poorly differentiated carcinomas tend not to survive as long as those with well-differentiated carcinomas. While patients with linitis plastica and signet ring tumors have long been considered to have a form of poorly differentiated cancer, this may not necessarily be the case. Instead, we may be looking at a totally separate histopathologic phenomenon in which many of these tumors would be considered to be quite well differentiated. Certainly, not every linitis plastica recurs after surgery, particularly when the peritoneum has not been broached.

The ratio of DNA content to total cell mass may also define the more immature cells. Unfortunately, the results of flow cytometry have not, to date, provided a definitive prognostic indicator in this disease.

THE EXTENT OF SURGERY

It has long been recognized that the operative risk for patients undergoing a distal subtotal gastrectomy is considerably less than that of patients treated by total gastrectomy. The difference is largely related to the increased risk of failure of the esophageal anastomosis to heal. Three factors are at the base of this problem. The longitudinal muscular structure of the esophagus, the diminished esophageal submucosa, and the lack of a peritoneal covering offer a reduced hold on sutures which can, at times, be difficult to place precisely. Technically, there is a potential that the jejunal limb may not reach the esophagus easily, limiting the potential of an anastomosis performed without tension on the suture line. Of at least equal importance, but less well recognized, is the fact that the normal blood supply of the lowermost portion of the esophagus comes from the celiac axis via cardial branches of the left gastric artery. At surgery, the left gastric artery is divided at its origin from the celiac axis to allow dissection of the lymphatics. Collateral circulation from above is poor because, in general, the blood supply of the midesophagus follows a circumferential pattern arising in short branches which come directly off the aorta. There is little longitudinal collateral circulation.

For cancers confined to the proximal stomach, a proximal gastrectomy allows a well-vascularized gastric pouch to be brought up into the mediastinum as high as the neck. When one examines 5-year survivals, it would appear that more patients treated by proximal gastrectomy are alive than are patients treated by total gastrectomy. These results do not necessarily imply indictment of the concept of total gastrectomy. Rather, they suggest that the total gastrectomies are generally performed for the patients with larger and more extensive tumors.

Controversies over the management of carcinomas of the proximal stomach and distal esophagus also include questions of the best incision. Many patients are elderly, have been smokers, and have a less than optimal cardiac status. If only a few extra centimeters of esophagus are needed to provide adequate (6-cm) clearance above gross tumor, a sternal split allows exposure to the esophagus to at least the level of the left inferior pulmonary vein, with enough space to allow exposure for performance of the anastomosis. The esophageal resection can be extended a bit higher but the exposure becomes less than optimal. Sternal split (usually angled into the third right interspace) carries minimal morbidity, compared to that of a thoracoabdominal incision. The traditional approach has utilized the left chest. However, the esophagus is not as well visualized from the left side, and the dissection can be carried no higher than the arch of the aorta. Even here, exposure for performance of the anastomosis is suboptimal.

Limitations of the extent of esophagus that can be resected are the major causes for incomplete resection with pathologic findings of tumor at the suture line. Generally, the tumor is in the submucosal lymphatics, emphasizing the importance of resection of at least 6 cm of "normal" esophagus above the uppermost level of the apparent tumor mass. From the right chest, esophageal resection can be extended up to the base of the neck, with an anastomosis constructed to the cervical esophagus, if necessary. Because the exposure of the posterior mediastinum is far superior from the right side, a thorough excision of lymph nodes that may or may not contain metastatic disease is possible from this side. This mediastinal dissection can include the preaortic lymph nodes which, in the case of cancers in the esophagus, are only at the level of the second echelon lymph nodes. Unfortunately, it has yet to be proven that this much more extensive dissection of the mediastinum improves the overall patient survival, even though, logically, it should. Because the long-term survival data developing among patients treated by the abdominocervical approach (which admittedly is not a "cancer operation" in the usual sense) is quite similar to that following the more extensive mediastinal dissections, it is possible that the presence of cancer in the preaortic lymph nodes is an indication of systemic disease.

The significantly poorer national results of surgery for cancers involving the proximal stomach, as compared to those in the distal stomach either suggest that the disease becomes systemic much earlier, or are an indictment of surgical technique.

Most gastrectomies for cancer include removal of the greater and lesser omentum, but generally the nodes along the superior border of the pancreas and the nodes in the celiac axis are left behind. While there is no evidence that resection of nodes in and around the superior mesenteric artery may improve survival, long-term survivals do occur in patients who have had celiac axis dissection and have involvement in one or more of the celiac axis lymph nodes.

The Japanese criteria for the surgery of gastric cancer define surgical resection in three classes: R1, R2 and R3, based on the extent of lymph node resection. Out of these criteria has developed the concept of the "elective" R2 and R3 resection. The concept suggests that patients in whom the last echelon of lymph nodes (N2 or N3) to be removed in their entirety, are free of metastases, when lower echelons (N1 in the case of the R2 dissection and N1 plus N2 in the case of the R3 dissection) contain metastases, have a markedly superior survival, particularly in the absence of peritoneal invasion. A preliminary review from an U.S. adjuvant study would tend to confirm the value of the elective "R2" dissection. Further data from any of the series of patients treated in the United States should establish the efficacy of R2-R3 resection as an elective procedure, confirming Japanese reports of the long-term survival value of extended lymphadenectomy.

Extension of primary gastric cancer into adjacent structures requires resection of the involved organ to preserve the potential for cure. In many cases, the surgeon opts, instead, to shave the tumor off the involved adjacent structure. Although occasionally the stomach is bound by fibrous adhesions to the adjacent structure, biopsy of the residual organ (e.g., pancreas) demonstrates cancer left behind in the vast majority of cases. Thus, when the tumor is shaved off the adjacent organ, cure is unlikely. However, the reduced potential for long-term survival when the adjacent structure must be removed, must be balanced against the added risk of these extended procedures. Once again, there are no hard data from which a definitive answer can be drawn in every case.

THE SPLEEN

Twenty years ago, a radical subtotal gastrectomy for cancer routinely included removal of the spleen. Usually the splenic vessels were ligated at the hilum and the spleen was connected on the specimen to the stomach by omental tissues, the short gastric vessels having been divided to leave a proximal pouch of stomach behind. Conceptually, lymph nodes at the hilum of the spleen were removed at this procedure, but unless the tumor arose along the greater curvature and contiguous with the spleen, these lymph nodes represented the second or third echelons of lymphatic defense. Unfortunately, the lymph nodes along the superior border of the pancreas and along the splenic artery were not removed. Neither were the lymph nodes adjacent to the head of the pancreas or behind the pylorus.

Currently, splenectomy is indicated only when lymph node metastases are detected at the hilum of the spleen, providing that the lymph nodes along the splenic artery are also removed; or for carcinomas of the fundus of the stomach or arising along the greater curvature, situations in which the splenic hilar lymph nodes might be considered first or, at most, second echelon level.

There is no evidence that removal of the spleen improves survival. Indeed, the results of a Japanese study would suggest that splenectomy might be detrimental to survival, although extent of the primary cancer was not considered. However, in Japan, most patients have early-stage cancers. Similar results were noted among patients in the control group of the adjuvant chemotherapy trial of the Gastrointestinal Tumor Study Group (GITSG), but the number of patients involved was too small for firm conclusions. It would take a randomized surgical study (an unlikely event) to establish whether splenectomy was really detrimental.

WHICH PATIENTS ARE CANDIDATES FOR ADJUVANT THERAPY?

Most traditional reports of the long-term outcome of patients treated by resection of gastric cancer have not evaluated survival based on the extent of the tumor. This question was addressed, at least with regard to the presence or absence of lymph node metastases, in the first surgical adjuvant trial of GITSG. For patients whose tumor had extended into the submucosa, muscularis, serosa, or beyond, but who had no lymph node metastases, 5-year survival exceeded 40%. For similar patients treated at Roswell Park, median survival is greater than 7 years. When one compares these results to the published reports from Japan, the differences are smaller than we might have expected.

In GITSG trials, the survival of patients with cancer in the distal stomach has been almost three times as long as that of patients with cancer of the proximal stomach or those in whom total gastrectomy was required. Except for the fact that proximal gastric cancer is still relatively uncommon in Japan, stage for stage the disease and results of its treatment are remarkably alike. To achieve the overall survivals similar to those being reported in Japanese studies, earlier diagnosis and more aggressive therapies will be necessary, including more rigorously defined extirpative procedures and, possibly, adjuvant therapy. Which patients should be considered as candidates for investigative trials of adjuvant therapy following a potentially curative gastric resection? In the absence of a proven treatment for advanced gastric cancer that significantly prolongs survival and includes a large number of objective complete responses (total disappearance of all known tumor), the risks associated with adjuvant therapy exceed the potential benefit for at least one-third of patients.

Candidates for adjuvant therapy include those patients whose cancers must be treated by proximal or total gastrectomy, grossly invade the serosa, or have shed cells into the peritoneum with a positive cytology in the peritoneal fluid. Patients treated by distal gastric resection in whom the second level lymph nodes contain metastases, in whom an "elective R3" resection has not been performed, and those treated by a less than an R2 resection, with any evidence of lymph node metastases, might also be considered for adjuvant therapy.

Patients whose tumors are confined to the gastric wall and have been treated by distal subtotal gastrectomy, with tumor-free margins, and patients in whom at least an R2 dissection was performed, with lymph node metastases confined to the immediate vicinity of the primary tumor, with no invasion of the peritoneum or of adjacent tissues, should not be exposed to adjuvant therapy. Roswell Park data suggest that for patients with one to three positive lymph nodes immediately adjacent to the tumor, treated by an elective R2 dissection, survival is little different from that of patients in whom the nodes are not involved.

Analysis of the results of treatment of patients with locally incurable gastric cancer, of the patterns of relapse in patients who have undergone curative resection, and of the failure of previous trials of surgical adjuvant therapy will lead to suggestions for future adjuvant therapies, including an emphasis on transperitoneal and lymph node metastases.

MANAGEMENT OF LOCALLY INCURABLE GASTRIC CANCER

Over the years, numerous reports have appeared to suggest that patients treated by a palliative resection for gastric cancer survive longer than those who do not. These reports have been unable to evaluate whether the failure to perform palliative resections was related to more advanced disease, and whether, had the resected patients been left with their stomachs intact, survival would have been any shorter. Nevertheless, these data provide a background against which therapies for patients in whom a surgical cure is not possible can be evaluated.

For patients who are treated by a palliative resection, the median survival is approximately 6 months. In patient subsets, such as those in whom the residual disease is a positive margin, or those whose only residual cancer is that left behind after the tumor is shaved off the pancreas, the medial survival may be 12 months or more. Nevertheless, no more than 3% of patients with residual disease can be expected to survive 5 years. Only 10% to 15% survive 2 years.

In 1974, GITSG examined a group of patients with locally unresectable disease, most, but not all, of whom had been treated by palliative resection. By definition, these patients had no distant metastases, in the liver or elsewhere, had no transperitoneal disease except in the immediate area of the stomach, and had no lymph node metastases outside of the upper abdomen. The concept was that all known disease could be encompassed in a radiation field smaller than 20 × 20 cm when visualized on an abdominal x-ray. The treatments involved a randomized comparison of chemotherapy using 5-fluorouracil and methyl-CCNU vs radiation therapy plus 5-fluorouracil followed by the same chemotherapy. Initial results suggested that the radiation therapy component of the combined modality arm had been detrimental to survival. Median survival for the group of patients treated with chemotherapy alone was 70 weeks, whereas the median survival of patients treated with radiation and chemotherapy was only half as long, 36 weeks.

The cause of many of the early deaths among patients with locally unresectable cancer treated by combined modality therapy was thought to be related to the omission of effective nutritional support during a very aggressive treatment program. Results of autopsies suggested that these patients had not died of progressive disease. Rather, death accompanied a clinical picture of marked weight loss, severe vomiting, diarrhea, and hematologic toxicity.

This trial was reanalyzed 4 to 5 years after the last patient had been entered. Among the patients who received combined modality therapy, 18% remained alive, whereas only 6% of those treated by chemotherapy alone survived 4 years or more. It must be remembered that this study was conducted at a time when the published 5-year survival for patients following resection of gastric cancer was approximately 20%. Because the study included only patients with known residual cancer, a therapeutic benefit was suggested. A subsequent study designed to confirm this lead, in which nutritional support was required during the period of aggressive therapy if caloric intake was inadequate, has been completed but awaits analysis.

Nevertheless, this preliminary study would suggest that residual disease in the pancreas, unresected tumor-bearing lymph nodes, and positive margins at the line of resection would be appropriately treated by a combination of radiation and chemotherapy provided that nutritional homeostasis is maintained.

PATTERNS OF FAILURE

As previously noted, gastric cancer spreads by four separate routes: by invasion of adjacent tissues, by metastases through the lymphatics to the lymph nodes, by invasion of tributaries of the portal veins to the liver, and by invasion through the peritoneal lining to distant peritoneal surfaces, including the ovary. While liver metastases are often considered the major cause of death, lymph node metastases and transperitoneal tumor dissemination are actually far more important. Autopsies on 260 patients who had died of metastatic gastric cancer at Roswell Park Memorial Institute, including 73 in whom there was recurrence of gastric cancer following an apparently curative resection, demonstrated that the patterns of metastatic dissemination in patients in whom no resection had been performed were similar to those seen in patients who had undergone a "curative resection" but whose cancer had recurred. There were some overlappings of the metastatic patterns. Generally, ovarian metastases were found in patients with peritoneal invasion, who subsequently would show metastases on other peritoneal surfaces. Patients with venous invasion developed metastases within the body of the liver. Most common were the patients with lymph node metastases, who showed a pattern of spread to lungs, bones, adrenals, and the brain. Patients with lymph node metastases were more likely to have peritoneal invasion and vice versa, whereas patients with liver metastases were more likely to have locally invasive tumors. The distinctiveness of these metastastic patterns could lead to speculation that two to four different tumors were being described. These cases had been drawn from the period before chemotherapy was commonly administered and thus do not reflect changes due to drug effects.

While we have not yet been able to detect a change in patterns of tumor spread associated with various chemotherapeutic regimens, the adjuvant trial of GITSG noted a decrease in the frequency of liver metastases among the patients who received chemotherapy (5-fluorouracil and methyl-CCNU), as compared to the concurrently randomized controls. This finding has been neither confirmed nor refuted by other adjuvant trials using the same drugs. Should this be a true positive result, future studies should be oriented toward other metastatic sites, such as intraperitoneal therapy or fat-soluble or particulate agents that could be taken up in the lymphatics.

WHY HAVE ADJUVANT THERAPIES FAILED?

To be effective in reducing the potential for recurrence, adjuvant therapy programs must have three properties:
1. The agent must reach the area of neoplastic disease.
2. The agent must be effective in killing the malignant cells.
3. The agent must be delivered at a time when the tumor load is at its minimum.

Adjuvant trials in the United States have generally lacked at least two of these prerequisites. For example, the trial of GITSG involved the drugs 5-fluorouracil and methyl-CCNU both of which are weak cytotoxic agents against gastric cancer cells. In addition, 5-fluorouracil has been shown not to penetrate lymph nodes and, when administered intravenously, reached the peritoneal cavity only in extremely low concentrations. Fewer data are available for the distribution of the nitrosourea, methyl-CCNU, an even less cytotoxic agent than 5-fluorouracil. In addition, treatment was usually begun at or near the end of the 6-week postoperative eligibility period, when one would expect the residual tumor mass to have at least doubled.

In contrast, the early Japanese trials used mitomycin C, often delivered intraperitoneally, usually on day of surgery and in the immediate postoperative period. Mitomycin C was supplemented by a fluorinated pyrimidine, but the entire course of chemotherapy was often completed by the time the patient left the hospital. These differences alone may be responsible for the apparent benefit of adjuvant therapy in Japanese trials. Mitomycin C, a modestly active cytotoxic agent against gastric cancer, was delivered to a major site of the cancer spread, the peritoneum, at a time when the residual cancer load was at its minimum, the immediate postoperative period.

Pilot trials of interest include the intraperitoneal administration of mitomycin C attached to activated charcoal, which provides a particulate substrate to be taken up through the lymphatics, and the intraperitoneal administration of fat-soluble immunostimulants (whose efficacy is unproven) which are absorbed into the lymphatics, thus ensuring delivery to major sites of potential residual tumor.

A proposed pilot trial in the United States would attempt to at least partially satisfy the requirements for effective therapy listed above. Intraperitoneal chemotherapy on the day of surgery and in the immediate postoperative period using mitomycin C and leukovorin-modulated 5-fluorouracil should provide at least a modicum of cytotoxic activity delivered to one major site of dissemination at the time when the tumor burden is at its lowest.

IMPROVING THE RESULTS OF CHEMOTHERAPY IN ADVANCED DISEASE

The problems faced in designing treatment programs for patients with advanced gastric cancer differ little from those for patients in whom a potentially curative resection has been performed. Major questions remain. Is "gastric cancer" one or several cancers? If more than one, how do these tumors differ in their responsiveness to cytotoxic agents? In the absence of more effective drugs, will modulating agents improve the efficacy of our current, very modest armamentarium? Should we not deliver antineoplastic therapy in a way to acheive significant drug concentration at the site of tumor?

Surgeons have long known that various gastric cancers behave differently. The prognosis of a patient with a fungating lesion on the greater curvature of the stomach is better than that of one with an ulcerating lesion on the lesser curvature. The prognosis for both was far better than that of a patient with an infiltrating carcinoma occupying most of the stomach wall and giving a "leather bottle" appearance to the organ. Pathologically, intestinal carcinoma most commonly occurs in polypoid lesions and on the greater curvature in patients whose normal mucosa shows intestinal metaplasia. Diffuse carcinoma typifies the poorer prognosis of linitis plastica. This pathologic classification of Lauren varied little from that of Mulligan and Rember who added a pylorocardial variant which frequently was an ulcerated lesion most commonly occurring along the lesser curavature. Do these represent three different cell types, three different cells of origin? When one considers the gastrin-secreting glands of the antrum, the acid- and pepsin-secreting glands of the body and fundus, and the mucus-secreting glands found diffusely throughout the organ, the possibility that these patterns of gross and microscopic pathology evolve into different patterns of disease dissemination and drug resistance cannot be overlooked. They must be tested as part of the design of future chemotherapy trials.

The relative cytotoxic inefficiency mandates the development of innovative approaches, with less reliance on the combination of 5-fluorouracil, Adriamycin, and mitomycin C. While this three-drug combination caused objective partial regressions of cancers in nearly 40% of patients with advanced disease, complete responses have been seen infrequently, and survival has not been prolonged. The apparent positive results in the initial trials of 5-fluorouracil and methyl-CCNU have not been confirmed. As adjuvant therapy, only one trial demonstrated benefit—that apparently confined to blood-borne metastases.

Recent studies have suggested a role for platinum and the nonpolyglutamating antifols such as triazinate. Pharmacologic modulation of fluorouracil by leucovorin has, in at least one study, improved the response rate over that expected from 5-fluorouracil alone. Most of the effective agents, the exception being doxorubicin (Adriamycin), appear to be potential modulators of 5-fluorouracil, in addition to their intrinsic cytotoxic potential. Thus, a modulating program might include nonpolyglutamating antifol preceding 5-fluorouracil, accompanied by cisplatin or a platinum analogue, which itself might be modulated by VP-16 (etoposide). The place of leucovorin would depend on whether it alters the cytotoxicity of the nonpolyglutamating antifol. A variation in need of confirmation is the combination of cisplatin, doxorubricin, and VP-16 reported from Germany. Eventually, five or six drug combinations, in which each agent not only has cytotoxic activity but also the potential to modulate the other component drugs (one might add doxorubicin as a noncross resistant agent or as a radiation potentiator), may impact on response and survival in a manner similar to the multiagent treatment of lymphoma. Long-acting drugs such as mitomycin C and the nitrosoureas may prove too toxic for repeated treatment, although the role of mitomycin C may be preserved by its value as an intraperitoneal cytotoxic.

Delivery of drugs to the site of the cancer has received insufficient attention. Intraperitoneal drug delivery can be effective treatment for microscopic disease and for tumor nodules with a diameter of 5 mm or less. For larger implants, drugs must be delivered systemically. It is likely that high concentration of the drug delivered intraperitoneally with resulting low systemic concentrations should be supplemented by additional drug given intravenously. Because intravenously administered drug results in low drug concentrations in the lymphatics, lymph node metastases require that a fat-soluble agent (such as nonpolyglutamating antifols) or a particulate agent (such as mitomycin C bound to charcoal) be administered by a route that will guarantee lymphatic drug delivery. Drugs bound in lipid microspheres would have theoretical advantages. An alternative would be an agent that could be administered orally and have reliable lymphatic absorption.

The Japanese enthusiasm for immunologic enhancing agents, while based in part on their minimal toxicity, suggests activity in these usually fat-soluble biologics. Intraperitoneal delivery of agents such as muramyl tripeptide (the active ingredient of Freund's adjuvant) should be assessed. Monoclonal antibodies of varying molecular weights attached to either radioactive or chemotoxic agents must be evaluated in terms of delivery of the antibody to the tumor and efficacy of the carried antineoplastic. Patients with malignant ascites may be ideal candidates for initial study of these agents because malignant cells are readily available.

SUMMARY

There can be little question that a new technique for earlier diagnosis of gastric cancer could significantly enhance the potential for cure. Improved comprehension of the carcinogenic process is a prerequisite for any screening test when the population at risk is poorly understood. As a result we must turn our clinical efforts toward a better understanding of the pathophysiology of gastric cancer to evaluate the long-known variations in growth patterns and histologies whose clinical significance is still unknown.

Aggressive studies of the modulating potential of various agents to enhance or alter cytotoxicity will require a series of carefully orchestrated phase I and phase II trials, examining the interrelationship of known potentially cytotoxic drugs, eventually leading to optimizing surface response studies. Ultimately gastric cancer will require an interdigitation of chemotherapeutic and immunologic agents combined with radiotherapy (which may be intraoperative or involve isotopes carried by single or combinations of monoclonal antibodies). The future role of surgery may change dramatically: effective drugs would be administered preoperatively, surgery serving to clean up residual disease and decrease the numbers of malignant cells to reduce the potential that postoperative therapy would be hampered by large numbers of drug-resistant cellular clones.

This chapter has examined reasons why gastric cancer can be considered a "difficult problem in gastroenterology." More questions have been raised than answered. A number of hypotheses have been offered to explain current treatment failures. It is hoped that the challenge of these hypotheses may stimulate a search for information that would remove gastric cancer from the "difficult problem" category.

Bibliography

1. Barrett NR: The lower esophagus lined by columnar epithelium. *Surgery* 1957; 41:881–894.
2. Charbit A, Malaise E, Tubiana M: Relation between the pathologic nature and the growth rate of human tumors. *Eur J Cancer* 1971; 7:307–315.
3. Douglass HO Jr, Lavin PT, Goudsmit A, et al: An Eastern Cooperative Oncology Group evaluation of combinations of methyl-CCNU, mitomycin C, Adriamycin, and 5-fluorouracil in advanced measurable gastric cancer (EST 2277). *J Clin Oncol* 1984; 2:1372–1381.
4. Douglass HO Jr, Nava HR: Gastric adenocarcinoma—Management of the primary disease. *Semin Oncol* 1985; 12:32–45.
5. Douglass HO Jr: Gastric cancer: Overview of current therapies. *Semin Oncol* 1985; 12(suppl 4):57–62.
6. Gastrointestinal Tumor Study Group: Controlled trial of adjuvant chemotherapy following curative resection for gastric cancer. *Cancer* 1982; 49:1116–1122.
7. Gastrointestinal Tumor Study Group: A comparison of combination chemotherapy with combined modality therapy for locally advanced gastric cancer. *Cancer* 1982; 49;1771–1777.
8. Goldie JH, Coldman AJ: The genetic origin of drug resistance in neoplasms. Implications for systemic therapy. *Cancer Res* 1984; 44:3643–3653.
9. Japanese Research Society for Gastric Cancer: The general rules for the gastric cancer study in surgery and pathology: Part I. Clinical classification. *Jpn J Surg* 1981; 11:127–139.
10. Lauren P: The two main histologic types of gastric carcinoma: Diffuse and so-called intestinal-type carcinoma. *Acta Pathol Microbiol Scand* 1965; 64:31–49.
11. Machover D, Goldschmidt E, Schwarzenberg L, et al: Treatment of advanced colorectal and gastric adenocarcinomas with 5-fluorouracil combined with high-dose leucovorin: An update, in Bruckner HW, Rustum YB (eds): *Advances in Cancer Chemotherapy. The Current Status of 5-Fluorouracil-Leucovorin Calcium Combination.* New York, Park Row, 1984, pp 55–64.
12. Mulligan RM, Rember RH: Histogenesis and biologic behavior of gastric carcinoma. *Arch Pathol* 1954; 58:1–25.
13. Nakajima T, Harashima S, Hirata M, et al: Prognostic and therapeutic values of peritoneal cytology in gastric cancer. *Acta Cytol* 1978; 22:225–229.
14. Nakajima T, Mitsumasa N: Adjuvant chemotherapy, immunochemotherapy and neoadjuvant therapy for gastric cancer in Japan, in Douglass HO Jr (ed): *Contemporary Issues in Clinical Oncology. Gastric Cancer.* New York, Churchill Livingstone, 1987, pp 125–143.
15. Oi M, Oshida K, Sugimura S: The location of gastric ulcer. *Gastroenterology* 1959; 36:45–64.
16. Paull A, Trier JS, Dalton D, et al: The histologic spectrum of Barrett's esophagus. *N Engl J Med* 1976; 295:476–480.
17. Preusser P, Wilke H, Achterrath W, et al: Advanced gastric carcinoma: A phase II study with etoposide (E), Adriamycin (A) and split course platinum (P) = EAP. *Proc Am Soc Clin Oncol* 1987; 6:(292)75.
18. Sarr MG, Hamilton SR, Marrone CG, et al: Barrett's esophagus: Its prevalence and association with adenocarcinoma in patients with symptoms

of gastroesophageal reflux. *Am J Surg* 1985; 149:187–193.
19. Skinner DS, Walther BC, Riddell RH, et al: Barrett's esophagus: Comparison of benign and malignant cases. *Ann Surg* 1983; 198:554–566.
20. Spechler SJ, Goyal RK: Barrett's esophagus. *N Engl J Med* 1986; 315:362–371.
21. Speyer JL, Sugarbaker PH, Collins JM, et al: Portal levels and hepatic clearance of 5-fluorouracil after intraperitoneal administration in humans. *Cancer Res* 1981; 41:1916–1922.
22. Stemmerman G, Hayashi T: The pathology of gastric cancer, in Douglass HO Jr (ed): *Contemporary Issues in Clinical Oncology. Gastric Cancer.* New York, Churchill Livingstone, 1987, pp 55–86.
23. Tubiana M, Malaise EP: Growth rate and cell kinetics in human tumours: Some prognostic and therapeutic implications, in Symington T, Carter RL (eds): *Scientific Foundations of Oncology.* Chicago, Year Book Medical Publishers, 1976, pp 126–136.
24. Witt TR, Bains MS, Zaman MB, et al: Adenocarcinoma in Barrett's esophagus. *J Thorac Cardiovasc Surg* 1983; 85:337–345.
25. Yamada K, Murphy GP, Douglass HO Jr: Comparison of intramural 5-fluorouracil and more conventional routes of drug administration on concentrations in gastric regional lymph nodes: A potential for trans-endoscopic adjuvant chemotherapy. *J Surg Oncol* 1979; 11:341–349.

III

Pancreas

12

Acute Pancreatitis:
When should slow resolution be cause for concern?
What is appropriate therapy for fulminant pancreatitis?

A

The gastroenterologist's view: FRANK BROOKS, M.D.

A clinical discussion of acute pancreatitis is certain to be limited in satisfying the needs of physicians caring for such patients because of the nature of the disease. First, there is no "gold standard" for the diagnosis. A histologic diagnosis would be most helpful, but this is available in only a minority of patients. The shortcomings of a clinical diagnosis are evident in the relatively high percentage of patients with fatal acute pancreatitis in whom the diagnosis was not suspected until laparotomy or autopsy. No laboratory tests are specific for acute pancreatitis.

Second, acute pancreatitis includes a spectrum of clinical illness and pathologic changes that vary from a mild illness characterized by abdominal pain and edema to an acute fatal illness with shock, renal failure, acute respiratory failure, and sepsis. The latter is less common but represents a severe challenge to the physicians and surgeons caring for them.

Third, acute pancreatitis can be the result of a variety of etiologic factors. Gallstone pancreatitis occurs in older patients and especially in women. In many inner-city hospitals, acute pancreatitis is attributed primarily to alcohol abuse in middle-aged men. However, many of these patients have had previous attacks of "acute pancreatitis" and indeed some students of pancreatitis believe that pancreatitis is a chronic disease in the alcoholic when first recognized. It is certainly true that many attacks of recurring acute pancreatitis in alcoholics subside within a few days with rest, analgesics, and abstinence.

Fourth, the last decade has witnessed a major effort, particularly by surgeons, to devise clinical and laboratory criteria to enable the physicians caring for these patients to stratify them in relation to their subsequent clinical course within 48 hours of admission and also after the first week. While a number of criteria have been identified, particularly after the first week, that separate those patients with severe pancreatitis, a relatively high percentage of patients with these same criteria will follow the course of mild to moderate pancreatitis.

Fifth and finally, it has not been possible in controlled clinical trials to demonstrate a clear-cut therapeutic efficacy of specific medical and surgical treatments of acute pancreatitis. This is the result of the wide spectrum of disease, the relatively small number of patients with severe acute pancreatitis seen in any one unit, and the shift in the nature of life-threatening complications between the first week (shock, renal failure, and acute respiratory failure) and the second week (sepsis). Nevertheless it seems likely that we are seeing more patients survive prolonged courses of severe acute pancreatitis than we did formerly.

THE CLINICAL DIAGNOSIS OF ACUTE PANCREATITIS

I have come to the conclusion that the most important factor in making the diagnosis of acute pancreatitis is a high index of suspicion. Most patients will present with abdominal pain, usually epigastric in origin. The onset occurs over hours; the pain is steady and lasts days rather than hours. Localizing physical signs are not prominent. However, the patient in shock, coma, or acute alcoholic intoxication may not complain of pain. Questions to identify risk factors are important[1] (see Table 12A–1). A previous history of attacks of acute pancreatitis in a middle-aged man with a history of years of excessive alcohol intake suggests the diagnosis of recurrent acute episodes in a patient with chronic alcoholic pancreatitis.

The presence of clinical jaundice suggests gallstone pancreatitis. Typical pain in a young woman with no history of alcohol abuse is consistent with familial pancreatitis. The presence of hyperlipidemia should be explored. Nonpenetrating abdominal trauma in a motor vehicle accident may lead to traumatic pancreatitis. Increasingly patients are being reported in whom medications are being identified as cause of acute pancreatitis; the medications include thiazide diuretics, azathioprine, and corticosteroids. The incidence of mild pain and hyperamylasemia after endoscopic retrograde cholangiopancreatography (ERCP) is high but fortunately clinical pancreatitis is uncommon. However, severe acute pancreatitis can occur. Hypercalcemia due to hyperparathyroidism or to parenteral alimentation may lead to acute pancreatitis. Postoperative acute pancreatitis is seen in patients undergoing surgery in the upper abdomen. Infectious pancreatitis is rare but the possibility of mumps pancreatitis must be kept in mind. Crohn's disease of the duodenum carries a risk of acute pancreatitis.

The association of hyperlipemia with acute pancreatitis is important, especially because the serum amylase may be normal. The mechanism by which hyperlipemia leads to pancreatitis is still unknown. A small percentage of patients with carcinoma of the pancreas may present with a syndrome of acute pancreatitis, but the underlying carcinoma soon makes itself evident.

THE PHYSICAL EXAMINATION IN ACUTE PANCREATITIS[2]

There are a few findings on physical examination that are virtually pathogno-

---

TABLE 12A–1.
Risk Factors for Acute Pancreatitis

Alcohol abuse
Gallstones
Familial pancreatitis: Hyperlipidemia
Nonpenetrating abdominal trauma
Drugs
ERCP
Hypercalcemia
Postsurgical pancreatitis—especially gastric, duodenal, and biliary tract surgery
Infectious pancreatitis
Crohn's disease of the duodenum
Hyperlipidemia
Carcinoma of the pancreas

monic of acute pancreatitis, for instance, such as ecchymoses of the flank (Grey Turner's sign), ecchymoses around the umbilicus (Cullen's sign), and multiple subcutaneous nodules of fat necrosis[2]. However, they occur so infrequently as to have little diagnostic value. On the other hand, findings of boardlike abdominal rigidity and decreased liver dullness and rapid progression of signs of an abdominal catastrophe favor the diagnosis of a ruptured viscus such as a perforated ulcer. Varying degrees of ileus are common, but colicky pain with high-pitched peristaltic sounds favor intestinal obstruction. Right upper-quadrant pain and jaundice may be due to both cholangitis due to stone and accompanying pancreatitis. Uppermost in the examiner's mind must be the determination not to overlook the diagnosis of a disorder that requires prompt laparotomy for diagnosis and successful treatment. Perhaps the most important course of action is frequent careful unhurried examination of the abdomen by the same examiners. Particularly unfortunate is the discharge from the emergency room with diagnosis of gastroenteritis only to have the patient brought back in extremis with acute hemorrhagic pancreatitis. For those patients with pain but less severe systemic signs, the major guide to the diagnosis is a high index of suspicion coupled with the presence of risk factors.

THE LABORATORY IN THE DIAGNOSIS OF ACUTE PANCREATITIS[3]

As noted earlier no laboratory tests are specific for acute pancreatitis.[3] Nevertheless, an elevated serum amylase has been the laboratory hallmark of pancreatitis. It is well-known that the percentage of patients with elevated amylase values will be higher if performed within 24 to 48 hours than later. The degree of elevation is also important in that values five to six times normal are more likely to represent acute pancreatitis, especially gallstone pancreatitis, than other types of abdominal catastrophes. However, it is clear that the correlation between the degree of elevation of amylase and the severity of the pancreatitis is poor. Persistent elevation of the serum amylase after a week or more suggests the presence of complications such as a pseudocyst or phlegmon.

Urinary amylase or amylase-creatinine clearance ratios are of little value in patients with normal serum values and are helpful mainly in the detection of macroamylase in those with elevated values. We now know that in normal sera there are two main isoamylases: a pancreatic and a salivary amylase. What is not yet clear is in how many patients with pancreatitis is the elevation of true pancreatic amylase masked by changes in the salivary amylase. Failures with the popular method using an inhibitor of salivary amylase have been reported.

There is also a variety of new methods for determining serum lipase, elastase, trypsin, phospholipase, and others. There is no proven advantage of one over others, but it is wise to use one other enzyme test where local experience is extensive as a check on the serum amylase.

Other laboratory procedures will be considered in the determination of prognosis and the presence of complications. X-ray films of the abdomen, including the diaphragm to check for free air indicating a perforated viscus, should be done early after admission. A left pleural effusion is common. Discovery of pancreatic calcification is indicative of chronic pancreatitis and favors recurrent acute exacerbations.

PREDICTING THE CLINICAL COURSE OF ACUTE PANCREATITIS

As indicated already, the diagnosis of acute pancreatitis, while important in accounting for the patient's symptoms and in avoiding risk factors for recurrence, is often of little help in identifying effective therapy. Many studies of mild-to-moderately-severe pancreatitis have been performed under randomized controlled conditions with nasogastric suction, glucagon, trypsin inhibitors, antibiotics, and anticholinergics without being able to distinguish between the agents and placebo. Almost all patients improved. Therefore it is of great importance to identify patients with severe pancreatitis and complications as soon as possible and to be able to predict those patients at great risk to develop these complications as the disease evolves. The data on the course of acute pancreatitis are conflicting. Part of this stems from the fact that surgeons tend to see the more severe cases of pancreatitis while internists and gastroenterologists see many patients with acute exacerbations of chronic alcoholic pancreatitis, which subside spontaneously in a few days. Therefore the frequency of severe acute pancreatitis and its mortality vary. However it is safe to say that the incidence is relatively low and the mortality is as high as 50%.

The terms acute hemorrhagic pancreatitis and acute necrotic pancreatitis are used synonymously with severe acute pancreatitis, while edematous pancreatitis is equated with mild acute pancreatitis. However these terms can only be confirmed by surgical exploration or perhaps in some patients by computerized axial tomography (CAT) scans. An increase in serum methemalbuminemia is not specific for acute pancreatitis.[4]

Criteria have been tested statistically in retrospective and prospective studies for their value in identifying patients with severe acute pancreatitis. Three such systems are listed in Table 12A–2.[5-7] Two depend on laboratory criteria and one on clinical criteria. When these criteria were tested by workers other than their originators, it was found that 94% to 100% of patients with severe acute pancreatitis met one or more of the criteria. However, only 30% to 35% of all patients meeting such criteria had severe pancreatitis.[8] In another report relying on CT scans,[9] the sensitivity was 75% to 81%, and the specificity was 57% to 75%. Prognostic indices were more reliable after 7 days than within the first 48 hours.[10]

It should be pointed out that most patients with acute pancreatitis do not develop recurrent attacks. Only 2% developed chronic pancreatitis in one study.[11] Sarles believes that chronic pancreatitis is not a sequel to acute pancreatitis.[11] The causes of death in acute pancreatitis are primarily related to the complications of the disease.[12]

COMPLICATIONS OF ACUTE PANCREATITIS

Most patients with severe acute pancreatitis follow a course in which shock, adult respiratory disease syndrome, acute renal failure, acute necrosis of the colon, and severe ileus or intestinal obstruction develop within the first week after the onset of the disease, while sepsis, pancreatic infection and abscess, and pseudocysts develop during the second and third weeks. However, a minority of patients will develop sepsis in the first week.[13]

Shock results primarily from a loss of fluid and protein into the bed of the pancreas in a fashion analogous to that of a severe burn. The importance of a myocardial depressant factor has not been confirmed. Development of the adult respiratory disease syndrome must be suspected when dyspnea and tachycardia occur and are confirmed by obtaining blood gases. Chest x-ray may show only atelectasis.

Acute renal failure is characterized by oliguria and a rising blood urea nitrogen (BUN). Hydration and repeated determination of serum electrolytes must be pursued vigorously. Acute necrosis of the colon and fistula formation may follow spread of the necrotic tissue high in proteolytic enzymes from the bed of the pancreas. Ileus is almost always present to some degree in severe acute pancreatitis, but gastric outlet or intestinal obstruction may develop.

Sepsis is the result of infection usually by enteric organisms of necrotic pancreatic tissue. Pus containing many white blood cells and confined within a fibrous wall is accepted as a pancreatic abscess. However, other patients may have an inflammatory mass with necrotic tissue from which bacteria may be cultured but without the presence of polymorphonuclear leukocytes or an abscess wall.[14] In others, cultures may be negative. The term pancreatic phlegmon may include both of the latter groups.[15] A pseudocyst is a cystic structure connecting with the pancreatic ducts but lined with inflammatory cells rather than epithelium. They may be single or multiple. Larger ones may be palpated as abdominal masses.

TABLE 12A–2.
Prognostic Criteria for Mild versus Severe Acute Pancreatitis*

On Admission	During or at 48 Hours After Admission
Data from Ranson[5] Age over 55 years White blood cell count greater than 16,000/mm^3 Blood glucose greater than 200 mg/dl Serum lactic dehydrogenase greater than 350 IU/L SGOT greater than 250 IU/L	*Data from Ranson*[5] Fall in hematocrit greater than 10% Rise in BUN greater than 5 mg/dl Serum calcium less than 8 mg/dl Arterial Po_2 less than 60 mm Hg Base deficit greater than 4 mEq/L Estimated fluid sequestration greater than 6,000 ml
	Data from Blamey et al.[6] Age greater than 55 years White blood cell count greater than 15,000/mm^3 Blood glucose greater than 175 mg/dl BUN greater than 42 mg/dl Arterial Po_2 less than 60 mm Hg Serum calcium less than 8.0 mg/dl Serum albumin less than 3.2 gm/dl Serum lactic dehydrogenase greater than 600 IU/L Serum oxalocetic or pyruvic Transaminase greater than 100 IU/L
	Data from Bank et al.[7] Cardiac: Shock, tachycardia greater than 130/min, arrhythmias, ECG changes Pulmonary: Dyspnea, rales, arterial Po_2 less than 50 mm Hg, adult respiratory distress syndrome Renal: Urine output less than 50 ml/hr rising BUN or serum creatinine Metabolic: Low or falling serum calcium, pH or albumin Hematologic: Falling hematocrit or disseminated intravascular coagulation Neurologic: Irritability, confusion Hemorrhage: Bloody peritoneal tap Tense abdominal distention: Ileus, moderate to severe ascites

*Data from Ranson JHC: Acute pancreatitis: Survival management, in Go VLW, Gardner D, Brooks FP, et al (eds): *The Exocrine Pancreas.* New York, Raven Press, 1986, pp 503–512; Blamey SL, Imrie CW, O'Neill J, et al: Prognostic factors in acute pancreatitis. *Gut* 1984; 25:1340–1346; and Bank S, Wise L, Gersten M: Risk factors in acute pancreatitis. *Am J Gastroenterol* 1983; 78:637–640.

Characteristically these patients continue to run a fever and maintain an elevated serum amylase. The cyst fluid contains a solution with a high amylase concentration. Some pseudocysts and pancreatic phlegmons resolve spontaneously over 4 to 6 weeks, but pseudocysts persisting longer or increasing in size are unlikely to do so.[16]

IMAGING IN ACUTE PANCREATITIS

CAT scan and ultrasound examinations have become important aids in diagnosing and in predicting the patients who will develop severe acute pancreatitis. The presence of paralytic ileus in acute pancreatitis limits the usefulness of ultrasound in determining the contour and consistency of the pancreas, but it can identify the presence of gallstones in the gall bladder. Unfortunately gallstones contributing to acute pancreatitis must enter the common bile duct. Stones could be identified in the feces of patients with gallstone pancreatitis. Such stones can be missed by ultrasound. In the diagnosis of pancreatic pseudocysts, ultrasound examination is the procedure of choice to detect the cystic character of the lesion.

The CAT scan is the most important imaging procedure to confirm the presence of an abnormal pancreas and detect the spread of necrosis and edema to adjacent structures. Enlargement of the pancreas, changes in density, and involvement of adjacent structures can be detected in the majority of patients (90% of necrotic pancreatitis and 79% of interstitial pancreatitis).[17] However, when the CAT scan was performed on admission and an abnormal pancreas was identified, 13% returned to normal within a week and 46% after 6 weeks.[18] So the CAT scan, like the prognostic criteria, identifies patients at risk for severe pancreatitis but also includes patients who eventually will be classified as having mild-to-moderate pancreatitis. However the CAT scan does add an objective measure of pancreatic disease and when used serially to follow patients will detect those who develop pancreatic abscess.

TREATMENT OF ACUTE PANCREATITIS

Treatment will depend on the severity of the pancreatitis, its etiology, and the presence of complications. For the internist this means that the mild attack of acute pancreatitis in the alcoholic may require only abstinence although this is notoriously difficult to achieve. The patient with acute gallstone pancreatitis may require surgical drainage of the common bile duct. In poor surgical risks, endoscopic sphincterotomy and extraction of any stones have been suggested. Drugs suspected of causing pancreatitis should be avoided, and hypercalcemia should be controlled.

The internist should be particularly alert to detect the adult respiratory syndrome, acute renal failure, and sepsis. For the first, blood gases are necessary and some authorities advise placement of a Swan-Ganz catheter. Vigorous measures of pulmonary toilet are indicated. Antibiotics are logically of value only in the presence of sepsis or infection or to prevent such complications in patients at high risk. Nasogastric suction is a traditional method of relieving pain. Demerol is preferred to morphine because of the actions of the latter on the biliary tree and its potential exacerbation of an ileus, but morphine may be needed to control the pain. Celiac ganglion block has its advocates for the relief of pain. In many units it is standard practice to follow patients with severe acute pancreatitis with a team consisting of both internists and surgeons. Once sepsis or necrosis involving the wall of the colon is suspected, the surgeon will have to intervene with a laparotomy. The value of peritoneal lavage early in the course of the disease is controversial,[19] indeed there are no controlled trials to indicate the value of medical or surgical measures in severe acute pancreatitis. However, the use of logical methods has been associated with recovery and in my opinion deserves continued practice until data from controlled trials become available.[20, 21]

Three representative case studies of patients with severe acute pancreatitis representing my personal experience with this disease over the last 8 years follow:

CASE STUDY NO. 1

A 73-year-old woman was admitted to the Hospital of the University of Pennsylvania (HUP) as a transfer patient from another hospital. Five days before admission to HUP she had an ERCP performed because of a suspicion of biliary tract disease. She developed severe abdominal pain and a serum amylase of 2000. Serum lipase was 500. Her white blood cell count rose to 12,000/mm.[3] Over the next few days she developed ecchymosis in the flank, her serum bilirubin rose to 5.2 mg/dl, and her serum glutamic oxaloacetic transaminase (SGOT) was 130 I U/L. Her serum calcium was 8.3 mg/dl. She became dyspneic and her resting P_{O_2} was found to be 34 mm Hg. She was transferred with a diagnosis of acute hemorrhagic pancreatitis and adult respiratory distress syndrome.

On admission to HUP she was writhing in bed with a temperature of 99.6 F, pulse of 104, and respiration of 26/minute. There were dry rales in the chest. Her skin was dry. She was diffusely tender in the right upper quadrant. The abdomen was distended and tympanitic with reduced peristaltic sounds. Initial laboratory tests showed a hemoglobin of 11.1 gm/100 ml, hematocrit 34%, white blood cell count of 16,600/mm^3.

Her blood glucose was 1.58 mg/dl, serum amylase 122 u/dl, serum creatinine 1.6 mg/dl, serum calcium 8.3 mg/dl, serum bilirubin 5.4 mg/dl, alanine aminotransferose (ALT) 45 U/L, aspartate aminotransferase (AST) 96 U/L, serum potassium 2.9 mEq/L. Chest x-ray showed patchy atelectasis. Her arterial P_{O_2} was 75 mm Hg while breathing room air. A CAT scan 2 days after admission showed diffuse enlargement of the pancreas with mottled density, peripancreatic edema, and extension of fluid into the paracolic gutters (Fig 12A–1). She was treated for acute respiratory disease syndrome ARDS and acute pancreatitis and placed on intravenous alimentation. At times she was confused and combative. Slowly she improved and was able to leave the hospital after 1 month. A CAT scan 30 months later showed much improvement (Fig 12A–2). Final diagnosis was acute hemorrhagic pancreatitis secondary to an ERCP.

CASE STUDY NO. 2

A 55-year-old white man was admitted to HUP as a transfer from another hospital where he had been admitted with a diagnosis of gallstones. Three weeks before admission to HUP he had a cholecystectomy and common duct exploration for gallstones. Two days

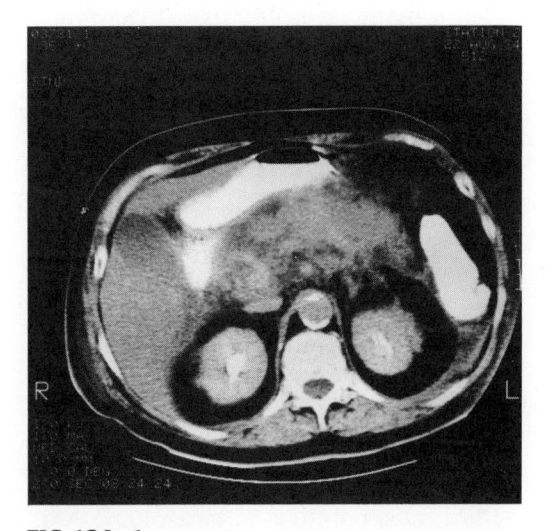

FIG 12A–1.
Case Study No. 1: Cat scan showing severe acute pancreatitis with enlargement of the pancreas, mottled density, and peripancreatic fluid. There is fluid in both paracolic gutters.

later his white blood cell count rose to 22,900/mm$_3$ ascites was noted, and an ultrasound examination showed a cystic mass in the pancreas.

Upon admission to HUP he was found to be hypotensive, to have a tachycardia with a rate of 130/minute

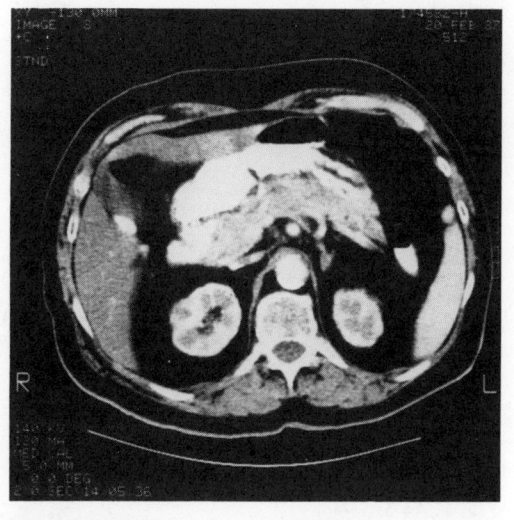

FIG 12A–2.
Case Study No. 1: A CAT scan 30 months later showing much improvement. At this time the patient had no symptoms of pancreatitis.

and a temperature of 100°F. There was a mass in the epigastrium. Laboratory studies showed a hemoglobin of 10.8 gm/dl, white blood cell count of 16,000/mm with 85% neutrophils, a serum calcium of 8.1 mg/dl, serum bilirubin 3.6 mg/dl, serum amylase 1080 IU/L, alkaline phosphatase 365 U/L, SGOT 25 U/L, serum glutamic pyruvic transaminase (SGPT) 45 U/L, and serum lipase 5.4 U/L. Chest x-ray showed a left pleural effusion. He developed melena and on endoscopy was found to have an acute superficial gastric ulcer. The pleural fluid had an amylase concentration of 249 units.

He gradually worsened and on the third hospital day a laparotomy was performed. A large peripancreatic abscess was found, and 2500 ml of pus were removed. Drains were placed in the pancreas. CAT scan of the pancreas showed acute necrotic pancreatitis. Two months later a cutaneous fistula draining the pancreatic duct, stomach, and colon was demonstrated on x-ray (Fig 12A–3). Culture of the pancreatic fluid grew out *Pseudomonas aeruginosa*. The patient was maintained on intravenous alimentation for 3 months before he was able to tolerate oral feedings. He gradually improved and was discharged 3 months after admission.

Six months later he developed epigastric pain and a large pancreatic mass, which on ultrasound proved to be a large pancreatic pseudocyst (Figs 12A–4 and 12A–5). A cystogastrostomy was performed and the patient recovered uneventfully. He has been free of recurrent pancreatitis for 7 years. The final diagnosis was severe acute necrotic pancreatitis with an abscess and later a pseudocyst following cholecystectomy for gallstones. There was no history of alcohol abuse.

CASE STUDY NO. 3

A 30-year-old white man was admitted to HUP as a transfer from another hospital. He had been admitted 3 days before with epigastric pain. There was a history of a similar attack of acute pancreatitis 5 years earlier. There was no history of alcohol abuse. On admission to HUP he was found to have a hard tender abdomen which was distended. Bowel sounds were reduced. Laboratory studies showed a serum amylase of 950 IU/L, a calcium of 6.6 mg/dl, a blood glucose of 232 mg/dl, and a BUN of 14 mg/dl. He had an arterial P_{O_2} at rest of 54 mm Hg. His condition deteri-

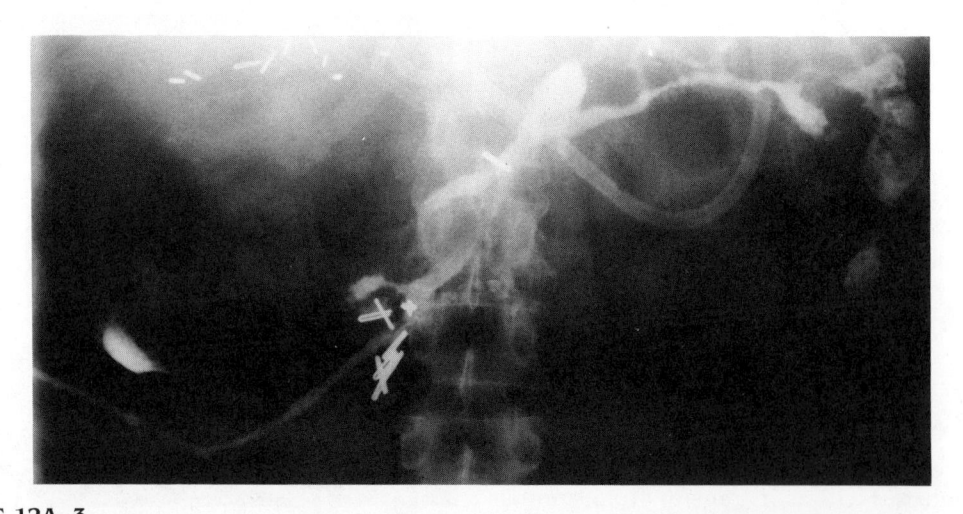

FIG 12A–3.
Case Study No. 2: Roentgenogram of the upper abdomen after the injection of contrast medium through a cutaneous fistula. Contrast material can be seen flowing into the pancreatic duct, the stomach, and the colon 2 months after the onset of acute pancreatitis.

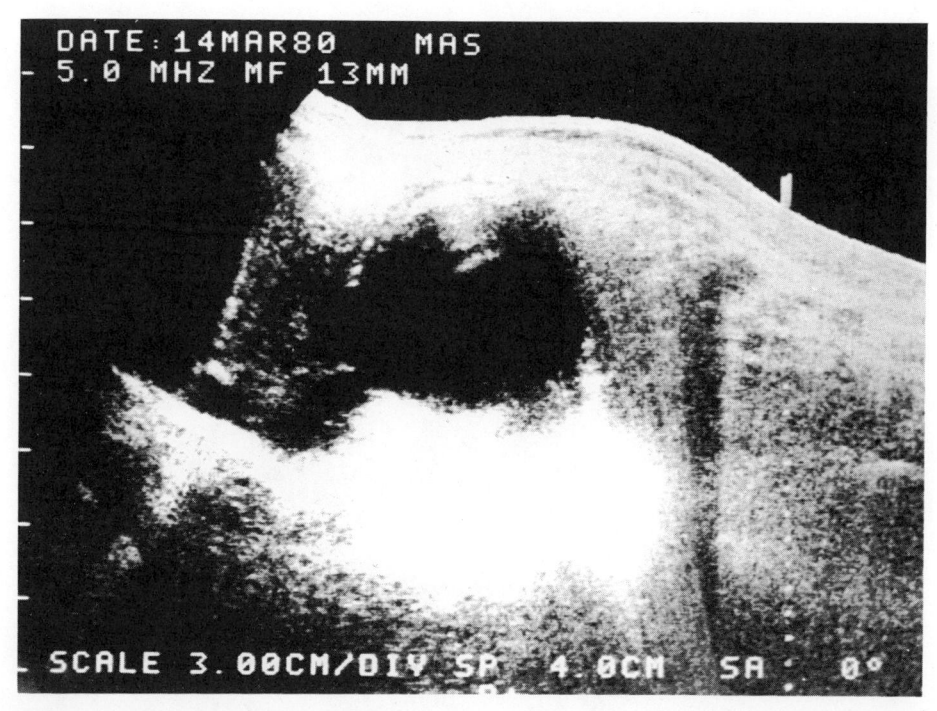

FIG 12A–4.
Case Study No. 2: Ultrasonogram showing a 15-cm pancreatic pseudocyst in the longitudinal plane 6 months after discharge from the original attack of pancreatitis.

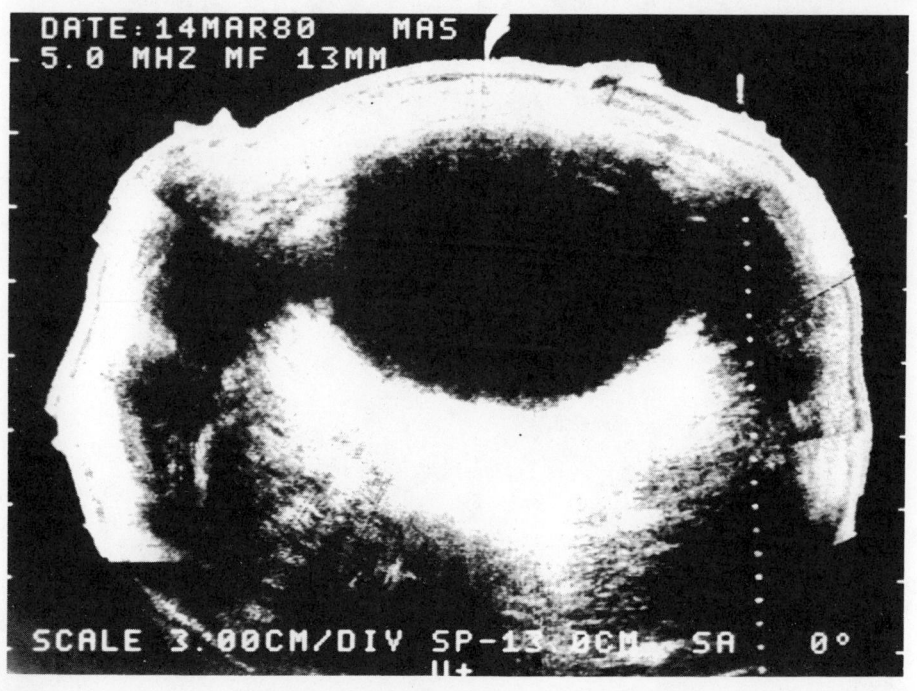

FIG 12A–5.
Case Study No. 2: Ultrasonogram in the circular plane showing the pseudocyst.

142 / PANCREAS

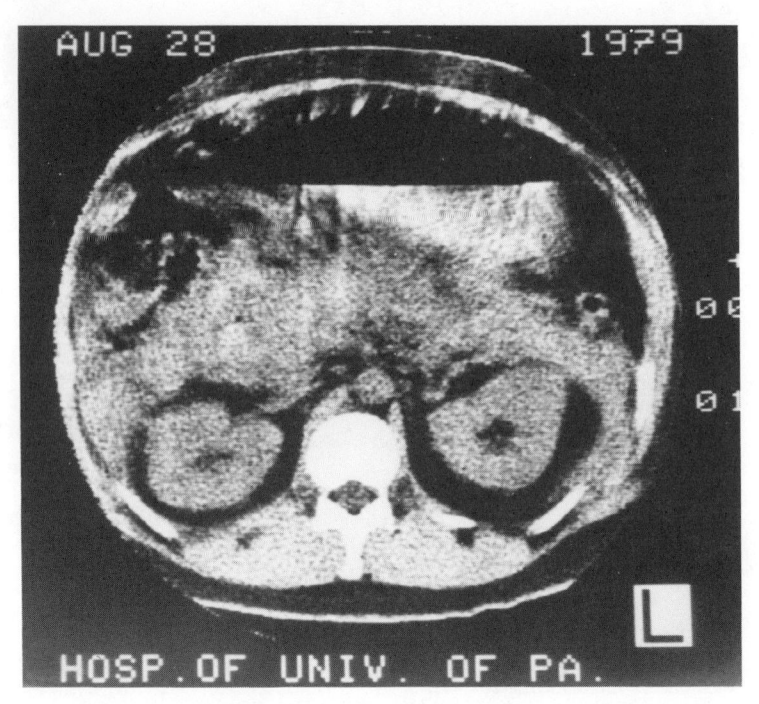

FIG 12A–6.
Case Study No. 3: CAT scan on admission showing an enlarged mottled pancreas and fluid around the left kidney. There is a mass in the tail of the pancreas.

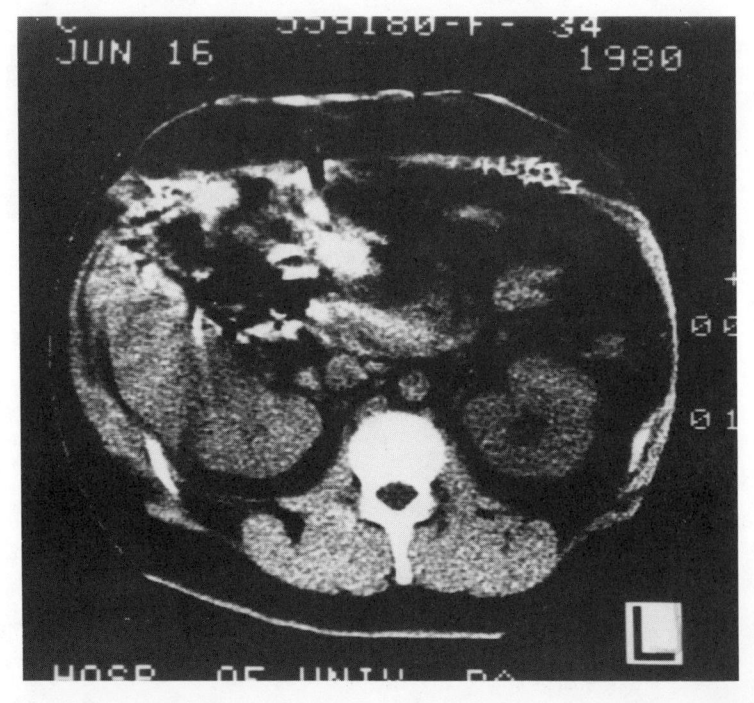

FIG 12A–7.
Case Study No. 3: CAT scan of the pancreas 10 months later. The pancreas is much smaller, and the fluid has disappeared.

orated, and a laparotomy was performed 2 weeks after admission. Extensive necrosis of the pancreas and erosion into the hepatic flexure was found. The surgeon performed debridement of the necrotic pancreas and retroperitoneal tissues, instituted sump drainage of the abdomen, and carried out a right hemicolectomy. The patient was placed on hyperalimentation. A CAT scan showed a large necrotic-appearing pancreas (Fig 12A-6). He continued to suffer from ARDS and later developed multiple cutaneous enteric fistulae. Two weeks after the laparotomy the abdomen had to be reopened and an abdominal abscess was drained. The patient slowly recovered. A CAT scan 10 months after the first showed much improvement (Fig 12A-7). The final diagnosis was severe acute idiopathic pancreatitis with necrosis of the hepatic flexure and an abdominal abscess. He left the hospital 4 months after admission. His subsequent course is unknown.

References

1. Brooks FP: *Diseases of the Exocrine Pancreas*. Philadelphia, WB Saunders, 1980, pp 5-39.
2. Banks PA: Acute pancreatitis: Clinical presentation in Go VLW, Garner JD, Brooks FP, et al (eds): *The Exocrine Pancreas*. New York, Raven Press, 1986, pp 475-480.
3. Levitt MD, Eckfeldt JH: Diagnosis of acute pancreatitis, in Go VLW, Gardner JD, Brooks FP, et al (eds): *The Exocrine Pancreas*. New York, Raven Press, 1986, pp 481-502.
4. Battersby C, Green MK: The surgical significance of methaemalbuminemia. *Gut* 1972; 12:995-1000.
5. Ranson JHC: Acute pancreatitis: Survival management, in Go VLW, Gardner D, Brooks FP, et al (eds): *The Exocrine Pancreas*. New York, Raven Press, 1986, pp 503-512.
6. Blamey SL, Imrie CW, O'Neill J, et al: Prognostic factors in acute pancreatitis. *Gut* 1984; 25:1340-1346.
7. Bank S, Wise L, Gersten M: Risk factors in acute pancreatitis. *Am J Gastroenterol* 1983; 78:637-640.
8. Cesar M, Marques A, Deas F, et al: Prognostic criteria in acute pancreatitis: A critical evaluation. *Gut* 1987; 28:A368.
9. London NJ, Neoptolemos JP, Bailey I, et al: Serial computed tomography (CT) scanning in acute pancreatitis. *Gut* 1987; 28:A369.
10. Garvin M, McMahon MJ: Serial objective measurement of severity in acute pancreatitis. *Gut* 1987; 28:A369.
11. Sarles H: Chronic pancreatitis: Etiology and pathophysiology, in Go VLW, Gardner JD, Brooks FP et al (eds): *The Exocrine Pancreas*. New York, Raven Press, 1986, pp 527-540.
12. Buggy BP, Nostrant TT: Lethal pancreatitis. *Am J Gastroenterol* 1983; 78:810-814.
13. Pemberton JH, Nagorney DM, Dogois RR: Pancreatic abscess, in Go VLW, Gardner JD, Brooks FP et al (eds): *The Exocrine Pancreas*. New York, Raven Press, 1986, pp 513-525.
14. Shearer MG, Dickson AP, Imrie CW, et al: Pancreatic pseudocyts and abscesses after acute pancreatitis. Report from multicenter study. *Gut* 1986; 27:A229-230.
15. Beger HG, Bittner R, Block S, et al: Bacterial contamination of pancreatic necrosis. *Gastroenterology* 1986; 91:433-438.
16. Shearer MG, O'Neil J, Imrie CW: Late follow-up of acute pancreatitis. *Gut* 1985; 26:A651.
17. Blick S, Maier W, Bittner R, et al: Identification of pancreas necrosis in severe acute pancreatitis: Imaging procedures versus clinical staging. *Gut* 1986; 27:1035-1042.
18. Sostre CF, Flournoy JG, Bova JG, et al: Pancreatic phlegmon: Clinical features and course. *Dig Dis Sci* 1987; 30(10):918-927.
19. Mayer AD, McMahon MJ, Corfield AP, et al: Controlled clinical trial of peritoneal lavage for the treatment of severe acute pancreatitis. *N Engl J Med* 1985; 312:399-404.
20. Ethan JT, Webster PD: The management of acute pancreatitis. *Adv Intern Med* 1980; 25:169-198.
21. Pellegrini CA: The treatment of acute pancreatitis: A continuing challenge (editorial). *N Engl J Med* 1985; 312:436-438.

B

The surgeon's view: CHARLES F. FREY and SIGISMUND S. PIKUL, II

THE NATURAL HISTORY OF PANCREATITIS

The common final pathway of acute pancreatitis, regardless of etiology, is the intraglandular activation of pancreatic enzymes resulting in inflammation and sometimes progression to autodigestion of the pancreas by its own excretory products (Table 12B–1). Trypsin is a prime suspect in both tissue lysis and as an activation factor of other highly destructive enzymes such as phospholipase A and elastase. Whether the process begins as an extracellular destruction of the acinar cell from proteolytic enzymes or intracellular destruction resulting from the mixing of intracellular lysosomes and zymogen granules is not known.[1,2] With the onset of inflammation, fluid is sequestered in the parenchyma and peripancreatic areas of the retroperitoneum, due to increased capillary permeability. This so-called pancreatic burn can accumulate many liters of exudate leading to hypovolemia and poor organ perfusion.

Acute Interstitial Pancreatitis

Morphology in the early stage of inflammation is one of an enlarged gland with glassy edema, a tense capsule and peripancreatic clear fluid. The process will not progress beyond this point in 80% of the patients with acute pancreatitis, and the disease can be classified in those patients as *acute interstitial pancreatitis* or edematous pancreatitis. Sterile inflammation and edema of the pancreas are the primary features, and peripancreatic fat necrosis may be found with acute interstitial pancreatitis.[1] With adequate resuscitation, almost all these patients improve without sequelae. The clinical pathologic manifestations of acute pancreatitis are summarized in Table 12B–2.

TABLE 12B–1.
Etiologic Associations of Acute Pancreatitis

Metabolic	*Ischemic*
Alcohol	Postoperative (cardiopulmonary bypass)
Hypercalcemia	
Hyperlipidemia	Atheroembolism
Drugs (azathioprine, sulphonamides, flurosemide, and others)	*Connective Tissue Disorders and Vasculitis*
	Systemic lupus erythematosus (SLE)
Scorpion venom	
Hereditary/genetic	Thrombotic thrombo-cytopenic purpura
Mechanical	
Cholelithiasis	Polyarteritis nodosa
Postoperative	*Infectious*
Trauma	Mumps
ERCP	Coxsackievirus
Pancreatic duct obstruction—tumor, *Ascaris* infection	Echovirus
	Mycoplasma
Pancreas divisum	
Duodenal obstruction	
Penetrating duodenal ulcer	

TABLE 12B–2.
Clinicopathologic Types of Acute Pancreatitis

Type	Description	CT Findings	Fine Needle Aspiration Findings	Treatment Strategy
Acute interstitial pancreatitis	Pancreatic edema/inflammation (fat necrosis	Enlarged gland	Bacteria negative	Supportive therapy Pain relief
Necrotizing pancreatitis	Peripancreatic pancreatic necrosis	Nonenhanced areas	Bacteria negative	Supportive therapy Resuscitation: fluids and antibiotics Operative resection only if hemodynamically unstable or pulmonary failure
Infected necrosis	Infected necrosis Invasive	Nonenhanced areas	Bacteria positive	Supportive therapy Resuscitation: fluids and antibiotics Debridement of necrosis mandatory Open drainage recommended
Pancreatic abscess	Walled off pus	Nonenhanced area, well defined, possibly cystic	Bacteria positive	Supportive therapy Resuscitation: fluid and antibiotics Operation or percutaneous drainage
Acute pseudocyst	Collection of enzymatic fluid, comminution of duct	Hypodense nonenhanced area	Bacteria negative	Wait 6–8 weeks Internal drainage or resection

Necrotizing Pancreatitis

Progression of the inflammatory process may occur, leading to pancreatic and peripancreatic necrosis of varying extent. It is poorly understood why edematous pancreatitis will progress to necrosis in selected patients, and there are many hypotheses proposed to explain this event. It is known that ischemia, from any cause, may be responsible for the transition from an edematous pancreas to necrotic pancreatitis.[3-5] Therefore, it follows, rapid adequate resuscitation with fluids to optimize perfusion of the pancreas and prevent ischemia is an essential component of therapy for these patients. Evidence from fine needle aspiration and surgical specimens in the first 7 days of severe acute pancreatitis indicates that sterile necrosis precedes infected necrosis.[6] We know that some patients with pancreatic necrosis will clinically improve, and their illness will resolve without sequelae.

Others develop infected necrosis, abscesses, and pseudocysts. *Necrotizing pancreatitis* is sterile inflammation in association with devitalized pancreatic and/or peripancreatic tissue. Morphologically, the necrosis is either patchy or diffuse, superficial or deep, parenchymal and/or peripancreatic, and may result in ductal damage and/or thrombosis of the splenic vein.[7] There is local activation of complement by trypsin and conversion of kallikrein to bradykinin and plasminogen to plasmin. The prostaglandins and clotting systems are also activated.[8, 9] A variety of other changes can occur consisting of an increased capillary leak, producing hypovolemia, leading to hypotension, diminished perfusion, stasis, venous thrombosis, and progressive ischemia of the pancreas. Systemic effects can occur, including pulmonary insufficiency from endothelial injury thought to be due to the actions of phospholipids[10] and diminished ventilation, due to elevation of the diaphragm and pleural effusions. Hyperglycemia,[11] hypocalcemia,[12, 13] myocardial depression,[14] renal insufficiency,[15] and hepatic failure[16, 17] are seen frequently in necrotizing pancreatitis. The systemic signs and symptoms that the patient develops in response to pancreatic necrosis form the basis for the physiologic signs of severity developed by Ranson,[18] Imrie,[12] and others.[19]

The presence of necrotizing pancreatitis in itself is not an indication for operation because many of these patients will survive without operation. However, in some instances, when the necrosis is extensive, the patient may develop pulmonary and/or hemodynamic instability. These patients benefit from operative intervention to excise the necrotic portion of the pancreas, followed by lavage of the remaining pancreas to remove all the locally generated acute phase reactants which are in high concentration about the pancreas.

The natural history of necrotizing pancreatitis is incompletely known. The number of patients with significant amounts of pancreatic necrosis and an absence of complications is unknown. We know only about the complications of necrotizing pancreatitis. Of those patients without pseudocysts, with necrotizing pancreatitis, only 40% to 50% will become infected.[20] Among the patients without infections, the percentage of patients who survive without sequelae is unknown. Some present months later with persistent pain and at that time are found to have a necrotic, uninfected sequestra of dead pancreas and peripancreatic fat or pseudocysts.

Infected Pancreatic and Peripancreatic Necrosis

In patients with necrotizing pancreatitis operated on by Beger,[20] he found 40% had secondary bacterial infections. He also found the incidence of infection increased with the extent of necrosis and peaked 2 to 3 weeks from the onset of symptoms. Some patients became infected as early as 3 to 4 days from the onset of symptoms. All patients with infected pancreatic necrosis require prompt operative intervention to remove the devitalized pancreatic and peripancreatic tissue. Percutaneous aspiration is useless in these circumstances. Classic purulence is often absent in these circumstances; rather, a thin, gray, turbid fluid exudes from the tissue planes. The infectious process is not walled off as in a pancreatic abscess, but more closely resembles an invasive fascitis, which can dissect and extend retroperitoneally behind the colon and small bowel mesentery. The only hope for survival in these patients is removal of the devitalized, infected tissue. The development of new areas of necrosis following debridement is characteristic of necrotizing pancreatitis and is due to the continued action of the bacteria and activated pancreatic enzymes, which progressively destroys previously viable tissue. In such patients, there is a need for reoperation to remove these newly created areas of devitalized, infected tissue.[15,16] Progression of infection, causing persistent sepsis the frequent need for reoperation and additional anesthetics, contributes to the morbidity and mortality associated with infected necrotizing pancreatitis. Recently, the open packing technique, popularized by Bradley,[21] has helped to reduce the need for reoperation and additional anesthetics. This technique is felt by some to be a factor in reducing the mortality associated with this infectious complication of pancreatitis.

Pseudocysts

Half of all patients with complications resulting from pancreatic necrosis develop pseudocysts. When the necrosis involves the parenchyma around and including a tributary or main pancreatic duct, extravasation of pancreatic fluid can occur. When this fluid, in continuity with the main pancreatic duct, becomes walled off by the pressure of surrounding structures it is the beginning of a pseudocyst, described best initially as a fluid collection.[7] If the fluid is not walled off in the abdomen, it becomes pancreatic ascites; if the fluid fistulizes into the chest, it becomes a pancreaticopleural or pericardial fistula.[22] Whether these early fluid collections persist or disappear, as occurs spontaneously in about 40% of patients, is largely dependent on whether proximal obstruction to the flow of pancreatic secretion exists and causes impedence to flow. Should the obstruction persist, ductal hypertension results which will perpetuate the pseudocyst, fistula, or ascites.

We have found markedly elevated pressure in cysts in continuity with the major pancreatic duct that have persisted for 6 to 8 weeks after the onset of symptoms— usually three to four times the normal pressure in the main pancreatic duct, which is 8 to 12 cm of water. Elevated pressures in pseudocysts are an indication there is proximal obstruction to outflow from the segment of the pancreas, elaborating the pancreatic secretion filling the cyst.

Pancreatic Abscess

A late complication of acute pancreatitis is pancreatic abscess. Pancreatic abscess is a collection of purulent material, in and around the pancreas, walled off and contained by inflammatory and fibrous tissue. Presentation is late in the course of acute pancreatitis, usually not appearing until 3 to 5 weeks after the onset of symptoms. In contrast, infected pancreatic necrosis generally presents earlier and usually has a higher morbidity and mortality rate with a higher incidence of systemic sepsis and multiorgan failure.[23] The loculated, walled-off pus contained in a pancreatic abscess may originate from liquefaction of necrotic material or a pseudocyst which becomes secondarily infected. It should be apparent the distinction between the infected pancreatic necrosis and pancreatic abscess is not always precise. Like the distinction between ulcerative colitis and granulomatous colitis, some cases have features of both and are difficult to classify. The distinction between infected pancreatic necrosis and abscess is most useful when applied to the management of patients with pancreatic infections. When there is particulate infected matter even in the face of surrounding gross pus, the patient should be treated by operation as though dealing with infected necrosis.

Sterile Sequestra

Peripancreatic necrosis may result in walled-off sterile fat sequestra. The necrotic fat enclosed by inflammatory walls, in the absence of bacteria or pus, may or may not cause symptoms. These loculations are not pseudocysts because they have no connection with the pancreatic ductal system and do not contain pancreatic juice. There is no need to intervene operatively unless these sequestra become symptomatic.[7]

DIAGNOSIS AND EARLY ASSESSMENT OF ACUTE PANCREATITIS

There are three steps in the diagnosis and early assessment of acute pancreatitis. First, one must confirm that pancreatitis is indeed present. Second, the etiology of the pancreatitis must be determined. The third step is to assess the severity of the pancreatitis.

Confirming the Presence of Pancreatitis

Clinical Presentation

The symptoms and signs of acute pancreatitis are nonspecific. Other disease processes, such as perforated peptic ulcer, acute cholecystitis, or intestinal ischemia, have similar presentation. The diagnosis of acute pancreatitis is one of exclusion in which the other causes of abdominal pain must be ruled out. In some patients, the diagnosis of acute pancreatitis is established at the time of laparotomy. Abdominal pain is the presenting complaint in greater than 90% of patients with acute pancreatitis and is usually epigastric in location. The pain may be diffuse and is typically characterized as steady, deep, and boring; ranging from mild to excruciating discomfort; and characteristically radiating to the back. The onset may be gradual over hours and days, but can be acute—waking the patient from sleep. Nausea and vomiting are present in 75% to 80% of patients. On physical examination, in mild cases of acute interstitial pancreatitis, the only findings may be epigastric tenderness on deep palpation. In 70% of cases, evidence of an ileus can be found, such as abdominal distention with hypoactive bowel sounds. Patients with necrotizing pancreatitis may present with hypovolemic shock, coma, abdominal distention, guarding tenderness, decreased bowel sounds, tachypnea, rapid shallow respiration, and pleural effusions, usually on the left side.[24] Oliguria, anuria, jaundice, tetany, or hyperglycemia may also be present. Rarely, retroperitoneal hemorrhage, indicated by periumbilical and flank ecchymoses (Cullen's and Grey Turner's signs), is noted.

Laboratory Identification of Patients with Acute Pancreatitis

Presently, there are no specific markers that consistently and correctly diagnose acute pancreatitis. The most commonly used tests to help support a diagnosis of acute pancreatitis are an elevated serum or urine amylase or serum lipase. These tests are nonspecific and, unless the clinician understands the reason for false-positive and false-negative examinations, can lead to misinterpretation (Table 12B–3). For example, false-positive test may be seen in patients with a perforated duodenal ulcer. Through the hole in the duodenum, pancreatic enzymes are extravasated into the peritoneal cavity where

TABLE 12B–3.
Causes of Hyperamylasemia

Pancreatic disease
Biliary tract disease
    Cholangitis
    Cholecystitis
Perforated ulcer or perforated viscus
Interstitial ischemia
Ruptured ectopic pregnancy
Aortic aneurysm
Renal failure
Diabetic ketoacidosis
Chronic liver disease
Salivary gland lesions—trauma, mumps, calculus
Drugs—opiates
Tumors—carcinoma of the lung, ovarian tumors
Macroamylasemia
Burns
Chronic alcoholism

they are picked up by the lymphatic system and returned through the thoracic duct elevating serum levels of amylase and lipase. A false-negative test can occur in a patient presenting with necrotizing pancreatitis. In the absence of viable acinar cells, an insufficient quantity of pancreatic enzymes may be produced to elevate serum levels even in the presence of ductal obstruction of the major pancreatic duct.

Other laboratory tests for acute pancreatitis have been proposed, including the measurement of amylase-to-creatinine clearance ratio, serum pancreatic isoamylase, trypsinogen level, and phospholipase A. These tests may be helpful in implicating pancreatitis as the cause of the patient's symptoms, but are less readily available, more expensive, and have not been shown conclusively in many clinical situations to be any more specific or accurate than the serum or urine amylase. Some recent studies have looked at immunoreactive pancreatic polypeptide (IPP) or carboxylic ester hydrolase (CEH) as specific serum markers for acute pancreatitis, but clinical trials are needed to confirm their accuracy and usefulness.

Laboratory findings that are not specific for acute pancreatitis but may be abnormal include hypocalcemia, leukocytosis, increased hematocrit due to hemoconcentration, hypokalemia, hyperglycemia, and elevated BUN. Evidence of hypoxia (PaO_2 < 60 mm Hg) is seen in up to 30% of patients with acute pancreatitis and is a warning of impending respiratory failure. An elevated serum creatinine or BUN in conjunction with oliguria or anuria indicates renal failure.

Radiologic Studies

Radiologic evaluation of a patient with abdominal pain should include a plain x-ray of the abdomen or KUB (kidney, ureter, and bladder) and a chest x-ray. In acute pancreatitis, the greatest value of a plain abdominal and chest film is for excluding other diagnoses, such as pneumoperitoneum associated with a perforated ulcer, air fluid levels seen with a small bowel obstruction, pneumobilia or gallstones, or a widened calcified aorta associated with aortic aneurysms. Plain abdominal films may show a classic sentinel loop in the left upper quadrant indicating a localized ileus, which is present in one third of patients with acute pancreatitis, or there may be pancreatic calcifications.

Ultrasound evaluation of the pancreas in acute pancreatitis is usually of little value because overlying gas associated with the accompanying ileus hinders the assessment of the pancreas. However, ultrasound is of great value in determining the etiology of pancreatitis.

The availability of computerized tomography (CT) scan has markedly improved our ability to identify patients with acute pancreatitis. Enlargement of the pancreas, peripancreatic fluid, or displacement of other organs may be seen.[25, 26] The CT scan also can be used in the assessment of the severity of pancreatitis. When used with vascular enhancement consisting of a bolus of contrast, areas of pancreatic necrosis are seen as regions of nonperfusion.[27]

Differential Diagnosis

The following disease states can have presentations similar to those of acute pancreatitis:
- Perforated peptic ulcer
- Acute cholecystitis
- Bowel obstruction
- Mesenteric and bowel ischemia
- Renal calculi
- Dissecting aortic aneurysm
- Myocardial infarction
- Right lower lobe pneumonia or lung abscess
- Hepatic abscess
- Retrocecal appendicitis

Each of these diseases should be excluded before assuming the diagnosis is acute pancreatitis, as many of them are correctable by surgical intervention.

Determining the Etiology of Pancreatitis

The most common causes of acute pancreatitis are alcohol, cholelithiasis, hyperlipidemia, and postoperative pancreatitis.

Together, they account for 75% to 95% of patients with acute pancreatitis. The incidence of each varies with the population sample and geographic area. A recent review of over 5,000 cases of acute pancreatitis by Ranson[28] found 55% were secondary to alcohol, 27% were related to cholelithiasis, and 19% were related to other or unknown causes.

Gallstone pancreatitis is a surgically correctable disease. All patients with pancreatitis should undergo ultrasound evaluation to determine the presence or absence of gallstones. Should gallstones be detected in patients with pancreatitis, these patients should not leave the hospital without correction of the biliary tract disease.[29] Experience has shown that it is like playing "Russian roulette" to discharge patients with gallstone pancreatitis without correcting their biliary pathology on the initial admission. Many patients with gallstone pancreatitis who are sent home without correction of their biliary disease do not return for treatment and as many as 30% of patients scheduled to be readmitted electively for cholecystectomy, return because of a recurrent attack within 3 months after their initial hospital admission for gallstone pancreatitis. The extra costs incurred by a second hospitalization cannot be justified in the face of scarce medical resources, when no improvement in morbidity and mortality can be demonstrated by a second hospitalization. Therefore, in 80% of patients with edematous pancreatitis, cholecystectomy should be performed promptly after the diagnosis of gallstone pancreatitis is established. Unless there are extenuating circumstances, the patient should not leave the hospital without cholecystectomy.[29]

Those patients with necrotizing pancreatitis, secondary to gallstones, will not benefit from cholecystectomy during their acute illness. The damage to the pancreas has already been done; the pancreas is already necrotic. Unless the patient has evidence of cholangitis or acute cholecystitis, life-threatening conditions in themselves, cholecystectomy should be postponed until the patient is hemodynamically stable or should be undertaken at the time of some other procedure made necessary by complications of the necrotizing pancreatitis.

Severity of Pancreatitis

Numerous schemes have been developed to assess the severity of pancreatitis based on the patient's physiologic response to the disease (e.g., Ranson,[30] Imrie,[31] and Bank[32]) (Table 12B–4). The physiologic and biochemical signs of severity are a reflection of the extent of pancreatic necrosis and the host's response to the necrosis. However, these physiologic signs, like the clinical assessment of the patient, have limitations. Most of Ranson's[28] criteria are not available for 48 hours after hospital admission, so that signs of severity do not provide a timely assessment of the presence or absence of pancreatic necrosis at hospital admission when it would be most important to initiate vigorous resuscitation on all patients with necrosis. Unfortunately, 39% of patients who will subsequently become critically ill may not, at the time of hospital admission, be identifiable on the basis of physiologic criteria or clinical assessment.[19] A further limitation of the signs of

TABLE 12B–4.
Signs of Severity of Pancreatitis*

On Admission
Age > 55 years
Blood glucose > 200 mg/dl
White count > 16,000/mm^3
LDH > 700 IU/L
SGOT > 200 Fraenkel units
First 48 Hours
Hematocrit decrease > 10 points
Serum calcium < 8 mg/dl
BUN increase > 5 mg/dl
Base deficit > 4 mEq/L
PaO$_2$ < 60 mm Hg
Fluid sequestration > 6 L

*From Ranson JCH, et al: Prognostic signs and the role of operative management in acute pancreatitis. *Surg Gynecol Obstet* 1974; 39(1):69–81.

severity is that they do not provide indications for or the time of operative intervention.

Another approach to severity is to search for markers of pancreatic necrosis. In patients in whom the diagnosis of pancreatitis has been established, elevation of acute phase reactants have been reported to be reliable indicators of necrosis in patients with pancreatitis at the time of admission. C-reactive protein is elevated[33] and alpha$_2$ macroglobulin levels depressed 30% or more[34] in necrotizing pancreatitis, but not in edematous or interstitial pancreatitis.[35] When alpha$_2$ macroglobulin levels are 30% of normal, both kinin and complement systems are activated.[36] Methemalbumin in the serum or peritoneal fluid is evidence of necrotizing pancreatitis.[37, 38] Peritoneal lavage can be performed within minutes of hospitalization. The presence of bloody or brownish fluid returns indicates necrotizing pancreatitis. Gram stain and cultures can also be obtained[39] (Fig 12B-1). Perhaps the most useful study in the early assessment of the patient with pancreatitis is the CT scan with vascular enhancement, which can be performed shortly after hospital admission[27] (Fig 12B-2). This study permits the identification of areas of nonperfused, necrotic pancreas. These areas of nonperfusion can be needle-aspirated, and the returns can be Gram stained and cultured.[6, 40] While it is unlikely that bacteria can be demonstrated the day or day after the onset of symptoms, Beger has shown that bacteria are present in the necrotic pancreas in some patients as early as 3 days after the onset of symptoms. This is much earlier than had been supposed.[20]

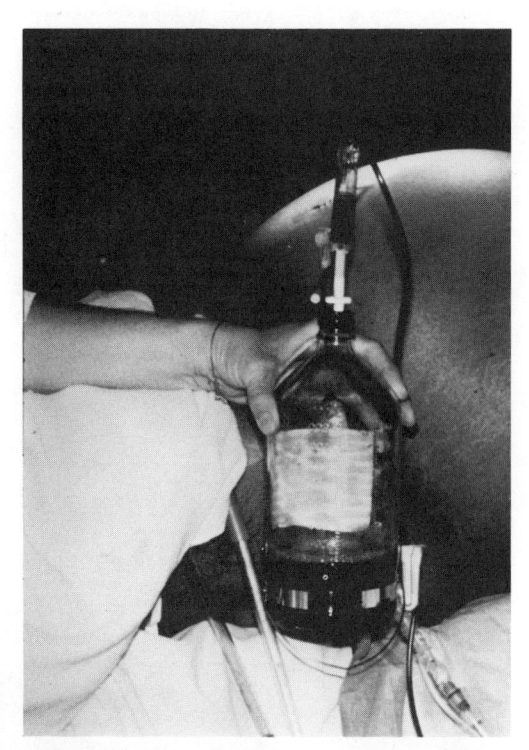

FIG 12B-1.
Diagnostic peritoneal lavage is a means of assessing the presence of necrotizing pancreatitis immediately available on hospital admission. Bloody or brownish fluid is indicative of necrotizing pancreatitis.

INITIAL TREATMENT

Initial treatment of acute pancreatitis is supportive and consists of placing the patient n.p.o. and providing fluid replacement, sedation, and nasogastric suction if the patient is vomiting. There is no evidence that gastric decompression by nasogastric sump-drainage puts the pancreas at rest sufficiently to shorten hospital stay. Nor are other methods of inhibiting pancreatic secretions helpful (e.g., glucagon[41] or somatostatin[42]). Therefore, if the patient is not vomiting, as is often the case in edematous pancreatitis, nasogastric suction is not required.[43] Fluid replacement is critical to a successful outcome in patients with pancreatitis. It is essential to correct hypovolemia and maintain adequate perfusion of the pancreas and other organs, such as the kidney, to prevent ischemic injury to these organs. Large volumes of electrolyte solutions may be required to restore normal urine flow in patients with necrotizing pancreatitis. The adequacy of fluid replacement can be assessed by measuring hourly urine flow, which should be between 30 and 60 ml/hour, and measuring right heart-filling pressures by means of a central venous pressure monitor. Serum

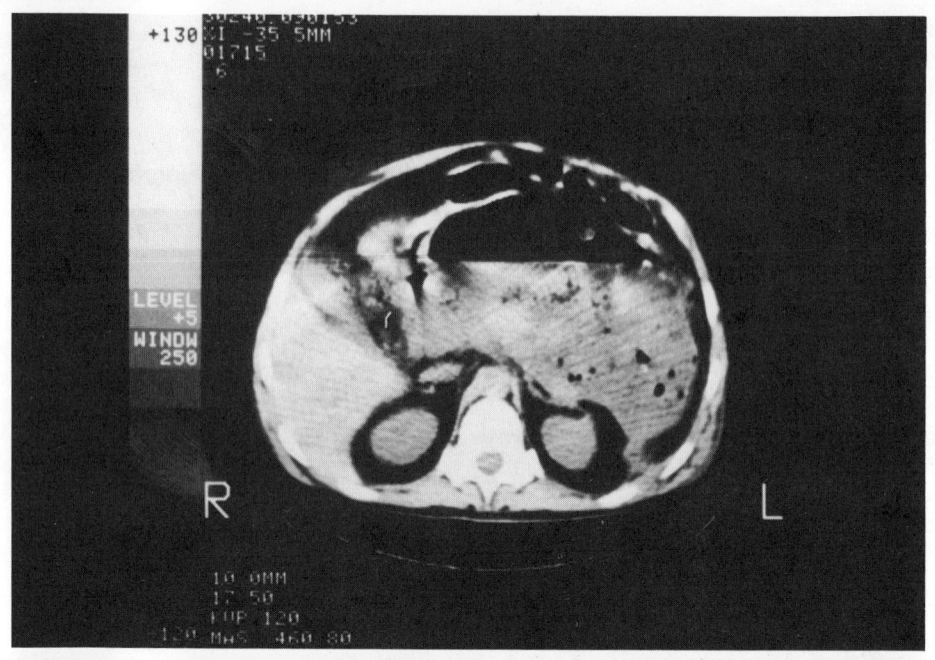

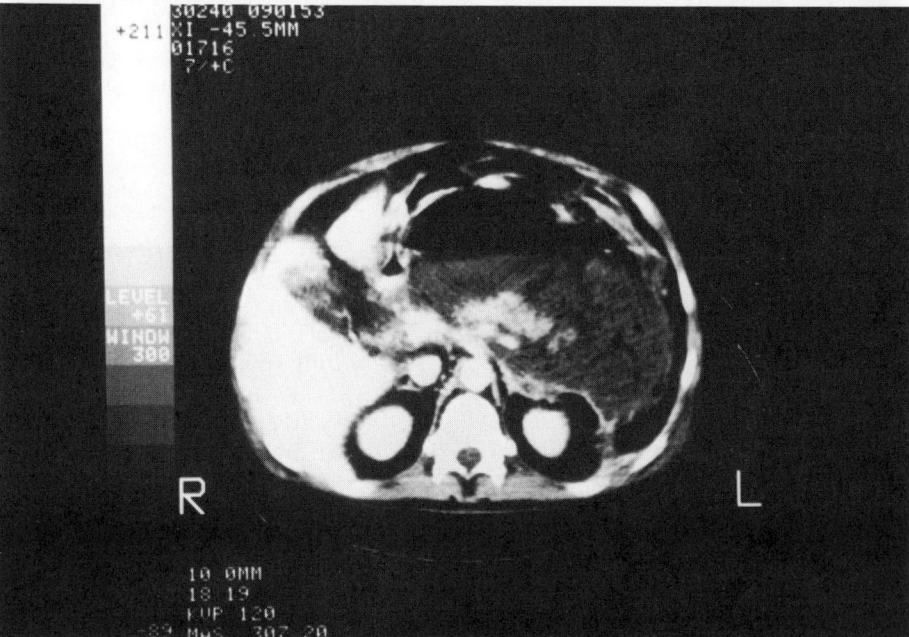

FIG 12B–2.
A, CT scan showing peripancreatic fluid and inflammation without definition of the pancreas.
B, CT scan with vascular enhancement showing hypodense areas of the neck and distal body and tail of the pancreas compatible with pancreatic necrosis. (These films were made available by the courtesy of Hans Beger, Professor and Chairman, Department of Surgery, Ulm University, Ulm, Germany.)

electrolytes should be closely monitored to detect the presence of hypocalcemia. Only ionized calcium needs to be measured because total serum calcium concentration is often misleading in the alcoholic patient who has a low serum albumin.[44] Ionized calcium values below 1.05 mEq/L require IV replacement therapy to prevent tetany, a rare complication of necrotizing pancreatitis.

Prevention of stress ulcers in patients should receive a high priority and prophylaxis instituted with H_2 blockers and antacids.[43] Hyperglycemia is often detected in patients with necrotizing pancreatitis and when present, requires insulin replacement.[11]

While broad spectrum antibiotics are of no proven value in 80% of patients with edematous pancreatitis and in the 10% of patients with pseudocysts or fluid collections, they should be used in an attempt to abort serious infections in patients with significant pancreatic necrosis. Studies of the role of antibiotics have been flawed. They have either not included patients at risk or used antibiotics proven not to be effective against many of the organisms common in infected pancreatic necrosis or pancreatic abscesses.[45–48]

Pulmonary function must be assessed frequently in all patients with necrotizing pancreatitis, who will often require ventilator management because of both impaired ventilation and damage to the lung due to the actions of phospholipase A and the loss of surfactant.[10, 49]

In the patient with necrotizing pancreatitis, nutritional support should be instituted as soon as the patient is hemodynamically stable. There is some evidence to suggest adequate nutrition might theoretically decrease the incidence of infected necrosis by decreasing permeability of the gut to bacterial invasion.[50] These patients will invariably have a prolonged ileus and may require parenteral nutritional support for long periods.[51]

Today, fewer patients with necrotizing pancreatitis are dying from the effects of shock and hypovolemia because of improved surgical intensive care unit care.

DEFINITIVE MANAGEMENT

Definitive management of patients with acute pancreatitis is based in part on the etiology of pancreatitis, the severity of pancreatitis, and the presence and nature of the complications of pancreatitis. All patients identified as having pancreatitis should undergo the following studies on the day of admission to the hospital: C-Reactive protein; alpha$_2$ macroglobulin; methemalbumin and either peritoneal lavage or CT scan to identify patients with significant pancreatic and peripancreatic necrosis. Unless this course is followed those patients who have significant pancreatic and peripancreatic necrosis but who clinically and on the basis of signs of severity (many of which are not available until 48 hours after onset of symptoms) may not appear initially to be seriously ill, will go unidentified. Most importantly some patients will not receive appropriate therapy on hospital admission commensurate with the severity of their illness. To optimize the care of the patient with pancreatic and peripancreatic necrosis, we feel it is essential to identify the presence of necrosis on the day of admission to the hospital. The passive approach of waiting several days or longer to identify many seriously ill patients because they are "not improving," or who after 2 to 3 days of hospitalization progressively develop three to four signs of severity, is unacceptable, now that we have tools available to identify pancreatic necrosis on the day of admission to the hospital. Pancreatologists should learn something from the field of trauma. We do not wait until the accident victim with suspected abdominal injury develops profound shock from blood loss, generalized peritonitis, or a perforated viscus, before initiating definitive therapy. To the contrary, with the accident victim, we perform peritoneal lavage in the emergency department moments after hospital admission to identify intra-abdominal bleeding or the presence of bowel contents. The incidence of complications following lavage for trauma is low, there are many negative lavages, but the procedure saves the lives of many accident victims because it identifies patients with severe injuries early and permits rapid resuscitation and definitive treatment to be initiated before generalized peritonitis and profound shock develop.

It may not be necessary to perform both peritoneal lavage and CT scan on every patient with acute pancreatitis because they provide similar information. Each hospital can determine which technique is most readily available, best tolerated by the patient, cost-effective, and acceptable to the physicians responsible for managing patients with pancreatitis. The advantages of CT scan are having a permanent record and a baseline from which changes can be detected by repeating the scan.

In those patients with a positive lavage or CT scan that shows fluid collections,[25, 52] marked swelling, or distortions of the normal anatomy of the pancreas, the CT scan should be repeated with vascular enhancement. The CT scan with vascular enhancement provides precise information regarding the extent and location of pancreatic necrosis.[27]

Interstitial or Edematous Pancreatitis

The studies enumerated above allow us to segregate patients into two groups. Those with interstitial or edematous pancreatitis that improves in 2 to 3 days after they are placed n.p.o. and given IV fluid replacement and appropriate pain relief; and those who, because of the presence of necrosis, will be expected to have a prolonged, and often complicated, course. Those patients with interstitial or edematous pancreatitis, if found to have their pancreatitis on the basis of gallstones, can undergo cholecystectomy before leaving the hospital. There is no increased risk to these patients if cholecystectomy is performed on the day of admission or within the next several days. In fact, many of these patients, as many as 60%, will show little evidence of pancreatitis at the time of cholecystectomy.[28] An operative cholangiogram should be performed on all patients with gallstone pancreatitis to eliminate the risk of leaving a retained common duct stone.

Pancreatic Necrosis

Those patients who, at the time of admission, are found to have evidence of pancreatic necrosis on the basis of C-reactive protein, alpha$_2$ macroglobulin, methemalbumin peritoneal lavage, or CT scan, should be moved to the intensive care unit and vigorously treated. From the very onset, they should have vigorous IV fluid therapy. The adequacy of replacement should be monitored by hourly urine output and central venous pressure, an assessment of right heart filling pressures. Large amounts of fluid may be required in these patients who may develop a profound capillary leak characteristic of necrotizing pancreatitis. We have given as much as 75 L of electrolyte solution over a 48-hour period to one critically ill anuric patient in order to maintain hemodynamic stability. This patient left the hospital alive 5 months later and was able to return to a normal life a year after recuperating from many of the complications associated with necrotizing pancreatitis.

All patients with necrotizing pancreatitis should, in our opinion, be started on broad spectrum antibiotic coverage against enteric organisms, because 40% will develop infectious complications.[20] Past studies on the efficacy of antibiotics in acute pancreatitis have claimed antibiotics to be ineffective in reducing morbidity and mortality. The designs of these studies were seriously flawed. The antibiotics used in the treatment arms of these studies would not have been expected to be effective against many enteric organisms.[45] Further, 90% of the patients in the control and treatment groups of these studies had edematous pancreatitis in which antibiotics would not be expected to be of any value. Of the 10 patients out of a hundred in these studies at risk of infection because of pancreatic or peripancreatic necrosis, we know less than half would have been expected to become infected in the absence of antibiotics. Analysis of these studies show the authors were comparing only two to three at-risk patients in the antibiotic treatment group.[45-48] Therefore, we feel the issue of the value of antibiotics in necrotizing pancreatitis has not been adequately evaluated. In the absence of a randomized, controlled study, common sense dictates the use of antibiotics in patients with pancreatic and peripancreatic necrosis in hopes of reducing the incidence of secondary infection in the necrotic pancreas.

Blood gases should be obtained if the respiratory rate is above 30; if blood gases show a PO_2 below 60 the patient should be subjected to endotracheal intubation and placed on a mechanical ventilator. Due to metabolic acidosis, breathing is rapid and deep. Not infrequently, high levels of positive end-expiratory pressure (PEEP) may be necessary in some patients with an ARDS type of picture. Insulin and glucose should be administered intravenously as needed. Ionized calcium levels should be obtained, and calcium supplements should be provided if depressed levels are observed. Total parenteral nutrition should be initiated when the patient is hemodynamically stable, because a long ileus may be anticipated in patients with necrotizing pancreatitis.

The presence of pancreatic necrosis is not an indication per se for operative intervention. Our therapeutic efforts are directed in such patients at preventing infection and at fluid resuscitation to perfuse the liver, kidneys, and pancreas optimally to prevent their failure and the extension of pancreatic necrosis. In a small percentage of patients with pancreatic necrosis, hemodynamic[53-55] and pulmonary function[54,56] may deteriorate progressively. In such patients, we recommend operative intervention.[57-59] These patients, along with those having infected necrosis, can be said to have fulminant pancreatitis. At operation, excision of the necrotic areas in the pancreas previously identified by CT scan with vascular enhancement, should be performed.[59] We combine excision with postoperative lavage of the lesser sac by through-and-through Davol catheters. We feel lavage of the lesser sac is far more efficacious in removing locally generated ferments containing high levels of complement, kinins, prostaglandins, and coagulation factors, than peritoneal lavage. Patients with pancreatic necrosis, requiring operative debridement of devitalized pancreas and peripancreatic fat, may be packed open as advocated by Bradley,[21] or the abdomen may be closed followed by through-and-through irrigations by lavage catheters placed from each side of the abdomen.

Infected Necrosis

According to Beger,[20] the patient with appreciable pancreatic necrosis has a 40% chance of becoming secondarily infected. Therefore, if the patient develops signs of sepsis, such as an increased capillary leak, manifested by an increase in fluid requirement or an increased need for insulin; deteriorating pulmonary or renal function; increased fever or leukocytosis usually after the third day of the disease; should arouse a high index of suspicion in the attending physician regarding the presence of secondary infection in the necrotic pancreas. The patient should be subjected to CT scan-guided needle aspiration of the pancreas and peripancreatic tissues and fluid collections.[6] Aspirated fluid should be Gram-stained and cultured. Should the Gram stain be positive, then prompt operative intervention is indicated to remove the necrotic pancreatic and peripancreatic tissue (Fig 12B-3). These patients cannot be adequately treated by percutaneous aspiration of solid particulate infected pancreatic and peripancreatic tissue. Pigtail catheter drainage of infected pancreatic necrosis instituted by CT scan or ultrasound guidance is doomed to failure due to the particulate nature of the necrotic tissue which inhibits its removal by small-diameter catheters.

If there is significant bleeding at the time of necrosectomy, we recommend splenectomy to avoid exsanguination from the splenic artery or vein, because vessel wall integrity may have been compromised by a combination of enzymatic and infectious necrosis. A characteristic feature of infected pancreatic necrosis is that, even after debridement of all devital-

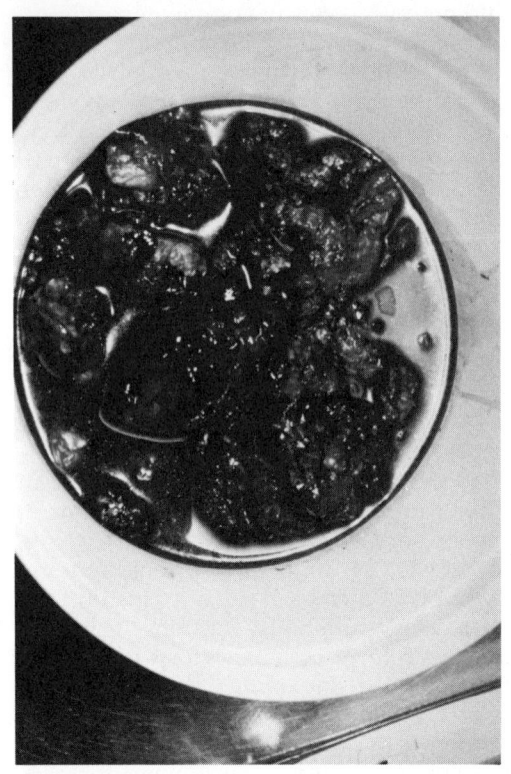

FIG 12B–3.
Infected necrotic pancreatic and peripancreatic tissue removed at operative debridement. This type of infection does not lend itself to percutaneous drainage.

ized pancreatic and peripancreatic tissue, new areas of necrosis will develop due to a combination of invasive infective organisms and activated pancreatic enzymes. These new areas of infected necrosis in the pancreatic and peripancreatic tissue will require reoperation for excision. For this reason, we favor an open drainage technique as popularized by Bradley.[21] His technique involves laying a nonadherent dressing over the pancreas, which has been debrided of all necrotic material. This nonadherent dressing should also cover the bowel. Packs are then placed within the dressings, creating a wide portal of entry to the retroperitoneum from the anterior abdominal wall. The patient can then be returned to the operating room in 2 to 3 days, at which time the packing is removed, and any additional necrotic pancreas or peripancreatic tissue is excised. The pack and nonadherent dressing can then be replaced. Usually after two or three of these sessions, or 6 to 8 days after the first operation, the bowel becomes fixed in placed and the patient does not have to be returned to the operating room to have the packing and dressings removed. When this stage in the healing process has been reached, debridement can be carried out at the patient's bedside in the surgical intensive care unit, without the need for a general anesthetic. Once the pancreatic bed is cleaned without the evidence of infection, the packing can be left out, and the abdomen can be loosely closed with stay sutures or allowed to granulate in. Surprisingly, many of the patients do not develop hernias. We have modified Bradley's technique. In addition to the open packing technique, we employ Davol catheters, inserted from each side of the abdomen, to obtain through-and-through drainage in the lesser sac by placing the catheters between the pancreas and the nonadherent gauze and pack. The open packing technique and the early identification of the patient with infected necrosis have led to a sharp reduction in the mortality of this dreaded complication of necrotizing pancreatitis. Bradley[21] reports the mortality in 21 patients to be 14%.

Pancreatic Abscess

Pancreatic abscess, which appears late in the course of necrotizing pancreatitis, differs only from infected pancreatic necrosis in that the extent of involvement of the pancreas is usually less, initially, and the purulent process is well walled off. Usually, the patient is less ill systemically, and the complication tends to occur later, after the onset of symptoms, than is the case with infected necrosis. Many of these patients do not have sufficiently severe systemic signs of necrosis for the term fulminant pancreatitis to be applied to them. The diagnosis of pancreatic abscess is easily established by CT scan or ultrasound guided aspiration with Gram stain and culture.[6] CT scan or ultrasound, in themselves, are not helpful in distinguishing between a pseudocyst and an abscess. Whether a pancreatic abscess arises from secondary infection of necrotic liquefied pancreatic and peripancreatic tissue, or from a secondarily infected pseudocyst, is unknown and probably not important in terms of management. Those patients who have well-defined, walled-off loculations of pus can be treated by either operative intervention and drainage or by percutaneous aspiration and drainage if the material is liquefied and does not plug off the drainage catheter.

As Braash pointed out in his 1975 report,[60] many patients with infected necrosis or pancreatic abscess may have sequelae and develop problems that fall under the heading of chronic pancreatitis. These include pain, main pancreatic duct strictures, discontinuity of the main pancreatic duct, and pseudocysts. For these reasons, all patients with pancreatic infections should be carefully followed for several years after their bout with infected pancreatic necrosis or abscess.

Pancreatic Pseudocyst and Peripancreatic Fat Sequestra

Patients with these conditions do not usually have extensive pancreatic necrosis. Usually, they have just enough parenchymal damage to expose a duct and create a vent for extravasation of pancreatic fluid in the face of proximal ductal obstruction. Seldom is the initial pancreatitis of such a severity to warrant application of the term fulminant pancreatitis. However, some misguided, eager interventionists can produce a fulminant morbid course in patients with fluid collections if they intervene inappropriately. In as many as 40% of patients with peripancreatic fluid collections, the collections will disappear spontaneously within 6 to 8 weeks after their appearance.[61] It is misguided and unnecessary in most patients with fluid collections for a radiologist to place drainage catheter for decompression of the collections at any time earlier than 6 to 8 weeks after the onset of symptoms. On the other hand, it is perfectly acceptable for the radiologist at anytime to aspirate fluid collections with a thin needle for purposes of determining if they are infected or not. However, leaving a pigtail catheter in these fluid collections is dangerous. The chances of initiating an infection where none previously existed through a catheter left in place is real. Catheters are a two-way street for infections. These infections may be life-threatening. When the catheter has been introduced at 2 to 5 weeks after the onset of symptoms, the fluid collection may not be walled off. Therefore the ensuing infection may not be limited just to the fluid collection, but may invade the entire retroperitoneum, resulting in a life-threatening infection. This practice of trying to drain fluid collections before 6 to 8 weeks is particularly reprehensible because the fluid collection might have disappeared spontaneously, and placement of a pigtail catheter exposes the patient to a totally unnecessary risk of serious infection. Aside from the risk of infection, chances of percutaneous drainage of a pseudocyst being successful is less than 50% in a mature cyst because of the continued production of secretions and persistence of obstruction of the proximal pancreatic duct, causing refilling of the cyst.[62]

The practice of endoscopic internal cyst-gastrostomy may be fraught with major risk to the patient.[63] The endoscopist cannot safely forestall or manage complications that could be life-threatening if he performs this procedure. Failure to create a window in an area of fusion of the cyst to the stomach will lead to extravasation of gastrointestinal contents into the retroperitoneum which could lead to peritonitis and death. The area of opening that the endoscopist can create is often insufficient to adequately decompress the cyst, and recurrence would be expected more often than not. Hemorrhage may occur from the cyst opening or from a pseudoaneurysm contained within the cyst. Either one of these problems would be difficult for the endoscopist to control.

References

1. Kloppel G, Dreyer T, Willemer S, et al: Human acute pancreatitis: Its pathogenesis in the light of immunocytochemical and ultra structural findings in acinar cells. Virchows Arch (Pathol Anat) 1986; 409:791–803.
2. Steer L, Meldolesi J: The cell biology of experimental pancreatitis. N Engl J Med 1987; 316:144–150.
3. Jones RT, Trump BF: Cellular and subcellular effects of ischemia on the pancreatic acinar cell. Virchows Arch (B) 1975; 199:325–336.
4. Nevalainen JJ, Anttinen J: Ultra structural and functional changes in pancreatic acinar cells during autolysis. Virchows Arch (B) 1977; 24:197–207.
5. Goodhead B: Vascular factors in the pathogenesis of acute hemorrhagic pancreatitis. Ann R Coll Surg Engl 1969; 45:80–97.
6. Gerzof SG, Banks PA, Spechler SJ, et al: Role of guided percutaneous aspiration in early diagnosis of pancreatic sepsis. Dig Dis Sci 1984; 29:950.
7. Frey CF, Bradley E, Beger H: Progress in acute pancreatitis: The necessity for clinicopathological definitions. Submitted for publication.
8. Lasson A, Laurell AB, Ohlsson K: Correlation among complement activation in protein inhibitors and clinical course in acute pancreatitis in man. Scand J Gastroenterol 1985; 20:335–345.
9. Farias LF, Frey CF, Holcroft JW, et al: Effect of prostaglandin blockers of ascites fluid in pancreatitis. Surgery 1985; 98:571–578.
10. Guice KS, Oldham KT, Wolfe RR, et al: Lung injury in acute pancreatitis: Primary inhibition of pulmonary phospholipid synthesis. Am J Surg 1987; 153:54–61.
11. Hallberg D, Theve NO: Observations during treatment of acute pancreatitis with insulin and glucose infusion. Acta Chir Scand 1974; 140:138–142.
12. Imrie CW, Allam BF, Ferguson JC: Hypocalcemia of acute pancreatitis: The effect of hypoalbuminemia. Curr Med Res Opin 1976; 4:101–116.
13. McMahon MJ, Woodhead JS, Hayward RP: The nature of hypocalcemia in acute pancreatitis. Br J Surg 1978; 65:216–218.
14. Lee WK, Fraser M, Lee C, et al: Depression of myocardial function during acute pancreatitis. Circ Shock 1981; 8:369–374.
15. Frey CF: Pathogenesis of nitrogen retention in pancreatitis. Am J Surg 1965; 109:747–755.
16. Frey CF, Brody GL: Relationship of azotemia and survival in bile pancreatitis in the dog. Arch Surg 1966; 93:295–300.
17. Roth E, Zoch G, Maurtiz W, et al: Metabolic changes of patients with acute necrotizing pancreatitis. Infusionsther Klin Ernahr 1986; 13:172–179.
18. Ranson JHC, Rifkind KM, Roses DF, et al: Objective of early identification of severe acute pancreatitis. Am J Gastroenterol 1974; 61:443–451.
19. McMahon JH, Playforth MJ, Pickford IR: A comparative study of methods for the prediction of severity of attacks of acute pancreatitis. Br J Surg 1980; 67:22–25.
20. Beger HG, Bittner R, Block S, et al: Bacterial contamination of pancreatic necrosis: A prospective clinical study. Gastroenterology 1986; 91:433–438.
21. Bradley EL, Fulenwider T: Open treatment of pancreatic abscess. Surg Gynecol Obstet 1984; 159:509–513.
22. Pottmeyer E, Frey CF: Pancreaticopleural fistulas. Arch Surg 1987; 122:648–654.
23. Frey CF, Lindenauer SM, Miller TA: Pancreatic abscess. Surg Gynecol Obstet 1979; 149:722–726.
24. Frey CF: Hemorrhagic pancreatitis. Am J Surg 1979; 137:616–623.
25. Siegleman SS, Copeland BE, Saba GP, et al: CT of fluid collections associated with pancreatitis. Am J Radiol 1980; 134:1121–1132.
26. Jeffrey RR, Federle MP, Cello JP, et al: Early computed tomographic scanning in acute severe pancreatitis. Surg Gynecol Obstet 1982; 154:170–174.
27. Kivisaari L, Somer K, Standertskjold-Nordenstam CG, et al: A new method for the diagnosis of acute hemorrhagic-necrotizing pancreatitis using contrast enhanced CT. Gastroenterol Radiol 1984; 9:27–30.
28. Ranson JH: Acute pancreatitis: Pathogenesis, outcome and treatment. Clin Gastroenterol 1984; 13:847–863.
29. Frey CF: A strategy for the surgical management of gallstone pancreatitis, in Beger HG, Buchler M (eds): Acute Pancreatitis. Berlin, Springer-Verlag, 1987, pp 242–250.
30. Ranson JCH, Rifkind KM, Roses DF, et al: Prognostic signs and the role of operative management in acute pancreatitis. Surg Gynecol Obstet 1974; 39(1):69–81.
31. Imrie CW: Observations on acute pancreatitis. Br J Surg 1974; 61:539–544.
32. Bank S, Wise L, Gersten M: Risk factors in acute pancreatitis. Am J Gastroenterol 1984; 78:637–640.
33. Mayer AD, McMahon MJ, Bowen M, et al: C-reactive protein: An aid to assessment and monitoring of acute pancreatitis. J Clin Pathol 1984; 37:207–211.
34. McMahon MJ, Bowen M, Mayer AD, et al: Relationship of alpha-2 macroglobulin and other antiproteases to the clinical features of acute pancreatitis. Am J Surg 1984; 147:164–170.
35. Buchler M, Uhl W, Malfertheiner P: Biochemical staging of acute pancreatitis, in Beger HG, Buchler M (eds): Acute Pancreatitis. Berlin, Springer-Verlag, 1987, pp 143–153.
36. Ohlsson K, Balldin G, Lasson A: Trypsin induced release of bradykinin and of C_3 fragments in man. Adv Exp Med Biol 1983; 156:1083–1090.
37. Winstone NE: Methemalbumin in acute pancreatitis. Br J Surg 1965; 52:804–808.
38. Geokas MC, Rinderknecht H, Walberg CB, et al: Methemalbumin in the diagnosis of acute hemorrhagic pancreatitis. Ann Intern Med 1974; 81:483–486.
39. Mayer AD, McMahon MJ: The diagnostic and prognostic value of operative lavage in patients

with acute pancreatitis. *Surg Gynecol Obstet* 1985; 160:507–512.
40. Hiatt JR, Fink AS, King W, et al: Percutaneous aspiration of peripancreatic fluid collections: A safe method to detect infection. *Surgery* 1987; 101:523–530.
41. Medical Research Council: Multicenter trial glucagon and apoprotinin: Death from acute pancreatitis. *Lancet* 1977; II:632–635.
42. Usadel K, Uberla KK, Leuschner V: Treatment of acute pancreatitis with somastostatin: Results of the multicenter double-blind trial. *Dig Dis Sci* 1985; 30:92.
43. Louidice TA, Lang J, Mehta H, et al: Treatment of acute alcoholic pancreatitis: The roles of cimetidine and nasogastric suction. *Am J Gastroenterol* 1984; 79:553–558.
44. Cooper MJ, Williamson RCN, Pollack AV: The role of peritoneal lavage in the prediction and treatment of severe acute pancreatitis. *Ann R Coll Surg Engl* 1982; 64:422–427.
45. Craig R, Pordal M, Myles E: The use of ampicillin in acute pancreatitis. *Ann Intern Med* 1975; 83:831.
46. Howes R, Zuidema GD, Cameron JL: Evaluation of prophylactic antibiotics in acute pancreatitis. *J Surg Res* 1975; 18:197.
47. Finch WT, Sawyers JL, Schenker S: A prospective study to determine the efficacy of antibiotics in acute pancreatitis. *Ann Surg* 1976; 183:667–671.
48. Stone HH, Fabian TC: Peritoneal dialysis in the treatment of acute alcoholic pancreatitis. *Surg Gynecol Obstet* 1980; 150:878.
49. Schuppisser JP, Grotzinger U, Osterwalder A, et al: The role of phospholipase A_2 in respiratory failure of acute pancreatitis. *Helv Chir Acta* 1984; 51:665–667.
50. Deitch EA, Winterton J, Li MA, et al: The gut as a portal of entry for bacticemia: Role of protein malnutrition. *Ann Surg* 1987; 205:681–691.
51. Goodgame JT, Fischer JE: Parenteral nutrition in the treatment of acute pancreatitis. *Ann Surg* 1977; 186:651–658.
52. Ranson JCH, Balthazar E, Caccavale R, et al: Computed tomography and the prediction of pancreatic abscess in acute pancreatitis. *Ann Surg* 1985; 201:656–665.
53. Beger HG, Krautzberger W, Bittner R, et al: Results of surgical treatment of necrotizing pancreatitis. *World J Surg* 1985; 9:972–979.
54. Bradley EL, Hall JR, Lutz J, et al: Hemodynamic consequences of severe pancreatitis. *Ann Surg* 1983; 198:130–133.
55. Ito K, Ramirez-Schon G, Shah PM, et al: Myocardial function in acute pancreatitis. *Ann Surg* 1981; 194:85–88.
56. Garcia-Szabo RR, Malik AB: Pancreatitis induced increase in lung vascular permeability. *Ann Rev Respir Dis* 1984; 129:580–583.
57. Lempinen M: Indications for surgery in extended pancreatic necrosis, in Beger HG, Buchler M (eds): *Acute Pancreatitis*. Berlin, Springer-Verlag, 1987, pp 305–309.
58. Gebhardt C: Indications for surgical intervention in necrotizing pancreatitis with extra pancreatic necrosis, in Beger HG, Buchler M (eds): *Acute Pancreatitis*. Berlin, Springer-Verlag, 1987, pp 310–313.
59. Beger HG, Bittner R, Buchler M, et al: Hemodynamic data pattern in patients with acute pancreatitis. *Gastroenterology* 1986; 90:74–79.
60. Camer SJ, Tan EGC, Warren K, et al: Pancreatic abscess. *Am J Surg* 1975; 129:426–431.
61. Bradley EL, Clements JL, Gonzalez AC: The natural history of pancreatic pseudocysts: A unified concept of management. *Am J Surg* 1979; 137:135–141.
62. Barkin JS, Smith FR, Pereiras R, et al: Therapeutic percutaneous aspiration of pancreatic pseudocysts. *Dig Dis Sci* 1981; 26:585–586.
63. Bradley EL: "Don't fix nothin that ain't broke." *Am J Surg* 1985; 149:197.

13

Common Duct Stones:
Does a patient with intact gall bladder require surgery after endoscopic removal of common duct stones?

STEPHEN E. SILVIS, M.D.

Choledocholithiasis represents a significant problem in modern clinical practice. The origin of these stones in individual patients is not clearly known. The evidence strongly supports the theory that the gallbladder is the source of the majority of common duct stones; however, stones clearly form within the bile duct. Primary bile duct stones are usually bilirubinate stones and are seen with stasis of the bile. In addition, they have been seen in patients with congenital absence of the gallbladder. In fact, the incidence of common bile duct stones is increased in patients with agenesis of the gallbladder.[1, 2] About 15% of patients with stones in the gallbladder also have stones in the bile duct. Conversely, 95% of common bile duct stones probably have their origins in the gallbladder.[3]

Many patients present with common bile duct stones months to years after cholecystectomy.[4] It is impossible to tell whether these are reformed stones or stones that were overlooked at the time of surgery. Often they are round, soft, earthy stones that have been thought by most observers to have arisen within the bile duct itself.[5, 6] In some instances there are several faceted stones that would appear to have arisen in the gallbladder and would have been asymptomatic for many years. In studies of Way,[7] it would seem that common bile duct stones may be asymptomatic for long periods of time, although an accurate knowledge of the natural history of choledocholithiasis is not well known. In patients following cholecystectomy, a sizable number present with common duct stones and do so within the first two years. Most observers believe that these stones were overlooked at the time of surgery. The common duct stones diagnosed three or four years after cholecystectomy are felt to be secondary stones that formed in the bile duct. There is a small incidence of recurrent stones that appears to be constant after cholecystectomy. A limited number of patients[6] continually reform stones within the bile duct; these require repeated therapy (Fig 13–1). Reasons for this stone formation are not apparent. Recurrent biliary infection and chronic stasis have, in at least some of these cases, been excluded. The origin of cholesterol stones is possibly the same as that previously discussed with regard to the gallbladder. Bilirubin stones are formed by deconjugation of bilirubin, secondary to infection within static bile, in partially obstructed ducts.[8–11]

CLINICAL MANIFESTATIONS OF CHOLEDOCHOLITHIASIS

Asymptomatic bile duct stones are being diagnosed more frequently as scanning techniques are used wherein common duct stones are visualized on a scan that

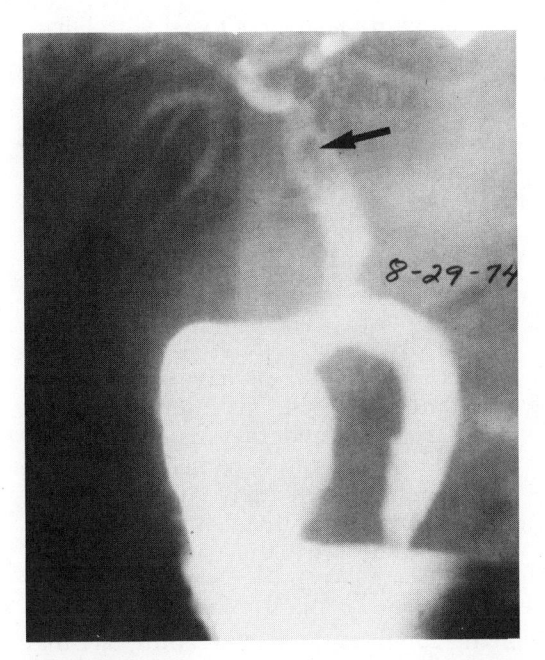

FIG 13–1.
This patient had a choledochoduodenostomy for common bile duct stones. He had had a cholecystectomy with exploration for common duct stones and then exploration for recurrent common duct stones. At the third exploration for duct stones the choledochoduodenostomy was performed. The patient is now being seen for common bile duct stones *(arrow)*. The choledochoduodenostomy and the ampulla both appear widely patent. These stones were removed with a balloon, and the patient has done well for 13 years. I do not understand why the stones reform; therefore, I anticipate that the patient is likely to have further problems. If these can be removed by simply cleaning the duct mechanically with balloons or baskets, that is the perferable method of treatment. Possibly the bile salts given the patient following this procedure influenced the reformation of stones, but there is not good evidence for this result.

was ordered for another reason. It is unclear whether all common duct stones should be treated when they are found, but it is probably advisable to do so. In the article by Way[7] approximately 50% of patients with common duct stones became symptomatic within 1 year, and in the study of silent gallstones from Malmo[12], about the same percentage developed symptoms within a two-year period. Although these data are not extensive, it seems apparent that all but extremely high-risk surgical patients should be treated when the stones are discovered because the morbidity of common duct obstruction is quite significant.

Biliary colic and/or jaundice are the most common indications of common bile duct stones. Patients may present with biliary colic in the absence of stones or jaundice. Infection within the biliary tree (cholangitis) may occur with common duct stones. However, it can occur with anything that obstructs or retards the flow of bile from the biliary tree such as benign or malignant strictures, compression of the bile duct, extrinsic masses, or parasitic infections within the bile duct. Although cholangitis is usually rather mild, there is a form of the disease described as suppurative cholangitis in which the patient is extremely ill. It is not a precisely defined entity because the presence of pus within the biliary tree does not indicate the clinical condition of the patient. It has been described as a syndrome known as Charcot's triad, consisting of pain, jaundice, chills, and/or fever. About 70% of the severely ill patients have all of the triad. Fever is present in 95%, pain in 90%, but clinical evidence of jaundice may be absent in up to 20% of the patients.[13–16] When suppurative cholangitis is suspected or established, prompt drainage of the biliary tree is essential. More mild forms of cholangitis will respond to nasogastric suction and antibiotic therapy.

Common bile duct stones are a well-defined cause of pancreatitis. The pancreatitis may present without signs of biliary disease. Alcoholic pancreatitis may present in combination with alcoholic liver disease, making it difficult at times to separate biliary from alcoholic pancreatitis.[17–19] This will be discussed further in the section entitled "Differential Diagnosis of Common Bile Duct Stones."

Less frequently, common bile duct stones may present as one of the remote complications of a disease such as liver abscess, which actually is a secondary result of the cholangitis produced by the bile duct obstruction. Obviously, any long-term obstruction of the common duct may produce biliary cirrhosis. This is an extremely unusual manifestation of common duct stones. In addition, elderly patients may present with weight loss with or without jaundice, anorexia, vague abdominal complaints, suggesting an abdominal malignancy, caused by common duct stones.

LABORATORY FINDINGS IN CHOLEDOCHOLITHIASIS

Asymptomatic common bile duct stone(s) may have entirely normal laboratory findings. Typical laboratory findings are that of increased direct reacting bilirubin in the range of 2 to 15 mgm%.[20] Values above 15 mgm% generally have associated liver disease or nearly complete obstruction. Serum alkaline phosphatase rises,[21] as does the 5-nucleotidase. The SGOT is usually only modestly elevated during stone obstruction. Occasionally very elevated transaminase is found immediately after high-grade obstruction.[22] These high SGOTs come down to approach normal rather quickly (i.e., within 1 or 2 days). The prothrombin time may be increased but is usually only slightly altered and it is corrected by the administration of intravenous vitamin K. The abnormal serum bilirubin may be quite brief in gallstone obstruction. The serum amylase frequently rises with the passage of a common duct stone. It also may be extremely transient. The blood counts are normal except in the presence of cholangitis when the white count may be markedly elevated.

DIFFERENTIAL DIAGNOSIS OF COMMON BILE DUCT STONES

A classic history and physical examination make the diagnosis of common duct stone(s) straightforward. However, a great many diseases may mimic the findings of ductal stones. The patient who has had the gallbladder removed will often describe the pain of common duct stones as similar to the attacks they suffered before their cholecystectomy. Renal and intestinal pain may be confused with biliary colic. Renal pain is usually in the flank and radiating down to the groin and to the inner aspect of the thigh. Intestinal colic is crampy and more midline, centering around the umbilicus, and frequently provokes emesis. The abdomen tends to distend with high-pitched bowel sounds. Hepatic abscess may be caused by choledocholithiasis. Amoebic or pyogenic hepatic abcesess may simulate cholangitis caused by choledocholithiasis. Patients with a solitary abscess have right upper-quadrant pain, which is often sudden in onset. Hepatic tenderness is quite apparent, and the liver may be palpable. It is a challenge to differentiate cholangitis and hepatic abscess with laboratory findings unless the abscess is visualized on ultrasound or CAT scan.

Important in the differential diagnosis of the common duct stone is the fact that the pain of acute myocardial infarction and the pain of biliary colic may at times be very similar. Slight jaundice may follow a myocardial infarction but is less common than with a biliary calculus. It usually does not appear until several days after the infarction rather than immediately, as in biliary calculus disease. Elevation of the SGOT may occur in both conditions. It rarely exceeds 100 to 150 units except when shock has supervened in myocardial infarction. Elevation of the SGPT will be noted in choledocholithiasis but does not occur in myocardial infarction.

Congestive heart failure can produce right upper-quadrant pain with distention of the liver, tenderness in that area, elevation of liver enzymes, and even jaundice. In patients with congestive heart failure, the temperature is normal and the white count remains normal. The patient usually has obvious signs of congestive heart failure, particularly findings of right-sided heart failure or tricuspid valve disease. The only difficult question is, does the patient have both biliary disease and congestive heart failure? It is occasionally difficult to separate the acute pancreatitis associated with common duct stone from acute pancreatitis of other etiology. This may require x-ray of the common duct to exclude a common duct stone before one may be absolutely certain of this differential diagnosis.[23-26]

DIAGNOSIS OF COMMON DUCT STONES

The ultimate diagnosis of common duct stones is their identification and removal either by surgery or endoscopic methods. Criteria for exploring the common duct at the time of surgery have been established in the surgical literature for many decades; these are: (1) history of cholangitis, (2) pancreatitis, (3) jaundice, (4) dilated common duct, and (5) palpable stones within the common duct.[27, 28] Many surgeons obtain operative cholangiograms before deciding to explore the common duct. Therefore, these are relative indications for common duct exploration.[29-31]

With the advent of ERCP[32-35] and good scanning techniques, the diagnosis of common duct stones can usually be made preoperatively. In Fig 13-2, ultrasound accurately delineates the size of the common duct and shows a stone within it. Ultrasound's reliability in identifying a stone is not good unless a clear shadow is seen.[35] The same can be said of CAT scans. One cannot be entirely sure whether this filling defect represents tumor or intraductal stone, but percentages would favor it being a stone. Figure 13-3 shows a plain film of the abdomen where calcified stones are clearly seen within the common bile duct and gallbladder. This definitively diagnoses the common duct stones. It is seen only with calcification of the outer rim of the biliary calculi.

There is now a consensus that the patient with jaundice should have cholangiographic demonstration of the cause of the jaundice prior to surgical treatment. This may be done by percutaneous transhepatic cholangiography (PTC) or by ERCP. The choice of test is based primarily on the local expertise and whether endoscopic retrograde sphincterotomy (ERS) will be done if a common duct stone is found. When dilated ducts are seen on ultrasound or CAT scanning techniques, PTC is almost certain to be successful. Bile duct dilatation does not influence the results of the ERCP. The only predictor of success or failure with ERCP would be the history of previous gastric surgery, particularly a Billroth II anastomosis. Then the success rate of ERCP drops to 65% to 80% from a 95% success rate in other situations.[36-40]

In both ERCP and PTC, care must be taken not to introduce air bubbles within the biliary tree. The air bubbles form around radiolucent filling defects that may be difficult to tell from common bile duct stones. In most situations they can be distinguished because stones will have at least one flattened edge. If the presence of a bubble artifact is questionable (Fig 13-4), it may be advisable to allow the duct to empty of contrast media and repeat the study, confirming the presence of a filling defect. Calculus will move down and bubbles will move up or coalesce if the patient is placed in the upright position. As one begins to fill the common duct, it is frequently wise to switch to less dense contrast media; otherwise small filling defects are likely to be hidden in the dense contrast.

Multiple faceted stones in the common duct clearly make the unequivocal diagnosis (Fig 13-5). At times, common duct stones may become impacted in the distal sphincter area. If this is a solitary common duct stone there may be a question of a distal tumor of the bile duct. On occasion, this cannot be resolved until either sphincterotomy with removal of the stone is accomplished or surgery with exploration of the area has been done.

TREATMENT OF COMMON DUCT STONES

Until very recently surgery represented the only successful therapy for common duct stone disease. Over the past decade numerous therapies have developed, which will be discussed in this chapter. The surgery for common duct stones is frequently done at the same time the cholecystectomy is performed. The gallbladder is removed and a longitudinal incision is made in the common duct, usually at

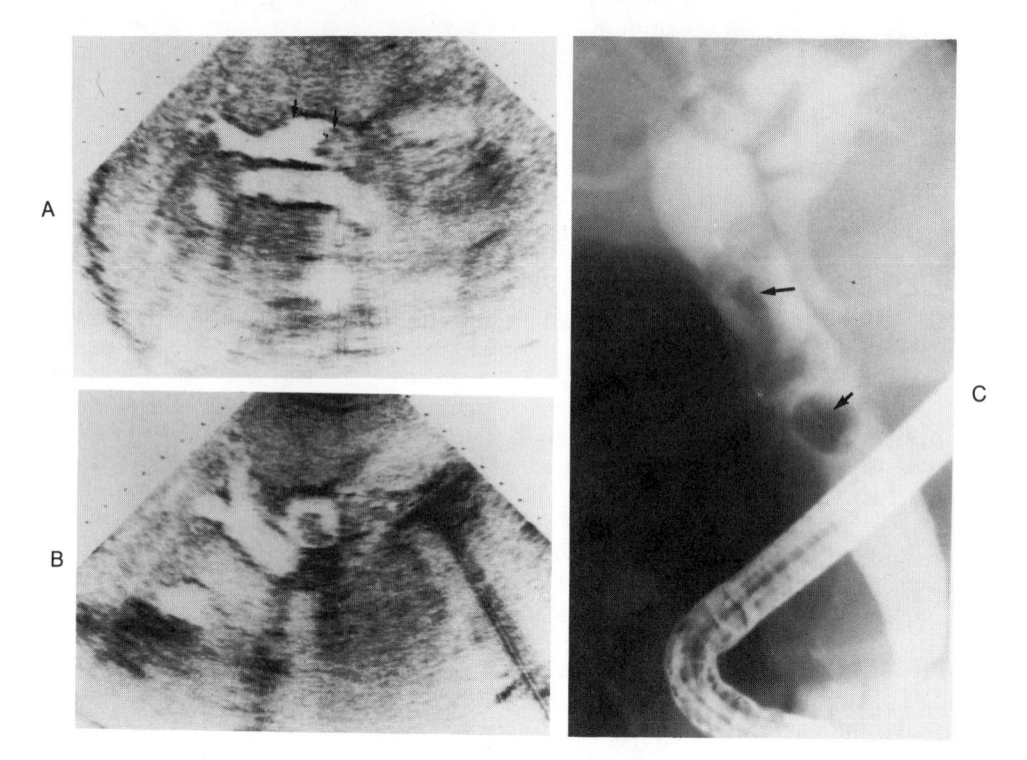

FIG 13–2.
The ultrasound of this patient shows a markedly dilated duct. **A,** The scan was done longitudinally to the common duct and shows a 2-cm duct *between the small arrows*. **B,** When this patient was scanned in a transverse diameter, an irregular filling defect shows within the dilated common bile duct, which appears to be floating within the duct. This is almost unequivocally a common bile duct stone. ERCP is indicated in this patient if the stone is to be removed by endoscopic sphincterotomy; if not, the diagnosis is firmly established. From the scan it was impossible to tell whether this was a single very large stone or a number of stones that were clustered together. Therefore, one could not give an opinion as to whether this could be removed by sphincterotomy or not. When measurements are made of the bile duct on ultrasound they are usually the common hepatic duct rather than the common bile duct. This clear representation of the common duct stone is seldom seen on ultrasonography. This is related to the fact that the stones are usually in the distal common duct which is retroduodenal. Air in the duodenum interferes with the ultrasound scanning technique. **C,** The cholangiogram of this patient demonstrates multiple calculi, the largest of which is about 1 cm (*long arrow*) above the balloon (*short arrow*). This film was taken after the sphincterotomy had been completed and as the stones were being extracted with a balloon. All of the stones were removed with the balloon. The patient had had a previous cholecystectomy and had no further symptoms in the following 4 years.

its midportion. The duct is probed with baskets and extracting forceps until no further stones can be removed. At this point a T-tube is inserted into the common duct and x-ray(s) taken to determine if stones are still present. When no more stones can be felt with forceps or by palpation, a T-tube cholangiogram is performed. If this test is negative, the patient is closed and a T-tube cholangiogram is repeated before it is removed, usually in about 2 weeks. Both Martin[41] and McSherry[42] have shown that common bile duct exploration adds significantly to the morbidity and mortality of cholecystectomy.

Fifteen years ago the first ERS was performed by Koch.[43, 44] During this period

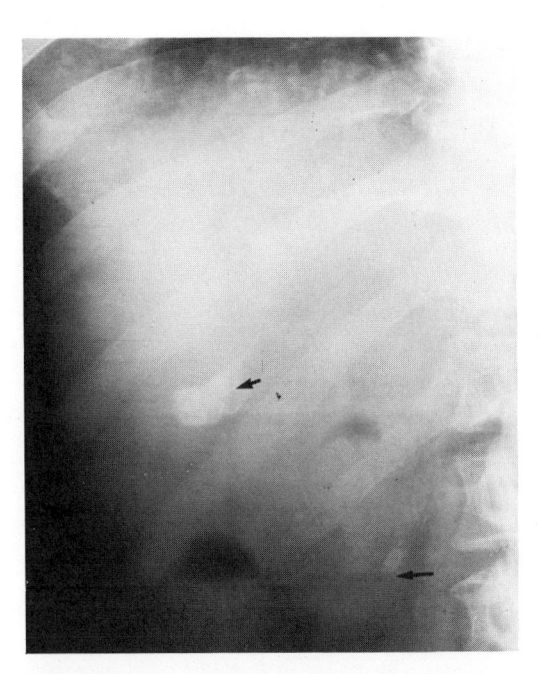

FIG 13–3.
This x-ray shows calcified stones in the gallbladder and common bile duct. Only a small percentage of stones are calcified, and they can be easily seen on the plain film of the abdomen. When the abdominal film is ordered for a problem not related to right upper-quadrant pain, it is then unclear whether these common duct stones *(long arrow)* are causing symptoms or not. The dense conglomeration of stones *(short arrow)* is undoubtedly within the gallbladder. Unless the patient has extremely severe coexisting disease, these stones should be removed. Evidence would suggest that removing the stones within the common duct is probably adequate treatment until symptoms are manifested from the stones inside of the gallbladder.

the success rate of the procedure has increased to 85% to 90%. ERS has become the procedure of choice for removing common duct stones.[33, 45–59]

Briefly, the ERS technique consists of passing a cannula, which has a short segment of wire exposed at the tip, into the common bile duct. This wire may be flexed by pulling on the handle at the proximal end to form a bowstring. The wire is retracted back into the duodenum so its position may be determined and aimed toward the duodenal lumen. Radiofrequency current is applied to the wire, and a cut is produced extending up through the papilla and into the distal common bile duct.

The size of the sphincterotomy should be tailored to the size of the stone. It is important to determine the length of the incision before the sphincterotomy is begun because once cutting begins edema develops, and it is much harder to determine landmarks. When cutting with the papillotome has reached the predetermined extent, the papillotome is flexed and the size of the orifice is measured. The length of the incision does not determine the diameter of the sphincterotomy because the duct runs tangentially through the duodenal wall.

If the sphincterotomy appears large enough, the papillotome is removed and replaced with a balloon. The first step is to measure the papillary orifice with a balloon the size of the largest common duct stone. If the balloon, which is the size of the stones, will pull through the sphincterotomy the stones can usually be removed. If the balloon does not come through and there is additional common bile duct in the duodenal wall, the balloon is removed and the sphincterotomy is extended. Extending the sphincterotomy probably increases the complication rate of both bleeding and perforation. Extensive edema may develop around the incision following the sphincterotomy. If one is unsuccessful in removing the stones at that time a nasobiliary tube may be inserted to allow drainage. After waiting 2 to 5 days for the edema to subside, a repeat attempt to remove the stones is often successful.

PROBLEMS IN PERFORMING ERS

Obviously the patient with abnormal coagulation represents a significant problem. If the defect is correctable, the procedure should be delayed. Hereditary coagulation defects must be corrected and maintained for 7 to 10 days because it takes some time for the sphincterotomy site to heal. When a coagulation defect is present, the increased risk of bleeding

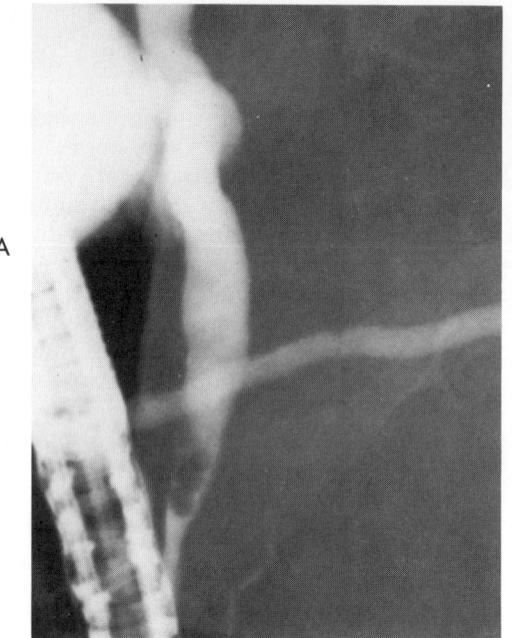

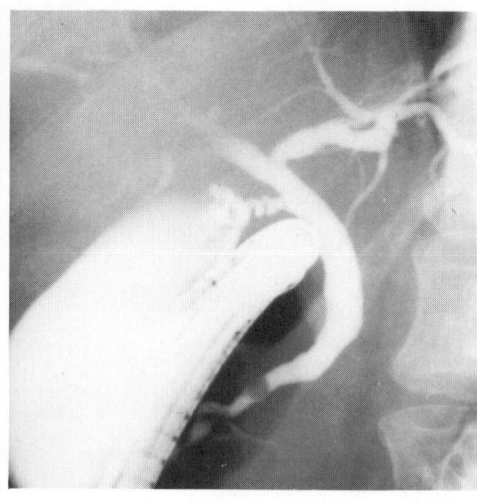

FIG 13–4.
This is a normal cholangiogram. **A,** There are small defects in the distal common bile duct which are round and uniform and have smooth edges; these have all the features of air bubbles. It is relatively easy to diagnose small stones because they usually have at least one edge that is flattened; this does not occur in air bubbles. However, some stones are entirely round, and in the presence of air bubbles, round stones can clearly be overlooked. **B** shows a single filling defect. It was difficult to determine whether it was a stone or an air bubble. In this case, the duct was allowed to empty and was then refilled, which demonstrated a normal duct.

must be weighed against the problem of the retained common duct stone. Usually coagulation problems can be corrected enough with fresh frozen plasma to perform the procedure. In the patient with end-stage liver disease and a common duct stone, the end-stage liver disease has a more serious prognosis than the common duct stone.

Sometimes there is a problem finding the papilla. With normal anatomy this is usually not difficult. In a small number of patients there is no longitudinal fold but only a small flat papilla that sits between the anatomical folds. The only way that these can be found is by carefully searching the medial duodenal wall for the papilla, and if bile is present following it back to the papillary orifice. Once these papilla have been found, they are quite easy to cannulate.

A gastric resection with either a Billroth I or II anastomosis makes the papilla more difficult to locate and to cannulate.[36–40] Frequently, a majority of the duodenal bulb has been resected. This places the papilla's location just beyond the Billroth I anastomosis. It is somewhat hard to see and is often difficult to get the scope to sit in exactly the right position for cannulation. Billroth I anastomosis is usually only a minor problem. A Billroth II requires passing the endoscope through the gastrojejunostomy and up the proximal limb to locate the papilla. As one is doing the cannulation and sphincterotomy, one must remember that everything is reversed. The endoscope is viewing up at the papilla rather than down at it in the usual position. It is quite easy for the sphincterotome to be entirely reversed and to be cutting down the duodenal wall, when in your visual field it appears to be in the proper position. Frequently,

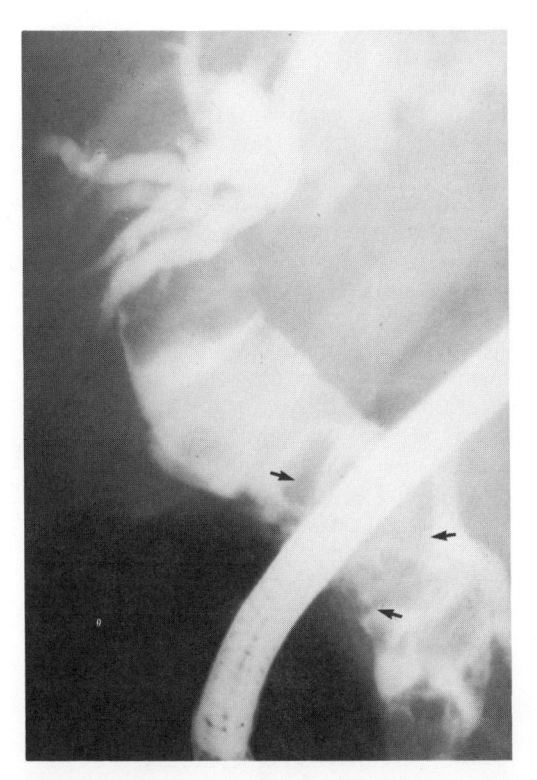

FIG 13–5.
This cholangiogram shows massive dilatation of the bile duct. The endoscope is approximately on the same plane as the bile duct; therefore, it can be used as a measuring device. The bile duct is over four times the size of the endoscope or greater than 4 cm in diameter. There are huge filling defects within the bile duct on this film. It is difficult to be certain which of these were single stones and which represented aggregation of multiple stones. Obviously, the filling defect behind the endoscope *(short arrows)* is too large to remove from the bile duct in a single piece. This was actually a soft conglomeration of stones and was removed with a standard sphincterotomy and a balloon extraction. The sphincterotomy was somewhat longer than usual; however, there was a long segment of intraduodenal common bile duct. Although no complications occurred in this patient, a long sphincterotomy probably has increased complications. Because we prefer not to make a long sphincterotomy these patients will be candidates for various methods of lithotripsy if they become effective.

almost the entire duodenal bulb has been resected at surgery, which leaves the papilla very close to the proximal closed end of the duodenum.

Sharp angulations of the duodenal limb may make it impossible to pass a scope up this limb, and the proximal limb may be too long for instrumentation. Because of all the problems with Billroth II anastomosis, the percentage of successful cannulations probably falls to about 80%, and the percentage of successful sphincterotomies decreases to 60% to 70%.[36–40] This should be borne in mind before the procedure is attempted so that both the referring physician and the patient realize that the prospect of failure is reasonably high.

Another problem in locating and cannulating the papilla is duodenal diverticula. Usually the papilla sits on the diverticular wall, and with careful searching it can be located. Rarely, the diverticula contains the papilla. The only way one can be certain of this is to visualize bile coming from the diverticulum. In these instances it cannot be visualized or cannulated. Most papilla sit on the rim where cannulation is possible, and if cannulation is successful, sphincterotomy usually can be performed (Fig 13–6). The diverticula probably form in the papillary area because the ducts pass through the wall and produce a weakness in the duodenal musculature. Remember that these diverticula are pseudodiverticula and have only mucosa in their wall. The endoscopist should not put instruments into the diverticulum because they can be easily perforated.[60, 61]

If the papilla can be identified it can almost always be cannulated. Obtaining the desired duct remains somewhat difficult in a small percentage of patients. The common bile duct is usually orientated cephalad and slightly to the left in the visual field. The pancreatic duct is orientated with the cannula going straight into the wall and directed slightly to the right in the visual field. These statements are true in about 85% to 90% of patients.[61] A small number of patients have reversal of the same phenomenon. Once the cannula is directed toward the common bile duct, contrast should be injected. It is satisfactory to visualize the common duct with

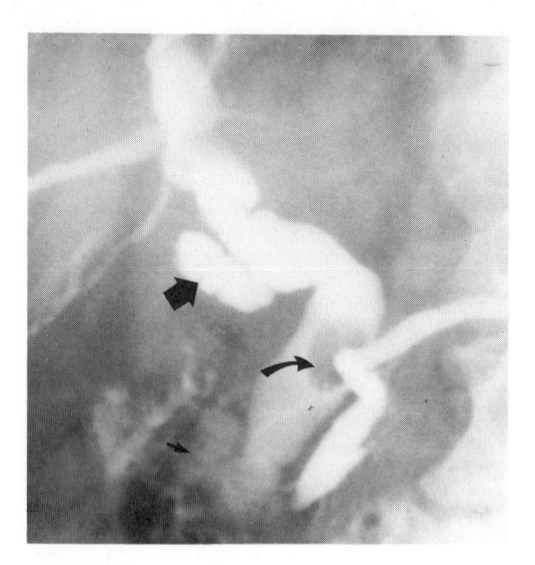

FIG 13–6.
This cholangiogram shows a slightly dilated common bile duct with a stone. The outline of a periampullary diverticulum is seen *(short arrow)*. The distal common bile duct runs alongside, but not actually in the diverticulum. If the sphincterotomy incision can be made on the ridge of the common bile duct, it can be performed safely even with the adjacent diverticulum. The long cystic duct stump *(long arrow)* is not a cause of symptoms unless it harbors biliary stones. The common duct stone *(large arrow)* is approximately 8 mm in diameter and was delivered through the distal segment of the bile duct by balloon traction. Periampullary diverticula usually occur where the duct perforates the duodenal wall. This causes the bile duct to be on the rim of the diverticulum.

the cannula impacted in the sphincter. The endoscopist determines the presence or absence of common duct stones, and their relative size is measured in comparison to the endoscope. Before sphincterotomy is attempted, one should review the risk and prospects for success.[62] If the stones are extremely large, a stricture is present, or the bile duct passes almost straight through the duodenal wall, the prospect of removing the stones by endoscopic sphincterotomy may be markedly reduced. Under these circumstances the patient should again be considered for surgical stone removal.

It is necessary to obtain a free cannulation prior to sphincterotomy. If this cannulation is difficult, it has become quite common to leave a wire in place so you can pass the papillotome over a wire. Usually, if a cannula cannot be passed freely into the bile duct, the papillotome will not pass; however, occasionally the papillotome will pass easily into the common duct when the cannulation was difficult. A number of instruments have been designed to assist in the difficult sphincterotomy when free cannulation cannot be obtained. The standard papillotome is a cannula with an exposed length of wire at the distal tip. The length of this wire varies from 20 to 30 mm. The handle on the proximal end allows variable bowing of the exposed wire. This exposed wire is directed from the common bile duct toward the duodenal lumen. A portion of the wire needs to be exposed within the duodenum, usually 10 to 15 mm of a 30-mm wire. Radiofrequency current is then passed through the wire to produce heating and cutting. This is done in a short incremental manner until the sphincterotomy has reached the predetermined size, which one has estimated to be large enough for the stones to be delivered from the bile duct.

The precut papillotome is designed to assist when the papillotome cannot be freely passed into the bile duct.[63] The wire comes out all the way to the tip of the cannula. It is passed up the papilla as far as possible, and then cutting is performed with radiofrequency current. The difficulty with this technique is to be certain that the papillotome is cutting toward the bile duct and will advance into the bile duct. Once the papillotome has cut into the bile duct, which has been confirmed on x-ray by the injection of radiopaque contrast, the sphincterotomy is done in the usual manner.

The fistulotomy instrument[64] is a cannula with a wire that can be advanced out the tip. The extended wire is used to do a precut of the sphincter when one can rather clearly define the common duct orifice, or to cut from the duodenal wall down into the bile duct where a clear bulge can be seen, to perform a choledochoduodenostomy. Once a small opening is made into the bile duct (confirmed by injecting radiopaque contrast), a standard papillotome may be used to complete the sphincterotomy. Both of these instruments probably carry increased risk, and the relative surgical risk needs to be weighed before they are used. The primary difficulty is not being able to cut freely into the bile duct, leaving an edematous area which may obstruct the bile duct and prevent completion of the procedure. This relative obstruction of the pancreatic and common bile duct may, at least theoretically, produce pancreatitis or biliary pancreatic sepsis. There have been incidences of cutting across the pancreatic duct with precut instruments, producing a pancreatic leak.

A recent development for cases where it is impossible to insert the papillotome has been a combined procedure:[65-67] (1) The invasive radiologist does a percutaneous transhepatic cholangiogram, passing a wire and then a basket down through the common bile duct into the duodenum. (2) The endoscopist inserts the sphincterotome into the basket. While the invasive radiologist retracts the basket, the endoscopist advances the papillotome until it is inserted into the common duct. The author has found this combined approach helpful in patients in whom the papilla is within the diverticulum or cannot be seen endoscopically. Once the sphincterotome is well up the common duct and flexed, it can be retracted and the papilla can be pulled out of the diverticulum. Frequently the sphincterotomy can then be done without difficulty. The other situations have been in patients with extremely tight papillae or when orientation on the papilla becomes impossible due to previous surgical procedures. Obviously, before a combined approach is performed, one must again consider the surgical risks. Patients who have had multiple surgical procedures into the upper abdomen may be surgically difficult, although the risks are probably not as greatly increased as we once thought.

We will briefly review the standard sphincterotomy.[61] The papillotome is passed into the duct; after slight flexion it is withdrawn until the wire is visualized in the duodenum. We need to be certain that the wire is pointing toward the duodenum and is oriented along the long axis of the common bile duct. It is well to determine how long a cut is desirable before one begins a sphincterotomy. This should be tailored to the size of the common duct stone. In addition, one should be able to see an impression of the common duct in the duodenal wall for the length that one wishes to make the sphincterotomy. Bulging of the bile duct into the wall after additional injection of contrast confirms bile duct position.

PROBLEMS OF THE LARGE COMMON BILE DUCT STONE

The average common bile duct stone is from 8 to 10 mm.[68] This is well within the range that can be removed readily by sphincterotomy. However, some stones reach sizes considerably beyond that and may be as large as 2 to 3 cm, which is clearly beyond the size that most sphincterotomies can be safely made.

My usual method of removing stones following sphincterotomy is by balloon extraction. Balloons that will inflate from 8 to 14 mm in diameter are currently available and are useful in measuring the size of the sphincterotomy as well as extracting the stones. There are two major problems when extracting stones with a balloon. If the duct is very large, the stone can slip around the balloon instead of being pulled down through the sphincterotomy, even when the opening is large enough to allow passage of the stone. The other is that the balloons tend to be rather fragile and frequently break, either in the sphincterotomy or by striking the scope. If the stones cannot be removed in a few attempts with balloon extraction it is common to place a nasobiliary tube in the duct, allow a 2 to 3-day period of time for the edema to subside, and then attempt extraction. Another problem is in a relative or absolute stenosis of the distal common duct. In Fig 13–7, the patient has what is probably a failure of the bile duct to dilate. The stone then lodges in the widely dilated portion. Often this distal

170 / PANCREAS

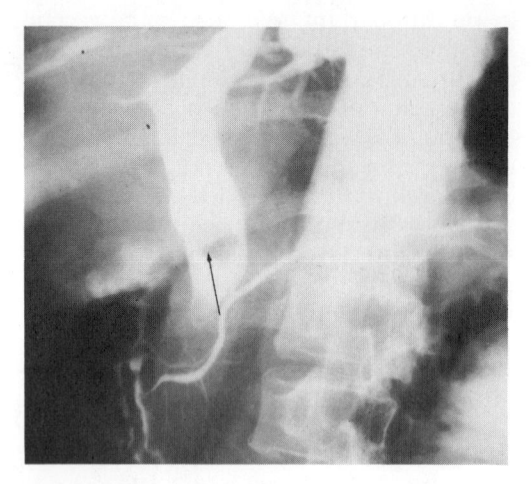

FIG 13–7.
This patient has had his gallbladder removed. There is a moderately dilated common bile duct with a regularly shaped stone in the distal duct *(long arrow)*. This is clearly differentiated from an air bubble because of its flat edges. Faintly seen is the distal common bile duct, which is not dilated. Frequently, common duct stones lodge in the bile duct above the pancreas causing obstructive jaundice. The distal segment of duct does not dilate. These stones can often be removed because the duct is not strictured, but instead has failed to dilate. When pressure is put on it to extract the stone, it will stretch to allow passage. On the other hand, this can represent a firm stricture, and the stone cannot be removed without first dilating the stricture. A sphincterotomy was made, and the stone was extracted with a balloon catheter.

duct is distensible and will yield, allowing the stone to be pulled through.[69] Patients with malignant strictures obviously can develop stones in the biliary stasis above the stricture (Fig 13–8). These should be recognized before the sphincterotomy is performed.

Mechanical lithotriptors[69–73] are a modification of the previously used Dormia baskets (Fig 13–9). The stone is entrapped in the wire basket, and the wires are pulled down under great pressure by the mechanical screw device to fracture the stone. The fragments of the stone are removed either with the basket or with a balloon. If the entire stone can be grasped in the mechanical lithotriptor, it can be crushed. Often only the edge of the stone can be grasped, and closing the basket may produce some shaving of the stone, reducing its size enough to remove the stone with a balloon.

The major problem with baskets and mechanical lithotriptors is trapping the stone within the basket. Frequently the basket will not open wide enough to catch the stone. Baskets having a plastic catheter can capture the stone. If the sphincterotomy is not wide enough to allow passage of both stone and basket, they may

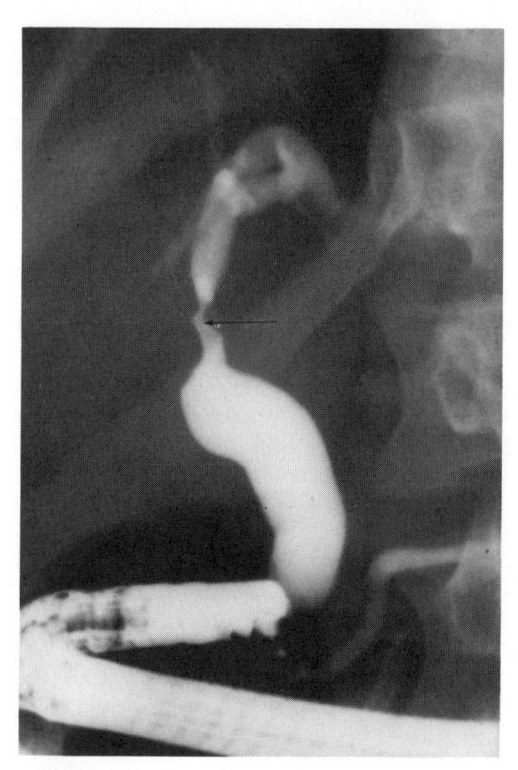

FIG 13–8.
This cholangiogram has a number of findings. There is a rather tight stricture in the common hepatic duct *(long arrow)*. Above this stricture is a filling defect representing a calculus. The distal common bile duct is dilated. At the terminus of the bile duct there is stricturing of both the bile duct and the pancreatic duct. These strictures represent metastatic carcinoma of the pancreas with calculus formation related to stasis, caused by the obstructing tumor. Obviously, calculi above malignant strictures should not be removed because the malignancy will reobstruct the duct. This patient required dilation of the stricture and stenting of the bile duct.

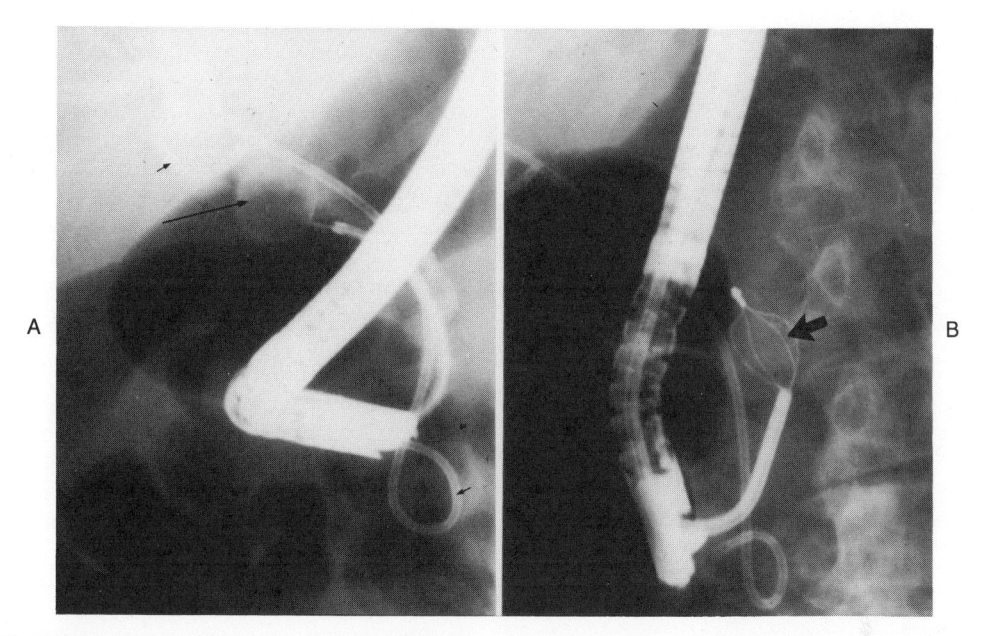

FIG 13–9.
This cholangiogram shows a large stone *(long arrow)*; at the time of the sphincterotomy it could not be extracted. Therefore, a pigtail stent *(short arrow)* was placed to allow drainage around the stone. **A,** a mechanical lithotriptor is being passed into the duct. **B,** the stone is captured within the mechanical lithotriptor *(large arrow)* and is being extracted. Afterward the pigtail stent was also removed. Allowing time for edema of the sphincterotomy to disappear will frequently facilitate the removal of very large stones. A small number of patients have been treated with the pigtail stent to bypass the stone(s). There is not extensive data on these patients, but they generally seemed to do quite well.

become impacted. If there is additional room to extend the sphincterotomy, the basket can be cut off and the endoscope removed. The endoscope is reinserted and a papillotome is passed alongside the basket to extend the sphincterotomy, allowing release of the entrapped basket. In some patients, surgical removal is necessary.

Electrohydraulic lithotripsy has been used for about a decade, primarily to fracture stones within the urinary tract.[74–76] Its basic principle is that of discharging a very short electrical spark of milliseconds duration into a fluid medium which produces an acoustic shock. This acoustic shock wave does not cause injury to structures that have elasticity, but will fracture crystalline structures such as calculi. A modified electrohydraulic lithotriptor that is passed through a catheter has been produced (Fig 13–10). This allows close contact with the stone but requires the balloon to keep the catheter away from the duct wall with short electrical discharges.[77–80] The fluid shock wave fragments the stone.

There is a small experience using extracorporeal focused electrohydraulic lithotripsy in common duct stones and in cholelithiasis. In common duct stones the work has been limited and the results are quite mixed. These expensive devices are not widely available, and at this time they must be considered experimental.[81–87]

Transhepatic use of electrohydraulic lithotripsy[88] has the distinct advantage of giving direct vision of the stone. It has been shown to be effective in only one case; it required a large tract, produced percutaneously into the bile duct.

Percutaneous transhepatic ultrasonic lithotripsy[89, 90] requires producing a straight tract which will admit a 12 French instrument. General anesthesia is necessary, and two reported cases were unsuccessful

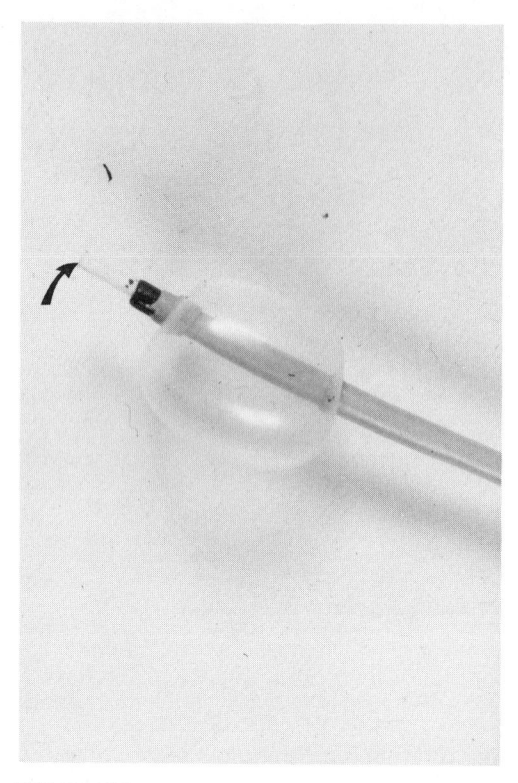

FIG 13–10.
This shows the tip of the electrohydraulic lithotriptor with the balloon inflated and the lithotriptor probe *(arrow)*. This bipolar probe transmits a very brief electric spark across the tip of the instrument. When it is placed in water an acoustical shock wave is generated that fractures nonelastic materials (such as stones) in its path. The catheter is necessary to inject contrast to visualize the stones and to inject saline to allow propagation of the shock waves. The presently available probe is a 9 F and requires a 4.2-cm channel scope. Maximum efficiency is reached when the lithotriptor probe is directly aligned and very close to the stone. However, it will fracture stones at a significant distance (6 to 10 mm) and also will fracture stones not directly in front of the probe.

because of failure to introduce the instrument.[89, 90] This procedure may cause rupture or leakage of the gallbladder which necessitates surgical intervention. It will take considerable observation and time to show that these procedures are better than surgical treatment.

A small number of cases report the use of a tunable dye wave laser that produces a very short impulse, which causes fracturing of a crystalline object.[91] This procedure requires direct vision of the stone through either a choledochoscope or through a scope passed up the papilla and into the bile duct. Most are done through a tract with a choledochoscope to visualize the stones. These must be considered experimental at the present time. Whether laser fracturing of gallstones will become widely useful has not yet been determined.

When sphincterotomy has been performed and a large stone has been demonstrated in the bile duct that cannot be removed by the usual methods, the physician must decide whether to do surgery, attempt to break it, or attempt to dissolve it. Monooctanoin has been used for a number of years. It is available clinically; however, it has only a 40% to 60% success rate, and a rather high percentage of the patients are intolerant to the diarrhea that may be produced.[92-98] Even in the patients who can tolerate the infusion of the monooctanoin through a transhepatic or nasobiliary catheter, usually 4 to 7 days are necessary to dissolve the stone.

Recent preliminary studies have described the dissolution of stones by perfusion of methyl-tert-butyl ether.[99-105] This methyl-tert-butyl ether dissolves gallstones in a few hours and does not injure the bile duct or gallbladder. Although not absorbed from the biliary tree, it is well absorbed from the small intestine. It injures the duodenum. The ether is an anesthetic producing sedation. At high levels, general anesthesia, irritation of the lung and bowel, hemolysis, and lowering of hematocrit occur. Methods must be developed to confine this material to the biliary tree before it can be generally effective in dissolving both bile and common duct stones.

COMPLICATIONS OF ERS[58, 61, 106–108]

Table 13–1 shows complications in a survey of 1,829 patients. Moderate bleeding (defined as bleeding that required no transfusions, required no surgery, and produced no mortality) was the most

TABLE 13–1.
ACUTE COMPLICATIONS OF ERS IN 1,829 CASES*

	Number	Percent (%)	Surgery	Death
Moderate bleed	35	1.9	0	0
Major bleed	21	1.1	3	2
Pancreatitis	56	3.1	4	0
Perforation	10	0.5	3	0
Cholangitis	16	0.9	2	1
Trapped basket	1	0.1	1	0
Acute cholecystitis	2	0.1	2	1
TOTALS	141	7.7	15	4 (0.2%)

*Data from Vennes JA, Silvis SE: Endoscopic retrograde sphincterotomy, in Silvis SE (ed): *Therapeutic Gastrointestinal Endoscopy*. New York, Igaku-Shoin, 1985, p 198.

common problem. Bleeding was considered severe when the patient became hypotensive or required transfusions. Three of these 21 patients in whom bleeding was severe required surgery and two died. The incidence of major bleeding was 1.1% of the total group. Pancreatitis occurred in 56 patients (3.1%), four of whom required surgery. The incidence of pancreatitis in endoscopic sphincterotomy is considerably higher than in endoscopic retrograde cholangiography, where it is usually somewhat under 1% of the cases. Cholangitis occurred in 16 patients (0.9%), two required surgery, and one died. There was one trapped basket and two acute cholecystitis in the group. One of the patients with acute cholecystitis suffered a fatal outcome. Overall mortality in the group was 0.2%, and the complication rate was 7.7%.

The majority of the problems were quite mild; however, acute pancreatitis can, on occasion, be extremely severe and four of these patients required surgery. Pancreatitis does not require surgery unless pseudocyst formation occurs. Severe arterial bleeding should have prompt surgery unless it can be stopped by immediate coagulation. If the bleeding patient is to be operated on, the operating surgeon should realize that the bleeding is probably coming from the apex of the sphincterotomy. Suture of this area must be done with care to avoid compromising the sphincterotomy opening. Perforation occurred in 10 patients (0.5%), three required surgery and there were no deaths. If the perforation is retroperitoneal, it is advisable to observe the patient while using nasogastric suction and antibiotics. If the perforation shows free air in the abdomen and the patient is entirely asymptomatic, a period of observation is indicated. If pain develops, the patient should have surgical exploration with drainage and an attempt at closure of the perforation. If the perforation is difficult to localize, peritoneal drainage is adequate treatment. Cholangitis can be prevented by adequate biliary drainage at the time of sphincterotomy. Acute cholecystitis following sphincterotomy requires cholecystectomy. The trapped basket must be removed because it will produce biliary stasis with high risk of cholangitis.

Long-term complications following stone removal are extremely uncommon.[61] Table 13–2 shows the long-term complications of 8,640 patients. There were 20 who had restenosis, 36 reformed stones, cholangitis with an unobstructed duct occurred in 10, for total complications of 66 (0.9%). Most of these long-term complications can be dealt with endoscopically by dilating or extending the sphincterotomy and by removing reformed stones or sludge in the unobstructed duct. If there is a question of further room to extend the sphincterotomy, the patient should probably be treated surgically with a biliary enteric bypass following stone removal.

**TABLE 13-2.
LONG-TERM COMPLICATIONS OF ERS FOR CHOLEDOCHOLITHIASIS (8,640 Procedures)***

	Choledocholithiasis
Restenosis	20
Reformed stones	36
Cholangitis with unobstructed duct	10
TOTAL	66 (0.9%)

*Data from Vennes JA, Silvis SE: Endoscopic retrograde sphincterotomy, in Silvis SE (ed): *Therapeutic Gastrointestinal Endoscopy*. New York, Igaku-Shoin, 1985, p 198.

Only in recent years has significant long-term follow-up become available. Almost all of this information is from survey data, which usually represent the minimal figure. A report by Cotton and Vallon[46] shows a considerably higher restenosis rate. Geenen and co-workers[109] and Staritz and co-workers[110] report modest reduction in the size of the sphincterotomy, which usually stabilized and did not progress on to a clinically significant stenosis.

GALLSTONES IN THE ETIOLOGY OF ACUTE PANCREATITIS

The relationship of biliary calculi and acute pancreatitis has been discussed since the report of Opie[111] in 1901. He reported that pancreatitis was related to obstruction of the main pancreatic duct. More recent studies have emphasized the role of biliary calculi passing through the sphincter of Oddi. Acosta[112] and Kelly[113] found stones in the stools of 85 of 96 patients with acute gallstone pancreatitis. Many gallstones passed the papilla in the first day after the acute attack. This finding explains why Acosta[112] found impacted stones in 63% of patients operated on in the first 48 hours and Kelly[113] found only five stones in 146 patients operated on the seventh day after the onset of pain.

There is always some uncertainty in the diagnosis of gallstone pancreatitis; both biliary calculi and chronic alcoholism are common in Western populations. The patient who has gallstones and pancreatitis generally is diagnosed as having biliary pancreatitis unless chronic alcoholism is very apparent. This pancreatitis usually subsides rather quickly. This is probably because most of the stones producing the pancreatitis pass through the sphincter of Oddi, and there are no other stones in the duct to produce recurrent obstruction. It is impossible to distinguish which patient will run a benign course and which will suffer severe pancreatitis. Initially, acute pancreatitis was considered a contraindication to ERCP. Numerous investigators have now shown that the flare of pancreatitis can be kept to a minimum. It is probably advisable not to fully opacify the pancreatic duct. If the pancreatic duct is visualized, the injection is discontinued. The cannula is then repositioned to obtain the desired common duct. Controversy exists regarding the best management of gallstone pancreatitis. Although the majority of these patients will recover, the disease may be severe and life threatening.

Endoscopists who treat these patients early in their illness are impressed with the dramatic improvement that occurs soon after stones are removed by ERS.[114-119] It is not established at this time whether ERS prevents the progression of pancreatitis. In my institution sphincterotomy is considered early in an attempt to reduce the pancreatic inflammation and obtain prompt relief of pain. The necessity for elective cholecystectomy to prevent further episodes of pancreatitis has not been well studied. It is likely that sphincterotomy will prevent these recurrences.

Common bile duct stones seen on T-tube cholangiogram after recent common duct exploration require a separate discussion.[120] These stones do not represent an urgent problem. The T-tube can be allowed to continue to drain or may be clamped, hoping that very small stones will pass. Should the patient have any pain or evidence of infection, the T-tube must be allowed to drain. The stones may be approached by mechanical extraction through the T-tube tract, as described by Burhenne[121] who has a 95% success rate with this technique. This requires a 6-week maturation of the tract and forceful dilation, often requiring several days, but it has a low morbidity. It works well for small stones (less than 8 mm in diameter).

Monooctanoin dissolution has been used with retained common duct stones by infusion through a T-tube. It usually requires inpatient infusions for 4 to 14 days; it has occasionally caused complications of sepsis which can be serious and frequently produces intolerable diarrhea. ERS can be done at any time but should be preceded by a period of watchful waiting. At times small stones can be induced to pass the papilla by cannulating with a balloon and dragging the stones through the intact papilla.[64, 70] This is almost never successful in stones larger than 8 mm which require ERS.

ERS AND STONE REMOVAL IN PATIENTS WITH AN INTACT GALLBLADDER[107, 122-127]

For the patient who is relatively ill with choledocholithiasis and has an intact gallbladder, sphincterotomy is indicated if there is no prior history of cholecystitis. It is difficult to distinguish acute cholecystitis from common duct stone(s) with suppurative cholangitis; however, in a patient with acute cholecystitis the tenderness is quite well localized in the right upper quadrant. In addition, symptoms of cholecystitis do not clear when the common duct stones are removed. If pain persists following removal of common duct stones when there was adequate drainage after sphincterotomy, prompt cholecystectomy must be performed for acute cholecystitis.

The majority of patients do very well after removal of common duct stones even with stones remaining in the gallbladder. The long-term management of this group is controversial. The initial endoscopic sphincterotomy was done only on those patients who were either acutely or chronically very ill. Many of these patients who were gravely ill had no trouble from their biliary tract disease, even though a diseased gallbladder with numerous stones had been left intact. Data have been slow to accumulate because elective cholecystectomy was frequently done after patients recovered from their acute illness because of the preconceived idea that it would be required because of recurrent symptomatology. The much larger group of patients were those who were chronically ill and were felt unlikely to tolerate a cholecystectomy. Therefore, they had surgery only if very severe symptoms occurred. However, these patients did not survive long periods of time due to severe nonbiliary diseases producing a high mortality.

Table 13-3 shows the current reports[108, 122-124] of follow-up on patients with intact gallbladder, having had the stones removed at sphincterotomy. There were a total of 399 patients of whom 19 (4.8%) had cholecystectomy. As an indication of the seriousness of the patient's associated disease, they had a 30.8% mortality related to other conditions but only one patient died of biliary disease. The range in follow-up was from 14 to 40 months. In the majority of patients the incidence of acute illness requiring cholecystectomy was very low, approaching the group with asymptomatic cholelithiasis reported by Gracie and Ransohoff.[128]

Age may be a factor in choosing whether to advise elective cholecystectomy or not. The younger patient obviously has more years in which to have trouble with residual gallstones, even though the recurrences per year are quite low. On the other hand, an acute attack of cholecystitis or suppurative cholangitis can be rather well tolerated by the young person, and the surgical treatment can be instituted when it becomes evident that

TABLE 13-3.
ERS FOR STONES IN PATIENTS WITH GALLBLADDER IN SITU

Author	Number of Cases	Follow-up (months)	Cholecystectomy	Died: Unrelated Cause	Died: Biliary Cause
Cotton[46]	112	40	6	39	0
Escourrou[107]	130	22	8	28	0
Adler[123]	37	14	3	9	0
Neoptolemos[124]	59	17	2	29	1
Martin[125]	61	24	0	18	0
TOTAL	399		19 (4.8%)	123 (30.8%)	1

definitive treatment is essential. In clinical practice, age is usually not a major factor because the majority of patients with common duct stones are beyond the sixth decade where age is not a significant factor in their selection for cholecystectomy.

Younger patients may have had acute gallstone pancreatitis. Many authors recommend elective cholecystectomy for these patients. The evidence for this is probably no better than for those who have had biliary colic. The primary reason for recommending it is either the severity of the attack that was treated by sphincterotomy, or the potential of a very severe attack of pancreatitis. Further studies are necessary to more accurately define the need for cholecystectomy.

The opposite question has been presented a number of times: Should sphincterotomy ever be performed to prevent recurrent common bile duct stones? This question usually refers to patients who have had rather classic attacks of common bile duct stone(s) after cholecystectomy or the patient who has had repeated attacks of gallstone pancreatitis. At the time these patients are studied by cholangiography and no stones can be identified. In both of these situations a prophylactic ERS can be justified only on the strength of the diagnosis that the patient has had recurrent attacks of common duct stones. Frequently this depends on the history of symptoms, and under those conditions alone, I would be reluctant to perform the procedure. When the history includes abnormal laboratory data at the time of the pain, I have, on occasion, performed a small endoscopic sphincterotomy. In these few instances finding small amounts of sludge within the duct made me rather confident that stones would reform if more adequate drainage had not been obtained.[129,130]

Stent placement and drainage[131] can be the treatment of choice in the patient who has very large stones that cannot be removed by any of the endoscopic methods and who is an extremely high surgical risk (Fig 13-9). In this situation a pigtail stent is placed so that one limb of the stent is above the stone and the other is in the duodenum. It is my feeling that this should be done only in the patient whose risk for a surgical procedure is high because the foreign bodies can produce recurrent biliary infection. Most authors have treated only a small number of patients in this manner and have the general impression that they are doing quite well. Long-term follow-up is often incomplete, the patients are very old and tend to be expiring from other causes, so the validity of the treatment over a long-term basis is ill-defined.

In summary, common duct stones are a frequent entity in Western culture. There is now a wide variety of treatment options for these problems. It is a valid assertion that endoscopic sphincterotomy is now the method of choice in the patients who have had their gallbladders removed. In patients with their gallbladders intact, it is the preferred treatment in the majority of patients although some would argue that in the younger, healthier patient, surgical removal would be the preferred form of therapy.

References

1. Chary S: Dissolution of retained bile duct stones using heparin. Br J Surg 1977; 64:347.
2. Golematis BC, Diamantis TN, Delikaris PG, et al: Intracholedochal sodium heparin in the management of retained common duct stones. Mt Sinai J Med 1980; 47:293.
3. DenBesten L, Doty JE: Pathogenesis and management of choledocholithiasis. Surg Clin North Am 1981; 61:893.
4. Hofmann AF, Schmack B, Thistle JL, et al: Clinical experience with monooctanoin for dissolution of bile duct stones: An uncontrolled multicenter trial. Dig Dis Sci 1981; 26:954.
5. Braasch JW, Fender HR, Bonneval MM: Refractory common bile duct stone disease. Am J Surg 1979; 139:526.
6. Madden JL: Primary common bile duct stones. World J Surg 1978; 2:465.
7. Way LW: Retained common duct stones. Surg Clin North Am 1973; 53:1139.
8. Tabata M, Nakayama F: Bacteria and gallstones: Etiological significance. Dig Dis Sci 1981; 26:218.
9. Madden JL, Vanderheyden L, Kandalatt S: The nature and surgical significance of common duct stones. Surg Gynecol Obstet 1968; 126:3.
10. Imamoglu K, Yonehiro EG, Perry JF Jr, et al: Formation of calculi following cholecystectomy attending partial occlusion of the common bile duct. Surg Forum 1957; 8:225.
11. Lygidakis NJ: Incidence and signficance of primary stones of the common bile duct in choledocholithiasis. Surg Gynecol Obstet 1983; 157:434.
12. Wenchert A, Robertson B: The natural course of gallstone disease: Eleven years review of 781 non-operated cases. Gastroenterology 1966; 50:376.
13. Boey JH, Way LW: Acute cholangitis. Ann Surg 1980; 191:264.
14. Thompson JL Jr, Tompkins RK, Longmire WP Jr: Factors in management of acute cholangitis. Ann Surg 1982; 195:137.
15. O'Connor MJ, Schwartz ML, McQuarrie DG, et al: Acute bacterial cholangitis: An analysis of clinical manifestation. Arch Surg 1982; 117:437.
16. Coelho JC, Buffara M, Pozzobon CE, et al: Incidence of common bile duct stones in patients with acute and chronic cholecystitis. Surg Gynecol Obstet 1984; 158:76.
17. Stone HH, Fabian TC, Dunlop WE: Gallstone pancreatitis: Biliary tract pathology in relation to time of operation. Ann Surg 1981; 194:305.
18. Kelly TR: Gallstone pancreatitis. Local predisposing factors. Ann Surg 1984; 200:479.
19. Kelly TR, Swaney PE: Gallstone pancreatitis: The second time around. Surgery 1982; 92:571.
20. Pellegrini CA, Thomas MJ, Way LW: Bilirubin and alkaline phosphatase values before and after surgery for biliary obstruction. Am J Surg 1982; 143:67.
21. Kiechle FL, Weisenfeld MS, Karcher RE, et al: Alkaline phosphatase in the assessment of choledocholithiasis before surgery. Am J Emerg Med 1985; 31:556.
22. Fortson WC, Tedesco FJ, Starnes EC, et al: Marked elevation of serum transaminase activity associated wtih extrahepatic biliary tract disease. J Clin Gastroenterol 1985; 7:502.
23. Siegel JH, Tone P, Menikeim D: Gallstone pancreatitis: Pathogenesis and clinical forms: The emerging role of endoscopic management. Am J Gastroenterol 1986; 81:774.
24. Neoptolemos JP, London N, Bailey I, et al: The role of clinical and biochemical criteria and endoscopic retrograde cholangiopancreatography in the urgent diagnosis of common bile duct stones in acute pancreatitis. Surgery 1986; 100:732.
25. Jones BA, Salsberg BB, Mehta, MH, et al: Common pancreaticobiliary channels and their relationship to gallstone size in gallstone pancreatitis. Ann Surg 1987; 205:123.
26. Lee MJ, Choi TK, Lai EC, et al: Endoscopic retrograde cholangiopancreatography after acute pancreatitis. Surg Gynecol Obstet 1986; 163:354.
27. Moss AA, Filly RA, Way LW: In vitro investigation of gallstones with computed tomography. J Comput Assist Tomogr 1980; 4:827.
28. Hampson LG, Fried GM, Stets J, et al: Common bile duct exploration: Indications and results. Can J Surg 1981; 24:455.
29. Wilson TG, Hall JC, Watts JM: Is operative cholangiography always necessary? Br J Surg 1986; 73:637.
30. Kitahama A, Kerstein MD, Overby JL, et al: Routine intraoperative cholangiogram. Surg Gynecol Obstet 1986; 162:317.
31. Reiss R, Deutsch AA, Nudelman I: Clinical significance of choledochal diameter and hyperbilirubinemia in acute cholecystitis. Int Surg 1985; 70:129.
32. Silvis SE, Rohrmann CA, Vennes JA: Diagnostic accuracy of endoscopic retrograde cholangiopancreatography in hepatic, biliary and pancreatic malignancy. Ann Intern Med 1976; 84:438.
33. Geenen JE, Vennes JA, Silvis SE: Resume on endoscopic sphincterotomy seminar. Gastrointest Endosc 1981; 27:31.
34. Lasser RB, Silvis SE, Vennes JA: The normal cholangiogram. Am J Dig Dis 1978; 23:586.
35. O'Connor HJ, Hamilton I, Ellis WR, et al: Ultrasound detection of choledocholithiasis: Prospective comparison with ERCP in the postcholecystectomy patient. Gastrointest Radiol 1986; 11:161.
36. Osnes M, Rosseland AR, Aabakken L: Endoscopic retrograde cholangiography and endoscopic papillotomy in patients with a previous Billroth II resection. Gut 1986; 27:1193.
37. Bedogni G, Bertoni G, Contini S, et al: Endoscopic sphincterotomy in patients with Billroth II partial gastrectomy: Comparison of three different techniques. Gastrointest Endosc 1984; 30:300.
38. Siegel JH, Yatto RP: ERCP and endoscopic papillotomy in patients with a Billroth II gastrectomy: Report of a method. Gastrointest Endosc 1983; 29:116.
39. Rosseland AR, Osnes M, Kruse A: Endoscopic

sphincterotomy (EST) in patients with Billroth II gastrectomy. *Endoscopy* 1981; 13:19.
40. Safrany L, Neuhaus B, Portocarrero G, et al: Endoscopic sphincterotomy in patients with Billroth II gastrectomy. *Endoscopy* 1980; 12:16.
41. Martin JK, Van Heerden JA: Surgery of the liver, biliary tract and pancreas. *Mayo Clin Proc* 1980; 55:333.
42. McSherry CK, Glenn F: The incidence and causes of death following surgery for nonmalignant biliary tract disease. *Ann Surg* 1980; 191:271.
43. Koch H, Classen M, Schaffner O, et al: Endoscopic papillotomy: Experimental studies and initial clinical experience. *Scand J Gastroenterol* 1975; 10:441.
44. Koch H, Rösch W, Schaffner O, et al: Endoscopic papillotomy. *Gastroenterology* 1977; 73:1393.
45. Ihre T, Lönn M, Kager L: Long-term effects of papillotomy. *Endoscopy* 1984; 16:109.
46. Cotton PB, Vallon AG: British experience with duodenoscopic sphincterotomy for removal of bile duct stones. *Br J Surg* 1981; 68:373.
47. Rösch W, Riemann JF, Lux G, et al: Long-term follow-up after endoscopic sphincterotomy. *Endoscopy* 1981; 13:152.
48. Classen M, Safrany L: Endoscopic papillotomy and removal of gallstones. *Br Med J* 1975; 4:371.
49. Zimmon DS, Falkenstein DB, Kessler RE: Endoscopic papillotomy for choledocholithiasis. *N Engl J Med* 1975; 293:1181.
50. Safrany L: Duodenoscopic sphincterotomy and gallstone removal. *Gastroenterology* 1977; 72:338.
51. Siegel JH: Endoscopic papillotomy in the treatment of biliary tract disease: 258 procedures and results. *Dig Dis Sci* 1981; 26:1057.
52. Passi RB, Raval B: Endoscopic papillotomy. *Surgery* 1982; 92:581.
53. Geenen JE: New diagnostic and treatment modalities involving endoscopic retrograde cholangiopancreatography and esophagogastroduodenoscopy. *Scand J Gastroenterol (Suppl)* 1982; 77:93.
54. Siegel JH: Endoscopy and papillotomy in diseases of the biliary tract and pancreas. *J Clin Gastroenterol* 1980; 2:337.
55. Cotton PB: Nonoperative removal of bile duct stones by duodenoscopic sphincterotomy. *Br J Surg* 1980; 67:1.
56. Kozarek RA, Sanowski RA: Nonsurgical management of extrahepatic obstructive jaundice. *Ann Intern Med* 1982; 96:743.
57. Safrany L, Cotton PB: Endoscopic management of choledocholithiasis. *Surg Clin North Am* 1982; 62:825.
58. Silvis SE: Current status of endoscopic sphincterotomy. *Am J Gastroenterol* 1984; 79:731.
59. Vennes JA: Management of calculi in the common duct. *Semin Liver Dis* 1983; 3:162.
60. Urakami Y, Kishi S, Seifert E: Endoscopic papillotomy (EPT) in patients wtih juxtapapillary diverticula. *Gastrointest Endosc* 1979; 25:10.
61. Silvis SE, Vennes VA: Endoscopic retrograde sphincterotomy, Silvis SE (ed): *Therapeutic Gastrointestinal Endoscopy*. New York, Igaku-Shoin, 1985, p 198.
62. Staritz M, Poralla T, Dormeyer HH, et al: Endoscopic removal of common bile duct stones through the intact papilla after medical sphincter dilation. *Gastroenterology* 1985; 88:1807.
63. Siegel JH: Precut papillotomy: A method to improve success of ERCP and papillotomy. *Endoscopy* 1980; 12:130.
64. Schapira L, Khawaja FI: Endoscopic fistulosphincterotomy: An alternative method of sphincterotomy using a new sphincterotome. *Endoscopy* 1982; 14:58.
65. Cohen H, Quinn M: Antegrade assistance for retrograde sphincterotomy using a new sphincterotome. *Gastrointest Endosc* 1986; 32:405.
66. Long WB, Schwarz W, Ring EJ: Endoscopic sphincterotomy assisted by catheterization antegrade. *Gastrointest Endosc* 1984; 30:36.
67. Robertson DAF, Ayres R, Haching CN, et al: Experience with a combined percutaneous approach to stent insertion. *Lancet* 1987; 2:1449.
68. Stave R, Osnes M: Endoscopic gallstone extraction following hydrostatic balloon dilatation of stricture in the common bile duct. *Endoscopy* 1985; 17:159.
69. Koch H, Rösch W, Walz V: Endoscopic lithotripsy in the common bile duct. *Gastrointest Endosc* 1980; 26:16.
70. Riemann JF, Seuberth K, Demling L: Mechanical lithotripsy of common bile duct stones. *Gastrointest Endosc* 1985; 31:207.
71. Demling L, Seuberth K, Riemann JF: A mechanical lithotripter. *Endoscopy* 1982; 14:100.
72. Staritz M, Ewe K, Meyer zum Büschenfelde KH: Mechanical gallstone lithotripsy in the common bile duct: In vitro and in vivo experience. *Endoscopy* 1983; 15:316.
73. Riemann JF, Seuberth K, Demling L: Mechanical lithotripsy through the intact papilla of Vater. *Endoscopy* 1983; 15:111.
74. Reuter HJ, Kern E: Electronic lithotripsy of ureteral calculi. *J Urol* 1973; 110:181.
75. Raney AM: Electrohydraulic lithotripsy: Experimental study and case reports with the stone disintegrator. *J Urol* 1975; 113:345.
76. Mitchell ME, Kerr WS Jr: Experience with the electrohydraulic disintegrator. *J Urol* 1977; 117:159.
77. Tanaka M, Yoshimoto H, Ikeda S, et al: Two approaches for electrohydraulic lithotripsy in the common bile duct. *Surgery* 1985; 98:313.
78. Sievert CE, Silvis SE: Evaluation of electrohydraulic lithotripsy on human gallstones. *Am J Gastroenterol* 1985; 80:854.
79. Silvis SE, Siegel JE, Katon RM, et al: Use of electrohydraulic lithotripsy to fracture common bile duct stones. *Gastrointest Endosc* 1986; 32:155.
80. Sievert CE, Silvis SE: Evaluation of electrohydraulic lithotripsy as a means of gallstone fragmentation in a canine model. *Gastrointest Endosc* 1987; 33:233.
81. Sackman M, Delius M, Sauerbruch T, et al: Extra-corporeal shock wave lithotripsy of gall-

stones: Results of 101 treatments. *Gastroenterology* 1987; 92:1608.
82. Burhenne HJ, Stoler JL: Minicholecystostomy and radiological stone extraction in high-risk cholelithiasis patients. *Am J Surg* 1985; 149:632.
83. Sauerbruch T, Delius M, Paumgartner G, et al: Fragmentation of gallstones by extracorporeal shock waves. *N Engl J Med* 1986; 314:818.
84. Staritz M, Floth A, Buess G, et al: Extracorporeal shock waves for gallstone fragmentation: First in vitro experience with a second generation device working without the conventional water bath. *Gastroenterology* 1987; 92:1652.
85. Staritz M, Floth A, Rambone A, et al: Extracorporeal shock waves (device of the second generation) for therapy of large common bile duct stones: Success and problems. *Gastroenterology* 1987; 92:1652.
86. Gelfand DW, McCullough DL, Myers RT, et al: Choledocholithiasis: Successful treatment with extracorporeal lithotripsy. *AJR* 1987; 148:1114.
87. Silvis SE: The role of lithotripsy in biliary stone disease. *Gastrointest Endosc* 1987; 33:328.
88. Ponchon T, Valette PJ, Chavaillon A: Percutaneous transhepatic electrohydraulic lithotripsy under endoscopic control. *Gastrointest Endosc* 1987; 33:307.
89. Hwang MH, Mo LR, Chen GD, et al: Percutaneous transhepatic cholecystic ultrasonic lithotripsy. *Gastrointest Endosc* 1987; 33:301.
90. Hwang MH, Mo LR, Yang JC, et al: Percutaneous transhepatic cholangioscopic ultrasonic lithotripsy (PTCS-USL) in the treatment of retained or recurrent intrahepatic stones. *Gastrointest Endosc* 1987; 33:303.
91. Lux G, Ell C, Hochberger J, et al: The first successful endoscopic retrograde laser lithotripsy of common bile duct stones in man using a pulsed neodymium-YAG laser. *Endoscopy* 1986; 18:144.
92. Palmer KR, Hofmann AF: Intraductal monooctanoin for the direct dissolution of bile duct stones: Experience in 343 patients. *Gut* 1986; 27:196.
93. Thistle JL, Carlson GL, Hofmann AF, et al: Monooctanoin, a dissolution agent for retained cholesterol bile duct stones: Physical properties and clinical application. *Gastroenterology* 1980; 78:1016.
94. Jarrett LN, Balfour TW, Bell GD, et al: Intraductal infusion of monooctanoin: Experience in 24 patients with retained common duct stones. *Lancet* 1981; 1:68.
95. Venu RP, Geenen JE, Toouli J, et al: Gallstone dissolution using monooctanoin infusion through an endoscopically placed nasobiliary catheter. *Am J Gastroenterol* 1982; 77:227.
96. Tritapepe R, Di Padova C, Pozzoli M, et al: The treatment of retained biliary stones with monooctanoin: Report of 16 patients. *Am J Gastroenterol* 1984; 79:710.
97. Sharp KW, Gadacz TR: Selection of patients for dissolution of retained common duct stones with monooctanoin. *Ann Surg* 1982; 196:137.
98. Train JS, Dan SJ, Cohen LB, et al: Duodenal ulceration associated with monooctanoin infusion. *AJR* 1983; 141:557.
99. Thistle JL, Nelson PE, May GR: Dissolution of cholesterol gallbladder stone (CGS) using methyl tert-butyl ether (MTBE). *Gastroenterology* 1987; 90:1775.
100. Allen MJ, Borody TJ, Thistle JL: In vitro dissolution of cholesterol gallstones: A study of factors influencing rate and a comparison of solvents. *Gastroenterology* 1985; 89:1097.
101. Allen MJ, Borody TJ, Bugliosi TF, et al: Rapid dissolution of gallstones by methyl tert-butyl ether: Preliminary observations. *N Engl J Med* 1985; 312:217.
102. Allen MJ, Borody TJ, Bugliosi TF, et al: Cholelitholysis using methyl tertiary-butyl ether. *Gastroenterology* 1985; 88:122.
103. Zakko SF, Hofmann AF: Microprocessor assisted solvent transfer system for infusion of methyl tert-butyl ether (MTBE) or other gallstone (GS) solvents into the gallbladder. *Gastroenterology* 1987; 92:1794.
104. Zakko SF, Hofmann AF, Schteingart C, et al: Percutaneous gallbladder stone dissolution using a microprocessor assisted solvent transfer (MAST) system. *Gastroenterology* 1987; 92:1794.
105. Di Padova C, Di Padova F, Montorsi W, et al: Methyl tert-butyl ether fails to dissolve retained radiolucent common bile duct stones. *Gastroenterology* 1986; 91:1296.
106. Dunham F, Bourgeois N, Gelin M, et al: Retroperitoneal perforations following endoscopic sphincterotomy: Clinical course and management. *Endoscopy* 1982; 14:92.
107. Escourrou J, Cordova JA, Lazorthes F, et al: Early and late complications after endoscopic sphincterotomy for biliary lithiasis with and without the gallbladder "in situ." *Gut* 1984; 25:598.
108. Leese T, Neoptolemos JP, Carr-Locke DL: Successes, failures, early complications and their management following endoscopic sphincterotomy: Results in 394 consecutive patients from a single centre. *Br J Surg* 1985; 72:215.
109. Geenen JE, Toouli J, Hogan WJ, et al: Endoscopic sphincterotomy: Follow-up evaluation of effects on the sphincter of Oddi. *Gastroenterology* 1984; 87:754.
110. Staritz M, Ewe K, Meyer zum Buschemfelde KH: Investigation of the sphincter of Oddi before, immediately after and six weeks after endoscopic papillotomy. *Endoscopy* 1986; 18:14.
111. Opie AE: Etiology of acute pancreatitis. *Bull Johns Hopkins Hospital* 1901; 12:182.
112. Acosta JM, Ledesma CL: Gallstone migration as a cause of acute pancreatitis. *N Engl J Med* 1974; 190:484.
113. Kelly TR: Gallstone pancreatitis. *Arch Surg* 1974; 109:294.
114. Van der Spuy S: Endoscopic sphincterotomy in the management of gallstone pancreatitis. *Endoscopy* 1981; 13:25.
115. Armstrong CP, Taylor TV, Jeacock J, et al: The biliary tract in patients with acute gallstone pancreatitis. *Br J Surg* 1985; 72:551.

116. Neoptolemo JP, London N, and Slater, ND: Prospective randomized study of ERCP and endoscopic sphincterotomy (ES) in acute pancreatitis. *Arch Surg* 1986; 121:697–702.
117. Safrany L, Cotton PB: A preliminary report: Urgent duodenoscopic sphincterotomy for acute gallstone pancreatitis. *Surgery* 1981; 89:424.
118. Lee MJR, Citoi TK, Lai ECS, et al: Value of ERCP in the identification of biliary causes of acute pancreatitis. *Gut* 1986; 27:228.
119. Rosseland AR, Solhaug JH: Early or delayed endoscopic papillotomy (EPT) in gallstone pancreatitis. *Ann Surg* 1984; 199:165.
120. O'Doherty DP, Neoptolemos JP, Carr-Locke DL: Endoscopic sphincterotomy for retained common bile duct stones in patients with T-tube in situ in the early postoperative period. *Br J Surg* 1986; 73:454.
121. Burhenne HJ: Percutaneous extraction of retained biliary tract stones: 661 patients. *Am J Roentgenol* 1980; 134:888.
122. Cotton PB: Follow-up after sphincterotomy for stones in patients with gallbladders. *Gastrointest Endosc* 1986; 32:157.
123. Adler D, Geenen JE, Venu R, et al: Is there a role for endoscopic sphincterotomy in patients with CBD stones and an intact gallbladder? *Gastrointest Endosc* 1983; 29:170.
124. Neoptolemos JP, Carr-Locke DL, Fraser I, et al: The management of common bile duct calculi by endoscopic sphincterotomy in patients with gallbladders "in situ." *Br J Surg* 1984; 71:69.
125. Martin DF, Tweedle DEF: Endoscopic management of common duct stones without cholecystectomy. *Br J Surg* 1987; 74:209.
126. Olaison G, Kald B, Karlqvist PA, et al: Routine cholecystectomy after endoscopic removal of common bile duct stones: An unnecessary procedure (Letter). *Endoscopy* 1987; 19:88.
127. Solhaug JH, Fokstuen O, Rosseland A, et al: Endoscopic papillotomy in patients with gallbladder in situ: Is subsequent cholecystectomy necessary? *Acta Chir Scand* 1984; 150:475.
128. Gracie WA, Ransohoff DE: The natural history of silent gallstones: The innocent gallstone is not a myth. *N Engl J Med* 1982; 307:798.
129. Popiela T, Karcz D, Marecik J: Endoscopic sphincterotomy as a therapeutic measure in cholangitis and as prophylaxis against recurrent biliary tract stones. *Endoscopy* 1987; 19:14.
130. Choi TK, Wong J: Endoscopic retrograde cholangiopancreatography and endoscopic papillotomy in recurrent pyogenic cholangitis. *Clin Gastroenterol* 1986; 15:393.
131. Siegel JH, Yatto RP: Biliary endoprostheses for the management of retained common bile duct stones. *Am J Gastroenterol* 1984; 79:50.

14

Pancreatic Pseudocyst and Abscess:
Is percutaneous drainage a reasonable option?

PETER A. BANKS, M.D.
STEPHEN G. GERZOF, M.D.

Percutaneous catheter drainage has been shown to be a safe, effective method of treating abdominal abscesses.[1] This chapter will define the role of percutaneous techniques in the treatment of pancreatic pseudocysts and pancreatic abscesses.

We should point out that our chapter title is incomplete in that a pancreatic abscess is only one of several infected pancreatic processes. The others are infected pancreatic pseudocyst, infected pancreatic fluid collection, and infected necrosis.[2,3] We would recommend the use of the term *pancreatic infection* rather than *pancreatic abscess* to refer to all infected pancreatic processes.

For the purpose of orientation, we will first provide anatomical definitions of these pancreatic processes based on specific CT criteria, and will then discuss the suitability of percutaneous techniques for each process. We will describe two percutaneous techniques capable of providing drainage. The first is percutaneous aspiration; the second is percutaneous catheter drainage (i.e., needle aspiration followed by the insertion of a pigtail catheter for continuous drainage).

ANATOMICAL DEFINITIONS OF ACUTE PANCREATITIS

Acute Interstitial Pancreatitis

Acute interstitial pancreatitis is characterized by acute intrapancreatic inflammation associated at times with peripancreatic inflammation and fat necrosis. CT scan typically shows a diffusely enlarged pancreas. By definition, there is scant if any pancreatic parenchymal necrosis. This appearance on CT scan has frequently been described as a "phlegmon" of the pancreas.[4,5] There has always been confusion and ambiguity about the meaning of this term, which provides no information as to whether the process is infected or contains areas of necrosis. Now, with the use of intravenous contrast enhancement, acute interstitial pancreatitis can be distinguished on CT from necrotizing pancreatitis,[6] and the term *phlegmon* may be outdated.

In acute interstitial pancreatitis, the administration of intravenous contrast shows uniform enhancement of the well-perfused pancreas. The absence of nonenhancing low attenuation areas by this technique excludes the presence of large foci of devitalized tissue or fluid.

In acute interstitial pancreatitis, bacteria are rarely if ever recovered from the pancreas, probably because there are no necrotic foci in which bacteria can thrive.

Necrotizing Pancreatitis

Necrotizing pancreatitis is more severe and is characterized by areas of devitalized pancreatic and/or peripancreatic tissue. These necrotic foci may be few in number and small in size or may involve large areas of the pancreas.[3,7] When intravenous contrast medium is administered, necrotic areas are not perfused and therefore do not enhance. They are thereby readily distinguished from well-perfused viable pancreatic tissue.

Areas of necrosis may also contain dark fluid composed of pancreatic secretion, old blood, and tissue fluid. Because fluid and necrosis may have an identical appearance on CT scan, it may not be possible to determine the relative proportions of each. At times there are considerable necrosis and a paucity of fluid,[7] or there may be copious fluid and less necrotic debris.

Necrotizing pancreatitis may be either sterile or infected. We[2] and others[8-11] have used CT-guided percutaneous aspiration with Gram stain and culture and found it to be a safe and accurate method for making this distinction (Fig 14–1).

Pancreatic Pseudocyst

Pancreatic pseudocysts are well-defined, smooth-walled, rounded fluid masses of low attenuation on CT scan[2] (Figs 14–2 through 14–4). Pseudocysts have been termed as either "acute" or "chronic."[12] An acute pseudocyst forms when pancreatic inflammation is severe and there is extravasation of enzyme-rich fluid through damaged pancreatic ducts. This fluid and variable amounts of blood and pancreatic debris then coalesce within

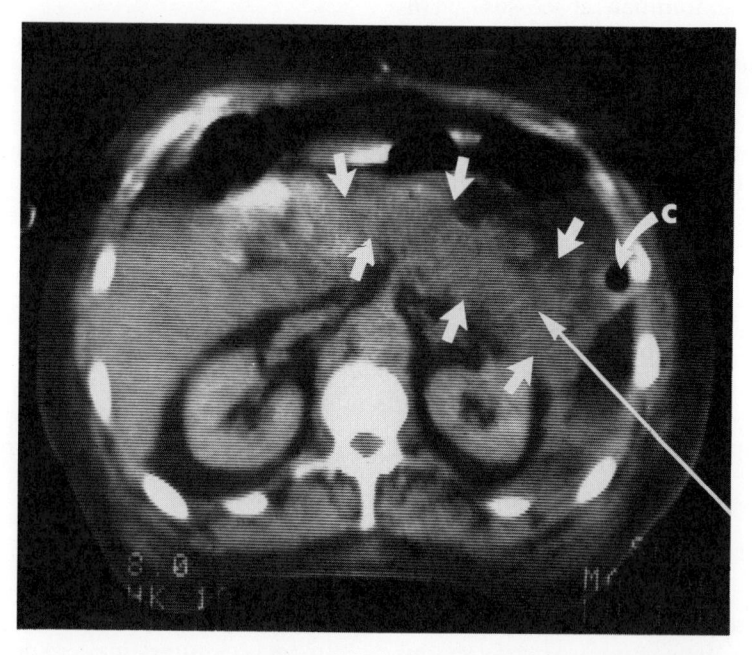

FIG 14–1.
Needle aspiration of infected necrosis. CT scan of the upper abdomen shows an ill-defined poorly marginated pancreatic inflammatory process *(white arrow)* involving the entire anterior pararenal space. Needle aspiration was performed from the left flank over the route of the *long white arrow* only after the position of the colon *(C)* was identified. Gram stain yielded gram-positive cocci and gram-negative rods. The patient underwent immediate operative debridement.

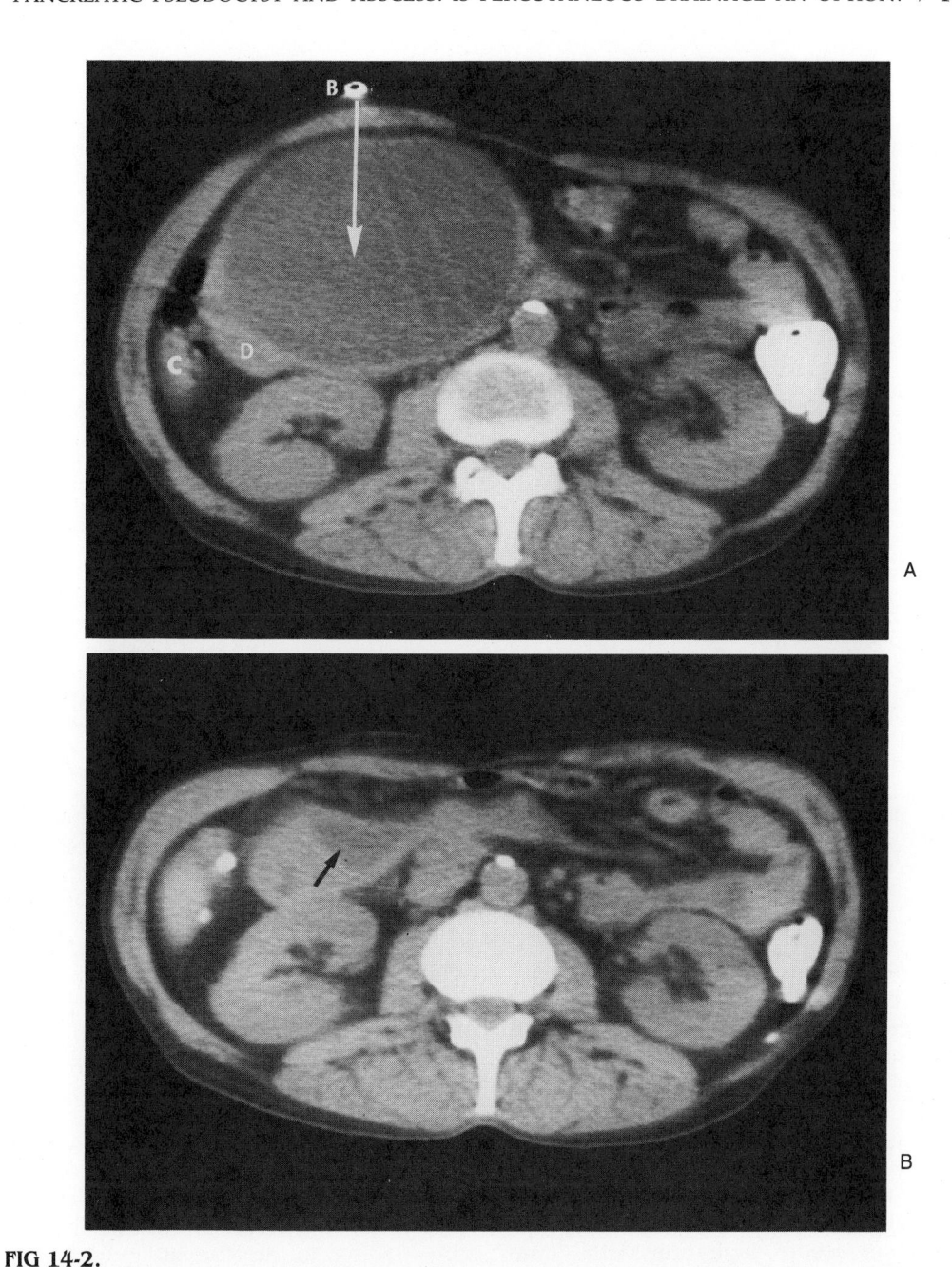

FIG 14-2.
Needle aspiration of sterile pseudocyst. **A,** there is a large well-defined 8 × 10 cm pseudocyst in the right side of the abdomen, which has sufficient internal pressure to bulge the anterior abdominal wall and displace the colon *(C)* and duodenum *(D).* To be certain that there was no small bowel compressed against the anterior abdominal wall by the pseudocyst and to avoid needle aspiration passing through a loop of bowel, we placed a barium mark *(B)* over the pseudocyst and repeated the CT scan. Once the safety of this diagnostic route *(white arrow)* was confirmed, needle aspiration was performed along the route of the *long white arrow.* Gram stain and culture were negative. **B,** Follow-up CT scan 5 minutes after removal of 670 ml of fluid shows complete collapse of the pseudocyst indicating considerable pliability of its inflammatory wall. There are only 10 to 15 ml of residual fluid *(arrow).*

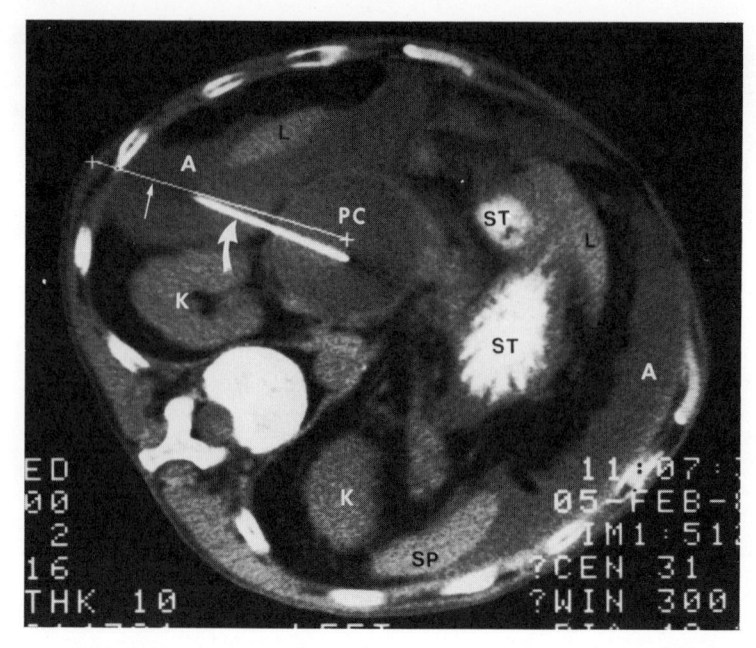

FIG 14-3.
Needle aspiration of sterile pseudocyst. CT scan of the upper abdomen shows marked ascites (A) throughout the upper abdomen. Diagnostic aspiration of the pseudocyst (PC) was performed by way of the right flank by rotating the patient to the left decuitus position. The planned route indicated by the computer cursor *(thin straight arrow)* passes through the ascites before entering the pseudocyst. The actual needle *(curved arrow)* follows the planned route almost exactly. The outer portion of the needle is not shown because it is just below the CT scan plane. Needle aspiration yielded slightly turbid fluid which on Gram stain and culture was sterile. The pseudocyst was aspirated completely and the needle was removed. ST = stomach, K = kidney, SP = spleen, L = lower margins of left and right lobes of liver.

a space demarcated by surrounding structures. Because of the presence of blood products and tissue debris, the fluid is frequently black or brown in color. Within a short time, a capsule of inflammatory reaction and fibrosis encircles the fluid, forming a round mass which can displace surrounding structures. An acute pseudocyst may be either sterile or infected. The distinction can easily be made by percutaneous needle aspiration with Gram stain and culture[2, 8-11] (Figs 14-2 through 14-4).

In comparison, a "chronic pseudocyst" is one that forms in a patient with known chronic pancreatitis (almost always secondary to alcohol abuse). It usually develops without an identifiable preexisting episode of acute pancreatitis. The patient usually describes the gradual onset of abdominal discomfort, which intensifies over several days or weeks. The chronicity of these symptoms or the development of a palpable mass usually prompts the patient to seek medical attention. Experience has shown that a pseudocyst that develops in this fashion is likely to have a mature capsule suitable for operative decompression at the time it is discovered.[12] The mechanism of a "chronic pseudocyst" appears to be increased intraductal pressure leading to rupture of a duct with leakage of pancreatic fluid that is eventually demarcated from surrounding structures by a capsule composed of inflammatory reaction. Because there may be scant acute inflammation of the pancreas, the fluid within a chronic pseudocyst is usually relatively clear, devoid of both blood products and necrotic debris. Chronic pseudocysts may also be sterile or infected.

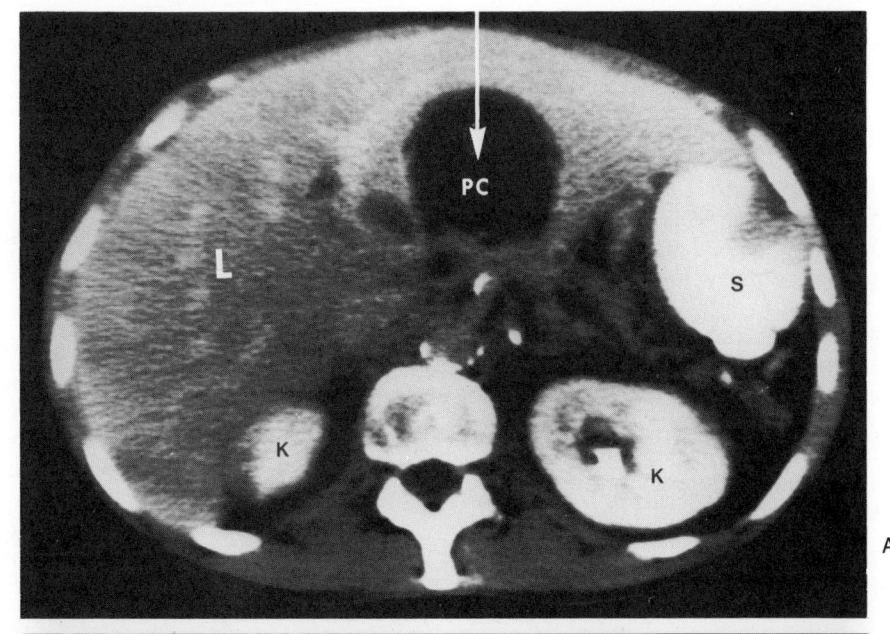

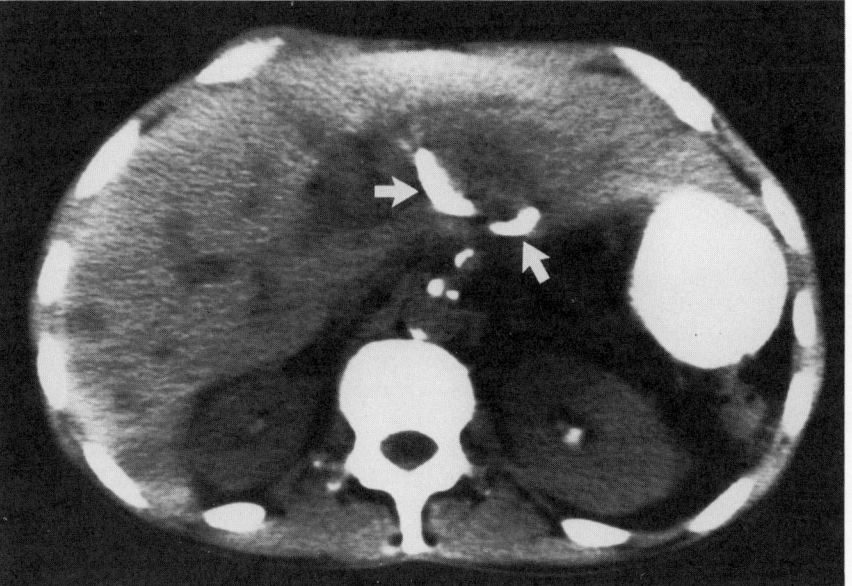

FIG 14–4.
Pigtail catheter drainage of infected pancreatic pseudocyst. **A,** CT scan of the upper abdomen in a patient with known pancreatitis who now has fever, leukocytosis, and increasing abdominal pain shows a well-defined 4 × 5 cm low-attenuation mass *(PC)* seemingly in an intrahepatic location. Serial scans showed it to be arising from the cephalad aspect of the pancreas and to have burrowed into the liver substance. L = liver, S = stomach. The kidneys *(K)* show marked contrast enhancement as does the liver parenchyma. Diagnostic needle aspiration was performed by a transhepatic route along the path of the *white arrow*. Five ml of creamy yellow fluid were obtained which showed numerous gram-negative bacilli on Gram stain. Percutaneous catheter drainage was recommended. **B,** An 8 F pigtail catheter was inserted by Seldinger technique. By using the course of the 20-gauge Teflon sleeve aspiration needle, a second entry into this infected pseudocyst was not required. Sixty ml of purulent material were drained initially. This CT scan immediately after drainage shows almost complete aspiration of the pseudocyst with the 8 F pigtail catheter *(arrows)* in good position. Note how the pigtail tip has promoted coiling of the catheter within the former pseudocyst cavity and prevented perforation of the far wall. After 24 hours, fluid, which had been somewhat viscous, was now thin, serous, and watery, and drained easily through the pigtail catheter. The patient defervesced, drainage gradually diminished over 7 days, and the catheter was removed 10 days after insertion. The patient did not require surgery and is well 2 years later.

Extrapancreatic Fluid Collection

An extrapancreatic fluid collection differs from a pancreatic pseudocyst on CT scan in that the collection is poorly defined and irregularly marginated.[2] It occurs when pancreatic fluid extravasates into the anterior pararenal space, posterior pararenal space, or lesser sac but does not coalesce into a round or oval structure. Extrapancreatic fluid collections may be either sterile or infected. The difference can be established by percutaneous aspiration with Gram stain and culture.[2]

Pancreatic Abscess

The term *pancreatic abscess* has frequently been used indiscriminately. First, as mentioned in the introduction, all infected pancreatic processes have generally been termed a *pancreatic abscess*. Second, proof of infection has not always been required. In some instances, bacteriologic studies have not been performed. Because enzymatic digestion of pancreatic and peripancreatic fat can produce a material of creamy consistency and yellow or brown color which looks like pus but is entirely sterile, the presence of infection *must* be confirmed by appropriate bacteriologic culture. In other instances, bacteriologic studies were performed but cultures proved to be negative. The rationale for considering a process that is bacteriologically sterile as a "pancreatic abscess" has been the notion that prior use of antibiotics may have temporarily inhibited bacterial growth. In our experience, the prior use of antibiotics has not been a factor in preventing the growth of bacteria within devitalized pancreatic and peripancreatic tissue.[2]

In accordance with the suggestion of Beger, we would define a pancreatic abscess in a way that distinguishes it from infected necrosis, infected pseudocyst, and infected peripancreatic fluid collections.[3,13] As such, a pancreatic abscess is a collection of frank pus in and around the pancreas that typically does not occur until approximately 5 weeks after the onset of pancreatitis. The exact pathophysiology is unclear. A pancreatic abscess could be a late sequela of either infected necrosis or infected pancreatic pseudocyst. Implied in this thinking is the notion that the fluid components of these processes are reabsorbed and are replaced by frank purulent material. A second mechanism for a pancreatic abscess is the placement of drains into the lesser sac or retroperitoneum during surgery for pancreatitis. Eventually, these drains serve as a pathway for the introduction of bacteria resulting in a localized purulent collection (Fig 14–5).

Generally, pancreatic abscesses have a very variable gross appearance, and the variation in CT appearance reflects this. They usually have an attenuation lower than normal pancreatic parenchyma but not as low as or homogeneous as water or bile. If hemorrhagic pancreatitis is a substrate for infection, the density may be higher. The margins are generally ill-defined initially, but may become better defined as inflammatory reaction contains the abscess (Fig 14–5). Gas bubbles may be seen and, when due to infected necrosis, are usually distributed throughout the abscess. When the gas is from prior surgery or an infected pseudocyst, bubbles are usually few in number and are well localized.

RADIOLOGIC TECHNIQUES

Indications for Needle Aspiration

There are three possible indications for needle aspiration: (1) diagnostic, to exclude sepsis; (2) therapeutic, to aspirate fluid collections or pseudocysts that have either become symptomatic or are large enough to eventually require surgical decompression; and (3) prophylactic, to decompress pseudocysts that, by virtue of their size or location, are at risk of rupturing, eroding into arteries, or causing biliary tract or bowel obstruction.

Technique of Needle Aspiration

CT is the imaging modality of choice for pancreatitis, and the scan should imme-

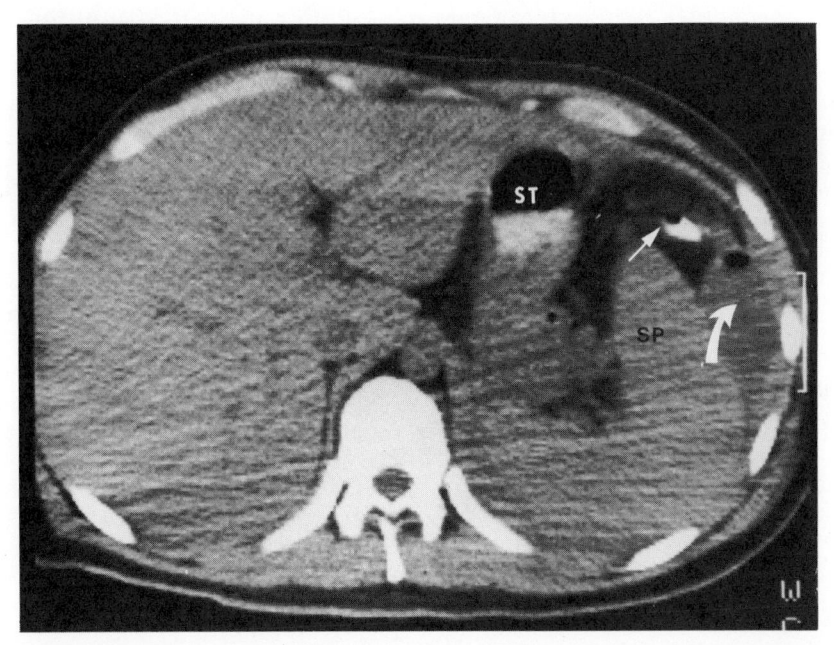

FIG 14–5.
Pigtail catheter drainage of pancreatic abscess. CT scan in a patient who had undergone previous debridement of infected necrosis now shows an abscess cavity in the left flank *(curved arrow)* containing an air bubble. After percutaneous aspiration revealed gram-positive cocci, a pigtail catheter was introduced and placed to gravity drainage. Drainage decreased progressively over the next 3 weeks, and the catheter was then removed. There has been no recurrence of abscess formation. Note adjacent portion of colon which contains gastrograffin and air bubble *(short straight arrow)*. ST = stomach, SP = spleen

diately precede each needle aspiration. CT provides a precise display of the extent and location of pancreatitis and the exact location of loops of bowel in relation to the pancreas. This display is of the utmost importance in planning a safe route to avoid bowel and thereby prevent iatrogenic infection.

CT scans should be performed supine with orally administered contrast medium to opacify stomach and bowel. The pelvis should be scanned at 2-cm intervals, because pancreatic inflammation may dissect widely not only in the cephalad but also in the caudad direction. Scans over the pancreas and over any inflammatory mass should be performed at 1-cm intervals. We use intravenous iodinated contrast medium when necessary to distinguish viable, perfused pancreatic tissue from fluid or necrotic tissue.

When the indication for needle aspiration is to differentiate sterile from infected pancreatitis, areas of low density by CT are the prime target. Once we plan a safe route, a barium mark is placed on the skin at the entry site. A CT scan is repeated at this level to confirm the site and the projected route. If necessary, minor adjustments can then be made with reference to the barium mark.

After sterile draping and under local anesthesia, a 4-mm incision is made with a No. 11 blade, and a 20-gauge Teflon sleeve needle is inserted along the projected route. Occasionally, when the route is close to bowel or when the course of the needle traverses normal pancreatic tissue, we use a 22-gauge Chiba needle. We remove only a small sample of fluid and send it for an immediate Gram stain, aerobic and anaerobic culture, and amylase determination. If the pancreatic process is a pseudocyst or fluid collection, we leave the Teflon sleeve in place for 5 to 10 minutes while the Gram stain is performed. In our experience, immediate Gram stain has been very reliable in distinguishing sterile from infected fluid.[2]

If the Gram stain shows no organisms, the remaining fluid is aspirated completely, and the Teflon sleeve is removed. If the fluid is infected, we usually insert a drainage catheter.

Indications for Pigtail Catheter Drainage

Potential uses of pigtail catheter drainage include the decompression of sterile and infected pseudocysts, sterile and infected fluid collections, and pancreatic abscesses.

Technique of Pigtail Catheter Insertion

The technique is a modification of the Seldinger technique adapted from angiography. It consists of using the Teflon sleeve of the aspirating needle to insert a guidewire into the pseudocyst. A dilator is advanced over the guidewire, and then an 8 F multiple side hole pigtail catheter is introduced. The pseudocyst is then evacuated by gentle manual suction, and the catheter is sutured to the skin to prevent dislodgement.

The catheter is connected to a bile bag so that fluid production by the pseudocyst can be measured. In general, we do not recommend periodic irrigation of the catheter with sterile saline because of the possibility of introducing infection during this irrigation. If the side holes of the pigtail catheter become occluded, as evidenced by abdominal pain, fever, and reaccumulation of fluid on CT scan, gentle irrigation with 5 to 10 ml of sterile saline is advised.

Usually, drainage volumes gradually decrease until the catheter drains less than 5 to 10 ml per day. At this point, the catheter can be removed.

PERCUTANEOUS DRAINAGE OF INFECTED NECROSIS?

It is difficult to distinguish sterile necrosis from infected necrosis by clinical criteria. Patients with sterile necrosis may appear septic with fever, leukocytosis, and abdominal pain.[2] Nor can CT differentiate between sterile and infected necrosis except when gas is present.[2] Occasionally, gas is also found in sterile pancreatitis if there is a pancreatic fistula or if loops of bowel become tethered into a mass.

In our practice, the clinical setting of severe pancreatitis coupled with fever and leukocytosis is an indication for immediate CT scan. If CT scan shows only interstitial pancreatitis, percutaneous aspiration is not performed. However, if CT scan shows pancreatic necrosis and/or fluid, diagnostic needle aspiration is performed to determine whether these areas are infected (Fig 14–1).

If the Gram stain or culture is positive for bacteria, the question frequently arises as to whether there is a role for percutaneous pigtail catheter drainage. We caution against this approach. Whereas infected pancreatic pseudocysts are almost entirely fluid and can be effectively (and often permanently) decompressed by percutaneous catheter drainage,[14] infected necrosis differs considerably. In some instances, infected necrosis contains only minimal fluid.[7] Even when there is considerable amount of infected fluid surrounding areas of pancreatic and peripancreatic necrosis, pigtail catheter drainage is still not advised. The reason for this caution is the fact that bacteria are not confined to the fluid component. The necrotic tissue itself is also teeming with bacteria.[15] Because the necrotic infected tissue is semisolid and too large to be aspirated through a pigtail catheter, wide operative debridement is required to eradicate infected necrosis.

The one potential indication of pigtail catheter drainage in infected necrosis is refractory shock and overwhelming clinical deterioration that preclude immediate surgery. In this circumstance, one might consider inserting one or more pigtail catheters to decompress the infected fluid component in anticipation of definitive surgery as soon as blood pressure stabilizes.[2,8]

PERCUTANEOUS DRAINAGE OF STERILE ACUTE PSEUDOCYST?

The natural history of an "acute pseudocyst" is uncertain. Because at least 30% resolve spontaneously, the role of percutaneous techniques is also uncertain and will remain so until a comprehensive study is performed in which percutaneous techniques are compared prospectively with the usual strategy of medical treatment for 4 to 6 weeks to allow the pseudocyst either to resolve or develop a mature capsule suitable for surgical decompression.

There are two potential methods for draining a sterile pseudocyst. The first is by simple percutaneous aspiration using a 20-gauge Teflon sleeve needle and removing the Teflon sleeve as soon as the entire volume of the pseudocyst has been aspirated (Figs 14–2 and 14–3). Because the collapsed pseudocyst remains in continuity with pancreatic ducts, it frequently reexpands with enzyme-rich fluid within a few hours or days. On occasion, aspiration has resulted in permanent closure of the pseudocyst[8,16]; in one study, aspirations repeated on multiple occasions eventually resulted in permanent closure of most pseudocysts.[17] Because of these successes, we are prepared to recommend needle aspiration on one or two occasions if a sterile pseudocyst is causing intractable severe pain or is expanding rapidly. This maneuver frequently relieves pain dramatically for at least a few days thereby reducing the need for narcotic medication. Rapid expansion may also be curbed, and symptoms from compression of a hollow viscus can be at least temporarily alleviated. We do not have a firm recommendation if a sterile pseudocyst is asymptomatic but is large enough to eventually require surgical decompression. It would seem reasonable to attempt needle aspiration on one or two occasions in an effort to avoid surgery if an experienced radiologist is available and a safe percutaneous route is assured. Additional experience will be required to determine whether this approach has merit.

The second method for draining a sterile pseudocyst is with the use of a pigtail catheter. In small series of patients, permanent closure has been noted in more than 50% of patients.[8,18–21] Pseudocysts that do not close permanently during pigtail catheter drainage are apt to develop a complication. The two most important complications are bleeding from the wall of the pseudocyst and introduction of bacteria resulting in secondary infection of the pseudocyst. These complications do not necessarily preclude eventual surgical decompression with anastomosis either to stomach or a loop of jejunum. Nonetheless, at the present time, we are not in favor of the use of a pigtail catheter as routine therapy for a sterile pseudocyst (Figs 14–2 and 14–3).

PERCUTANEOUS DRAINAGE OF STERILE CHRONIC PSEUDOCYST?

The role of percutaneous techniques for the treatment of a sterile chronic pseudocyst is uncertain. Because a chronic pseudocyst is caused by increased intraductal pressure, percutaneous efforts at decompression will likely fail. In our judgment, there has not been sufficient experience in this setting to recommend either percutaneous aspiration or percutaneous pigtail catheter drainage.

PERCUTANEOUS DRAINAGE OF INFECTED ACUTE PSEUDOCYST?

The usual treatment of an infected pseudocyst has been external surgical drainage because of the understandable reluctance to perform an anastomosis to an adjacent hollow viscus in a septic field. Several investigators have recently shown that most infected acute pseudocysts can be permanently closed by pigtail catheter drainage and antibiotics without need for surgery[8,14,19–21] (Fig 14–4). The reason for successful pigtail catheter drainage of infected pseudocysts as compared to variable results with drainage of sterile pseudocysts is not known. In our opinion, there has been sufficient success with pigtail catheter drainage to recommend this approach as a reasonable option for infected acute pseudocysts.

PERCUTANEOUS DRAINAGE OF INFECTED CHRONIC PSEUDOCYST?

There has not been sufficient experience with this technique to assess its efficacy. We would attempt percutaneous pigtail catheter drainage but would rely on surgical decompression if this technique failed.

PERCUTANEOUS DRAINAGE OF EXTRAPANCREATIC FLUID COLLECTION?

Because an extrapancreatic fluid collection is not marginated by a fibrous capsule as in the case of a pseudocyst, particular caution should be applied to interventional techniques lest bacteria be introduced into an entire retroperitoneal space. With this in mind, we recommend percutaneous aspiration with Gram stain and culture in order to distinguish between a sterile and infected fluid collection. If the process is found by Gram stain to be sterile, we do not recommend the use of a pigtail catheter but would simply aspirate the fluid and remove the Teflon sleeve. If the process is found by Gram stain to be infected, our limited experience is that either pigtail catheter drainage or surgical drainage is helpful.[2]

PERCUTANEOUS DRAINAGE OF PANCREATIC ABSCESS?

CT-guided percutaneous needle aspiration with Gram stain and culture is an accurate method to determine whether a collection is sterile or infected. If sterile, we would not recommend catheter drainage. If infected, on the basis of our experience (Fig 14–5) and that of others,[8] pigtail catheter drainage is likely to be effective therapy and is recommended to eradicate a pancreatic abscess.

SUMMARY

In our experience, CT-guided percutaneous aspiration with Gram stain and culture has proven to be a safe accurate method of distinguishing sterile from infected pancreatic processes and is recommended for this purpose. Needle aspiration is recommended for evacuating a pancreatic pseudocyst or extrapancreatic fluid collection once it is found to be sterile by Gram stain. The role of needle aspiration as definitive therapy for these sterile processes has not as yet been defined. Percutaneous catheter drainage is effective therapy for infected pancreatic pseudocysts and pancreatic abscesses. The role of catheter drainage as definitive therapy for a sterile pseudocyst remains unclear. Percutaneous catheter drainage should not be attempted to treat infected necrosis unless overwhelming sepsis precludes immediate surgery.

References

1. Gerzof SG, Robbins AH, Johnson WC, et al: Percutaneous catheter drainage of abdominal abscesses, a 5 year experience. *N Engl J Med* 1981; 305:653–657.
2. Gerzof SG, Banks PA, Robbins AH, et al: Early diagnosis of pancreatic infection by computed tomography-guided aspiration. *Gastroenterology* 1987; 93:1315–1320.
3. Beger HG, Bittner R, Block S, et al: Bacterial contamination of pancreatic necrosis: A prospective clinical study. *Gastroenterology* 1986; 91:433–438.
4. Warshaw AL: Lowering the level of uncertainty in late pancreatitis (editorial). *Gastroenterology* 1987; 93:1434–1437.
5. Sostre CF, Flournoy JG, Bova JG, et al: Pancreatic phlegmon, clinical features and course. *Dig Dis Sci* 1985; 30:918–927.
6. Block S, Maier W, Bittner R, et al: Identification of pancreatic necrosis in severe acute pancreatitis: Imaging procedures versus clinical staging. *Gut* 1986; 27:1035–1042.
7. Banks PA, Gerzof SG, Sullivan JG: Central cavitary necrosis: Differentiation from pancreatic pseudocysts on CT scan. *Pancreas*, 1988; 3:83–88.
8. van Sonnenberg E, Wittich GR, Casola G, et al: Complicated pancreatic inflammatory disease:

Diagnostic and therapeutic role of interventional radiology. *Radiology* 1985; 155:355–340.
9. Crass RA, Meyer AA, Jeffrey RB, et al: Pancreatic abscess: Impact of computerized tomography on early diagnosis and surgery. *Am J Surg* 1985; 150:127–130.
10. Hiatt JR, Fink AS, King W III, et al: Percutaneous aspiration of peripancreatic fluid collections: A safe method to detect infection. *Surgery* 1987; 101:523–530.
11. Barkin JS, Pereiras R, Hill M, et al: Diagnosis of pancreatic abscess via percutaneous aspiration. *Dig Dis Sci* 1982; 27:1011–1014.
12. Crass RA, Way LW: Acute and chronic pancreatic pseudocysts are different. *Am J Surg* 1981; 142:660–663.
13. Bittner R, Block S, Buchler M, et al: Pancreatic abscess and infected pancreatic necrosis: Different local septic complications in acute pancreatitis. *Dig Dis Sci* 1987; 32:1082–1087.
14. Gerzof SG, Johnson WC, Robbins AH, et al: Percutaneous drainage of infected pancreatic pseudocysts. *Arch Surg* 1984; 119:888–893.
15. Banks PA, Gerzof SG, Chong F, et al: Does infected necrosis require surgical debridement? (abstract). *Dig Dis Sci* 1987; 32:1159.
16. Barkin JS, Smith FR, Pereiras R: Therapeutic percutaneous aspiration of pancreatic pseudocysts. *Dig Dis Sci* 1981; 26:585–587.
17. Colhoun E, Murphy JJ, MacErlean DP: Percutaneous drainage of pancreatic pseudocysts. *Br J Surg* 1984; 71:131–132.
18. Banks PA, Gerzof SG: Role of percutaneous aspiration in the treatment of pancreatic pseudocysts, in Sato T, Yamauchi H (eds): *Pancreatitis.* Tokyo, University of Tokyo Press, 1985, pp 199–204.
19. Karlson KB, Martin EC, Fankuchen EI, et al: Percutaneous drainage of pancreatic pseudocysts and abscesses. *Radiology* 1982; 142:619–624.
20. Torres WE, Evert MB, Baumgartner BR, et al: Percutaneous aspiration and drainage of pancreatic pseudocysts. *AJR* 1986; 147:1007–1009.
21. Nunez D Jr, Yrizarry JM, Russell E, et al: Transgastric drainage of pancreatic fluid collections. *AJR* 1985; 145:815–818.

15

Pain of Chronic Pancreatitis:
What are the management options?

W. GARDNER ROWELL, M.D.
PHILLIP P. TOSKES, M.D.

The morbidity from chronic pancreatitis usually manifests itself in two ways, steatorrhea with weight loss or pain. While the former problem is well understood and the treatment straightforward, the pathophysiology of pain in chronic pancreatitis is not, and treatment is often frustrating, straining the patient–physician relationship and sometimes resulting in narcotic addiction. Many theories on the pathogenesis of the pain associated with chronic pancreatitis have arisen but, with the exception of the pain related to a pseudocyst, none have withstood critical examination. Drainage of a pseudocyst will often bring dramatic relief of pain. If no pseudocyst is found, two clinical patterns emerge:
1. Some patients will demonstrate no abnormalities on ERCP and an abnormal secretin test
2. Other patients will have dilated ducts or strictures detected by ERCP.

Traditionally, treatment of the latter group has been thought to be amenable to surgery with the procedure of choice being pancreatic duct decompression.[1] Subsequently, Bornman and co-workers published a paper that failed to show any relationship between dilated ducts or strictures found at ERCP and pain in patients with chronic calcific pancreatitis.[2] Patients who were free from pain for more than 1 year had the same degree of abnormalities at ERCP as did those with persistent pain. In a series of 101 patients with suspected or definite chronic pancreatitis, the Copenhagen pancreatitis study group found no correlation between the presence of dilated ducts observed at ERCP and the intensity of pain as indicated by the patients.[3] Close examination of those series that claim excellent results with duct decompression brings out several points:
1. Many patients actually had a pseudocyst drained, which should afford relief from pain
2. Often relief from pain was closely associated with abstinence from alcohol and probably was not related to the surgical procedure
3. The relief from pain actually may have been a result of progressive pancreatic exocrine impairment

In fact, in one study where patency rate following pancreaticojejunostomy was assessed by ERCP, there was no correlation between patency and pain relief.[4] Duct dilation seen in advanced chronic pancreatitis may not be a consequence of proximal obstruction or strictures but rather the consequence of epithelial destruction associated with severe fibrosis. These studies suggest that factors other than ductal obstruction or narrowing may be important in the genesis of the pain of chronic pancreatitis.

Despite the lack of understanding of the pathogenesis of pain in chronic pancreatitis, there are several management options available to the clinician in treating these patients. These options fall under the categories of supportive care, medical management, surgical management, and miscellaneous interventions.

SUPPORTIVE CARE

Supportive care for chronic pancreatitis has traditionally consisted of analgesics, small, frequent low-fat meals, abstinence from alcohol, and pancreatic enzyme therapy if steatorrhea was present. Because of the addictive potential of narcotic analgesics with long-term use, we tend to use non-narcotic analgesics for pain such as a combination of acetaminophen and propoxyphene (Darvocet-N 100). In our experience, the use of strong narcotic analgesics for the pain of chronic pancreatitis invariably results in narcotic addiction with continued pain. Small, frequent low-fat meals are prescribed in hopes of causing less pancreatic stimulation along with an adequate daily caloric intake and a reduction in steatorrhea. There is some evidence that a diet excessively low or high in fat content increases the risk for the development of pancreatitis and on that basis some clinicians have recommended a moderate (fat) intake.[5] We do not routinely recommend this diet. Although it is well documented that pancreatic pain may continue following the cessation of all alcohol intake, common sense dictates that abstinence be followed by all patients with chronic pancreatitis, regardless of the etiology.

MEDICAL MANAGEMENT

Anecdotal reports of pain relief in patients with chronic pancreatitis receiving pancreatic enzyme formulations for steatorrhea led to the suggestion that the oral administration of pancreatic enzymes might decrease the abdominal pain associated with chronic pancreatitis. To date three placebo-controlled clinical trials using pancreatic enzyme formulations to treat abdominal pain in patients with chronic pancreatitis have been reported.[6-8] Two of these studies,[6,7] including the one from our own medical center, demonstrated pancreatic extract to be efficacious in relieving abdominal pain—particularly in female patients with chronic pancreatitis without steatorrhea whose pancreatitis was largely of the idiopathic variety. In the one negative study,[8] an enteric-coated microsphere formulation (Pancrease) was used, which may have failed because this preparation may not release its enzymes until it goes beyond the duodenum—the feedback sensitive part of the intestine.[9]

It appears that pancreatic serine proteases (trypsin, chymotrypsin, elastase) inhibit pancreatic exocrine secretion, putting the pancreas at rest and affording relief of pain. These clinical observations fit with a large amount of data in experimental animals that indicate that the presence of serine proteases in the lumen of the proximal small intestine somehow inhibits the release of cholecystokinin (CCK) and down-modulates pancreatic enzyme secretion.

In a recent study, we provided the first data that proteases in the lumen of the proximal small intestine modulate pancreatic exocrine secretion in patients with chronic pancreatitis and in normal subjects.[7] Large quantities of bovine pancreatic proteases perfused acutely into the duodenum or administered by mouth chronically were demonstrated to suppress pancreatic exocrine output in patients with chronic pancreatitis with mild-to-moderate exocrine impairment (defined as a peak bicarbonate concentration between 55 and 80 mEq/L on the secretin test and normal fat absorption) and in age- and sex-matched controls. The group in which this phenomenon was best demonstrated was comprised of middle-aged women with idiopathic chronic pancreatitis. These patients also showed the greatest pain relief when given pancreatic extract therapy. Interestingly, patients with more advanced chronic pancreatitis (pancreatic insufficiency with peak bicarbonate concentrations <50 mEq/L and steatorrhea), usually alcohol related, did not demonstrate suppression of pancreatic secretion with proteases nor did they tend to respond to pancreatic extract therapy for their abdominal pain.

That double-blind crossover study confirmed the report by Isaksson and Ihse that chronic pancreatic extract therapy reduces the frequency and severity of recurrent abdominal pain in patients with chronic pancreatitis.[6] However, Isaksson and Ihse's study used a 7-day crossover design, which may have been too short for evaluation of the response because of the variability of pain in patients with chronic pancreatitis. In addition, our experience indicates the benefit of pancreatic extract on certain objective maldigestive parameters may carry over for several days. It is noteworthy that in the Isaksson and Ihse study, the best response to enzyme therapy occurred in female patients with idiopathic chronic pancreatitis. Of the 19 patients they evaluated, 10 were "good responders" to pancreatic extract and 9 were "poor responders." Although they did not quantitate steatorrhea in their patients, it is interesting to note that the best results in our study were seen in patients with normal fecal fat excretion (usually women with idiopathic chronic pancreatitis), and the worst results were seen in patients with steatorrhea (i.e., severe pancreatic impairment).

Large doses of pancreatic extract are required to effect feedback inhibition of pancreatic secretion. It has been our experience that Viokase, eight tablets with meals and at bedtime, is the best enzyme regimen available at the present time. If this fails to achieve pain relief we add $NaHCO_3$, 650 mg before and after each dose, to protect the enzymes from destruction during gastric transit. If patients are unable to take $NaHCO_3$ tablets due to the high sodium load, an H_2 receptor antagonist or one of the enteric-coated enzyme preparations may be used (Table 15–1). Due to the delayed dissolution of currently available enteric-coated enzyme preparations, the proximal duodenum tends to be bypassed and therefore feedback inhibition may not occur, resulting in unsatisfactory pain relief from these preparations in some patients. We are currently investigating more potent enzyme preparations with optimal microsphere size and different enteric coatings, which may be more appropriate for patients with pain secondary to chronic pancreatitis.

In spite of the need to take 32 tablets per day at an expense of approximately $75 per month, our experience has been that there is remarkable patient compliance with the pancreatic extract program. Furthermore, narcotic usage is greatly curtailed or abolished. These clinical observations seem to be specific. In uncontrolled clinical observations over a 5-year period, we have noted no effect on the abdominal pain in patients who had irritable bowel syndrome, gastritis, acid-peptic disorders, or primary psychoneurosis.

TABLE 15–1.
Our Approach to the Use of Pancreatic Extract

Pancreatic extract
   Schedule: Before meals (and at bedtime if the patient experiences pain)
   Dose:
      Viokase®   8 capsules at each time
      or Cotazym®   6 capsules at each time
      or Ilozyme®   4 capsules at each time
      or Pancrease®   3 capsules at each time (enteric coated)

If no significant improvement occurs with extract alone add:
Sodium bicarbonate*†
   Schedule: Before and after each meal (and at bedtime if the patient experiences pain)
   Dose: Sodium bicarbonate 650 mg ac and pc (and 1300 mg hs if needed)

*We have not noted hypercalcemia or milk-alkali syndrome with this dose of sodium bicarbonate.
†We do not recommend concomitant treatment with sodium bicarbonate and enteric-coated enzyme preparations because increased gastric pH may cause premature release and inactivation of enzymes.

SURGICAL MANAGEMENT

Patients who fail maximal medical therapy should undergo ERCP, and those who have dilated ducts may be candidates for a surgical ductal decompression procedure. Short-term pain relief may be achieved in up to 80% of patients, although long-term results are closer to 50%.[1] Furthermore, successful ductal decompression does not halt the progression to exocrine or endocrine insufficiency and, as mentioned earlier, some have failed to find a correlation between long-term surgical patency and pain relief.[4, 10] For those patients who fail medical management and have a normal caliber or narrowed main pancreatic duct, subtotal pancreatectomy (with removal of 95% of the gland) has been recommended by some clinicians. Exocrine and endocrine supplementation will be required following such extensive resection.

Other interventions that have been used in an attempt to relieve pain in patients with chronic pancreatitis include celiac plexus block and total rest of the gastrointestinal tract by keeping the patient on no oral nutrient intake while maintaining their nutritional needs by total parenteral nutrition. Both of these modalities are temporizing procedures at best.

In a recent series of 36 patients (13 with pancreatic cancer and 23 with chronic pancreatitis), celiac plexus block gave very disappointing results in the patients with chronic pancreatitis.[11] Although valuable in providing pain relief to the cancer patients, the effects in patients with chronic pancreatitis were unpredictable and short-lived. Perhaps the failure of the nerve block was due to the inflammation and fibrosis around the celiac plexus, which could limit the diffusion of the alcohol used for the nerve block.

It should also be emphasized that such nerve blocks are not without significant morbidity (i.e., serious neurologic damage, impotence, and hyperesthesia of the lower extremities). The generally poor results and potential serious complications have greatly dampened our enthusiasm for celiac plexus block in patients with pain secondary to chronic pancreatitis.

Total pancreatectomy leads to severe metabolic disturbances, and this is one of the reasons this surgical approach has not been used very frequently in patients with the pain of chronic pancreatitis. Consequently, the adjunctive use of pancreatic autotransplantation is being evaluated for patients with chronic pancreatitis. The experience to date with islet cell infusion into the portal vein has been disappointing—both from the perspective of not being able to make recipients insulin independent and because of severe complications, such as disseminated intravascular coagulation and acute portal hypertension.

In a very limited number of patients, total pancreatectomy followed by segmental or whole organ pancreatic autotransplantation has resulted in pain relief and insulin independence for a follow-up period of 2 to 18 months. If such a procedure is shown to be worthwhile, pancreatic resection may be performed earlier in the course of chronic pancreatitis before there has been extensive damage to the endocrine pancreas.

MISCELLANEOUS INTERVENTIONS

Finally, our laboratory has stressed the importance of elevated blood levels of CCK in the pathogenesis of the pain of chronic pancreatitis. Following the administration of large doses of pancreatic extract to patients with chronic pancreatitis, not only does pain decrease, but blood levels of cholecystokinin fall toward normal levels.[12] This is most impressive in the patients with mild-to-moderate exocrine impairment and severe pain (i.e., those with idiopathic chronic pancreatitis). It may be that pancreatic stimulation is constantly occurring in these patients secondary to the elevated blood CCK levels. In this regard, a new CCK antagonist, L364–718 (Merck Inc), may be important in treating the pain of these patients. This newly developed benzodiazepinelike peripheral CCK receptor antagonist is the most potent CCK antagonist known. L364–718 is also effective as a CCK antagonist when given orally. Our laboratory[13]

```
                    Recurrent Abdominal Pain
                              ↓
                    Diagnostic Evaluation
                    ┌─────────┴─────────┐
                 Negative              Positive
                    ↓              (end of evaluation)
              Secretin test
           ┌────────┴────────┐
        Negative           Positive
   (end of evaluation)        ↓
                  Viokase, 32 tablets/day × 30 days
                   ┌────────────┴────────────┐
              Pain relief           Unsatisfactory pain relief
         (end of evaluation)                  ↓
                                       Add NaHCO₃
                              ┌────────────┴────────────┐
                         Pain relief         Unsatisfactory pain relief
                    (end of evaluation)                  ↓
                                                       ERCP
                                              ┌──────────┴──────────┐
                                         Dilated ducts         Ducts not dilated
                                              ↓                      ↓
                                       Peustow procedure            TPN
                                                               Celiac block
                                                           Pancreatic Resection
```

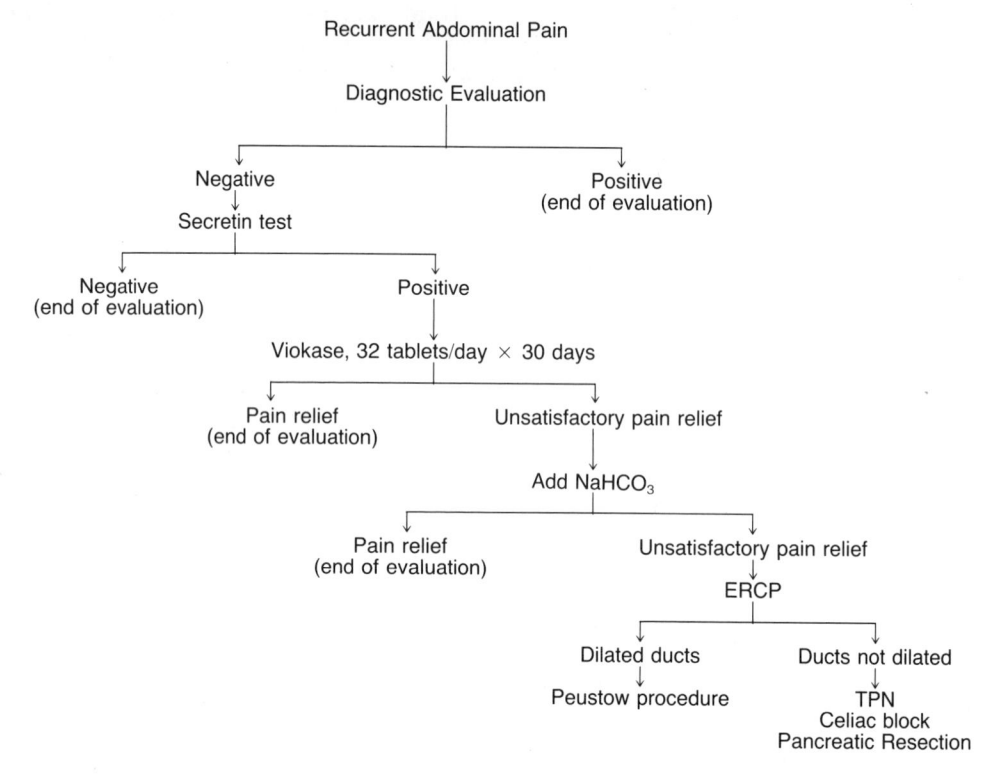

FIG 15–1.

has shown this inhibitor to be quite effective in suppressing pancreatic enzyme secretion when administered intraduodenally to rats. It may be that this CCK receptor antagonist may decrease pancreatic stimulation secondary to CCK, thereby "resting" the pancreas and affording pain relief.

SUMMARY

In conclusion, the major advancement in the treatment of the patient with pain from chronic pancreatitis has been the ability to down-modulate pancreatic secretion using oral pancreatic enzymes. Presumably this results in artificial "pancreatic rest," which relieves pain in approximately 80% of patients with idiopathic pancreatitis and 25% of patients with alcoholic pancreatitis. Traditionally, those patients with dilated ducts have been thought to respond to surgical decompression but recent data make one question the effectiveness of surgery in this setting. It is possible that progression of the disease process ultimately results in pain relief unrelated to the surgical procedure.[14] The final determination in that regard awaits a randomized controlled study. In the meantime, we feel that the flow diagram in Fig 15–1 represents the most reasonable approach to patients with chronic pancreatitis and pain.

References

1. Moosa AR: Surgical treatment of chronic pancreatitis: An overview. *Br J Surg* 1987; 74:661–667.
2. Bornman PC, Marks IN, Girdwood AH, et al: Non-correlation of ERCP findings to abdominal pain in patients with chronic pancreatitis. *Br J Surg* 1980; 67:425–428.

3. Reimer JA, Matzen P, Malchow-Moller A, et al: Pattern of pain, duet morphology and pancreatic function in chronic pancreatitis. Scand J Gastroenterol 1984; 19:334–338.
4. Kugelberg CH, Wehlin L, Arnesjo B, et al: Endoscopic pancreatography in evaluating results of pancreaticojejunostomy. Gut 1976; 17:267–272.
5. Dubree JP, Sarles H: Multicenter survey of the etiology of pancreatic disease. Relationship between the relative risk of developing chronic pancreatitis and alcohol protein and lipid consumption. Digestion 1978; 18:337–350.
6. Isaksson G, Ihse I: Pain reduction by an oral pancreatic enzyme preparation in chronic pancreatitis. Dig Dis Sci 1983; 28:97–102.
7. Slaff J, Jacobson D, Tillman CR, et al: Protease-specific suppression of pancreatic exocrine secretion. Gastroenterology 1984; 87:44–52.
8. Halgreen H, Thorsgaard Pedersen N, Worning H: Symptomatic effect of pancreatic enzyme therapy in patients with chronic pancreatitis. Scand J Gastroenterol 1986; 21:104–108.
9. Dutta S, Hubbard V, Appler M: Critical evaluation of the therapeutic efficacy of a pH sensitive enteric-coated pancreatic enzyme preparation in the treatment of exocrine pancreatic insufficiency secondary to cystic fibrosis. Dig Dis Sci, (in press).
10. Warshaw AL, Popp JW, Schapiro RH: Long-term patency, pancreatic function, and pain relief after lateral pancreaticojejunostomy for chronic pancreatitis. Gastroenterology 1980; 79:289–293.
11. Leung JWC, Bowen-Wright M, Aveling W, et al: Coeliac plexus block for pain in pancreatic cancer and chronic pancreatitis. Br J Surg 1983; 70:730–732.
12. Slaff JI, Wolfe MM, Toskes PP: Elevated fasting cholecystokinin levels in pancreatic exocrine impairment: Evidence to support feedback regulation. J Lab Clin Med 1985; 105:282–285.
13. Rowell W, Scott M, Curington C, et al: Studies of pancreatic exocrine secretion using L364-718, a potent new orally effective CCK receptor antagonist (abstract). Gastroenterology 1987; 92:1712.
14. Ammann RW, Hanner B, Furagalli I: Chronic pancreatitis in Zurich, 1963–1972. Digestion 1973; 90:404–415.

16

Pancreas Divisum:
Do the authorities now agree?

GLEN A. LEHMAN, M.D.

Pancreas divisum (PDiv) is being recognized more frequently in clinical medicine as the use of ERCP increases. The "difficult problems" relating to this diagnosis that will be addressed in this chapter are: (1) techniques used to obtain detailed information about the dorsal pancreas by minor papilla cannulation, (2) how to separate clinically significant (symptomatic) from coincidental PDiv, and (3) treatment plans for PDiv.

EMBRYOLOGY AND DEFINITIONS

Pancreas divisum (PDiv) is a congenital variant of pancreatic ductal anatomy in which ductal systems of the dorsal and ventral pancreatic buds fail to fuse (Fig 16–1,B). Normally the anterior portion of the pancreatic head, nearly the entire pancreatic body, and the entire pancreatic tail develop from the dorsal pancreatic bud, whereas the posterior part of the pancreatic head and uncinate process develop from the ventral pancreatic bud. The dorsal pancreas therefore gives origin to three fourths or more of the pancreatic parenchyma and drains its exocrine secretion out of the relatively small minor papilla orifice. It is hypothesized that this relative obstruction to flow through the minor papilla predisposes to pain and pancreatitis. One third of PDiv patients have no apparent pancreatic ductal system that communicates with the major papilla. When this occurs, the embryologic ventral pancreas drains cephalad into the dorsal system and out the minor papilla (Fig 16–1,E). Nearly 10% of PDiv patients have a minute duct connecting the ventral and dorsal pancreas[1] (Fig 16–1,C). This condition is termed incomplete PDiv, although functionally the entities remain the same.

INCIDENCE OF PANCREAS DIVISUM

Autopsy series have reported incidence of PDiv from 4% to 12.5% (Table 16–1, page 200). The mean from series of greater than 1000 autopsies was 6.8%. There are data that show a lower incidence of PDiv in Orientals and blacks.[2] Approximately one third of annular pancreas patients have coexistent PDiv.[3]

ERCP DIAGNOSIS AND MINOR PAPILLA CANNULATION

In the vast majority of instances PDiv will be diagnosed by ERCP when a short delicate ventral pancreas ductal system that arborizes into terminal fine branches over a 5- to 50-mm distance is seen. The ventral ductogram is usually "normal" except for its small size, although there is a low incidence of chronic pancreatitis, tumor, pseudocyst, and so forth. During ventral ductography acrinarization commonly occurs, causes transient pain, but

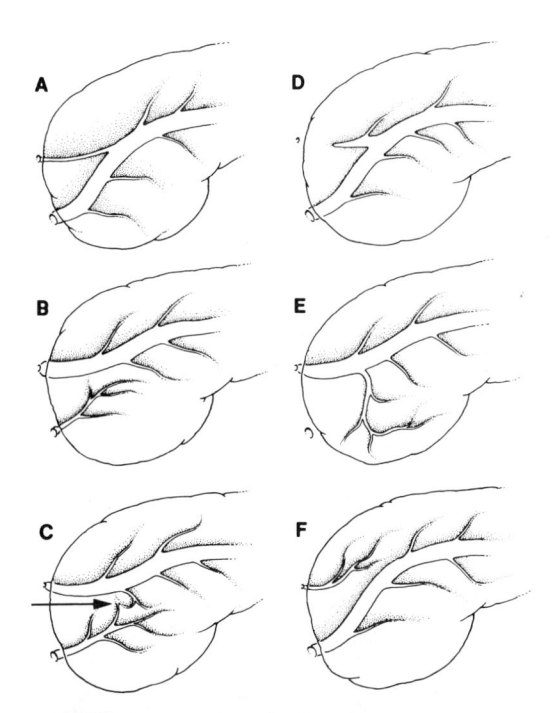

FIG 16–1.
Variant pancreatic ductal anatomy. **A,** the most common pancreatic ductal anatomy with the main pancreatic duct draining by the major papilla and the accessory pancreatic duct communicating with the main pancreatic duct and draining into the minor papilla. **B,** typical pancreas divisum with the dorsal pancreatic duct being the main pancreatic duct and draining exclusively by way of the minor papilla. The ventral pancreas is a small ductal system draining by way of the major papilla. **C,** same as B except the dorsal and ventral ductal systems communicate by way of a small communicating branch. **D,** same as A except accessory pancreatic duct is incomplete and does not communicate with the minor papilla. **E,** dorsal dominant variant of pancreas divisum in which the entire pancreas drains into the dorsal ductal system and out the minor papilla (i.e. the ventral pancreas drains cephalad into the dorsal ductal system). **F,** similar to D except the accessory pancreatic duct communicates only with minor papilla and does not communicate back to the main ductal system. This "reversed pancreas divisum" is functionally insignificant.

rarely causes significant pancreatitis. When a ventral pancreas is filled with contrast, the dorsal pancreas remains nonvisualized unless minor papilla cannulation is undertaken. Because the dorsal pancreas represents the majority of the pancreatic mass, minor papilla cannulation is the key to defining the remainder of the potential pancreatic pathology (i.e., the original goal for the ERCP). Approximately one third of PDiv patients will have no ventral pancreas visualized by major papilla cannulation.[4] Additionally, many centers experience a 5% to 15% major papilla pancreatogram failure rate. Whenever major papilla cannulation fails, minor papilla cannulation is needed.

The minor papilla is generally located approximately 2 cm cephalad and slightly anterior to the major papilla. The minor papilla appearance is usually similar to the major papilla except that it is considerably smaller and has no longitudinal fold. Alternatively, the minor papilla may be very inconspicuous and appear as a tiny dimple or papule with almost no elevation. The minor papilla is optimally viewed with the endoscope bowed along the greater curvature of the stomach with approximately 100 cm of instrument inserted into the patient (Fig 16–2). If the minor papilla cannot be identified or its orifice cannot be clearly seen, intravenous secretin (1 unit per kilogram) can be given to induce visible flow of pancreatic juice from the minor papilla.[5] In PDiv the majority of juice flows out the minor papilla, and the minor papilla orifice becomes more evident.

Minor papilla cannulation can occasionally be performed with a tapered-tip 5 F catheter, but this is the exception. In most instances a needle-tipped catheter[5,6] is needed. I have had best results using a 23-gauge blunted needle extending 2 mm beyond a *tapered-tipped* catheter. The tapered tip of the catheter is very helpful, because the needle tip is not hidden. The needle must protrude far enough from the catheter to be visible during cannulation. Alternatively, an 0.018-inch-diameter guidewire through a 3 F catheter combination may be used to cannulate deeply. Contrast medium is injected after guidewire withdrawal. Such needle catheters and 3 F catheters with guidewires are commercially available (Wilson Cook, Inc., Winston-Salem, North Carolina 27105).

It is *critical* to identify the orifice of the minor papilla before attempting to probe

TABLE 16–1.
Autopsy Frequency of Pancreas Divisum

First Author and Year	Site	Total Cases	Pancreas Divisum (%)	Pancreatic Disease Excluded
Kleitsch (1955)	US	48	6 (12.5%)	Not stated
Birnstingl (1959)	UK	150	7 (4.7%)	Yes
Berman (1960)	US	143	8 (5.4%)	No
Hand (1963)	US	50	4 (8%)	Yes
Dawson (1961)	Canada	120	9 (7.5%)	Not stated
Rienhoff (1946)	US	100	4 (4%)	Yes
Smanio (1969)	Brazil	200	13 (6.5%)	Not stated
Baldwin (1911)	US	75	5 (6.5%)	Yes
Milbourn (1960)	Sweden	167	15 (9.0%)	Yes
TOTAL		1063	72 (6.8%)	

and cannulate with the needle catheter. Such catheters can quickly traumatize the tissue and obscure the opening. If secretin has been given, it is often hard to fill the pancreatic tail with contrast during active juice flow (Fig 16–2). Attempts to fill the entire tail in a vigorously secreting gland probably increase the incidence of pancreatitis and should be avoided. I recommend attempting to cannulate without secretin and reserving its use to patients in whom the orifice cannot be otherwise identified. These methods can achieve an 80% to 90% cannulation rate.

Table 16–2 shows findings in our series of 74 ERCP dorsal ductograms in 84 PDiv patients. Structural abnormalities were present in 22% of the cases and consisted most often of chronic pancreatitis changes. Cotton[7] and Warshaw[8] also detected dorsal duct abnormalities in 25% of PDiv cases. Patients with a history of pancreatitis are more likely to have dorsal duct abnormalities than patients being

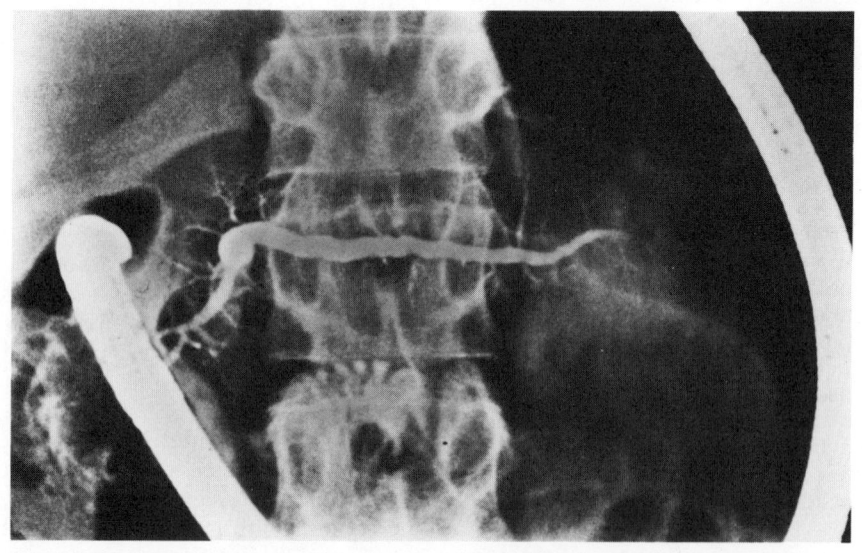

FIG 16–2.
Minor papilla cannulation with the endoscope positioned along the greater curvature of the stomach. Secretin was given, and the pancreatic tail was intentionally not completely filled. Minor chronic pancreatitis changes are present in this 16-year-old female.

TABLE 16–2.
ERCP Dorsal Ductography Abnormalities in 74 Pancreas Divisum Cases (Dorsal Ductography Successful 74/84* Cases)

	Number of Patients†
Chronic pancreatitis	
Advanced	6
Mild	6
Pseudocysts	2
Intraductal stones	4
Body/tail agenesis	1
Pancreatic cancer	1
Delayed drainage‡	31

*Includes ten patients with incomplete PDiv; in four patients minor papilla cannulation was required to adequately fill the dorsal pancreas.
†Three patients with two structural abnormalities.
‡Ten minutes if no secretin; >5 minutes if secretin given.

evaluated for pain alone. Additional information from dorsal ductal contrast injection can be gained by measuring the contrast drainage time and the patient's response to duct injection (i.e., pain). No series of unequivocally asymptomatic PDiv patients has been studied to define "normal drainage time" or "normal pain response." Nevertheless, if 10 minutes is somewhat arbitrarily taken as the upper limit of normal for PDiv drainage time (when no secretin or narcotics are given), 42% of patients in our series showed slow drainage. All patients with abnormal ductograms also had delayed drainage.

PANCREAS DIVISUM—A *CAUSE* OF SYMPTOMS OR *COINCIDENTAL* FINDING?

PDiv occurs in approximately 6% to 7% of the general population, but only a very small portion of these persons will ever have symptoms referrable to the pancreas or biliary tree and undergo ERCP. In other words, the majority of PDiv patients remain asymptomatic throughout life. Does PDiv predispose to pancreatitis?

Statistical Association

From a statistical standpoint, if minor papilla obstruction causes obstructive pancreatitis, then the incidence of PDiv in patients with pancreatitis (especially "idiopathic" pancreatitis) should be higher than the incidence of PDiv in the general population or in patients undergoing ERCP for reasons other than pancreatitis. Series[7–10] totalling several hundred patients found PDiv two or three times more often in idiopathic pancreatitis patients than in patients without pancreatitis or pancreatitis with specific etiologies. Two large series[11,12] tallying over 450 PDiv patients have not confirmed this statistical association between PDiv and pancreatitis. In our series of 84 patients with PDiv, we found PDiv to be present in 24% of patients with idiopathic pancreatitis in contrast to 8% ($p < 0.05$) of patients with pancreatitis from other causes.

How can the discrepancies among series be explained? Almost certainly there are differences in the definitions of "idiopathic" and "alcoholic" pancreatitis used. Referral patterns vary (i.e., certain centers receive greater numbers of failed ERCP, idiopathic pancreatitis, or PDiv patients). Racial factors may exist. Because PDiv is unquestionably coincidental in certain ERCP patients, this serves to dilute patient numbers in whom it may be (or is) etiologic.

I believe there are sufficient data to conclude that PDiv is associated with clinically significant minor papilla stenosis and obstructive pancreatic pain or pancreatitis. In any large series of PDiv patients however, PDiv will not be the cause of symptoms in many of the patients.

Diagnostic Criteria

Table 16–3 lists studies and trials which may be used to differentiate PDiv patients with clinically significant minor papilla orifice narrowing from those who do not. The sensitivity and specificity of these studies are being evaluated, but many uncertainties remain.

TABLE 16–3.
Findings Suggestive of Pathologically Significant Minor Papilla Narrowing in Pancreas Divisum

Major Criteria
1. Chronic pancreatitis changes in dorsal pancreas associated with a normal ventral pancreas (ductogram, CT scan and/or histology)
2. Symptom resolution (temporary versus long-term) with dorsal duct decompression (stenting, sphincterotomy, or other surgical therapy)

Minor Criteria
1. Pain with dorsal pancreas contrast injection
2. Delayed dorsal ductogram drainage time
3. Dorsal pancreatic duct dilation with secretin administration as monitored by ultrasound
4. Abnormal manometry of minor papilla or dorsal pancreatic duct
5. Abnormal secretin stimulated dorsal pancreatic juice analysis
6. Resistance to passage of probe ≤ 0.75 mm in diameter (intraoperative)

Major Criteria

Dorsal Pancreatitis. The diagnostic finding that most strongly incriminates the relative minor papilla stenosis of PDiv as a cause for symptoms is the identification of changes of chronic pancreatitis in the dorsal portion of the gland coexistent with a normal ventral pancreas. This combination of abnormal dorsal and normal ventral pancreatogram findings is present in approximately 25% of ERCP cases in which dorsal ductal information is available.

Temporary Stent Trial. Another means to separate symptomatic from asymptomatic PDiv is temporary trial stenting of the minor papilla at ERCP. Although only limited data are available, preliminary findings indicate that 60% to 90% of symptomatic PDiv patients stented had temporary relief of their symptoms from stenting.

Minor Criteria

Pain provocation upon injection of the dorsal pancreatic duct suggests a pancreatic origin of the patient's pain. Evaluation of the pain response in a sedated patient is admittedly difficult. I avoid narcotics (if possible) to facilitate this observation and to avoid narcotic stimulation of any sphincter musculature present.

Drainage time of contrast media injected into the main pancreatic duct (without PDiv) is generally considered abnormal if longer than 10 minutes. I have empirically applied this value to the dorsal pancreas and consider drainage time longer than 5 minutes abnormal if secretin was given.

The *secretin ultrasound* test was reported by Warshaw[13] as a noninvasive method to evaluate the dorsal pancreatic duct diameter during vigorous exocrine secretion. Ductal dilation was interpreted as evidence for pathologically significant minor papilla narrowing. He reported an excellent predictive value for this test in that patients who dilated their duct responded favorably to surgical pancreatic duct decompression, whereas patients who did not dilate their duct did not respond favorably. Bolondi[14] reported that the main pancreatic duct dilated after secretin stimulation in normal subjects without PDiv. Cotton's summary[15] of limited European experiences failed to confirm Warshaw's data. Further studies are needed to clarify the value of this method.

Minor papilla manometry has been performed on a very limited number of PDiv patients. A basal sphincter zone and phasic waves have been observed. Staritz[16] reported that symptomatic PDiv patients had dorsal pancreatic duct pressures of 23.7 mm Hg in contrast to main pancreatic duct pressures of 10.8 mm Hg in normal non-PDiv patients. I have measured minor papilla and dorsal duct pressures by triple-lumen, low-compliance, water-perfused 5 F catheter methods in six PDiv patients who had recurrent symptoms after surgical sphincteroplasty. Basal "sphincter" pressures measured 72 to 180 (mean 100) mm Hg. Dorsal duct pressures were 12 to 27 (mean 21) mm Hg. No phasic waves were seen. These basal sphincter pressures were interpreted as elevated, and most patients had fewer symptoms after stenting or repeat sphincteroplasty.

Secretin-stimulated dorsal pancreatic juice collection has been reported by Keith[17] who found abnormal exocrine secretion in four of four PDiv patients tested (despite normal dorsal ductograms). Cotton[7] noted that abnormal secretory testing correlated with abnormal dorsal ductography.

Probe patency. At surgery, a minor papilla orifice that does not easily admit at least a 0.75 mm lacrimal probe[17] is considered stenotic. Using this criterion, Warshaw[8] noted that patients with a stenotic minor papilla were much more likely to get pain relief after sphincteroplasty than patients without stenosis. Whether such probe evaluation can be applied to ERCP remains to be evaluated.

Although the diagnostic predictive value of the minor criteria have not been adequately evaluated, I use these criteria as evidence for or against placement of a trial stent.

THERAPY OF PANCREAS DIVISUM

Medical

Many people with PDiv will be asymptomatic or have such minor symptoms that no pancreatic therapy is needed. If therapy is needed the most conservative approach would be medical. It seems reasonable to suggest a chronic pancreatitis regimen consisting of anticholinergics, low-fat diet, and pancreatic enzyme replacement in an effort to decrease pancreatic secretion (i.e., quantity of juice flow through the minor papilla). A randomized study is currently in progress comparing such medical therapy to endoscopic stenting. If the patient's symptoms warrant a more aggressive approach or medical therapy fails, endoscopic or surgical therapy should be considered.

Endoscopy

Endoscopic therapy includes minor papilla dilatation, stenting, and sphincterotomy. Dilatation alone with 5–10 F catheters may give transient pain relief or provoke pancreatitis. I don't recommend use of dilatation alone. Most stenting data[18–20] available to date are only in abstract form. Technically, the procedure involves cannulation of the minor papilla with an 0.018 to 0.035-inch-diameter guidewire within a #3–5 F tapered catheter system. The minor papilla may then be dilated up to 5–10 F with push-type catheters. Once dilated, a 2- to 7-cm-length 5–10 F straight, barbed stent is then left to bridge the minor papilla. The optimal length, composition, flexibility, contour, diameter, and number of side holes of such stents have not been defined. Short-term improvement in symptoms or pancreatitis was observed by Geenen[20] in 17 of 19 patients, by Seigel[18] in 25 of 29 patients, and 12 of 16 PDiv patients from our own series. To date long-term success with stents has been suboptimal with occlusion of stents in 2 to 6 months being common and recurrence of pancreatitis being frequent once stents occlude or fall out. Geenen replaced stents at 6-month intervals.

Seigel[18] reported that eight patients whose symptoms temporarily improved by stenting had more sustained relief with surgical duct decompression. Patients who did not have pain relief with stenting (three patients) did not improve after surgical decompression either. At this point, minor papilla stenting appears to provide temporary benefit only, although detailed long-term studies are needed. Use of stent trials to select patients who will respond to minor papilla sphincterotomy or sphincteroplasty appears reasonable, although larger series and longer follow-up are also needed.

Some of the factors that affect stent trials are patient selection criteria (pain only versus pancreatitis), whether abnormal or normal dorsal ducts are stented, ultimate stent occlusion with debris, transient increased pain, and pancreatitis from stent placement and placebo effect.

Minor papilla sphincterotomy at endoscopy has undergone very limited trials. Extreme caution must be exercised as more than a 3- to 4-mm cut probably includes pancreatic tissue. An initial report[21] with a small series of patients was largely unsuccessful, although such aggressive maneuvers as snare removal of the minor papilla and biopsy excision of the minor papilla were included. Preliminary reports from Europe[22, 23] of more typical short sphincterotomies have been more promising with nearly three-quarters of patients having symptom relief. The cut may be made with a standard short-wire sphincterotome, a precut sphincterotome, or with a needle-knife cutting above a stent. Mild pancreatitis is generally provoked, although serious pancreatitis has not yet been reported by minor papilla sphincterotomy. The follow-up has generally been less than 24 months and inadequate to determine the restenosis rate. I have performed 12 minor papilla endoscopic sphincterotomies with good-to-excellent relief of pain or pancreatitis in nine (mean follow-up 15 months). Placement of a stent before or after sphincterotomy is recommended to prevent occlusion of the orifice from edema. Because of potential risks, minor papilla sphincterotomy cannot be recommended for general use until further experience is obtained.

Surgery

The surgical approaches to PDiv are predominately those of ductal decompression. The simplest procedures are minor papilla sphincterotomy and sphincteroplasty[8, 17, 24] Approximately 100 such operations have now been reported in the literature. Outcomes have been only modestly successful with approximately two thirds of these patients having good or excellent results. Patients who had documented prior bouts of pancreatitis but not advanced chronic pancreatitis responded best to sphincteroplasty. Recurrence of pancreatitis or pain from restenosis of the minor papilla has been a significant problem in 10% to 30% of cases.[8, 25] Reported follow-up has generally been limited to 1 to 3 years. Placement of intraoperative intraductal stents to help maintain long-term ductal patency needs further evaluation. Severe acute pancreatitis including hemorrhagic pancreatitis and death have occurred postoperatively; therefore, the decision to operate must be weighed *very carefully*. The data on symptom relief from surgical intervention are not easily interpreted because most surgeons agree that the gallbladder should be removed if it is still present. A portion of the clinical responders might therefore be patients with subtle gallbladder disease as the cause for their pain.

Additionally, the combination of minor and major papillae sphincteroplasties has been advocated by several surgical centers. The rationale for this is based on the clinical judgment that one still cannot be sure which papilla is the culprit in symptom production and that a high frequency of major papilla (sphincter of Oddi) dysfunction is reported in PDiv.[24, 26]

More aggressive pancreatic decompressive procedures or resective procedures may be warranted if the patient has incapacitating symptoms, advanced chronic pancreatitis, or if minor papilla sphincteroplasty fails.[27]

SUMMARY

PDiv patients with gallstones, tumors, peptic ulcer disease, or other obvious causes for their symptoms (Fig 16–3) should be treated accordingly (and the PDiv should be ignored). PDiv patients with mild-to-moderate symptoms (including pancreatitis) are best treated with watchful waiting and a medical regimen. PDiv patients with severe symptoms or pancreatitis should be aggressively evaluated. If no other etiology is found, ductal decompressive therapy on a trial or permanent basis should be strongly considered.

Further studies are needed to determine how accurately we can select patients who will respond to duct decompressive therapy. Additionally, the long-term efficacy of endoscopic and surgical duct decompressive therapy awaits evaluation.

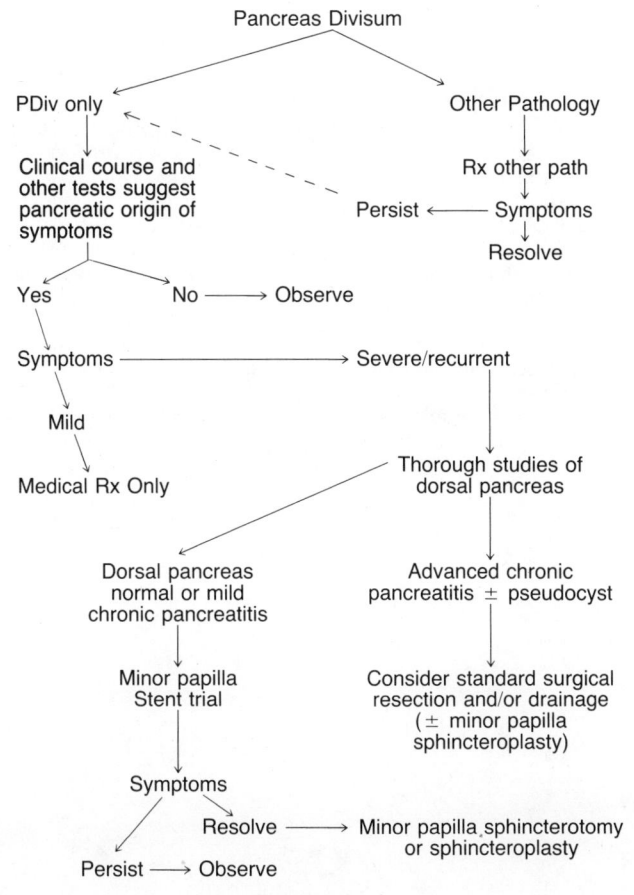

```
                        Pancreas Divisum
                       /       |        \
                      /        |         \
            PDiv only          |          Other Pathology
                ↓              |               ↓
        Clinical course and    |          Rx other path
        other tests suggest    |               
        pancreatic origin of   |    Persist ← Symptoms
        symptoms               |               ↓
                ↓              |           Resolve
           Yes    No → Observe
            ↓
        Symptoms ─────────────→ Severe/recurrent
            ↓                           ↓
          Mild                  Thorough studies of
            ↓                   dorsal pancreas
       Medical Rx Only         /        ↓
                              /          
                   Dorsal pancreas    Advanced chronic
                   normal or mild    pancreatitis ± pseudocyst
                   chronic pancreatitis      ↓
                          ↓           Consider standard surgical
                   Minor papilla      resection and/or drainage
                   Stent trial        (± minor papilla
                          ↓            sphincteroplasty)
                     Symptoms
                    /        \
              Resolve ────→ Minor papilla sphincterotomy
                /              or sphincteroplasty
        Persist → Observe
```

FIG 16-3.

References

1. Tulassay Z, Papp J, Farkas IE: Diagnostic aspects of incomplete pancreas divisum. *Gastrointest Endosc* 1986; 32(6):428.
2. Smanio T: Proposed nomenclature and classification of the human pancreatic duct and duodenal papillae. *Int Surg* 1969; 52(2):125-134.
3. Lehman GA, O'Connor KW: Coexistence of annular pancreas and pancreas divisum–ERCP diagnosis. *Gastrointest Endosc* 1985; 31(1):25-28.
4. McHenry R, O'Connor KW, Kopecky K, et al: Pancreas divisum: Incidence of abnormalities at dorsal ductography (DDG) and ventral ductography (VDG). *Gastrointest Endosc* 1986; 32(2):157.
5. O'Connor KW, Lehman GA: An improved technique for accessory papilla cannulation in pancreas divisum. *Gastrointest Endosc* 1985; 31:13.
6. Dunham F, Deltenre M, Jeanmart J, et al: Special catheters for ERCP. *Endoscopy* 1981; 13:81-85.
7. Cotton PB: Congenital anomaly of pancreas divisum as a cause of obstructive pain and pancreatitis. *Gut* 1980; 21:105-114.
8. Warshaw AL, Richter J, Shapiro RH: The cause and treatment of pancreatitis with pancreas divisum. *Ann Surg* 1983; 198(4):443-452.
9. Gregg JA: Pancreas divisum: Its association with pancreatitis. *Am J Surg* 1977; 134:539-543.
10. Kruse A: Fourth European Congress of Gastrointestinal Endoscopy Symposium: "Diagnosis of management of pancreatic disease." *Endoscopy* 1981; 13:51.
11. Delhaye M, Engelholm L, Cremer M: Pancreas divisum: Congenital anatomic variant or anomaly? *Gastroenterology* 1985; 89:951-958.
12. Mitchell CJ, Lintott DJ, Ruddell WS, et al: Clinical relevance of an unfused pancreatic duct system. *Gut* 1979; 20:1066-1071.
13. Warshaw AL, Simeone J, Schapiro RH, et al: Objective evaluation of ampullary stenosis with ultrasonography and pancreatic stimulation. *Am J Surg* 1985; 149:65-72.
14. Bolondi L, Gaiani S, Gullo L, et al: Secretin administration induces a dilatation of main pancreatic duct. *Dig Dis Sci* 1984; 29:802-808.
15. Cotton PB: Pancrease divisum—curiosity or culprit? *Gastroenterology* 1985; 89(6):1431-1435.
16. Staritz M: Intraductal pressure measurements in

pancreas divisum. Presented at Cleveland Clinic Meeting, March 1987.
17. Keith RG, Shapero TF, Saibil FG: Treatment of pancreatitis associated with pancreas divisum by dorsal duct sphincterotomy alone. *J Surg* 1982; 25(6):622–626.
18. Seigel JH, Pullano M, Cooperman A: Endoscopic therapy for acquired pancreatitis: An effective long term treatment modality. 5 year follow-up (abstract) *Am J Gastroenterol* 1987; 82:973.
19. Knapp AB, Zimmon DS: Endoscopic stents as diagnostic aids in patients with pancreatitis secondary to pancreas divisum (abstract). *Gastrointest Endosc* 1986; 32(2):159.
20. Geenen JE: Endoscopic therapy in select types of pancreatic disease. Presented at St. Luke's Hospital, Racine, WI, October 1987.
21. Cotton PB: Endoscopic cannulation and sphincterotomy at the accessory papilla in pancreas divisum. *Gastrointest Endosc* 1979; 25(1):37.
22. Soehendra N, Kempeneers I, Nam V CH, et al: Endoscopic dilation and papillotomy of the accessory papilla and internal drainage in pancreas divisum. *Endoscopy* 1986; 18:129–132.
23. Sahel J, Sarles H: Treatment of pancreatic pain and pancreatitis due to pancreas divisum (abstract). *Gastroenterology* 1983; 84:1292.
24. Madura JA, Fiore AC, O'Connor KW: Pancreas divisum detection and management. *Am Surg* 1985; 51(7):353–357.
25. Gregg JA, Monaco AP, McDermott WV: Pancreas divisum results of surgical intervention. *Am J Surg* 1983; 145:488–492.
26. Gregg J, Solomon J, Clark G: Pancreas divisum and its association with choledochal sphincter stenosis. *Am J Surg* 1984; 147:367–371.
27. Blair AJ, Russell CG, Cotton PB: Resection for pancreatitis in patients with pancreas divisum. *Ann Surg* 1984; 200(5):590–594.

17

Pancreatic Cancer: What is a reasonable approach?

MARTIN H. KALSER, M.D., PH.D.

An early aggressive approach by experienced gastroenterologists and surgeons to the diagnosis and therapy of exocrine pancreatic cancer is mandatory if the past dismal course of this disease is to be improved. This approach contrasts markedly with a widespread perception that any therapy, including surgery, of any pancreatic cancer is associated with poor results.[1] The implication, therefore, is that once the diagnosis is definite, treatment of such a lesion should be palliative. Yet resective surgery for early disease, in selective cases, can have a 20% 5-year survival rate in experienced medical centers.[2,3] The key factor is early clinical staging of the lesion with recognition of those cases that are potentially curable or amenable to therapy. In this chapter we will try to point out this type of approach.

INCIDENCE

Overall pancreatic exocrine cancer is the fifth most common cause of cancer death in the United States (the fourth most common in males and the sixth in females). In most Western countries, the overall incidence averages about 9.5 per hundred thousand population. The true incidence has increased in the past four to five decades about three- to fourfold.[4] This incidence, which is increasing, again argues for an aggressive and hopeful rather than a do-nothing and hopeless approach.

APPROACH

An approach with potential for successful outcome involves (1) a high degree of suspicion by the physician first seeing the patient with suggestive symptoms, (2) referral to a diagnostic center sophisticated in pancreatic maladies, (3) follow-up with a qualified pancreatic surgeon in selected cases, and (4) combined adjuvant therapy managed by an oncologist. It remains a truism that in a proportion of patients with pancreatic malignancy, therapy is not beneficial and can be associated with miserable side-effects. Distinguishing accurately which patients may be amenable to therapy can be done clinically almost on the initial visit if one understands the natural course of this disease. It is also imperative that management begin immediately. The key factor is the location of the malignancy in the pancreas and its proximity to the common duct.

CLASSIFICATION

Exocrine pancreatic cancer includes two distinct diseases, based on the location of the tumor. There is much difference in clinical presentation, treatment, and prognosis with each type. Lesions to the head of the pancreas, in general, present earlier and are more amenable to specific therapy. Lesions to the body and tail are entirely different in their presentation and

CANCER OF THE HEAD OF THE PANCREAS

Clinical Presentation

The presenting symptoms of head lesions are jaundice, abdominal pain, and weight loss.

Jaundice is the main symptoms of head lesions, occurring in about 60% to 70% of cases.[5] In the overwhelming majority, the jaundice is of the extrahepatic, obstructive type. It may be very insidious, with the patient only noting darkening of the urine or yellowness in the sclera. Pruritis is often an accompaniment and indeed may be the initial complaint. While 62% of patients with carcinoma of the head of the pancreas are jaundiced when first seen, the more selected subgroup are those who have painless jaundice (Table 17–1). In one large series, about three quarters of the successfully resected lesions were in patients presenting with painless jaundice.[5] Overall, about one third of patients with painless jaundice, due to carcinoma of the pancreas, can have a successful resection of the lesion. This is quite encouraging for pancreatic carcinoma, although it may not be as good as statistics for other types of gastrointestinal malignancies. Jaundice with pain is much more common, and, although resectable lesions may have painful jaundice, the overall resectability and potential for cure is much less in patients with cancer of the head of the pancreas and pain.

Overall, *pain* as a presenting symptom with an abdominal component is almost universal. Over 90% of patients have pain, either abdominal alone (45%) or abdominal with radiation to the back (45%). Only 8% to 10% have back pain alone (Table 17–2).

Weight loss of varying degees is also a very common symptom upon presentation. It is primarily the result of decreased caloric intake due to pain and jaundice. Occasionally malassimilation due to obstruction of the pancreatic duct with decreased intraduodenal pancreatic enzymes or prolonged hyperglycemia can be a contributing factor to the weight loss.

Laboratory

The complete blood count is most likely to be normal with anemia rarely occurring in advanced cases in which there may be some gastrointestinal blood loss secondary to invasion of the gastrointestinal duodenal mucosa from an expanding pancreatic neoplasm.

The major changes, however, are in the tests of hepatic function and disease with a cholestatic profile. There is elevation of the direct and total serum bilirubin, hepatic alkaline phosphatase, GGTP, 5-nucleotidase, and leucine aminopeptidase, and minimal elevation of the transaminases. In hepatic metastatic disease, jaun-

TABLE 17–1.
Incidence of Jaundice in Pancreatic Cancer Patients*

Site of Cancer	Patients Jaundiced (%)
Head of pancreas	62
Body and tail of pancreas	16
All cases	48

*Adapted from Kalser MH, Barkin J, MacIntyre JM: Pancreatic cancer. Assessment of prognosis by clinical presentation. *Cancer* 1985; 56:397–402.

TABLE 17–2.
Incidence of Pain in Pancreatic Cancer Patients*

Absent	21%
Present	79%
Abdominal alone	35%
Back alone	8%
Combined	36%

*Adapted from Kalser MH, Barkin J, MacIntyre JM: Pancreatic cancer. Assessment of prognosis by clinical presentation. *Cancer* 1985; 56:397–402.

dice is not commonly present, and the abnormalities are in the hepatic alkaline phosphatase and transaminases.

Carcinoembryonic antigen (CEA) can be elevated by jaundice, metastatic hepatic disease, and a large pancreatic tumor mass.[6] It has no value as an early diagnostic tool. Extrahepatic jaundice in itself can have an elevated CEA in the range of 10, which reverses when the biliary obstruction is surgically relieved. Values between 5 and 25 may be seen with a large primary mass or recurrent disease as well as minimal hepatic metastatic involvement. The various analogues of CEA have the same diagnostic significance without any specific advantage in diagnosis.

CANCER OF THE BODY AND TAIL OF THE PANCREAS

Pancreatic exocrine malignancy in the body and tail of the pancreas is truly the helpless situation commonly associated with all pancreatic carcinomas. The relative good news is that only one third of all pancreatic exocrine cancers are in this location. The guarded prognosis results from the fact that the lesion is much larger by the time it is diagnosed as compared to lesions adjacent to the common duct. The medium area of these lesions when diagnosed has been reported to be 30 cm^2 representing a 6 × 5 cm mass. Because the location is removed from the common duct, jaundice is unusual and is certainly not an early symptom or sign such as seen in early lesions of the head of the pancreas. Pain and weight loss are the major presenting complaints in patients with carcinoma of the body or tail.[5]

Clinical Presentation

Jaundice occurs as a presenting symptom only in one sixth (16%) of carcinomas of the body or tail as opposed to two thirds (67%) of head lesions (i.e., four times as frequent a finding in head lesions). Rarely is the jaundice painless. Hepatic and biliary involvement in these cases is most often the result of metastases or a large mass pressing on the porta hepaticus.

Pain, as in lesions of the head of the pancreas, has an abdominal component in four of five cases. In half of these, the abdominal pain radiates to the back. Back pain alone without an abdominal component is unusual and occurs in less than 10%.

Weight loss is usually quite marked.

Patients aged sixty and older, presenting predominantly with abdominal and/or back pain, anorexia, and weight loss, must be evaluated for possible cancer of the body or tail of the pancreas.

Other presentations can occur, but these are extremely unusual. These include acute cholecystitis, acute pancreatitis, acute gastrointestinal hemorrhage, thromboembolic phenomenon, spinal back pain, and polyarthritis. Depression is not too rare as a secondary symptom. Primary depression may also be associated with anorexia, weight loss, and functional abdominal pain. This clinical presentation may be very similar to carcinoma of the distal pancreas. A thorough work-up is needed to rule out pancreatic mitosis in these patients.

Physical examination is minimally contributory, unless there is widespread hepatic metastasis, in which case the palpable liver with hard nodules readily gives the diagnosis. Otherwise, a palpable mass in the epigastrium, representing the tumor, is not commonly perceived. Splenomegaly resulting from involvement and thromobosis of the splenetic vein is also unusual.

Laboratory Findings

Laboratory findings are primarily the result of hepatic involvement resulting in these cases from metastatic disease, or direct invasion of the porta hepaticus by the tumor. The serum bilirubin is minimally, if at all, elevated. However, the alkaline phosphatase and transaminases are abnormal, primarily due to hepatic metastatic involvement or involvement of the porta hepaticus. The serum pancreatic enzymes, amylase and lipase, are most often normal and do not add anything to the diagnosis. Similarly urinary amylase and amylase clearance do not help. The CEA is more likely to be elevated because of the hepatic metastases or the large size of the tumor.[6] The diagnostic interpretation is the same as that described for lesions located in the head of the pancreas, namely that values above 25 are indicative of hepatic metastasis.

DIAGNOSIS

Imaging

CT and ERCP are the primary proven diagnostic tools. Ultrasound (US) of the pancreas and magnetic resonance imaging (MRI) at some institutions may be of similar value. The value of noninvasive imaging will vary depending on the expertise of the staff of each individual institution. While US and CT have been reported to have similar accuracy in the diagnosis of pancreatic disease,[7] CT although a bit more costly, is the better diagnostic tool in this situation. The relative disadvantages of US are that the body and tail are not always adequately visualized and that gastrointestinal gas may interfere with the image, necessitating repeating the examinations. CT, using oral and intravenous contrast, affords state-of-the-art imaging of the total pancreas. CT also has the capability of demonstrating small hepatic metastasis. MRI does not offer any advantages over CT. Other noninvasive imaging techniques, such as biliary scintography or liver spleen scan, are not of any value. Similarly various studies of the hollow gut are useless when this entity is suspect. With imaging of the pancreas, the most definitive finding is that of a discrete, definable mass. However, enlargement of one part or all of the gland may be suspicious for a tumor. Normally on CT the head of the pancreas is 3 cm in diameter, body is 2.5 cm, and the tail is 2 cm. Increased diameter with clinical suspicion warrants further studies, particularly ERCP.

ERCP is the most definitive, nonoperative diagnostic procedure available. Again, this requires an experienced endoscopist and a radiologist experienced in pancreatic disease. Even in the best of hands, however, the pancreatic duct may not be visualized in 15% of the patients. Visualization of the common duct is also of value in determining if it is dilated. The characteristic finding on ERCP is a "cut off" sign in which the pancreatic duct does not fill beyond the lesion.

Percutaneous Pancreatic Aspiration Cystology

In this procedure, a thin needle is passed through the anterior abdominal wall under CT or US guidance into a mass in the pancreas. The mass is then aspirated, and the aspirate is evaluated cytologically for malignant cells.

This technique is reserved for inoperable cases in which resection is deemed impossible because of the size of the lesion or a metastatic disease and in which bypass surgery, either biliary or duodenal, is not indicated.

Laparotomy

Exploratory abdominal laparotomy for the diagnosis of pancreatic neoplasm is rarely, if ever, needed and should only be attempted in a very isolated situation. An added diagnostic difficulty with this procedure is that with the exposure of a pancreatic mass at laparotomy, biopsy of a suspicious area may not show malignancy, even if the mass is malignant. This is because a biopsy may show only the chronic inflammation that surrounds the malignancy and not the tumor. The ultimate diagnosis is by examination of the pancreatic tumor by serial section after its removal. The one situation in which exploratory laparotomy for pancreatic cancer sometimes occurs is when there is difficulty in distinguishing an enlarged pancreas with chronic pancreatitis from one with a malignancy. This occurs when a patient has known chronic pancreatitis and develops a persistent deteriorating course and the diagnostic approach as mentioned above is inconclusive. Pancreatic resection in such a case, on occasion, may be necessary with a definitive diagnosis established only on pathologic examination of the resected specimen.

STAGING

Definition

Pretreatment staging allows selection of cases that can be predicted with a fair degree of accuracy to respond to therapy and allow selection of potential successful treatment.[5]

There are three stages:
Stage I is probably resectable disease
Stage II is nonresectable but localized nonmetastatic disease.
Stage III is widespread disease.
Stage I should be considered as potentially curable; stage II responds to therapy; stage III, at the present time, does not respond to any specific therapy.

Stage I

The main finding in stage I is the relatively small lesion (9 cm^2) in the head of the pancreas on preoperative screening without evidence of metastases. The most suggestive clinical presentation is painless jaundice, although abdominal pain with jaundice and characteristic imaging findings still warrant classification as stage I. It can not be emphasized too strongly that this is a potentially resectable and curable lesion in this stage. While stage I is at present reserved for lesions of the head of the pancreas, with early diagnosis small masses of the body and or tail may eventually also be classified as stage I.

Stage II

Stage II includes a larger lesion (16 cm^2 or greater) without liver metastasis on imaging, CT, US, or MRI. These are locally unresectable lesions overwhelmingly located in the head of the pancreas. The most frequent clinical presentation is jaundice with abdominal pain that radiates to the back in about half of the cases. Survival in these patients is improved with radiation and/or chemotherapy.

Stage III

Stage III describes a hopeless disease that doesn't respond to any known treatment. Imaging techniques show metastatic disease and a large tumor. In one large series the medium area was 30 cm^2. These are mostly located in the body and/or tail.

Performance Status

Performance status is defined by the Eastern Cooperative Oncological Group (ECOG) helps predict the response to therapy and general prognosis. The ECOG performance criteria are:

0 = fully ambulatory and symptom free
1 = fully ambulatory but with symptoms
2 = confined to bed less than 50% of the day
3 = confined to bed more than 50% of the day
4 = confined to bed all of the time

Prognosis and survival vary directly with the performance status within each stage and with each treatment. Thus, patients in stage III disease who have ECOG performance status of 0 or 1 do much better and live longer than those who initially are status 2 or 3. Similarly with stages I and II with therapy, the better the performance status, the better the prognosis and survival.

TREATMENT

Surgical Resection

Surgical resection is the most desirable treatment. When the preoperative and initial surgical evaluation discloses a lesion under 16 cm^2 (preferably 9 cm^2) without metastatic disease, the surgeon should be prepared to mobilize the head of the pancreas and resect. Surgeons who do not have experience and expertise in pancreatic surgery *should not attempt* the initial abdominal exploration in these patients. Because the overwhelming number of lesions are in the head, a Whipple's type resection, leaving part of the body and tail of the pancreas, is the procedure of choice. The patient is not left with an insulin-dependent diabetes. At one time total pancreatectomy was advocated in the belief that there were microscopic nests of malignancy throughout the gland. However, it has been adequately demonstrated that survival is not increased with total pancreatectomy.[8] Patients with cancer cells in the margin of the resective gland have less chance of survival than those in whom the margin and lymphatics are free of disease.[2]

Surgical Bypass

Biliary bypass is the more common procedure because of obstructive jaundice, although duodenal bypass for intraduodenal luminal obstruction may also be necessary. For bilary bypass without resection of the pancreas, a choledocho rather than a cholecysto bypass to the gut lumen is preferred, being more dependable albeit more difficult to do. However, only the most adept surgeons should attempt surgery of the pancreas. A gastrojejunostomy with bypass of the duodenum is mandatory if the patient has symptoms of gastric outlet obstruction with impaired gastric emptying, nausea, or vomiting. In fact, combined bypass of both the distal common duct and duodenum has been advocated when there is obstruction of one or the other. The present evidence is that bypass surgery in jaundiced patients does prolong life and should be done when indicated.

Combined Radiation and Chemotherapy[9,10]

Combined radiation and chemotherapy is the nonsurgical treatment. Radiation or any chemotherapeutic agent alone is not as effective as the combined approach. Radiation is given to the maximum dose of 6000 rads in a fractionated course. The details are left to the radiation therapist. Both 5-fluorouracil and Adriamycin have been used in conjunction with radiation therapy. Chemotherapy agents are constantly undergoing protocol evaluation, therefore the exact details of administration of these agents are best left to the medical oncologist.

Indications for the use of combined therapy are (1) as adjuvant therapy following resection of the tumor and (2) in patients with localized nonmetastatic disease. Survival and perhaps the cure rate are improved when adjuvant therapy is given to patients who have attempted curative resection of the pancreas. Survival is also prolonged as compared to controls with combined radiation and chemotherapy in patients with stage II localized nonmetastatic disease. Are the side effects of therapy with the relatively limited prolongation of life worth giving the therapy? Side effects vary greatly from patient to patient, and only the patient and his physician can determine if combined therapy should be continued.

PROGNOSIS AND SURVIVAL

The overall prognosis is poor, and survival is limited as compared to malignancies of the hollow gut. Yet survival and indeed the number of 5-year cures are significant in patients who have resection of an early carcinoma of the head of pancreas.

Survival in the natural history of pancreatic cancer is directly related to the stage of the disease, although overall median survival is discouraging at present. Medium survival of stage I patients was reported to be 73 weeks; for stage II patients it was 33 weeks; and for stage III patients it was only 10 weeks. These figures, particularly for stage III, are discouraging.[5]

Treatment can influence survival. In stage I patients, adjuvant combined radiation and chemotherapy significantly prolonged survival after resection of the tumor, as compared to those not receiving this therapy. Five-year survival in this group was reported to be 20% in the resected and adjuvant treated patients.[3] Although the number of cases was very small, 5-year survival was projected to approach 50% in those in whom the malignant changes histologically were confined completely to the pancreas. Combined radiation (4000 or 6000 rads) and chemotherapy (5-FU) were found to prolong survival to a significantly greater degree than radiation therapy alone.[9]

CONCLUSIONS

Exocrine pancreatic cancer remains a very recalcitrant disease: The incidence is progressively increasing and there is a dismal prognosis compared to other malignancies of the gut. An enlightened aggressive approach can offer prolongation of life and even cure to selected patients with this disease. Success is dependent on early suspicion and the involvement of sophisticated and experienced diagnosticians, surgeons, and oncologists immediately after a patient presents with suggestive symptoms. Unfortunately, community hospitals do not have the expertise, and referral to an appropriate pancreatic center is mandatory if we are to have success in the treatment of at least some of these cases. The middle-age patient, presenting with obstructive jaundice, particularly if it is painless jaundice, should initiate the appropriate chain of events. With very early diagnosis, resective surgery, and combined radiation and chemotherapy, the survival rate for this disease can be significantly improved.

References

1. Herman RE, Cooperman AM: Current concepts in cancer: Cancer of the pancreas. *N Engl J Med* 1979; 301:482–485.
2. Kalser MH, Ellenberg SS: Pancreatic cancer adjuvant combined radiation and chemotherapy following curative resection. *Arch Surg* 1985; 120:899–903.
3. Douglass HO Jr, Stablein DM, Kalser MH, et al: *Confirmation by the Gastrointestinal Tumor Study Groups that Survival Following Potentially Curative Resection of Pancreatic Cancer is Improved by Multidisciplinary Post Operative Therapy in Adjuvant Therapy of Cancer V.* New York, Grune & Stratton, 1987.
4. Silverberg E: Cancer statistics. *Cancer* 1980; 80:23–44.
5. Kalser MH, Barkin J, MacIntyre JM: Pancreatic cancer. Assessment of prognosis by clinical presentation, *Cancer* 1985; 56:397–402.
6. Kalser MH, Barkin J, Redlhammer D, et al: Circulatory carcinoembryonic antigen in pancreatic carcinoma. *Cancer* 1978; 42:1468–1471.
7. Barkin J, Vining D, Miale A Jr, et al: Computerized tomography, diagnostic ultrasound and radionuclide scanning. Comparison of efficacy in pancreatic cancer. *JAMA* 1977; 238:2040–2042.
8. Edis, AJ, Kiernon PD, Taylor WR: Attempted curative resection of ductal carcinoma of the pancreas. *Mayo Clin Proc* 1980; 55:532–536.
9. Moertel CG, Frytal S, Hahn RG, et al: Therapy of locally unresectable pancreatic carcinoma. *Cancer* 1981; 48:1705–1710.
10. Gastrointestinal Tumor Study Group: Therapy of locally unresectable carcinoma of the pancreas. Comparison of combined modality therapy (chemotherapy plus radiotherapy) to chemotherapy alone. In manuscript.

IV

Liver

18

Intractable Ascites:
What should be done?

JOHN T. GALAMBOS, M.D.

The patient with intractable ascites should be differentiated from the intractable patient with ascites. The former is a patient with cirrhosis whose ascites cannot be diuresed by standard diuretic therapy and limited sodium intake and who does not have chylous, malignant, or infected ascites. In contrast, the intractable patient with ascites is the one who cannot be managed outside the hospital, but who can be diuresed in the hospital with some form of diuretic therapy, bed rest, and limited sodium intake. Intractable ascites in a cirrhotic patient is the manifestation of the late stages of chronic liver disease and hepatic failure.

Excessive sodium retention is the primary problem of the early stage of ascites. In its later stages, avid renal sodium retention is accompanied by vasomotor changes characterized by decreased systemic vascular resistance, rising cardiac output, and decreasing "effectiveness" of the rising circulating plasma volume. As a rule, patients with intractable ascites have impaired renal function, decreased renal blood flow, and renal cortical ischemia as the decreased renal blood flow is shunted toward the inner cortex and medulla. This deprives the long cortical nephrons of effective glomerular filtration. These cortical nephrons are the most efficient ones to excrete sodium chloride.

It is useful to differentiate functional renal failure (which usually is reversible) and hepatorenal syndrome (which is not). Functional renal failure is characterized at first by increased but "normal" serum creatinine. However, normal values are normal in normal people. A "normal" BUN or creatinine may be abnormal in malnourished cirrhotic patients with decreased lean body mass (manifested by decreased 24-hour urine creatinine/height ratio) and poor protein intake. Functional renal failure occasionally develops gradually and spontaneously as part of the natural history of cirrhosis, or it may be precipitated. The treatment, therefore, depends on the cause. The precipitating causes include diuretic therapy, paracentesis, systemic infection, asymptomatic bacterial peritonitis, hemorrhage, and other severe systemic events such as heart failure, trauma, and so forth. Standard diuretic therapy can accelerate functional renal failure, which can progress to an irreversible, terminal stage of hepatic and renal failure. The hepatorenal syndrome has no clinical, laboratory, physiologic, or pathologic explanation and has no known therapy. A clinically important point is that a reversible functional renal failure can rapidly progress to the irreversible hepatorenal failure.

A good understanding of the mechanisms that contribute to changes of systemic and renal hemodynamics and renal failure helps the physician devise a strategy to improve renal (and hepatic) function and to alleviate ascites in these patients. The control mechanism of renal hemodynamics and function in cirrhosis is complex and is affected both by physiologic compensatory responses and by the various "therapeutic" measures. Certain generalizations can be made.

PATHOPHYSIOLOGY

Increased sympathetic activity is suggested by elevated *norepinephrine* plasma concentration in cirrhotic ascitic patients. The elevated norepinephrine levels have a positive correlation with renin activity and aldosterone levels and a negative correlation with urinary sodium excretion.[1] Patients with cirrhosis who develop intractable ascites show a down-regulation of their beta$_2$ receptors.[2] The increased sympathetic activity of these ascitic patients is best explained by the perceived decrease of the effectiveness of the plasma volume. Transient increase of central blood volume by immersion in water produces natriuresis and diuresis, but does not suppress plasma norepinephrine.[3] Prolonged elevation of plasma volume by insertion of a LeVeen shunt returns plasma catecholamines to normal.[4]

Major changes in the *renin-angiotensin* system were described in patients with ascites and cirrhosis. This topic was recently reviewed.[5] In general, in patients with intractable ascites plasma renin activity is increased while renin substrate is decreased. However, the degree of changes in this system is variable. Indeed, even in the same patient under apparently similar clinical conditions renin levels may vary. On the other hand, I observed similar abnormalities of plasma renin activity in different clinical conditions in ascitic cirrhotic patients (i.e., high renin activity was seen in both "intractable" and "responsive" ascites). Another problem in the interpretation of peripheral plasma renin activity is that intracellular renin can produce angiotensin I, and angiotensin II may also act within the cell.

The only natural substrate of renin is angiotensinogen, which is synthesized and secreted by hepatocytes. In a regional vascular bed, renin generates 80% to 90% of angiotensin I, which is hydrolyzed by its converting enzyme to the active angiotensin II, which in turn has to bind to its specific receptor to effect vascular caliber.[6]

The octapeptide of angiotensin II is the active hormone of the renin-angiotensin system. It affects the kidney, the adrenals, and a variety of other organs.[7] In the kidney its primary effect is vasoconstriction, which explains a decrease of renal blood flow and glomerular filtration rate. The predominance of efferent arteriolar constriction causes an increase of filtration fraction. The preferential efferent arteriolar vasoconstriction is probably due to a preferential afferent arteriolar vasodilating effect of certain renal prostaglandins.[8] Angiotensin II also increases proximal tubular sodium reabsorption and exerts a negative feedback effect on renin secretion.

Angiotensin II and potassium are potent stimuli of *aldosterone* production both in vitro and in vivo. Potassium is a specific stimulus to the zona glomerular. Indeed, aldosterone biosynthesis is affected at multiple loci by potassium status. Other stimuli are ACTH and serotonin.[9] From a clinical point of view it is important to remember that potassium administration increases the rate of aldosterone synthesis and secretion to a degree similar to that of the renin-angiotensin system.[10]

Aldosterone secretion is under maximum dopaminergic inhibition, which can be overridden by angiotensin II and potassium. Metoclopramide, a dopamine antagonist, significantly increases plasma aldosterone concentrations in standard therapeutic doses as it antagonizes dopamine inhibition of aldosterone secretion directly at the cellular level.[11,12]

Aldosterone acts in the distal nephron. It causes sodium retention and potassium excretion in normal humans. The former effect may be "escaped," but the latter continues regardless of the presence or absence of sodium retention. Aldosterone also promotes H$^+$ secretion and can cause alkalosis.

Hyperaldosteronism is common in cirrhosis with ascites. Changes of aldosterone concentrations induced by altering plasma volume are mediated by the renin-angiotensin system.[13] Although it is usually assumed that plasma concentration of aldosterone is correlated with the presence and severity of ascites, it does not parallel the clinical status of cirrhotic patients. This problem is compounded by recent observations that not only aldosterone itself but its metabolites within the kidney may regulate receptor-mediated sodium transport.[14] Another confounding variable is the suggested increase of renal tubular sensitivity to aldosterone in cirrhosis. At any rate, hyperaldosteronism is not essential for the maintenance of ascites but seems to play a role in its accumulation.[15]

Atrial natriuretic factor (ANF), a peptide hormone, can induce diuresis, natriuresis, and relaxation of vascular smooth muscle. Its role in water and sodium retention in cirrhosis is not clear. The relationship between immunoreactivity and biologic activity is not established. The reported observations on ANF and ascites in cirrhosis are not in general agreement. Whether sodium intake, potassium intake, physical activity, or drugs affect plasma ANF levels and can explain the discrepancies in the published observations is not clear.[16] ANF, like renin and aldosterone, responds rapidly to changes of plasma volume.[17]

The precise role of *prostaglandin (PG)* on renal function in ascitic cirrhotic patients is not known. The best explanation of available observations is that PGs have little if any effect as long as renal blood flow and function are normal. Vasodilator PGs are increased as a compensatory mechanism against potent vasoconstrictors such as vasopressin, angiotensin II, and norepinephrine. Increased renal PG production of the A, E, and I (prostacyclin) series exerts a protecting effect on renal blood flow and glomerular filtration and promotes natriuresis.[18,19] Conversely, the failure of this compensation is characterized by a decline of the vasodilating PGs and a rise of renal thromboxanes; this is seen as hepatorenal failure develops. There is no good evidence, however, that thromboxanes in the kidney play a role in the production of renal failure in cirrhosis.[19] Consistent with this hypothesis are the clinical observations that nonsteroidal anti-inflammatory drugs (NSAID) promote sodium retention and interfere with diuretic therapy of ascitic cirrhotic patients. The direct effect of PGs on renal tubular sodium transport is controversial.

Antidiuretic hormone (ADH) activity and *arginine vasopressin (AVP)* plasma concentrations are elevated in decompensated cirrhotic patients with ascites. One of the best explanations for this increase is nonosmotic stimulation of ADH release by a critical decrease of the "effective" blood volume.[20]

Unlike angiotensin II, a moderate pressor dose of vasopressin causes an increase of the ratio of systemic to renal vascular resistance and increases renal blood flow despite a decrease of cardiac output. This selective protection of renal vasomotor tone seems to be due to vasopressin-induced release of vasodilator PGs in the kidney.[21]

Water excretion is impaired in decompensated cirrhosis. This can lead to dilutional hyponatremia—a condition that can develop spontaneously but more frequently, is caused, by injudicious diuretic therapy. The inability of these patients to excrete a water load normally is the mechanism of hyponatremia. One of the most important reasons for the impaired water excretion is the marked decline of the proportion of the glomerular filtrate delivered to the distal nephron where free water can be generated. A contributing reason is the ADH-induced enhanced reabsorption of water in the most distant segments of the nephron. Both of these mechanisms lead to oliguria.

At this junction it is important to emphasize that patients with ascites and abnormal renal function also have hepatic insufficiency. It is easy to overlook changes in hepatic functional capacity, which are difficult to measure. Clinical measurements of hepatic function are not readily available for the physician in clinical practice. Indeed, even in sophisticated university hospitals these liver function tests are usually not available for the day-to-day management of patients. Clinically close monitoring of renal function and quantitating renal failure are possible because of technical reasons. Important as it is, the degree of renal failure should not obscure the fact that the major underlying problem is hepatic failure and that ascites is only a symptomatic manifestation of the metabolic and circulatory abnormalities caused by the liver disease. It is well known that cirrhotic patients with progressive renal failure have a worse prognosis than ascitic patients with stable or improving renal function. Indeed, plasma renin concentrations and urinary sodium excretions predicted the survival of nonazotemic cirrhotic patients.[22] However, the prognosis of cirrhotic patients with ascites is just as predictable when elevations of plasma bilirubin or prothrombin time instead of creatinine are considered. These sick cirrhotic patients with ascites do not die *because* of renal failure; they die *with* renal failure, *because* of hepatic failure. No one needs to die because of renal failure. Anephric patients can be effectively managed with peritoneal or hemodialysis. Cirrhotic patients cannot be kept alive with dialysis once hepatorenal syndrome develops. When the kidneys of these patients are transplanted to recipients with normal livers, reasonably good renal function and diuresis are demonstrated in most of the recipients.[23]

THERAPY

Therapy of *intractable ascites* may conflict with the therapy of a *patient with ascites*. Although the two cannot be rigidly separated, these are discussed separately. The usual emphasis on sodium restriction and drug therapy of ascites is easy to understand: it is easier to restrict intake and force diuresis than to improve nutrition and reverse hepatic failure.

Therapy of Ascites

Medical Therapy

Sodium Restriction. The more severe the sodium restriction, the more likely the patient will gradually lose ascites and the less likely that the extracellular fluid volume will increase. An ideal diet contains no more than 20 mEq of sodium a day. While this type of diet may be acceptable for well-nourished and affluent patients, most patients with cirrhosis and ascites are malnourished. A sodium-free diet is expensive and unpalatable. Because it has been shown that nutritional rehabilitation improves the effectiveness of diuretic therapy,[24] sodium restriction should be tempered with the provision of optimum protein, calorie, and trace nutrient intake. A practical compromise is a 2-gm sodium diet which enables the patient to consume a reasonably tasty and attractive diet without a surcharge for special sodium-free foods. Because anorexia is frequently associated with refractory ascites, a proportion of the 2 gm of sodium in the diet is not even consumed.

Fluid Restriction. Cirrhotic patients with intractable ascites usually have decreased serum osmolality (if they are not azotemic) and hyponatremia. The serum sodium usually is between 126 and 135 mEq/L. It seems that the "osmostat" in these patients is reset because these patients are asymptomatic despite substantial reduction of their plasma sodium concentrations. Increasing the sodium concentrations in the plasma by a few milliequivalents with severe fluid restriction provides no perceptible benefit to these patients; on the other hand, it inflicts a great deal of unnecessary discomfort. Worse than that, fluid restriction prevents patients whose anorexia prevents them from eating a nutritionally adequate diet, from consuming supplemental nutrition such as a liquid formula diet. The few exceptions are patients who are excessive water drinkers; in these patients fluid restriction is essential. In the majority of patients with hyponatremia, rigid fluid restriction is more likely to be punitive than beneficial.

Most of the patients with hyponatremia and ascites have normal or increased total body sodium, and the hyponatremia is due to excessive water retention. Mild-to-modest depressions of plasma osmolality and sodium concentrations are well tolerated, and treatment is not needed unless hyponatremia becomes severe (sodium < 125 mEq/L). Severe hyponatremia may be treated with restricted fluid intake. This, however, is slow to reverse the condition if it has a clear-cut beneficial effect at all. Another form of therapy in patients with intractable ascites is 30 to 90 gm of urea per day if the bilirubin is under 6 mg/dl and the BUN is low. This therapy was effective in a small group with or without water restriction and with or without diuretics.[25]

If the patient with intractable ascites has a creatinine clearance over 35 ml/min, I usually am successful in increasing the low serum sodium concentration with the rapid IV infusion of 50 gm of mannitol once or twice a day. This even permits continued IV hyperalimentation with 2 L of sodium-free solution in most but not all patients by reversing progressive hyponatremia.[26, 27]

If severe hyponatremia develops in an ascitic patient with more severe renal failure, it can be treated with paracentesis (see below).

Intravenous Therapy. If oral diuretics are ineffective or produce progressive azotemia, then IV diuretic therapy may be effective. This therapy can produce rapid diuresis without increasing BUN concentration. Indeed, it may reverse prerenal azotemia.

Exclusion criteria are: creatinine clearance less than 35 ml/min or an inability to tolerate sudden expansion of plasma volume (heart failure, recent variceal hemorrhage, and so forth).

To prevent excessive potassium loss, pretreatment with spironolactone to increase urinary Na/K > 1 is required. Otherwise, the patient is given 10 mg. of amiloride just before IV infusion starts. Then, 250 ml of 5% albumin is given IV at 180 ml/hr; than furosemide 40 mg is given IV; then 250 ml of 20% mannitol is infused at 300 ml/hr or faster. Electrolytes, BUN, creatinine and weight, as well as intake and output, are monitored. If the patient diureses but the BUN is rising, this usually is correctable by increasing albumin infusion to 500 ml. If the serum sodium is too low or decreases, this usually improves if 20% mannitol infusion is increased to 500 ml. If diuretic response is poor, it may improve if 10 mg of metolazone is given just before the albumin infusion and if the furosemide dose is increased.

Large-Volume Paracentesis. Paracentesis always removes ascites, although attempts to do a paracentesis are not always successful. The tap must not be made over the epigastric vessels, next to scars, or over skin vessels. In malnourished cirrhotic patients, a catheter tract often leaks ascites after the paracentesis is completed. Albeit unplanned, it may be helpful, nevertheless, and it should be considered in therapeutic logistics. A leak is more likely to develop and stops more slowly if the tap is over the "linea alba" and is less likely if the "safest" spot is used (i.e., two thirds of the distance from the umbilicus to the left iliac crest). If a post-paracentesis leak develops, I use an ileostomy bag and measure ascitic fluid leak. I have not encountered bacterial peritonitis more often after paracentesis with leaks than without a leak.

Large-volume paracentesis is safe if posttherapy reduction of plasma volume is prevented.[17, 28] The removal of "all" the ascitic fluid is just as safe and is more cost-effective than removing it piecemeal. If the patient has overt edema, then 5 to 6 L of ascites can be removed without deterioration of renal function even if no IV plasma is given. In nonedematous patients, 125 ml of 5% albumin or fresh plasma is given for each liter of ascites removed and can be infused as one unit every 6 hours. Daily BUN concentrations, weight, and careful observation of neck veins can be used as indices of adequacy or excessiveness of IV plasma therapy. Infusion of too much plasma or albumin accelerates the reaccumulation of ascites; too little increases BUN and flattens neck veins.

In the case of chylous ascites due to cirrhosis or abdominal surgery, repeated paracentesis accompanied by a 30-gm fat, 2-gm sodium diet usually is successful. Chylous ascites, like malignant ascites, cannot be diuresed.

The most rapid, efficient, and safe way to correct severe *hyponatremia* is a large-volume paracentesis, which eliminates the increases of total body sodium, followed by IV hypertonic NaCl to raise the reduced serum sodium concentration to half way toward normal. For example, in a 60 kg nonedematous patient (after paracentesis), the plasma sodium concentration is 118 mEq/L. The estimated total body water is 40 L. Because sodium and an anion are the major osmoles in the extracellular fluid (ECF), an increase of sodium concentration toward normal must be calculated in regard to total body water and not only ECF volume (estimated ECF = 14 L). To increase sodium plasma concentration halfway to normal (to 130 mEq/L), 480 mEq of sodium are needed. As a practical matter, 500 ml of 5% NaCl (431 mEq of sodium) can be infused at 60 ml (52 mEq sodium)/hr. During this period other IV fluids are discontinued, and oral fluid intake is restricted to the equivalent of the estimated insensible water loss and urine output. This therapy never induced a neurologic syndrome.[29]

If the patient has progressive *functional renal failure*, then paracentesis is accompanied by monitoring central venous pressure (CVP) or preferably by Swan-Ganz monitoring. "Renal" doses of dopamine (less than 5 µg/kg/min) are infused, and plasma volume is vigorously increased with fresh plasma (or 5% albumin) to a CVP of 17 to 20 ml saline, depending on the patient's tolerance. Pulmonary congestion is monitored by repeated auscultations of the chest, measures of pulmonary artery and capillary wedge pressures, and chest x-rays to detect and correct pulmonary edema if it develops.

Surgical Therapy

The insertion of one of the peritoneal venous shunts (PVS) theoretically is equivalent to a continuous paracentesis and ascitic fluid reinfusion-induced expansion of the plasma volume. The results are good if the patient does not become infected, does not have variceal hemorrhage, does not develop untoward side effects such as a reaction to ascitic fluid reinfusion, and if the mechanics continue to function well. Unfortunately, the benefits do not parallel the indications: The sicker the patient, the worse the outcome; the less the patient needs the device (i.e., the refactory patient), the better the outcome. In general, the duration of hospitalization is shorter and the interval between discharge and rehospitalization is longer in patients with a PVS than those on standard diuretic therapy. There is little if any difference in the survival rate; the mortality rate is high due to advanced liver disease in both surgically and medically treated cirrhotic patients with resistant ascites. Consequently, the outcome of intractable ascites depends mainly on the course of liver disease and only to a lesser degree on the complications of ascites or its therapy.

Therapy of the Patient with Intractable Ascites

Supportive Care

It is axiomatic that all treatable complications of cirrhosis and hepatic failure should be corrected as best one can. This is beyond the scope of my brief. Recognition and prednisolone therapy of aggressive chronic active hepatitis, at times even in hepatitis B with positive hepatitis Be antigen (HBeAg), can reverse the course of intractable ascites. Malnutrition is common in cirrhosis with intractable ascites. Hyperalimentation is beneficial in these patients. Enteral hyperalimentation is the most cost-effective method if the patient has very small or no esophageal varices.[24] The standard enteral feeding tube predictably caused variceal hemorrhage the second or third week of therapy (at times sooner) despite the use of the combination of the standard "antiulcer" agents. I consider esophageal varices a contraindication for prolonged nasogastric intubation.

Peripheral or central hyperalimentation is preferable in patients with varices in the esophagus. Peripheral hyperalimentation consists of a P-900[27, 30] solution, which provides 35 to 45 gm of amino acids and intralipid. The nutritional benefits are similar to that of central hyperalimentation (total parenteral nutrition—TPN) if the patient consumes over 700 calories in the diet.

Specific Therapy

Because the development of truly *intractable ascites* is the manifestation of an advanced stage of liver disease and carries a very poor prognosis for a useful life, the best "therapy" of these patients is liver transplant if the mechanism of the underlying liver disease cannot be corrected. Patients with nonalcoholic cirrhosis (particularly those with primary biliary cirrhosis or sclerosing cholangitis), hepatic vein occlusion, or cryptogenic cirrhosis (and probably also those with chronic active hepatitis), should be evaluated by a liver transplant team. Unnecessary delay of liver transplant may reduce the chance of survival of the perioperative period. Alcoholic cirrhosis can also be considered if prolonged abstinence can be documented and alcoholism can be considered "cured."

References

1. Bichet DG, Van Putten VJ, Schrier RW: Potential role of increased sympathetic activity in impaired sodium and water excretion in cirrhosis. *N Engl J Med* 1982; 307:1552–1557.
2. Gerbes AL, Remien J, Jüngst D, et al: Evidence for down-regulation of beta-2-adrenoceptors in cirrhotic patients with severe ascites. *Lancet* 1986; i: 1409–1411.
3. Epstein M, Larios O, Johnson G: Effects of water immersion on plasma catecholamines in decompensated cirrhosis. *Miner Electrolyte Metab* 1985; 11:25–34.
4. Blendis LM, Sole MJ, Lossing A, et al: The effect of peritoneovenous shunting (PVS) on blood and urinary catecholamines in hepatic ascites (abstract). *Hepatology* 1985; 5:960.
5. Navar LG, Rosivall L: Contribution of the renin-angiotensin system to the control of intrarenal hemodynamics (editorial review). *Kidney Int* 1984; 25:857–868.
6. Morris BJ: New possibilities for intracellular renin and inactive renin now that the structure of the human renin gene has been elucidated (editorial review). *Clin Sci* 1986; 71:345–355.
7. Reid IA: The renin-angiotensin system and body function. *Arch Intern Med* 1985; 145:1475–1479.
8. Heller J, Horáček V: Angiotensin II: Preferential efferent constriction? *Renal Physiol* 1986; 9:357–365.
9. Fraser R, Brown JJ, Lever AF, et al: Control of aldosterone secretion (editorial review). *Clin Sci* 1979; 56:389–399.
10. Fagard R, Cattaert A, Lijnen P, et al: Responses of the systemic circulation and of the renin-angiotensin-aldosterone system to ketanserin at rest and exercise in normal man. *Clin Sci* 1984; 66:17–25.
11. Carey RM, Thorner MO, Ortt EM: Effects of metoclopramide and bromocriptine on the renin-angiotensin-aldosterone system in man. Dopaminergic control of aldosterone. *J Clin Invest* 1979; 63:727–735.
12. Carey RM, Thorner MO, Ortt EM: Dopaminergic inhibition of metoclopramide-induced aldosterone secretion in man. Dissociation of responses to dopamine and bromocriptine. *J Clin Invest* 1980; 66:10–18.
13. Epstein M (ed): *The Kidney in Liver Disease*, ed 2. New York, Elsevier Biomedical, 1983.
14. Morris DJ: Further studies on aldosterone metabolism. *Ann Clin Lab Sci* 1986; 16:94–102.
15. Sellars L, Shore AC, Mott V, et al: The renin-angiotension-aldosterone system in decompensated cirrhosis: Its activity in relation to sodium balance. *Q J Med* 1985; 56:485–496.
16. Gerbes AL, Arendt RM, Paumgartner G: Atrial natriuretic factor. Possible implications in liver disease (editorial). *J Hepatol* 1987; 5:123–132.
17. Simon DM, McCain JR, Bonkovsky HL, et al: Effects of therapeutic paracentesis on systemic and hepatic hemodynamics and on renal and hormonal function. *Hepatology* 1987; 7:423–429.
18. Laffi G, La Villa G, Pinzani M, et al: Altered renal and platelet arachidonic acid metabolism in cirrhosis. *Gastroenterology* 1986; 90:274–282.
19. Rimola A, Ginés P, Arroyo V, et al: Urinary excretion of 6-keto-prostaglandin $F_1\alpha$, thromboxane B_2 and prostaglandin E_2 in cirrhosis with ascites. *J Hepatol* 1986; 3:111–117.
20. Bichet D, Szatalowicz V, Chaimovitz C, et al: Role of vasopressin in abnormal water excretion in cirrhotic patients. *Ann Intern Med* 1982; 96:413–417.
21. Yared A, Kon V, Ichikawa I: Mechanism of preservation of glomerular perfusion and filtration during acute extracellular fluid volume depletion. Importance of intrarenal vasopressin-prostaglandin interaction for protecting kidneys from constrictor action of vasopressin. *J Clin Invest* 1985; 75:1477–1487.
22. Arroyo V, Bosch J, Gaya-Beltrán J, et al: Plasma renin activity and urinary sodium excretion as prognostic indicators in nonazotemic cirrhosis with ascites. *Ann Intern Med* 1981; 94:198–201.
23. Koppel MH, Coburn JW, Mims MM, et al: Transplantation of cadaveric kidneys from patients with hepatorenal syndrome. Evidence for the functional nature of renal failure in advanced disease. *N Engl J Med* 1969; 280:1367–1371.
24. Smith J, Horowitz J, Henderson JM, et al: Enteral hyperalimentation in undernourished patients with cirrhosis and ascites. *Am J Clin Nutr* 1982; 35:56–72.

25. Decaux G, Mols P, Cauchie P, et al: Treatment of hyponatremic cirrhosis with ascites resistant to diuretics by urea. *Nephron* 1986; 44:337–343.
26. Galambos JT, Hersh T, Fulenwider JT, et al: Hyperalimentation in alcoholic hepatitis. *Am J Gastroenterol* 1979; 72:535–541.
27. Nasrallah SM, Galambos JT: Aminoacid therapy of alcoholic hepatitis. *Lancet* 1980; ii:1276–1277.
28. Ginés P, Arroyo V, Quintero E, et al: Comparison of paracentesis and diuretics in the treatment of cirrhotics with tense ascites. Results of a randomized study. *Gastroenterology* 1987; 93:234–241.
29. Sterns RH, Riggs JE, Schochet SS Jr: Osmotic demyelination syndrome following correction of hyponatremia. *N Engl J Med* 1986; 314:1535–1542.
30. Isaacs J, Millikan W, Stackhouse J, et al: Parenteral nutrition of adults with a 900 milliosmolar solution via peripheral veins. *Am J Nutr* 1977; 30:552–559.

19

Transplantation: Who? When? Where?

DAVID H. VAN THIEL, M.D.

Liver transplantation has proven to be clinically useful and often life-saving in a variety of irreversible acute and chronic liver diseases for which no satisfactory medical therapy is available.[1-10] The initial application of liver transplantation in a clinical situation was reported by Starzl in 1963.[1] The gradual development of the surgical procedure and its application has been an outstanding example of the utilization of evolving biomedical advances in patients who otherwise have little or no hope of survival.

A major milestone in the development of liver transplantation was the introduction of cyclosporine A in 1974 as an immunosuppressant. An important subsequent surgical advance has been the addition of venous bypass during the anhepatic phase of the operation. This procedure reduces intraoperative bleeding, renal dysfunction, and the risk of postoperative infectious complications caused in part by portal hypertension and prolonged congestion and stasis in the splanchnic bed and lower extremities.[5,6,11,12] Additional improvements in the surgical procedure include use of portal vein grafts, development of alternative methods of arterialization of the liver graft, and introduction of the intraoperative cell saver to reduce the blood transfusion requirement associated with the procedure.[13-15]

This work was supported in part by grants from: NIAAA AA 06601 and NIDDK AM 32556

In general, the results of liver transplantation have been best in children, in whom long-term survival of greater than 5 years may be as high as 85% to 90%. Results of liver transplantation in adults have been less favorable but nonetheless are still quite impressive, with long-term survival depending on many factors, including the patient's age, clinical status at the time of transplantation, and underlying diagnosis. Five-year survival rates in several series of adult patients range from 55% to 85%.[16,17] These results are particularly impressive when it is recalled that the alternative of medical therapy for these patients yields 1-year survival rates of only 0 to 30%.[1-10]

CANDIDACY FOR ORTHOTOPIC LIVER TRANSPLANTATION

The indications for which liver transplantation has been and continues to be performed have been expanding steadily since 1981 when the current era of improved survival, attributed in part to the introduction of cyclosporine and the team approach to liver transplantation, began.[1-10] The liver diseases for which orthotopic liver transplantation is indicated can best be grouped into four major categories: chronic advanced irreversible liver disease, hepatic malignancies, fulminant hepatic failure, and inborn errors of metabolism.

The decision to transplant patients with

chronic irreversible disease or fulminant hepatic failure is not particularly difficult. The survival without transplantation is usually less than 1 year.[1, 3, 4, 18-21] The major problem with the application of liver transplantation to patients with hepatic malignancy is tumor recurrence. The vast majority of such patients experience a recurrence within 1 to 4 years after successful transplantation.[22-24] Improvements in patient selection procedures, particularly the identification and management of extrahepatic disease, and the use of liver transplantation in combination with aggressive antitumor chemotherapy or biologic response modifiers may improve the long-term survival of patients transplanted for this indication.

The most exciting and rapidly expanding area of clinical liver transplantation is the application of liver transplantation to the problem of inborn errors of metabolism involving cell surface receptors, organelle dysfunction, or enzyme deficiencies. Many of the infants and children with these diseases lack histologically evident hepatic disease as demonstrated by standard microscopic evaluations of liver biopsy material and routinely used biochemical tests of liver injury and function.[25-35] The availability and success of liver transplantation in these patients are changing the approach to these unusual problems. For example, it would no longer be acceptable to subject a child with homozygous type II hyperlipoproteinemia to a brief life of progressive atherosclerotic disease, repeated myocardial infarction, coronary artery revascularization surgeries, and even heart transplantation to ameliorate a problem that liver transplantation reverses by providing low-density lipoprotein (LDL) receptors.[28, 35] The same logic applies to children with the Crigler-Najjar syndrome and to children with various urea cycle enzyme deficiencies.[32] Specifically, children with the Crigler-Najjar syndrome and urea cycle enzyme deficiencies identified before the development of irreversible neurologic impairment are cured by liver transplantation.[32-34] Similarly, children with glycogen storage diseases (particularly type I and IV), tyrosinemia, and protoporphyria need not suffer the inevitable and often irreversible consequences of their metabolic errors, because liver transplantation provides a cure.[26, 27, 30, 34] Based on the experience to date, one might reasonably argue that once the diagnosis of a fatal metabolic liver disease is established in a child, liver transplantation should be performed as soon as an appropriate donor organ can be identified.

Because the prognosis for an individual awaiting a liver transplantation varies considerably depending on the indication for the procedure as well as the severity of the disease and its associated complications at the time of transplantation, all individuals considered potential liver transplantation candidates should undergo a protocol evaluation. Such protocol evaluations serve five major goals:

1. Establishment of a specific, well-supported diagnosis
2. Documentation of the severity of the disease
3. Identification and possible preoperative modification of the complications of the disease that may adversely affect survival with or without transplantation
4. Estimation of the long-term prognosis of the patient with and without orthotopic liver transplantation in order to establish a realistic risk–benefit ratio
5. Development of a database at each transplantation center that allows for continual updating of statistics regarding survival and prognosis and that will allow for the comparison of results obtained among centers for individual diseases.

Once patients have been identified as potential candidates for liver transplantation, they should be carefully evaluated for the presence of specific indications to determine the optimal timing of the procedure. Broad indications for liver transplantation include hepatic failure, hepatic cancer that cannot be otherwise resected yet remains localized to the liver, metastatic neoplastic disease limited to the liver (rare), and metabolic liver disease for which no adequate therapy is currently

TABLE 19–1.
Indications for Orthotopic Liver Transplantation

I. Advanced chronic liver disease
    Predominantly cholestatic diseases
        Primary biliary cirrhosis
        Primary sclerosing cholangitis
        Biliary atresia
        Familial cholestatic syndromes
    Predominantly hepatocellular disease
        Chronic viral-induced liver disease
        Chronic drug-induced liver disease
        Alcoholic liver disease
        Idiopathic autoimmune liver disease
    Predominantly vascular disease
        Budd-Chiari syndrome
        Veno-occlusive disease
II. Hepatic malignancies that are not resectable
    Hepatocellular carcinoma
    Cholangiocarcinoma
    Rare nonhepatocellular or bile ductular tumors that arise within the hepatic parenchyma
    Isolated hepatic metastatic disease
        Carcinoid
        Pancreatic islet cell tumor
        Others
III. Fulminant hepatic failure
    Viral hepatitis
        A, B, D, non-A, non-B, EBV, other
    Drug-induced liver disease
        Halothane
        Gold
        Disulfiram
        Acetaminophen
        Others
    Metabolic liver disease
        Wilson's disease
        Reye's syndrome
        Organic acidurias
IV. Metabolic liver disease
    Alpha$_1$-antitrypsin deficiency
    Wilson's disease
    Homozygous type II hyperlipoproteinemia
    Crigler-Najjar syndrome type I
    Erythropoietic protoporphyria
    Urea cycle deficiencies
    Glycogen storage diseases type I and IV
    Tyrosinemia
    Hemochromatosis

available (Table 19–1). The indications of hepatic failure used to identify appropriate candidates for the procedure from among a group of potential candidates are shown in Table 19–2. In general, these manifestations reflect advanced excretory, synthetic, or metabolic abnormalities of liver disease or advanced symptomatic liver disease that preclude the likelihood of either short-term (less than 6 months) or meaningful long-term survival.

After a candidate has been identified and evaluated for the presence of indications for liver transplantation, a careful screening evaluation should be performed to find any contraindications (Table 19–3). As might be expected, the list of *absolute* contraindications has progressively declined and the list of relative contraindications has expanded as liver transplantation has become more widely performed.

TABLE 19–2.
Clinical and Biochemical Indications for Liver Transplantation Candidacy

---

I. Acute liver failure
    Bilirubin   > 10–20 mg/dl and
    Prothrombin time   increasing
                            > 10 sec above control
                                and increasing
    Progressive encephalopathy of at least grade 3
II. Chronic liver disease
    A. Cholestatic liver disease
        Bilirubin > 10–15 mg/dl
        Intractable pruritus
        Intractable bone disease
    B. Hepatocellular liver disease
        Albumin < 2.5 gm/dl
        Hepatic encephalopathy
        Prothrombin time > 5 sec above control
    C. Factors common to both types of liver disease
        Hepatorenal syndrome
        Recurrent spontaneous bacterial peritonitis
        Intractable ascites
        Recurrent episodes of biliary sepsis
        Development of a hepatocellular carcinoma

Several problems have been deleted from the original listing of contraindications.[1, 2] These include the presence of advanced chronic renal disease, chronic alcoholism, portal vein thrombosis, and age greater than 60 years (in an individual with adequate cardiopulmonary function). Patients with chronic renal disease can be transplanted successfully if combined organ transplants (liver and kidney)

TABLE 19–3.
Contraindications for Liver Transplantation

Absolute contraindications
  Active sepsis outside the hepatobiliary tree
  Metastatic hepatobiliary malignancy
  Advanced cardiopulmonary disease
  AIDS
Relative contraindications
  Advanced chronic renal disease
  Age greater than 60 years
  Portal vein thrombosis
  Cholangiocarcinoma
  Hypoexemia with intrapulmonary right to left shunts
  HBgAg and HBeAg positivity
  Prior portacaval shunting procedure
  Prior complex hepatobiliary surgery
  HIV positivity without clinical AIDS

---

are performed.[36] Hepatorenal syndrome has been successfully reversed following liver transplantation.[37] Furthermore, patients with portal vein thrombosis have been successfully transplanted with thrombectomy and portal vein reconstruction.[38] Liver transplantation has been successfully performed in patients who have had previous splenorenal shunts.[39] The upper age limit of candidates for orthotopic liver transplantation has increased progressively from age 40 in 1981 to age 76 in a patient transplanted in Pittsburgh.[40]

As success with liver transplantation has increased, the management of patients with liver disease who might become candidates for liver transplantation has changed also, particularly in the area of surgical management of biliary disease and of portal hypertension. Prior abdominal surgery increases the technical difficulties experienced by the surgeon during the recipient hepatectomy phase of the liver transplant procedure.[1, 2, 17] The problems caused by prior abdominal surgery result primarily from the development of adhesion-associated neovascularity in an individual with portal hypertension. These adhesion-associated shunts lead to increased operative blood loss and greatly increased blood product consumption. Moreover, the surgical placement of biliary stents to achieve biliary drainage and bile duct reconstructive procedures often leads to adhesions and scarring, which will render subsequent biliary reconstruction difficult if liver transplantation is performed. While prior abdominal surgery does not preclude liver transplantation, a history of surgery may adversely affect the relative desirability of transplantation thereby influencing both the timing and likelihood of success.

As the success with liver transplantation exceeds the long-term survival of patients with portacaval shunts constructed because of variceal bleeding, the rationale for performing such shunting procedures needs to be reconsidered. Fortunately, coincident with the advent of liver transplantation, the increasing availability and success of variceal sclerotherapy have led to a major shift in the approach to varices away from surgery and toward nonsurgical means of controlling bleeding.[41-44]

An important consideration is the ability of the patient to comprehend the magnitude and implications of liver transplantation. The need for lifelong monitoring of immunosuppressant therapy must be understood and accepted. A pretransplantation psychiatric evaluation as well as provision of extensive educational material for the patient and family is often helpful.

DISEASE-SPECIFIC INDICATIONS FOR LIVER TRANSPLANTATION

Major results of the developing experience with liver transplantation have been the identification of several disease-specific indications for the procedure and attempts to develop even more specific indices regarding prognosis both before and following liver transplantation. The following is a compilation of some of the current disease-specific indications and prognostic factors in liver transplantation.

Primary Biliary Cirrhosis

Patients with primary biliary cirrhosis are considered especially good candidates for liver transplantation.[1-10, 45] The majority of these patients are middle-aged women with no evidence of other major organ failure. Indications for liver transplantation include progressive jaundice (bilirubin greater than 10 to 15 mg/dl), recurrent hemorrhage from esophagogastric varices, uncontrollable ascites, progressive osteodystrophy, intractable pruritus, malnutrition and wasting, and hepatic encephalopathy.

Progress has been made in identifying prognostic factors useful in deciding which patients with primary biliary cirrhosis are at increased risk of dying and are therefore potential candidates for liver transplantation.[46-49] For example, in one study of patients with primary biliary cirrhosis, five variables were identified as indicative of a poor prognosis: high serum bilirubin, increasing age, presence of cirrhosis, low serum albumin, and central lobular cholestasis on liver biopsy.[47]

The question whether primary biliary cirrhosis recurs in the allograft liver is an important yet unanswered one.[24, 45, 50-53] The histologic lesions of primary biliary cirrhosis and those of chronic hepatic allograft rejection and graft-versus-host disease involving the liver are quite similar. With careful evaluation of the histopathology, characteristics distinguishing between recurrent primary biliary cirrhosis and chronic rejection can often be identified (Table 19-4). Nonetheless, similarities in the pathologic appearances have suggested that primary biliary cirrhosis, like liver graft rejection, may result from a T-

TABLE 19-4.
Histologic Features that Distinguish Chronic Rejection from Recurrent Primary Biliary Cirrhosis

Primary-biliary-cirrhosis
  Portal infiltrate with lymphocytes
  Fibrosis with cirrhosis
  Granuloma
  Active periportal piecemeal necrosis
  No endothelialitis
  No arterial disease
Rejection
  Mixed portal inflammatory cells, eosinophils, lymphocytes, and polymorphonuclear cells
  No cirrhosis—but often fibrosis
  Active portal and hepatic vein endothelialitis
  Subendothelial foam cells often with arterial thrombosis
  Little or no periportal piecemeal necrosis
  No granuloma

cell-dependent immune-mediated liver disease in which the immune response is directed against the bile ducts.[54]

Primary Sclerosing Cholangitis

Patients with advanced liver disease from primary sclerosing cholangitis are generally excellent candidates for liver transplantation.[2, 55] Most of these patients are young men between the ages of 20 and 40 years, often with no other major organ disease except inflammatory bowel disease (usually ulcerative colitis).[56] Indications for liver transplantation for primary sclerosing cholangitis include progressive jaundice (bilirubin greater than 10 to 15 mg/dl), recurrent bleeding from esophagogastric varices, advanced ascites, progressive osteodystrophy, intractable pruritus, and hepatic encephalopathy.[2, 55] This listing is essentially identical to that outlined for patients with primary biliary cirrhosis. Patients with primary sclerosing cholangitis, however, are at risk of developing bile duct carcinoma and must be evaluated carefully for bile duct carcinoma prior to liver transplantation even though the presence of such a tumor often cannot be excluded preoperatively. In patients with primary sclerosing cholangitis and ulcerative colitis, the exclusion of occult colonic carcinoma is also mandatory prior to liver transplantation.

Consideration of operative risk must take into account any previous surgical procedures, such as placement of biliary stents, U tubes, Roux-en-Y choledochojejunostomy, or total colectomy for ulcerative colitis. Endoscopically placed bile duct stents have less effect on later liver transplantation, and when possible should be considered in patients with primary sclerosing cholangitis who are likely to become liver transplantation candidates in the future.

In the past, biliary tract surgery performed in attempts to establish drainage often resulted in relapsing biliary and/or hepatic sepsis. Not unexpectedly such sepsis adversely affects prognosis both before and after liver transplantation. Patients with primary sclerosing cholangitis who have had prior surgical procedures and resultant biliary sepsis before transplantation have only a 50% to 65% survival rate at 1 year as compared to a 1-year survival rate as high as 70% to 80% in those without prior surgical procedures.[55]

Previous colectomy and ileostomy do not preclude liver transplantation but increase the operative risk and may lead to major problems with abdominal contamination, particularly if the ileostomy site is high in the right upper quadrant and has to be relocated.

The issue of possible reoccurrence of primary sclerosing cholangitis in the transplanted biliary system remains unsettled. Radiologically demonstrated biliary tract findings identical to those of primary sclerosing cholangitis have been reported following liver transplantation. Most of these abnormalities result from operative damage to the bile duct or its arterial supply resulting in bile duct ischemia. Such bile duct lesions have been reported in liver transplantation recipients with and without prior primary sclerosing cholangitis and, therefore, cannot be assumed to represent recurrent disease per se.

Chronic Acute Hepatitis and Cirrhosis

Patients with idiopathic (autoimmune) chronic active hepatitis and cirrhosis and with signs of advanced hepatocellular failure, such as hypoalbuminemia (less than 2.5 gm/dl), intractable ascites, hypoprothrombinemia (greater than 5 seconds above control), bleeding from esophagogastric varices, and recurrent advanced grades of hepatic encephalopathy, are candidates for hepatic transplantation.[1-10]

Only a single case of recurrent chronic active hepatitis of the autoimmune type has been reported following liver transplantation.[57] Whether this case represents recurrent disease or an immune-mediated attack against the transplanted organ not related to the primary disease process remains uncertain.[24, 57]

The role of liver transplantation in patients with chronic hepatitis B, especially those who are HBeAg positive, is unclear.[58, 59] Recurrence of hepatitis B following transplantation has been reported in almost all such patients.[59] Whether patients who are HBsAg positive and have anti-HBe are more favorable candidates for liver transplantation is currently unknown.

Patients with chronic non-A, non-B hepatitis who have advanced cirrhosis with hepatic failure or bleeding from esophagogastric varices are candidates for liver transplantation.[60] Whether non-A, non-B hepatitis recurs in the transplanted liver remains to be established.[58]

Fulminant Hepatic Failure

Liver transplantation has been performed successfully for fulminant and subacute hepatic failure due to viral hepatitis, drug toxicity, and unknown causes (presumably non-A, non-B hepatitis).[61, 62] Most of these patients have been in stage 3 or stage 4 hepatic coma before liver transplantation, and most, if not all, have required respiratory support.

The prognosis for patients with fulminant hepatic failure is quite guarded and depends on the ability of the liver transplantation and ICU teams to keep the patient alive, identify an appropriate donor in sufficient time, and perform the transplantation procedure with minimal warning or preparation. Nonetheless, the survival figures for such cases in whom liver transplantation has been performed are quite encouraging. In one center, survival at 1 year was 55% as compared to 20% or less for those who did not survive to the time of transplantation or who were managed medically.[61, 62] The observation that patients with fulminant hepatitis B who undergo transplantation can recover without recurrent hepatitis B infection in the new organ has encouraged several groups to transplant more such patients.[58]

Patients with fulminant non-A, non-B hepatitis have been transplanted. However, unlike the situation with fulminant hepatitis B, several patients with putative non-A, non-B hepatitis have had an episode of recurrent acute hepatitis in the allograft 4 to 6 weeks following successful transplantation.[61] Despite the recurrent hepatitis, many patients with chronic non-A, non-B hepatitis who have been transplanted have survived without evidence of either progressive hepatic dysfunction or prolonged hepatitis.

Hepatic Vein Thrombosis (Budd-Chiari Syndrome)

Hepatic vein thrombosis (Budd-Chiari syndrome) may present as a rapidly evolving illness or develop gradually over several months.[63, 64] Hepatic vein thrombosis may develop without an apparent underlying cause or as a complication of an illness known to cause vascular thrombosis. It occurs predominantly in two separate age groups: young adult women with or without evidence of a myeloproliferative disease, and middle-aged adult males who frequently have no evidence of an underlying disorder.[63, 64] Young female patients have been transplanted successfully.[38] Such individuals require lifelong anticoagulation following successful liver transplantation. If there is evidence of a primary myeloproliferative disease, these patients should be treated for the underlying disorder.[65]

Wilson's Disease

Patients with fulminant hepatic failure or advanced cirrhosis from Wilson's disease should be considered for liver transplantation.[66, 67] The survival for patients with Wilson's disease and decompensated cirrhosis treated medically is generally quite unfavorable. As a result, Sternlieb has suggested that liver transplantation be considered in any patient with Wilson's disease in whom fulminant hepatocellular necrosis has occurred or in those in whom signs of hepatocellular decompensation develop despite 2 to 3 months of chelation therapy.[66]

Follow-up evaluation of patients who have undergone transplantation for Wilson's disease indicates excellent rehabilitation occurs, with a 5-year survival rate of 70%. Preliminary studies evaluating copper kinetics in such patients have suggested that, as in the case of homozygous type II hyperlipoproteinemia, liver transplantation reverses the basic defect which is an inadequate mechanism for the disposal of copper.

Alcohol-Induced Liver Disease

Whether to employ liver transplantation in patients with end-stage alcohol-induced disease has been an area of considerable concern and controversy.[68] Major reasons for reluctance in proceeding to liver transplantation have included concern the alcoholic patient will resume excessive alcohol use following transplantation and the rather poor results in the few patients with alcoholic liver disease thus far transplanted—approximately a 20% 1-year survival.[16] My approach has been to consider patients for transplantation who have a proven record of abstinence (6 months or more) and evidence of irreversible liver disease. As part of the preoperative evaluation, these patients are carefully investigated for evidence of other alcohol-related disorders, such as infection, chronic pancreatitis, cardiomegaly, and neurologic deficits. In no contraindications are found and the patient is an otherwise suitable candidate, transplantation appears appropriate.

Pediatric Liver Diseases

Biliary Atresia

On average, 25% of the estimated 300 children who would benefit from a liver transplant yearly in the United States[69] die while waiting for a suitable donor.[70, 71] This fact is not entirely due to a lack of potential donor organs. Patients with extrahepatic biliary atresia account for more than half the children who have undergone liver transplantation worldwide.[69–73] This disorder is characterized by discontinuity of bile drainage from the liver to the duodenum because of partial or complete absence of extrahepatic bile ducts. The incidence of the disorder varies among different ethnic groups from 0.6 to 1/10,000 live births. In the past, less than 5% of infants with biliary atresia survived beyond 2 years. A marked change in the prognosis occurred after the introduction of the Kasai procedure (hepatic portoenterostomy) in 1959. Bile flow is reestablished in 40% to 80% of cases. This variation depends on a number of factors such as patient age (results have been better when the child operated on is 1 to 2 months of age) and the surgeon's skill and experience. The 5-year survival with a normal bilirubin is 33%. However, many, if not all, patients develop cirrhosis with portal hypertension by the age of 5 years[71, 73] and the remaining two/thirds of children exhibit relentless progressive cholestasis and eventually terminal liver failure.

Most patients who have had liver transplantation have had one or more failed Kasai procedures and are between 2 and 4 years of age at the time of transplantation. Because of the difficulties in obtaining adequate numbers of *pediatric* livers suitable for transplantation, particularly livers which would be appropriate for very small children, it is currently accepted practice for children with extrahepatic biliary atresia to undergo at least one attempt at operative biliary drainage (Kasai procedure) before proceeding to liver transplantation. Whether a second attempt should be made in the case of a failed first Kasai procedure is controversial. Such drainage procedures may be at least temporarily effective in slowing the progression of the disease and allow a very small child with liver disease to grow, thereby expanding the pool of potential donor organs available. Current data also suggest that liver transplantation in a child with a failed Kasai procedure is no more difficult or costly in terms of survival, blood usage, and operating time than such an operation in a child without previous abdominal surgery.[74]

Paucity of Interlobular Bile Ducts

In most large series of children with a paucity of interlobular bile ducts, the majority have had the syndromic form, arteriohepatic dysplasia or Alagille's syndrome, which is characterized by chronic cholestasis (91%), characteristic facies (95%), cardiovascular abnormalities (85%), vertebral anomalies (81%), and posterior embryotoxon (88%). Only 5% of these children with the syndromic form are reported to die from causes directly attributable to liver disease; however, recurrent episodes of cholestasis are quite common. The major indications for liver transplantation in these children are pruritus, bone disease, the complications of portal hypertension, and hepatocellular carcinoma.[75] The major contraindication to liver transplantation in these children is the cardiovascular abnormalities found in about 12% of these children.

In addition to the syndrome of interlobular bile duct deficiency, there are several different familial cholestatic syndromes. These disorders represent a diverse and ill-defined group of autosomal recessive cholestatic diseases. Affected children usually present with cholestasis and a variable deterioration of synthetic liver function. Instead of having markedly elevated levels of gamma-glutamyl transpeptidase and cholesterol, the majority of these children have normal or low levels of this enzyme.

Alpha$_1$-Antitrypsin Deficiency

Alpha$_1$-antitrypsin is a potent protease inhibitor (Pi) produced primarily in the liver.[76] The severe deficiency state (phenotype PiZZ) was first noted to be associated with neonatal cholestasis and chronic liver disease in 1969.[77, 78] PiZZ deficiency is found in 0.02% to 0.06% of newborns, with many of these progressing to chronic liver disease.[76-79] This phenotype is also associated with the development of pulmonary emphysema in young adults. Liver transplantation results in the acquisition of the donor Pi phenotype and normal circulating levels of alpha$_1$-antitrypsin.[80]

The indications for liver transplantation in these children include chronic cholestasis that does not recede and severe hepatic synthetic defects. It is currently believed that early transplantation will reduce the prevalence of chronic lung disease in the adult life of such patients.

Hereditary Tyrosinemia

Children with hereditary tyrosinemia pose a dilemma with regards to when transplantation should be considered. The natural history of this metabolic disorder divides affected individuals into two main groups: those who present early in life with a fulminant course and rapid deterioration of their liver function and those with a more indolent course.[81] Infants with early onset of liver failure would obviously benefit from liver transplantation as soon as the diagnosis is established. Children with a more chronic course often have a prolonged symptom-free interval with few problems related to their liver disease. The risk of developing hepatoma, however, is omnipresent in such cases. In a review of 43 patients, 37% developed hepatocellular carcinomas at a median age of 4 years.[82] These children often have multiple regenerative nodules within their livers, which makes it quite difficult to identify the hepatomas by ultrasound or CT scanning techniques.[83] Ideally, these children should be transplanted early before metastases preclude transplantation.[84] In general these children do very well after transplantation; the metabolic abnormality, however, may not be entirely corrected.[85-87]

PREDICTIVE FACTORS FOR POSTOPERATIVE PROBLEMS

In addition to recognizing disease-specific differences in survival following liver transplantation, it is also important to recognize certain preoperatively determined clinical parameters to predict those patients who are at increased risk for postoperative problems, especially infections.[88-90] Because infection is the leading cause of death following liver transplantation, many of these same preoperative predictors of infection also help to identify patients at increased risk for death following otherwise successful surgery.[88] Specifically, preoperative levels of total serum bilirubin, immunoglobulin levels, white blood cell and polymorphonuclear leukocyte counts, and serum creatinine levels are all increased ($p < 0.001$) in patients who develop postoperative bacterial infections as compared to those who do not.[88] Stepwise discriminant analysis of 27 variables revealed that the preoperative level of the serum creatinine is the most reliable risk factor for bacterial infection in the immediate postoperative period. The next most important variable in terms of increased risk of postoperative infection was the polymorphonuclear leukocyte count followed by the serum immunoglobulin G level and the degree of elevation of serum bilirubin.[88]

When death is the independent variable in the discriminant analysis of postoperative parameters, the factors most predictive of an untoward event are, in order: serum creatinine level, bilirubin level, hepatic encephalopathy, ascites, white blood cell count, polymorphonuclear cell count, and the helper-to-suppressor T-cell ratio.[88]

Preexisting renal dysfunction has been found to be a very important prognostic parameter in patients being considered for liver transplantation.[90] Two major types of postoperative renal impairment are seen in liver transplant recipients. Early renal dysfunction occurs during the first week after transplantation, with a peak incidence on the third and fourth postoperative day. Some evidence of early renal failure occurs in about half the patients and presumably reflects, in many instances, cyclosporine toxicity. In addition, hepatocellular liver disease, preoperative hepatic encephalopathy, ascites, and hypoalbuminemia, as well as intraoperative arterial hypotension have been found to be important independent predictors of early postoperative renal impairment in liver transplant recipients.

Late-onset renal impairment (onset after the first postoperative week) has a less favorable prognosis than does early-onset renal failure.[90] Factors associated with late-onset renal failure include shock, graft failure, and use of nephrotoxic agents such as cyclosporine, aminoglycosides, and amphotericin. In many patients, several adverse prognostic factors are present, and the prognosis is especially unfavorable. Clearly, these observations provide strong empiric support for the continued use of preoperative protocols in evaluating and managing liver transplantation patients.

IMMUNOSUPPRESSIVE DRUGS: REGIMENS USED IN LIVER TRANSPLANTATION PROGRAMS

Cyclosporine

This cyclic endecapeptide was first described as having immunosuppressive properties by Borel in 1976.[91] It inhibits generation of interleukin-2 (Il-2) production in vitro, thereby decreasing the proliferation of T cells bearing Il-2 receptors, as well as other T-cell-dependent factors.[92,93] The major limiting factor in its use is nephrotoxicity.[94] Unfortunately, many liver transplant recipients already have compromised renal function, which is compromised further by the operation and the use of nephrotoxic antibiotics pre- and postoperatively. The unusually high number of associated lymphomas associated with the use of cyclosporine reported initially[95] has been shown to occur at a rate no greater than with conventional immunosuppression (approximately 0.5%).[96] Other side effects of the drug include a poorly defined cholestasis, hypertrichosis, gingival hyperplasia, hand tremors and painful burning paresthesias of the palms and soles, encephalopathy, benign fibroadenomas of the breast, and regional flushing. Some abdominal discomfort and/or diarrhea after ingestion of the drug may be seen in the initial months in patients with incomplete fat absorption, due to the oil base used in the commercial preparation. Allergic reactions to the drug have also been attributed to the oil base, because they do not recur with use of the intravenous solution. Hypertension may be exacerbated or caused by cyclosporine but can usually be relatively easily controlled with the use of captopril. With time and a reduction in cyclosporine dosage, hypertension usually resolves.

Immediately before surgery, liver transplant recipients are given cyclosporine (2 mg per kilogram body weight intravenously over 1 to 2 hours).[1, 5, 17] Postoperatively the patients are continued on cyclosporine at the same dose every 8 hours, and cyclosporine trough levels are monitored. As soon as the patient is taking liquids by mouth, a combination of oral and intravenous cyclosporine is instituted; this dual route of administration is continued until hepatobiliary and gastrointestinal function returns fully. Therefore, the switch from intravenous to oral cyclosporine therapy alone is gradual. Once the patient is taking all medications orally, cyclosporine is given at specific times, usually twice a day, to allow for continued ease of monitoring trough blood levels of the drug. The ultimate goal is to administer the lowest possible dose of cyclosporine that will maintain normal graft function. This is usually accomplished by maintaining a cyclosporine trough level (whole blood) greater than 200 ng/ml and usually below 400 ng/ml by high pressure liquid chromatography (HPLC) and between 600 and 1000 ng/ml by radioimmunoassay (RIA).

Corticosteroids (Glucocorticoids)

Glucocorticoids appear to act at several levels of the immune response, by decreasing cellular class II or HLA Dr antigen expression, by inhibiting interleukin-2 production, and by being cytolytic.[97, 98]

Methylprednisolone is used initially and is given in progressively declining amounts over a 5-day period as follows:
- 50 mg intravenously every 6 hours for four doses
- 40 mg intravenously every 6 hours for four doses
- 30 mg intravenously every 6 hours for four doses
- 20 mg intravenously every 12 hours for two doses

and 10 to 20 mg per day therafter. Presumed rejection episodes (preferably confirmed by liver biopsy) are initially managed by a "bolus corticosteroid recycle" consisting of a 0.5 to 1.0 gm of methylprednisolone bolus, followed by 200 mg, 160 mg, 120 mg, 80 mg, and 40 mg given intravenously on consecutive days.

Antilymphocyte and Antithymocyte Globulins

Rejection episodes unresponsive to bolus steroid recycle therapy are treated with antilymphocyte globulin (Atgam) or, more recently, with monoclonal antithymocyte globuin (OKT3).[99, 100] Skin testing and determination of humoral antibodies to animal proteins are required before using either of these globulins. Moreover, premedication with a combination of H_1-receptor antagonists (usually diphenhydramine) and glucocorticoids (Solu-Cortef) given parenterally 30 minutes before the globulin preparation may help prevent untoward reactions. Both globulins are typically given intravenously once a day for 7 to 10 days. Bronchospasm, chest and joint pains, nausea, vomiting, and diarrhea can occur with the use of either antilymphocyte or antithymocyte globulin. The development of acute respiratory symptoms in a patient given these agents requires that the drug be stopped or that additional glucocorticoids and, occasionally, epinephrine be administered.

Other Immunosuppressive Agents

To prevent "rebound" rejection, which occasionally occurs after completion of a course of antilymphocyte or antithymocyte globulin, either azathioprine (50 to 100 mg/day) or cyclophosphamide (25 to 50 mg/day) is given for several days or weeks in combination with cyclosporine and prednisone. Both agents interfere with DNA synthesis within rapidly dividing cells. Such triple therapy can be useful also to reduce the dose of cyclosporine A required. Bone marrow suppression is the major side effect of these agents' use and can affect all blood cell elements; this side effect limits their use. Cholestatic jaundice with hepatic injury and development of fibrosis can be seen in patients on prolonged high doses of azothioprine.[101, 102] Veno-occlusive disease of the liver also can be an untoward consequence of the use of azothioprine. The patient's leukocyte and platelet counts must be followed in patients who are taking either azathioprine or cyclophosphamide because both these agents are myelotoxic.

GRAFT REJECTION

Clinically, rejection is manifested by malaise, fever, graft tenderness, jaundice, and a variable increase in the serum level of liver injury tests.[103] Bile, as observed by T-tube drainage, becomes less viscous and lighter in color. An episode of rejection can be expected to occur 5 to 10 days after transplantation and is most often successfully managed, as described above, with a "bolus corticosteroid recycle."

Early (acute) hepatic allograft rejection is characterized histopathologically by the presence of a lymphocytic endothelialitis of the hepatic arterioles, portal veins, and terminal hepatic venules.[104–109] In addition, the portal areas are expanded with a mixture of mature lymphocytes and an even greater number of lymphoblastoid cells. These cells appear to be most numerous in and about the bile ducts and bile ductules. As the rejection process continues, the endothelialitis becomes less evident, while the portal areas become more expanded with a mixed inflammatory infiltrate of lymphoblastoid cells, eosinophils, polymorphonuclear leukocytes, and mature lymphocytes. Bile ducts and proliferating bile ductules are progressively destroyed. Ultimately, with chronic rejection, the bile duct paucity syndrome (vanishing bile ducts) appears in which the number of identifiable ducts is progressively reduced.[104–109] With advanced chronic rejection, portal-to-portal bridging fibrosis and subintimal accumulation of foamy macrophages are seen in the larger radicles of the hepatic arteries.

RETRANSPLANTATION

When early (acute) graft rejection reaches the point of severe hepatic dysfunction or when late (chronic) rejection with vanishing bile ducts becomes severe, retransplantation is utilized.[109] Retransplantation, rather than successive cycles of increasing immunosuppressive therapy, is performed to avoid prolonged use of excessive immunosuppressive drugs, which often results in the frequently fatal development of renal failure or sepsis from bacterial, viral, and/or fungal agents.

Once the decision to retransplant a patient is made, the immunosuppressive regimen is reduced to a minimal level or discontinued altogether. This reduction in immunosuppressive therapy is designed to reduce the risk of infection prior to or associated with retransplantation and can be initiated as soon as the decision to retransplant is made. The need to resort to the difficult decision of retransplantation appears to have been reduced with the introduction of the use of OKT3; nonetheless, retransplantation is still necessary in approximately 20% to 25% of all patients who are transplanted in some centers.[109]

Urgent retransplantation is necessary in cases of primary graft failure or hepatic artery thrombosis associated with graft failure or sepsis (see below).

THE POSTOPERATIVE PERIOD

The post-transplant period may be complicated by three major problems: technical difficulties related to surgery, which usually present in the immediate postoperative course; infection, either viral or bacterial; and rejection, which is usually evident by 7 to 14 days after transplantation.

Initially, the patient is managed on a respirator in the intensive care unit for 12 or more hours postoperatively. A vigorous urine output is maintained, and the coagulation status of the patient is monitored and corrected as necessary.

Graft function is monitored using a variety of parameters. Standard liver tests such as AST, bilirubin, and alkaline phosphatase are elevated for 3 to 4 days but should begin to fall rapidly if graft function is good. Worsening of either the hepatocellular enzymes or coagulation status should initiate efforts to evaluate the vascular status of the graft looking for thrombosis or anastomotic stenoses.

Virtually all patients who have successful transplants have some degree of postoperative hypertension and many require intensive medical therapy for this particular problem. The cause of this hypertension is probably multifactorial. Elevated renin and catecholamine levels are usually found, and renal toxicity from a variety of drugs (especially CSA) is also present in these patients.

Pulmonary problems often complicate the immediate postoperative period. These include ARDS, pulmonary edema, and atelectasis. Temporary paralysis of the right hemidiaphragm is a relatively common occurrence in very small patients and contributes to their ventilatory problems. Vigorous chest physiotherapy and early bronchoscopy in the case of persistent atelectasis are essential to the respiratory management of these children.

The post-transplant patient is at significant risk for infection for several reasons. Most are severely debilitated at transplant, all receive immunosuppression and a large number of blood products, and all have indwelling venous and arterial catheters in the initial postoperative period.

Viruses are frequent causes of infection; cytomegalovirus is the most common. Acute Epstein-Barr virus (EBV) infection has been documented also.

Central nervous system complications with multiple etiologies often result in increased intracranial pressure. It has recently been suggested that postoperative neurologic complications occur frequently (33%) with the most frequent being seizures.[110] In the past, neurologic complications were the result of air embolism, cerebral hemorrhage, hypotension, or severe electrolyte and metabolic changes around the time of operation. Postoperative neurologic complications include cerebral abscess and meningoencephalitis. Recent data suggest that cyclosporine may be contributing to these neurologic complications. Monitoring electrolytes, especially calcium and magnesium, is important because medical therapy can prevent seizures on this basis.

Not all instances of graft dysfunction that occur after liver transplantation result from rejection. Early (days to weeks) graft dysfunction may result from primary graft failure as a result of graft ischemia or reoxygenation injury, or from one or another technical problems such as hepatic artery thrombosis or dehiscence of the biliary anastomosis. Primary graft failure can present in a dramatic fashion. Instead of recovering rapidly following transplantation, the patient decompensates, and overt hepatic failure develops, manifested as progressive coma, abnormal liver injury tests, coagulopathy, oliguria, acidosis, hyperkalemia, and hypoglycemia. Urgent retransplantation is the only means of saving such patients.

Technical complications of surgery usually result from problems with either the biliary or arterial reconstructions.[1, 111-113] Persistent jaundice, particularly with bile leaking from abdominal drains, strongly suggests a problem with the biliary anastomosis. Both abdominal US and CT should be obtained in such cases to look for an extrabiliary collection of fluid (bile) or bile duct dilatation.[114] If the patient has a T-tube, a cholangiogram should be obtained.[115, 116] A bile leak requires reexploration and repair. An obstructed bile duct may be drained percutaneously and subsequently treated surgically, endoscopically, or radiologically, depending on its location and the available expertise of the center.

Hepatic arterial thrombosis usually presents with the sudden onset of fever, rapid deterioration of liver biochemical tests, and, often, bacteremia caused by an enteric organism. When doubt exists regarding arterial thrombosis, either a Doppler ultrasound or an arteriographic study is indicated.[116-119] Hepatic artery thrombosis has three general patterns of presentation: (1) acute hepatic infarction with sepsis and fulminant hepatic failure, which mandates immediate retransplantation; (2) a delayed bile leak resulting from ischemic necrosis of the common bile duct at, or just distal to, the site of the anastomosis, which requires retransplantation rather than attempts at biliary tree repair; and (3) relapsing bacteremia, which can occasionally be treated with prolonged intravenous antibiotics and percutaneous needle drainage of identifiable abscesses.[112, 115, 116] If the patient remains febrile and fails to respond to such therapy, retransplantation is required.[109]

Occasionally, cyclosporine hepatotoxicity should be considered as a possible cause of persistently abnormal liver injury tests and cholestasis in an otherwise recuperating liver transplant recipient. The diagnosis of cyclosporine hepatotoxicity is very difficult (and often impossible) to establish and should only be considered when cyclosporine levels are quite high and other evidence for cyclosporine toxicity such as nephrotoxicity, hypertension, and tremulousness is evident. Management consists of markedly reducing (or discontinuing) cyclosporine and observing the course of the patient while monitoring the cyclosporine levels. In patients with T-tubes, lowering of cyclosporine levels can be hastened simply by draining the bile.[120]

INFECTIOUS COMPLICATIONS OF LIVER TRANSPLANTATION

Viral (herpes simplex, cytomegalovirus, and EBV) and other opportunistic infections such as *Legionella* and *Pneumocystis carinii* may present as hepatic dysfunction, malaise, fever, dyspnea, or fatigue in liver transplant patients, and should be considered whenever a transplant patient who has been doing well suddenly develops new symptoms.[121, 122] Herpes simplex virus infection can be treated with oral acyclovir (5 mg/kg) every 8 hours or by an intravenous infusion for 10 to 14 days. Cytomegalovirus can be treated with dihydroxymethylpropoxy-methylguanine (DHPG).[123, 124] *Legionella* infection is treated with erythromycin. *Pneumocystis carinii* infection may be treated with trimethoprim-sulfamethoxazole. It should be remembered that both *Legionella* and *Pneumocystis* may produce dyspnea and hypoxemia in the absence of radiologic evidence of a pulmonary infiltrate.

In some transplant programs, acyclovir is administered to all patients for 2 to 3 weeks in the immediate postoperative period. Other programs have resorted to the long-term chronic use of a single daily dose of trimethoprim-sulfamethoxazole daily to prevent *Pneumocystis* infection.

EVALUATION OF LATE LIVER DYSFUNCTION

Episodes of late liver dysfunction characterized by elevated serum levels of gamma glutamyl transpeptidase and alkaline phosphatase with or without hyperbilirubinemia may occur weeks to months after transplantation. If such dysfunction does not improve after one or two courses of bolus corticosteroid recycling, the biliary tree should be studied by either an endoscopic retrograde or a transhepatic cholangiogram. Indirect methods for evaluating the biliary system, such as the use of ultrasound, CT scanning, or nuclear medicine scanning, may fail to detect common duct stones or anastomotic strictures of the biliary tree. Liver biopsy is often helpful in identifying the cause of the liver injury.[104, 105, 107] The failure to make the correct diagnosis may result in inappropriate treatment. Such an incorrect diagnosis and treatment often lead to excessive immunosuppression, sepsis, and death. In all such cases, biliary obstruction must be assumed to be the cause of hepatic dysfunction until a direct method of biliary tract visualization has specifically excluded biliary obstruction as the cause of the hepatic dysfunction.

QUALITY OF LIFE FOLLOWING LIVER TRANSPLANTATION

The vast majority of children who survive liver transplantation return to school at or near the grade level expected for their age. Most adults who survive liver transplantation return to work. Many begin to have families,[125-127] and most are considerably better adjusted than are groups of patients with other chronic nonlethal medical illnesses.[128] In fact, the quality of life for most survivors of liver transplantation is similar to that for the normal population.[9, 17, 128]

References

1. Starzl TE, Iwatsuki S, Van Thiel DH, et al: Evolution of liver transplantation. *Hepatology* 1982; 2:614–636.
2. Van Thiel DH, Schade RR, Starzl TE, et al: Liver transplantation in adults. *Hepatology* 1982; 2:637–640.
3. McMaster P, Jurewicz WA, Gunson BK, et al: The current state of liver and pancreas transplantation. *Scand J Gastroenterol* 1985; 117:69–79.
4. Keating JJ, Johnson RD, Johnson PJ, et al: Clinical course of cirrhosis in young adults and therapeutic potential of liver transplantation. *Gut* 1985; 26:1359–1363.
5. Williams R, Blackburn A, Neuberger J, et al: Long-term use of cyclosporin in liver grafting. *Q J Med* 1985; 57:897–905.
6. Starzl TE, Iwatsuki S, Shaw BW Jr, et al: Liver transplantation in the cyclosporin era. *Prog Allergy* 1986; 38:366–394.
7. Darby H, Selden C, Hodgson HJ: Prolonged survival of cyclosporine-treated allogeneic hepatocellular implants. *Transplantation* 1986; 42:325–326.
8. Jenkins RL: The Boston Center for Liver Transplantation (BCLT). Initial experience of a new surgical consortium. *Arch Surg* 1986; 121:424–430.
9. Tzakis AG, Gordon RD, Makowka L, et al: Clinical considerations in orthotopic liver transplantation. *Radiol Clin North Am* 1987; 25:289–297.
10. Pichlmayr R, Ringe B, Lauchart W, et al: Liver transplantation. *Transplant Proc* 1987; 19:103–112.
11. Shaw BW Jr, Martin DJ, Marquez JM, et al: Venous bypass in clinical liver transplantation. *Ann Surg* 1984; 200:524–534.
12. Griffith BP, Shaw BW Jr, Hardesty RL, et al: Veno-venous bypass without systemic anticoagulation for transplantation of the human liver. *Surg Gynecol Obstet* 1985; 160:270–272.
13. Shaw BW Jr, Iwatsuki S, Bron K, et al: Portal vein grafts in hepatic transplantation. *Surg Gynecol Obstet* 1985; 161:66–68.
14. Shaw BW Jr, Iwatsuki S, Starzl TE: Alternative methods of arterialization of the hepatic graft. *Surg Gynecol Obstet* 1984; 159:490–493.
15. Dzik WH, Jenkins R: Use of intraoperative blood salvage during orthotopic liver transplantation. *Arch Surg* 1985; 120:946–948.
16. Scharschmidt BF: Human liver transplantation: Analysis of data on 540 patients from our four centers, in Gips CH, Krom RAF (eds): *Progress in Liver Transplantation*. Boston, Martinus Nijhoff Publishers, 1985, pp 249–266.
17. Busuttil RW, Goldstein LI, Danovitch GM, et al: Liver transplantation today. *Ann Intern Med* 1986; 104:377–389.
18. Christensen E, Schlichting P, Anderson PK, et al: A therapeutic index that predicts the individual effects of prednisone in patients with cirrhosis. *Gastroenterology* 1985; 88:156–165.
19. Christensen E, Bremmelgaard P, Bahnsen M, et al: Prediction of fatality in fulminant hepatic failure. *Scand J Gastroenterol* 1984; 19:90–96.
20. Karvountzis GG, Rederer AG: Relation of alpha fetoprotein in acute hepatitis to severity and prognosis. *Ann Intern Med* 1974; 156–160.
21. Scotto J, Opolon P, Eteve J, et al: Liver biopsy and prognosis in acute liver failure. *Gut* 1973; 14:927–933.
22. Iwatsuki S, Gordon RD, Shaw BW Jr, et al: Role of liver transplantation in cancer therapy. *Ann Surgery* 1985; 202:401–407.
23. Starzl TE, Iwatsuki S, Shaw BW Jr, et al: Treatment of fibrolamellar hepatoma with partial or total hepatectomy and transplantation of the liver. *Surg Gynecol Obstet* 1986; 162:145–148.
24. Portmann B, O'Grady J, Williams R: Disease recurrence following orthotopic liver transplantation. *Transplant Proc* 1986; 18:136–141.
25. Hood JM, Koep LJ, Peters RL, et al: Liver transplantation for advanced liver disease with alpha-1-antitrypsin deficiency. *N Engl J Med* 1980; 302:272–275.
26. Malatack JJ, Finegold DN, Iwatsuki S, et al: Liver transplantation for type I glycogen storage disease. *Lancet* 1983; 1:1073–1075.
27. Groth CG, Ringden O: Transplantation in relation to the treatment of inherited disease. *Transplantation* 1984; 38:319–327.
28. Bilheimer DW, Goldstein JL, Grundy SM, et al: Liver transplantation to provide low-density-lipoprotein receptors and lower plasma cholesterol in a child with homozygous familial hypercholesterolemia. *N Engl J Med* 1984; 311:1658–1664.
29. Sokol RJ, Francis PD, Gold SH, et al: Orthotopic liver transplantation for acute fulminant Wilson disease. *J Pediatr* 1985; 107:549–552.
30. Tuchman M, Freese DK, Sharp HL, et al: Persistent succinylacetone excretion after liver transplantation in a patient with hereditary tyrosinaemia type I. *J Inherited Metab Dis* 1985; 8:21–24.
31. Rakela J, Kurtz SB, McCarthy JT, et al: Fulminant Wilson's disease treated with postdilution hemofiltration and orthotopic liver transplantation. *Gastroenterology* 1986; 90:2004–2007.
32. Wolff H, Otto G, Giest H: Liver transplantation in Crigler-Najjar syndrome. A case report. *Transplantation* 1986; 42:84–86.
33. Kvittingen EA, Jellum E, Stokke O, et al: Liver transplantation in a 23-year-old tyrosinaemia patient: Effects on the renal tubular dysfunction. *J Inherited Metab Dis* 1986; 9:216–224.
34. Van Thiel DH, Gartner LM, Thorp FK, et al: Resolution of the clinical features of tyrosinemia following orthotopic liver transplantation for hepatoma. *J Hepatol* 1986; 3:42–48.
35. Hoeg JM, Starzl TE, Brewer HB: Liver trans-

plantation for treatment of cardiovascular disease: Comparison with medication and plasma exchange in homozygous familial hypercholesterolemia. *Am J Cardiol* 1987; 59:705–707.
36. Margreiter R, Kramar R, Huber C, et al: Combined liver and kidney transplantation (letter). *Lancet* 1984; 1:1077–1078.
37. Wood RP, Ellis D, Starzl TE: The reversal of the hepatorenal syndrome in four pediatric patients following successful orthotopic liver transplantation. *Ann Surg* 1987; 205:415–419.
38. Lerut J, Tzakis AG, Bron K, et al: Complications of venous reconstruction in human orthotopic liver transplantation. *Ann Surg* 1987; 205:404–414.
39. Equivel CO, Klintmalm G, Iwatsuki S, et al: Liver transplantation in patients with patent splenorenal shunts. *Surgery* 1987; 101:430–432.
40. Starzl TE, Todo S, Gordon R, et al: Liver transplantation in older patients. *N Engl J Med* 1987; 316:484–485.
41. Terblanche J, Northover JM, Bornman P, et al: A prospective controlled trial of sclerotherapy in the long term management of patients after esophageal variceal bleeding. *Surg Gynecol Obstet* 1979; 148:323–333.
42. Clark AW, MacDougall BRD, Westaby D, et al: Prospective controlled trial of injection sclerotherapy in patients with cirrhosis and recent variceal hemorrhage. *Lancet* 1980; 2:552–554.
43. MacDougall BRD, Westaby D, Theodossi A, et al: Increased long term survival in variceal haemorrhage using injection sclerotherapy. Results of a controlled trial. *Lancet* 1982; 1:124–127.
44. Yassin VM, Sherif SM: Randomized controlled trial of injection sclerotherapy for bleeding esophageal varices. An interim report. *Br J Surg* 1983; 70:20–22.
45. Esquivel CO, Benardos A, Demetris AJ, et al: Liver transplantation for primary biliary cirrhosis in 76 patients during the cyclosporine era. *Gastroenterology* 1988; 94:1207–1216.
46. Christensen E, Crowe J, Doniach D, et al: Clinical pattern and course of diseases in primary biliary cirrhosis based on an analysis of 236 patients. *Gastroenterology* 1980; 78:236–246.
47. Christensen E, Neuberger J, Croue J, et al: Beneficial effect of azathioprine and prediction of prognosis in primary biliary cirrhosis. *Gastroenterology* 1985; 89:1084–1091.
48. Christensen E, Schlichting R, Andersen PK, et al: The Copenhagen Study Group for Liver Diseases. Updating prognosis and therapeutic effect evaluation in cirrhosis with Cox's multiple regression model for true dependent time variables. *Second J Gastroenterol* 1986; 21:163–174.
49. Christensen E, Schlichting P, Fauerholdt L, et al: Changes of laboratory variables with time in cirrhosis: Prognostic and therapeutic significance. *Hepatology* 1985; 5:843–853.
50. Fennell RH Jr: Ductular damage in liver transplant rejection: Its similarity to that of primary biliary cirrhosis and graft-versus-host disease. *Pathol Annu* 1981; 16:289–294.
51. Neuberger J, Portmann B, MacDougall BR, et al: Recurrence of primary biliary cirrhosis after liver transplantation. *N Engl J Med* 1982; 306:1–4.
52. Jones EA: Primary biliary cirrhosis and liver transplantation (editorial). *N Engl J Med* 1982; 306:41–43.
53. Van Thiel DH, Gavaler JS: Recurrent disease in patients with liver transplantation: When does it occur and how can we be sure? *Hepatology* 1987; 7:181–184.
54. Kaplan M: Primary biliary cirrhosis. *N Engl J Med* 1987; 316:521–528.
55. Marsh JW Jr, Iwatsuki S, Makowka L, et al: Orthotopic liver transplantation for primary sclerosing cholangitis. *Ann Surg* 1988; 207:21–28.
56. LaRusso NF, Wiesner RH, Ludwig J, et al: Primary sclerosing cholangitis. *N Engl J Med* 1984; 310:899–903.
57. Neuberger J, Portmann B, Calne R, et al: Recurrence of autoimmune chronic active hepatitis following orthotopic liver grafting. *Transplantation* 1984; 37:363–365.
58. Demetris AJ, Lasky S, Van Thiel DH, et al: Pathology of hepatic transplantation. A review of 62 adult allograft recipients immunosuppressed with a cyclosporine steroid regimen. *Am J Pathol* 1985; 118:151–161.
59. Demetris AJ, Jaffe R, Sheahan DG, et al: Recurrent hepatitis B in liver allograft recipients: Differentiate between viral hepatitis B and rejection. *Am J Pathol* 1986; 125:161–172.
60. Alter HJ: Resolved and unresolved issues in non-A, non-B hepatitis, in Williams R, Maddrey WC (eds): *Liver.* Butterworths, London, 1984, pp 165–198.
61. Peleman RR, Gavaler JS, Van Thiel DH, et al: Orthotopic liver transplantation for acute and subacute hepatic failure in adults. *Hepatology* 1987; 7:484–489.
62. Iwatsuki S, Esquivel CO, Gordon RD, et al: Liver transplantation for fulminant hepatic failure. *Semin Liver Dis* 1985; 5:325–328.
63. Maddrey WC: Hepatic vein thrombosis (Budd-Chiari syndrome): Possible association with the use of oral contraceptives. *Semin Liver Dis* 1987; 7:32–39.
64. Mitchell MC, Boitnott JK, Kaufman S, et al: Budd-Chiari syndrome: Etiology, diagnosis and management. *Medicine* 1982: 61:199–218.
65. Seltman HJ, Dekker A, Van Thiel DH, et al: Budd-Chiari syndrome recurring in a transplanted liver. *Gastroenterology* 1984; 84:640–643.
66. Sternlieb I: Wilson's disease: Indications for liver transplant. *Hepatology* 1984; 4:155–175.
67. Sokol RG, Francis PD, Gold SH, et al: Orthotopic liver transplantation. Acute, fulminant Wilson disease. *J Pediatr* 1985; 107:549–552.
68. Atterbury CE: The alcoholic in the lifeboat. Should drinkers be candidates for liver transplantation? *J Clin Gastroenterol* 1986; 8:1–4.
69. Gantner JC Jr, Zitelli BJ, Malatac JJ, et al: Orthotopic liver transplantation in children. Two years experience with 47 patients. *Pediatrics* 1984; 74:140–146.
70. Zitelli B, Malatack J, Gartner J Jr, et al: Evaluation of the patient for liver transplantation. *Pediatrics* 1986; 78:559–564.

71. Alagille D, Valayer J, Odievre M, et al: Long-term follow-up in children operated on by corrective surgery for extrahepatic biliary atresia, in Kasai M (ed): *Biliary Atresia and Its Related Disorders.* New York, Elsevier, 1983, pp 233–243.
72. Iwatsuki S, Shaw BW Jr, Starzl TE: Liver transplantation for biliary atresia. *World J Surg* 1984; 8:51–56.
73. Bernard O, Alvarez F, Brunnelle F, et al: Portal hypertension in children. *Clin Gastroenterol* 1985; 14:45–51.
74. Cuervas-Mons V, Rimola A, Van Thiel DH, et al: Does previous abdominal surgery alter the outcome of pediatric patients subjected to orthotopic liver transplantation? *Gastroenterology* 1986; 90:853–857.
75. Kaufman SS, Wood PR, Shaw BW Jr, et al: Hepatocarcinoma in child with the Alagille syndrome. *Am J Dis Child* 1987; 141:698–703.
76. Sharp HL: The current status of alpha-1-antitrypsin, a protease inhibitor, in gastrointestinal disease. *Gastroenterology* 1976; 70:611–621.
77. Odievre M, Martin JP, Hadchouel M, et al: Alpha-1-antitrypsin deficiency and liver disease in children: Phenotypes, manifestations, and prognosis. *Pediatrics* 1976; 57:226–232.
78. Sharp HL, Bridges R, Krivit W, et al: Cirrhosis associated with alpha-1-antitrypsin deficiency: A previously unrecognized inherited disorder. *J Lab Clin Med* 1969; 73:934–940.
79. Psacharopoulos H, Mowat A, Cook P, et al: Familial factors and the severity of liver disease in genetic deficiency of alpha-1-antitrypsin (PiZZ). *Arch Dis Child* 1981; 56:803–808.
80. Hood J, Koep P, Peters R, et al: Liver transplantation for advanced liver disease with alpha-1-antitrypsin deficiency. *N Engl J Med* 1980; 302:272–274.
81. Larochelle J, Mortezai A, Belanger M, et al: Experience with 37 infants with tyrosinemia. *Can Med Assoc J* 1967; 97:1051–1057.
82. Weinberg A, Mize C, Worthen H: The occurrence of hepatoma in the chronic form of hereditary tyrosinemia. *J Pediatr* 1976; 88:434–440.
83. Day D, Letourneau J, Allan B, et al: Radiographic evaluation of the liver in hereditary tyrosinemia. *AJR*, in press.
84. Starzl TE, Zitelli B, Shaw B Jr, et al: Changing concepts: Liver replacement for hereditary tyrosinemia and hepatoma. *J Pediatr* 1986; 106:604–608.
85. Flatmark A, Bergan A, Sodal G, et al: Does liver transplantation correct the metabolic defect in hereditary tyrosinemia? *Transplant Proc* 1986; 18:67–69.
86. Tuchman M, Freese DK, Sharp HL, et al: Contribution of extrahepatic tissues to biochemical abnormalities in hereditary tyrosinemia type I: Study of three patients after liver transplantation. *J Pediatr* 1981; 110:399–404.
87. Van Thiel D, Gartner L, Thorp F, et al: Resolution of the clinical features of tyrosinemia following orthotopic liver transplantation for hepatoma. *J Hepatol* 1986; 3:42–48.
88. Cuervas-Mons V, Millan I, Gavaler JS, et al: Prognostic value of preoperatively obtained clinical and laboratory data in predicting survival following orthotopic liver transplantation. *Hepatology* 1986; 6:922–927.
89. Cuervas-Monn V, Martinez AJ, Dekker A, et al: Adult liver transplantation: An analysis of the early causes of death in 40 consecutive cases. *Hepatology* 1986; 6:495–501.
90. Rimola A, Gavaler JS, Schade RR, et al: Effects of renal impairment on liver transplantation. *Gastroenterology* 1987; 93:148–156.
91. Borel J, Feurer C, Magree C, et al: Effect of the new antilymphocytic peptide cyclosporine A in animals. *Immunology* 1977; 32:1017–1021.
92. Hess AD, Tutschka PJ, Pu Z, et al: Effect of cyclosporine A on human lymphocytes *in vitro* IV. Production of T cell stimulatory growth factors and development of responsiveness to these growth factors in CsA-treated primary MLR cultures. *J Immunol* 1982; 128:360–366.
93. Kahan B: Cyclosporine: The agent and its actions. *Transplant Proc* 1986; 17(suppl):5–11.
94. Iwatsuki S, Esquivel C, Klintmalm G, et al: Nephrotoxicity of cyclosporine in liver transplantation. *Transplant Proc* 1985; 17(suppl 1):191–194.
95. Caine RY, Rolles K, White DJ, et al: Cyclosporine A initially as the only immunosuppressant in 34 recipients of cadaveric organs, 32 kidneys, 2 pancreases, and 2 livers. *Lancet* 1979; I;1033–1035.
96. Penn I: Lymphomas complicating organ transplantation. *Transplant Proc* 1983; 15:2790–2793.
97. Dupont E, Wybran J, Toussaint A: Glucocorticosteroids and organ transplantation. *Transplantation* 1984; 37:331–334.
98. Hockland M, Larsen B, Heron I, et al: Corticosteroids decrease the expression of beta-2 microglobulin and histocompatibility antigen on human peripheral blood lymphocytes *in vitro. Clin Exp Immunol* 1981; 44:239–244.
99. Esquivel CO, Fung JJ, Markus B, et al: OKT3 in the reversal of acute hepatic allograft rejection. *Transplant Proc* 1987; 14:2443–2446.
100. Fung JJ, Demetris AJ, Porter KA, et al: Use of OKT3 with cyclosporine and steroids for reversal of acute kidney and liver allograft rejection. *Nephron*, in press.
101. Bjorkman D, Hammond E, Lee R, et al: Methotrexate induced hepatic fibrosis: An immunofluorescent and electromicroscopic study. *Gastroenterology* 1987; 92:1720–1726.
102. Zimmerman HJ: *Hepatotoxicity.* New York, Appleton-Century-Crofts, 1978, pp 528–533.
103. Esquivel CO, Jaffe R, Gordon RD, et al: Liver rejection and its differentiation from other causes of graft dysfunction. *Semin Liver Dis* 1985; 5:369–374.
104. Snover DC, Sibley RK, Freese DK, et al: Orthotopic liver transplantation: A pathological study of 63 serial liver biopsies from 17 patients with special reference to the diagnostic features and natural history of rejection. *Hepatology* 1984; 4:1212–1222.
105. Eggink HF, Hofstee N, Gips CH, et al: Histopathology of serial graft biopsies from liver

transplant recipients. *Am J Pathol* 1984; 114:18–31.
106. Si L, Whiteside TL, Van Thiel DH, et al: Lymphocyte subpopulations at the site of "piecemeal" necrosis in end stage chronic liver diseases and rejecting liver allografts in cyclosporine-treated patients. *Lab Invest* 1984; 50:341–347.
107. Hubscher SG, Clements D, Elias E, et al: Biopsy findings in cases of rejection of liver allograft. *J Clin Pathol* 1985; 38:1366–1373.
108. Snover DC, Freese DK, Sharp HL, et al: Liver allograft rejection. An analysis of the use of biopsy in determining outcome of rejection. *Am J Surg Pathol* 1987; 11:1–10.
109. Shaw BW Jr, Gordon RD, Iwatsuki S, et al: Retransplantation of the liver. *Semin Liver Dis* 1985; 5:394–401.
110. Adams DH, Ponsford S, Gunson B, et al: Neurologic complications following liver transplantation. *Lancet* 1987; 1:949–952.
111. Tzakis AG: The dearterialized liver graft. *Semin Liver Dis* 1985; 5:375–376.
112. Starzl TE, Iwatsuki S, Esquivel CO, et al: Requirements in the original technique of liver transplantation. *Semin Liver Dis* 1985; 5:349–356.
113. Tzakis AG, Gordon RD, Shaw BW Jr, et al: Clinical presentation of hepatic artery thrombosis after liver transplantation in the cyclosporine era. *Transplantation* 1985; 40:667–671.
114. Letourneau JG, Day DL, Frick MP, et al: Ultrasound and computer tomographic evaluation in hepatic transplantation. *Radiol Clin North Am* 1987; 25:323–331.
115. Segel MC, Zajko AB, Bowen A, et al: Hepatic artery thrombosis after liver transplantation: Radiologic evaluation. *Am J Roent* 1986; 146:137–141.
116. Segel MC, Zajko AB, Bowen A, et al: Doppler ultrasound as a screen for hepatic artery thrombosis after liver transplantation. *Transplantation* 1986; 41:539–541.
117. Zegel HG, Cole-Beuglet C, Carpenter G: Pre- and post-operative hepatic transplant evaluation by ultrasound and computerized tomography. *J Clin Ultrasound* 1981; 9:101–103.
118. Wozney P, Zajko AB, Bron KM, et al: Vascular complications after liver transplantation: A 5-year experience. *Am J Roent* 1986; 147:657–663.
119. Brown RK, Memsic LDF, Busuttil RW, et al: Accurate demonstration of hepatic infarction in liver transplant recipients. *J Nucl Med* 1986; 27:1428–1431.
120. Andrews W, Iwatsuki S, Shaw BW Jr, et al: Bile diversion and cyclosporine dosage. *Transplantation* 1985; 39:338–341.
121. Rubin RH: Infection in renal and liver transplant recipients, in Rubin RH, Young LS (eds): *Clinical Approach to Infection in the Compromised Host.* New York, Plenum Medical Book Co., 1981, pp 553–605.
122. Wood RP, Shaw BW Jr, Starzl TE: Extrahepatic complications of liver transplantation. *Semin Liver Dis* 1985; 5:377–384.
123. Collaborative DHPG Treatment Study Group: Treatment of serious cytomegalovirus infections with 9-(1,3-dihydroxy-2-propoxymethyl) guanine in patients with AIDS and other immunodeficiencies. *N Engl J Med* 1985; 314:801–805.
124. Bach MC, Bagwell SP, Knapp NP, et al: 9-(1,3-dihydroxy-propoxymethyl) guainine for cytomegalovirus infections in patients with the acquired immunodeficiency syndrome. *Ann Intern Med* 1985; 103:381–382.
125. Schmid R, Newton JJ: Childbirth after liver transplantation (letter). *Transplantation* 1980; 29;432–435.
126. Penn I, Makowski EL, Harris P: Parenthood following renal and hepatic transplantation. *Transplantation* 1980; 30:397–400.
127. Penn I, Makowski EL: Parenthood in kidney and liver transplant recipients. *Transplant Proc* 1981; 13:36–39.
128. Tarter RE, Van Thiel DH, Hegedus AM, et al: Neuropsychiatric status after liver transplantation. *J Lab Clin Med* 1984; 103:776–782.

20

Chronic Hepatitis:
What are the newer approaches to management?

SHEILA SHERLOCK, D.B.E., M.D.

DEFINITION

Chronic hepatitis is usually defined as a chronic inflammatory disease of the liver lasting for at least 6 months.[1] The 6-month criterion prevents premature diagnosis after an acute attack of viral hepatitis, when hepatic histology is that of an unresolved hepatitis and is difficult to interpret. In the absence of a history of an acute attack, it is not so necessary to wait 6 months and diagnosis may be earlier, although a follow-up of 6 months is wise before chronicity is deemed certain.

Classically a distinction is made between chronic persistent hepatitis, in which inflammation is confined to the portal zone (zone 3) and the limiting plate between liver cell columns and portal zones is intact (Fig 20–1), and chronic active hepatitis, in which portal zones are expanded by a cellular, largely mononuclear infiltrate and the limiting plate is eroded by so-called piecemeal necrosis (Fig 20–2). Cirrhosis, defined as widespread nodular formation and fibrosis with destruction of a zonal architecture, may coexist with chronic hepatitis. Whatever the type of chronic hepatitis, the same underlying liver histology is seen. Superimposed are features relative to the etiology (Table 20–1).

PRESENTATION

The patient comes to the clinician through general circumstances, symptoms, physical signs, or abnormal serum biochemical tests. The most important general symptom is fatigue. Physical signs include jaundice, vascular spiders (rarely), a large or small liver, and splenomegaly. Suggestive abnormal biochemical test results are a modestly raised serum bilirubin level, increased transaminases and gammaglobulin values, and a moderately raised serum alkaline phosphatase. The next step is to test for serum hepatitis B surface antigen (HBsAg); management depends on whether this is positive or negative (Fig 20–3).

SUGGESTIVE CLINICAL PROFILE

Chronic hepatitis B is suggested by the ethnic origin of the patient, homosexuality, drug abuse, or a likely contact with blood of patients carrying hepatitis B (Table 20–1). The patient may present because of fatigue. Serum transaminases may be found at a routine medical check or by biochemical screening for some unrelated condition. Hepatitis B may be diagnosed at the time of blood donation.

243

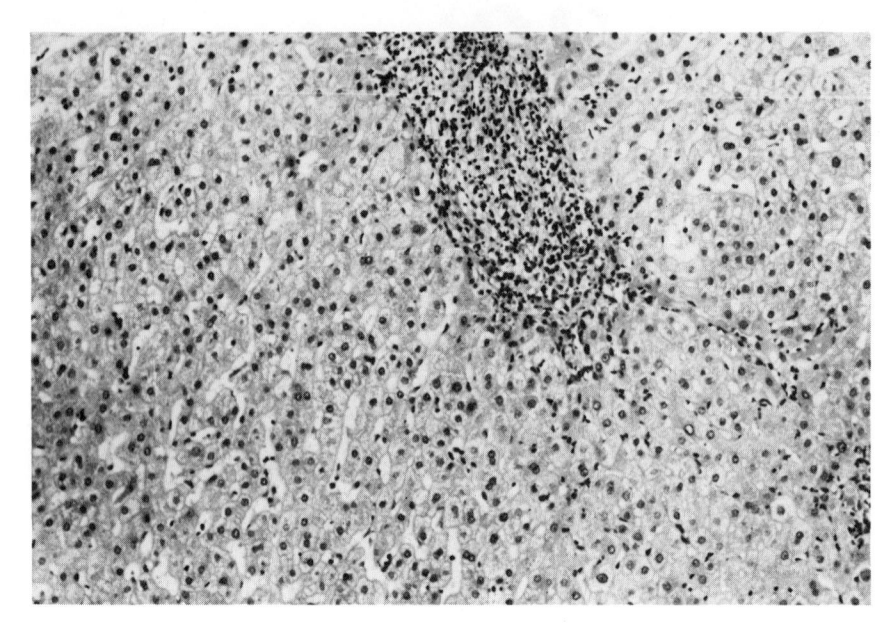

FIG 20–1.
Chronic persistent hepatitis. The portal zone is expanded with inflammatory, largely mononuclear, cells. The limiting plate of liver cells is preserved. Stained hematoxylin and eosin.

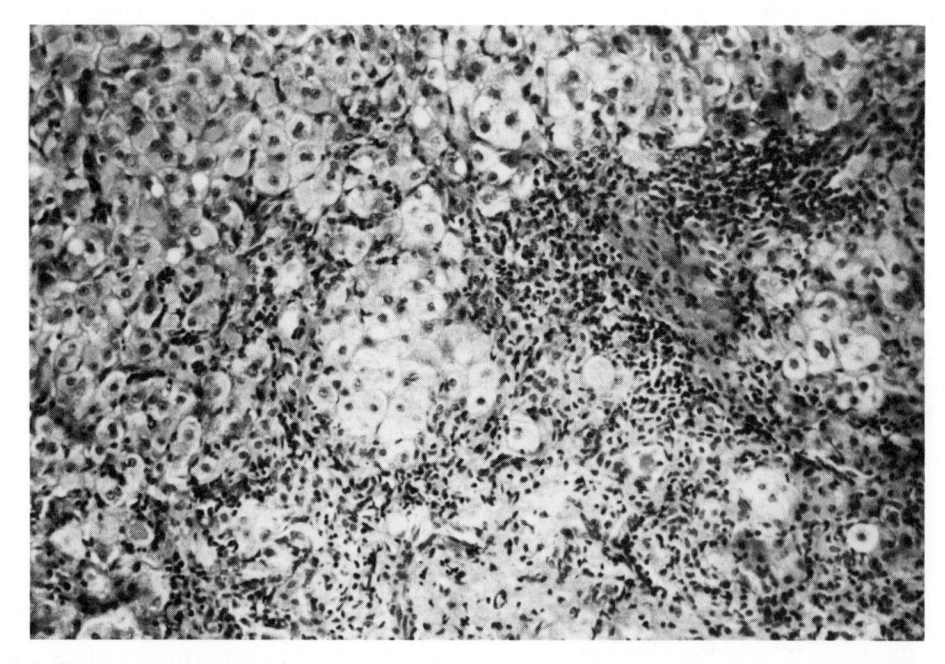

FIG 20–2.
Chronic active hepatitis (severe). Note isolation of liver cells into rosettes, fibrosis, piecemeal necrosis, and many inflammatory, largely mononuclear, cells. Stained hematoxylin and eosin.

TABLE 20–1.
Classification of Chronic Hepatitis

Etiology	Predominant Age	Predominant Sex	Associations	Diagnostic tests
Hepatitis B	All	M	Immigrants from Orient, Africa, Mediterranean Health-care workers, homosexuals, drug abusers, immunosuppressed	HBsAg, HBc, HBeAg, anti-HBe, HBV DNA, anti HDV
Hepatitis, non-A, non-B	All	Equal	Blood transfusion Blood products Drug abuse	None
Autoimmune	14–25 and postmenopausal	F	Multisystem (diabetes, arthralgia, hemolytic anemia, nephritis)	ANA +ve 70% SMA +ve 70% Serum gamma globulin high "Florid" liver histology
Wilson's disease	10–30	Equal	Family history Hemolysis Neurologic signs	Kayser-Fleischer rings, serum copper, ceruloplasmin, urinary copper, liver copper
Drug	Middle aged and elderly	F	INAH, methyl dopa, furantoin, dantrolene, antithyroid drugs	History, liver histology

246 / LIVER

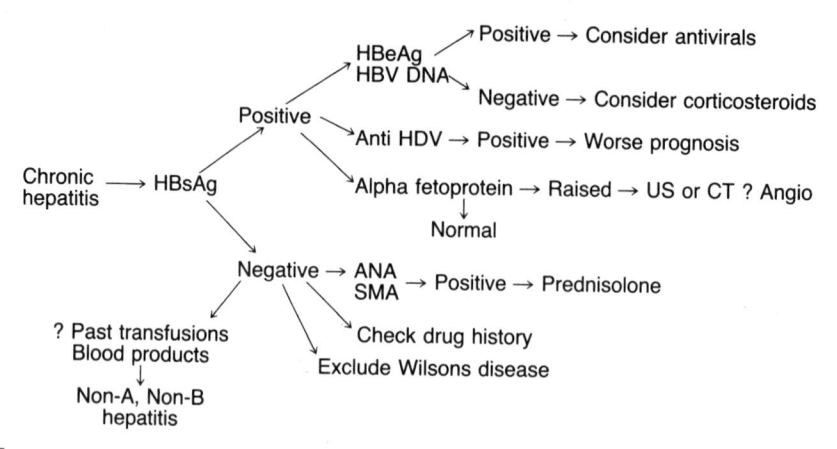

```
                                    ┌→ Positive → Consider antivirals
                              HBeAg ┤
                              HBV DNA
                              ┌─────→ Negative → Consider corticosteroids
                    Positive ─┤
                              ├→ Anti HDV → Positive → Worse prognosis
                              │
                              └→ Alpha fetoprotein → Raised → US or CT ? Angio
Chronic   ──→ HBsAg                            ↓
hepatitis                                    Normal

                    Negative → ANA  → Positive → Prednisolone
                              SMA
              ┌─────────┘       ↘
      ? Past transfusions      Check drug history
      Blood products        Exclude Wilsons disease
              ↓
         Non-A, Non-B
          hepatitis
```

FIG 20-3.
The management of chronic hepatitis depending on whether the patient is hepatitis B surface antigen (HBsAg) positive or negative.

In a known hepatitis B carrier, a relapse with jaundice and high transaminase values may indicate superadded infection with delta virus.[2]

The history of receiving a blood transfusion or blood products, however distant, suggests non-A, non-B hepatitis. The patient may bring a chart recording up and down serum transaminase levels over many months or years.

Autoimmune chronic active hepatitis should be expected in women, usually aged 15 to 25 years, in whom amenorrhea is usual, or in women about the menopause age. The patient is mildly jaundiced and nourished with vascular spiders. Splenomegaly is usual. Serum aspartate transaminase and gamma globulin levels are very high (Fig 20-4). Associated features may include fever, arthralgias, lymphadenopathy, and Coombs' positive hemolytic anemia (Table 20-2).

Drug-related chronic active hepatitis most frequently affects older persons, often women. The patient has usually been taking the drug for more than 1 month. Drugs incriminated include isoniazid, methyl dopa, dantrolene, ketoconazole, but any drug should be suspected.

Wilson's disease usually presents before the age of 25, sometimes with hemolysis and ascites. A family history must be obtained; siblings may have suffered or died from liver disease. There may be parental consanguinity. Kayser-Fleischer corneal rings are usually, but not always, present. Neurologic features such as slurred speech or tremor may be present or absent in young people with hepatic Wilson's disease. Serum ceruloplasmin and copper values are reduced, and 24-hour urinary copper is increased. If a liver biopsy is performed, the copper content must be quantitated and is increased.

LABORATORY TESTS

The expected profile of serum biochemical tests is total bilirubin variably raised, high serum transaminases, albumin normal or low, gamma globulin raised, and alkaline phosphatase moderately raised.

Hematology tests should include a hemoglobin level. The white cell and platelet count may be low if the spleen is enlarged. However reduced the platelet count may be, clinical bleeding is unusual

Patient	Examination	Biochemical	Antibodies	Diagnosis
Female 15–25 >45	Vascular spiders Splenomegaly →	Gammaglobulin ↑↑ Transaminases ↑↑ Bilirubin ↑ →	Nuclear 80% Smooth muscle 70% →	Autoimmune chronic hepatitis

FIG 20-4.
Features suggesting chronic active hepatitis of autoimmune type.

TABLE 20–2.
Associated Lesions in 81 Cases of Autoimmune Chronic Active Hepatitis

Purpura	2
Erythemas	4
Arthralgia	9
Lymphadenopathy	2
Pulmonary infiltrates	7
Pleurisy	2
Rheumatic heart disease	4
Ulcertaive colitis	5
Diabetes	3
Hashimoto's thyroiditis	2
Renal tubular defects	3
Lupus kidney	3
Hemolytic anemia	1

and splenectomy should never be performed for this secondary hypersplenism.

Prothrombin time may be disproportionately increased in the autoimmune group.

Every patient should have a test for hepatitis B surface antigen. Further management depends on the result (Fig 20–3).

THE ROLE OF LIVER BIOPSY (TABLE 20–3)

Liver biopsy is essential to confirm the diagnosis, to assess activity, to determine the presence or absence of cirrhosis, and to indicate a possible etiology.[3]

The biopsy should be performed only if the prothrombin time is not more than 3 seconds prolonged over control, and the partial thromboplastin time (PTT) is normal. Platelets should exceed 80,000. Infusion of fresh frozen plasma and platelets is essential if biopsy is to be performed in those with abnormal blood clotting. If it is necessary to perform a liver biopsy in such patients, it can be done under laparoscopic, CT, or ultrasound control. A trucut needle is used, and a gel foam plug may be injected through the outer cannula after the inner cutting needle and biopsy specimen have been removed. Biopsy by the transjugular route is an alternative in patients with abnormal clotting.[4]

Outpatient liver biopsy is particularly useful in patients with suspected chronic hepatitis who have normal blood coagulation. It considerably lessens the cost and adds to the convenience of the patient.

Experienced histopathologists are required for interpretation.[5] Chronic hepatitis is a patchy disease, and sampling difficulties add to the problems of the pathologist. Accuracy of diagnosis is proportional to the size of the specimen and probably 15 mm with five portal tracts is necessary for accurate interpretation.[6] However, samples of smaller length are often sufficient to exclude chronic active hepatitis. A stain for connective tissue, such as Mallory's trichrome or reticulin, is essential if cirrhosis is to be diagnosed.

Activity is assessed by the extent of periportal piecemeal necrosis and inflammation and the preservation or otherwise of the limiting plate. The extent of the intralobular focal necrosis and inflammation may be even more important than the periportal changes in predicting an unfavorable course.[7] Bridging necrosis and fibrosis may be portal–central or portal–portal. This finding is serious and a probable marker of progression to cirrhosis.[8] The overall appearances may be quite similar in the various types of chronic

TABLE 20–3.
Suggestive Liver Histology in Chronic Hepatitis

Type	Features
B	Usually mild
	Ground-glass cells
	Orcein positive
Delta	Delta antigen in hepatocytes
Non-A, non-B	Fat
	Lobular component
Drug	Eosinophils, fat, granulomas
Wilson's disease	Ballooned hepatocytes, glycogenic nuclei, fat

hepatitis, and so be unhelpful in giving the etiology. However, there are some suggestive patterns (Table 20-3).

The chronic hepatitis associated with hepatitis B infection is likely to be mild, the appearances being intermediate between chronic persistent hepatitis and chronic active hepatitis. A more active picture, with a particularly prominent lobular component, focal hepatocyte necrosis, and cellular infiltration, is seen as a patient converts from the replicative (HBeAg and HBV DNA positive) to the integrated (HBeAg and HBV DNA negative) stages.[5] Hepatitis B surface antigen may be demonstrated within the hepatocyte as ground-glass cells or by orcein staining.

A particularly active chronic hepatitis is seen in hepatitis B carriers with superadded delta virus infection. This may be confirmed by using immunoperoxidase-linked anti-delta, when delta antigen is demonstrated in the hepatocyte nuclei.

Changes suggesting a chronic hepatitis due to non-A, non-B viruses are not diagnostic but are only suggestive. They include fatty change, prominent intralobular mononuclear infiltration, lymphoid aggregates, acidophil bodies and evidence of damage to bile duct epithelium.

Autoimmune chronic active hepatitis is associated with a particularly active histologic picture. Aggressive septum formation isolates groups of liver cells as rosettes. Piecemeal necrosis, plasma cells and lymphocytic infiltration are prominent. Cirrhosis frequently coexists.

The chronic active hepatitis of Wilson's disease is marked by ballooned liver cells, clumped cytoplasmic glycogen, and glycogenic vacuolation of the nuclei. Fatty change is usual. Sometimes, the picture of acute alcoholic hepatitis, including Mallory's hyaline, is seen. Stains for copper are unreliable, but quantitative estimations show raised levels, and this investigation should always be performed.

Drug-related chronic hepatitis is suggested by bridging while eosinophilic infiltration, granulomas, and fat may also be seen.

TREATMENT

Chronic HBV Hepatitis

The patient must be counseled about personal infectivity. Close family, and especially sexual contacts and children, after screening for serum HBsAg, anti-HBc, and anti-HBs, should be considered for hepatitis B vaccination. Alcohol excess should be avoided because it enhances the effects of HBV carriage.

Many factors determine treatment in the HBsAg-positive patient.[9] Most patients with chronic hepatitis B lead normal lives; strong reassurance will prevent introspection by the patient. The patient should avoid becoming excessively fatigued, but bed rest is not helpful. Physical fitness is encouraged by graduated exercises.

A distinction must be made between the replicative and the integrated stages of the disease. During the phase of acute viral replication, the patient's serum is positive for HBeAg and HBV DNA. At some stage, the hepatitis B viral genome becomes an integral part of the host's genome so that viral genes are transcribed along with those of the host. The hepatocytes secrete HBsAg, but serum HBeAg is absent, anti-HBe develops, and HBV DNA can no longer be detected. Treatment is aimed at controlling infectivity, eradicating the virus, and preventing the development of cirrhosis and hence, possibly, hepatocellular carcinoma. It is unusual with any treatment to actually rid the patient of the hepatitis B virus. In the replicative stage, reduction or cessation of inflammatory necrosis of hepatocytes may be achieved by successful antiviral therapy.[9,10] In these patients, alpha interferon, whether lymphoblastoid or recombinant, must be considered. The full course is 5–10 million units/m^2 intramuscularly three times a week for 12 weeks (Fig 20-5). Side effects include malaise, fever, and small decreases in white cell and platelet counts. A positive response is shown by loss of HBeAg and HBV DNA and a transient rise in transaminases as infected cells are lysed. Ultimately liver

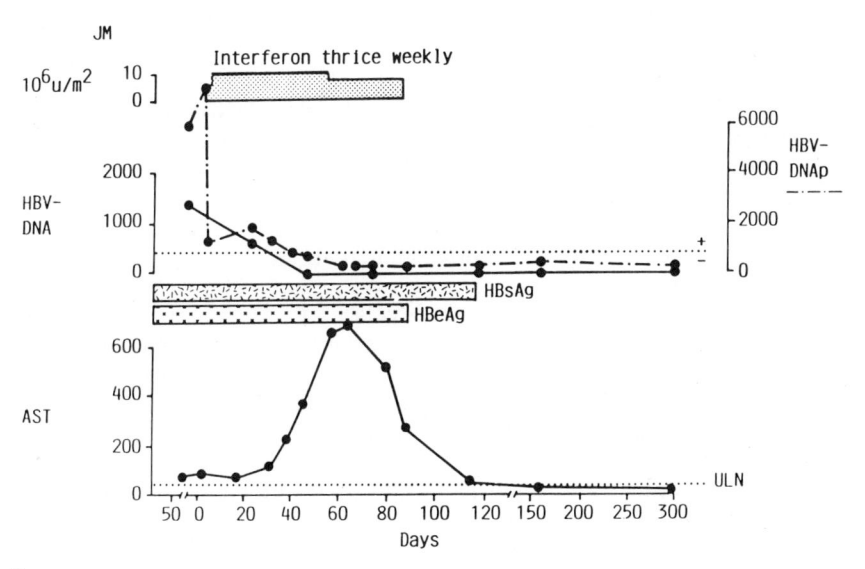

FIG 20–5.
Interferon was given three times a week for 12 weeks to this hepatitis B surface antigen (HBsAg) and hepatitis "e" antigen (HBeAg) positive patient with chronic hepatitis. HBV DNA and HBV DNR fell to undetectable levels as did HBsAg and HBeAg. There was a rise in serum aspartate transaminase (AST, GOT) which then fell to below the upper limit of normal (ULN). This result can be expected in 60% to 70% of treated patients although it is rare for HBsAg to become undetectable. (Thomas HC, Scully LJ: Antiviral therapy in hepatitis B infection. *Br Med Bull* 1985; 41:374–380.

biopsy appearances show less inflammation and hepatocellular necrosis. Serum HBeAb appears after about 6 months. It is unusual for HBsAg to be cleared unless the patient is treated very soon after acquiring the disease.

Antiviral treatment must be considered for the HBe antigen-positive patient, who is likely to disseminate hepatitis B (Table 20–4). Those seen early after infection; the young, the heterosexual, and those compliant with prolonged intramuscular therapy are particularly suitable. Those with active disease as shown by high transaminases and liver biopsy appearances are more likely to respond. In well-chosen patients, a 70% response rate can be expected. A good candidate is a person with a clear exposure who develops an acute attack of hepatitis B and remains HBsAg- and HBeAb-positive after 6 months. Corticosteroids enhance viral replication, and, after withdrawal, an immunologic rebound results in a fall of viral markers including HBV DNA. Immunocompetence is restored, and cells expressing target viral antigens are destroyed.[11] Better results are obtained if a full course of interferon is given following the corticosteroids.[12] This routine however, can be dangerous; enhancing the immune response by corticosteroids followed by withdrawal may lead to hepatocellular failure. Therefore, this therapy should not be used for ill patients with severe liver disease evi-

TABLE 20–4.
Factors Determining Response of Patients with Chronic Hepatitis B to Antiviral Therapy

Good response	Female
	Heterosexual
	Compliant
	Recent infection
	High serum transaminases
	"Active" liver biopsy
Bad response	Homosexual
	HIV positive
	Disease acquired early
	Oriental

denced by such features as jaundice or ascites.

Apart from general measures, there is no well-defined treatment for the HBeAg- and HBV-negative patient in the integrated stage of the disease. If the patient is symptomless or has only mild symptoms, conservative measures are all that should be offered. Advanced age and concomitant disease such as diabetes or a history of many years of nonprogressive liver disease also contraindicate treatment. Such patients should have clinical and biochemical tests every 6 months with liver biopsies, as indicated, to assess progress.

In some anti-HBe patients, perpetuation of the chronic hepatitis may be immunologically mediated. Such patients with negative tests for HBV DNA must be considered for prednisolone if they are symptomatic and if liver biopsy shows chronic active hepatitis with or without cirrhosis. Prednisolone is started in a dose of 30 mg for 1 week, and reduced to a maintenance dose of 10 to 15 mg daily continued for 3 months. If there is no clinical or biochemical evidence of benefit, the drug is stopped; if there is improvement, it may be continued, usually for about 2 years. Such therapy must in no way be regarded as ideal; it is indicated only for rapidly progressive disease or failure of other available treatment. Life may be prolonged.

There is no established treatment for the hepatitis Delta virus-positive patient. Alpha-interferons have been tried for these patients, but with equivocal results. It is possible that prolonged, low doses of alpha-interferons may be useful, but the results of large, prospective controlled trials are awaited.

Patients who are HBsAg positive with chronic hepatitis or cirrhosis, especially if male and more than 45 years old, should be screened regularly so that hepatocellular carcinoma may be diagnosed early when surgical resection may prove possible. It is suggested that serum alpha-fetoprotein be measured and ultrasound examination performed at intervals of 6 months.

Chronic Non-A, Non-B Hepatitis

In the absence of any serologic marker to make an exact diagnosis or to monitor therapy, it is difficult to know the correct management of chronic hepatitis due to non-A, non-B viruses. Preliminary results in an uncontrolled trial have suggested that treatment with recombinant alpha-interferon may reduce serum transaminase levels and improve hepatic histology.[13] It is possible therefore that interferon, given long-term in low doses, may control disease activity in some patients. Results of a multicenter controlled trial and particularly the advent of a definitive marker to monitor results are awaited.

Autoimmune Chronic Active Hepatitis

Drugs that alter immunologic processes, especially prednisolone, are particularly effective.[14] Benefit is seen particularly in the first 2 years. Well-being is increased, appetite improves, fever and arthralgias are controlled. Biochemical changes are less constant, although serum bilirubin, transaminase, and gamma globulin levels usually fall, and serum albumin concentrations rise. The effect on hepatic histology is variable and unconvincing. Certainly progression from chronic hepatitis to cirrhosis does not seem to be prevented.

If the patient is symptomatic and has very high serum transaminase and gamma globulins and a wildly active chronic hepatitis on liver biopsy, the decision to start prednisolone is easy. If symptoms are mild or absent, and biochemical tests only modestly impaired, but the liver biopsy shows a definite chronic active hepatitis, the decision is less easy. Clinical judgment, a vague term, must be invoked.

The usual dose is 30 mg prednisolone for 1 week, reducing to a maintenance dose of 10 to 15 mg daily. The initial course lasts 6 months. If a remission has ensued—judged clinically, biochemically and, if possible, by a further liver bi-

TABLE 20–5.
Chronic Active Hepatitis

Duration of prednisolone therapy is at least 2 years until
ANA −VE
Bilirubin
γ Globulin } are normal
Transaminase
Liver biopsy inactive
Usually more than 2 years

opsy—the drug should be tapered off slowly over a period of about 2 months. In general, however, prednisolone therapy extends over 2 to 3 years and often longer, sometimes for life (Table 20–5). Premature withdrawal leads to relapse.[15] Although control is usually reestablished, there are occasional fatalities. It is indeed difficult to decide when to withdraw therapy. Long-term, low-dose prednisolone maintenance is probably preferable. Alternate-day prednisolone therapy is not recommended because the incidence of serious complications is higher, and histologic remission is less frequent. More serious complications include diabetes, bone thinning, and serious infections. None is usually a problem if the dose of prednisolone is not more than 15 mg daily. If 20 mg prednisolone daily has not produced a remission, azathioprine (Imuran), 50 to 100 mg daily, may be added. It is not given routinely. Other indications include gross cushingoid features, associated diseases such as diabetes, or other side effects developing at doses required to induce a remission. Azathioprine should never be given alone.

Ten-year survival with treatment is 63%.[14] About one third of patients achieve a 5-year remission rate, while two-thirds relapse and have to be retreated. In half of those who have a remission, it will be sustained, especially if the chronic hepatitis is diagnosed early, and if immunosuppression is adequate. Relapse does not affect the long-term prognosis, although retreatment has more side effects. Corticosteroid therapy prolongs life, but most patients eventually reach the end stage of cirrhosis.

Drug-Related Chronic Active Hepatitis

A drug etiology should be considered in any patient presenting with chronic hepatitis. Clinical and biochemical improvement follows withdrawal. Therefore all drugs that the patient is receiving, if not actually life-saving, should be stopped until the nature of the chronic hepatitis is established. Recovery follows stopping the drug; however, fatal subacute hepatic necrosis may ensue if therapy is continued after the hepatic reaction has commenced.

Wilson's Disease

Initially, penicillamine in doses of 1 to 2 gm daily are mandatory. The maintenance dose is about 1 gm daily and should not on any account be discontinued. Fatal liver disease can follow noncompliance even after 20 years of successful penicillamine treatment.[16]

Oral zinc is given to block the intestinal uptake of copper. Dose is 50 mg elemental zinc (as the acetate salt) three times a day *between* meals.[17] It can be given in the initial stages but should not replace penicillamine as long-term therapy.

PREGNANCY

Women who present with chronic hepatitis are often young. Fertility is low but with treatment, menses return, and these women may become pregnant; this should not be contraindicated. Liver function may deteriorate during pregnancy but, after delivery, soon returns to its previous level. The fetal loss rate is about 33%, and the baby may be born prematurely but will be normal. The coexistence of liver disease with pregnancy should not per se indicate termination. Management must be in a specialist obstetric unit with the back-up of a hepatology department. In the autoimmune group, corticosteroids must be continued during pregnancy.

Babies of an HBsAg-positive woman, whether she is HBeAg positive or not, must receive hepatitis B immune globulin and the first dose of hepatitis B vaccine at the time of birth. The full course of vaccine is then completed.

In patients with Wilson's disease, penicillamine should be continued during pregnancy

THE ROLE OF HEPATIC TRANSPLANTATION

Obviously transplantation should not be done at the stage of chronic hepatitis but only when late cirrhosis has developed.[18] Age, psychosocial status, economics, infections, and previous upper abdominal surgery are among the preoperative considerations.

Transplant of the cirrhotic liver is difficult, for reasons related to portal hypertension and poor blood clotting. Removal of a small cirrhotic liver may be difficult. Recurrence of the original disease is likely with hepatitis B and delta infections. The position of recurrence of non-A, non-B hepatitis is uncertain. Patients with autoimmune chronic active hepatitis and cirrhosis may show a return of their disease.

Transplantation may be indicated in patients with Wilson's disease. Copper metabolism returns to normal after a transplant. The procedure must be considered in those with fulminant Wilson's disease, in those who fail to improve after 3 months continous penicillamine, and in those who relapse when noncompliant with therapy.

References

1. Sherlock S: Chronic hepatitis, in *Diseases of the Liver and Biliary System*, ed 7 Oxford, Blackwell Scientific Publications, 1985, pp 295–330.
2. Lok ASF, Lindsay I, Scheuer PJ, et al: Clinical and histological features of Delta infection in chronic hepatitis B virus carriers. *J Clin Pathol* 1985; 38:530–533.
3. Sherlock S, Dick R, van Leeuwen DJ: Liver biopsy today: The Royal Free Hospital experience. *J Hepatol* 1984; 1:78–85.
4. Lebrec D, Goldfard G, Degott C, et al: Transvenous liver biopsy—An experience based on 1000 hepatic tissue samplings with this procedure. *Gastroenterology* 1982; 83:338–340.
5. Scheuer PJ: *Chronic Hepatitis in Liver Biopsy Interpretation*, ed 4. London, Bailliere Tindall, 1988, pp. 113–130.
6. Schlichting P, Holund B, Poulsen H: Liver biopsy in chronic aggressive hepatitis. Diagnostic reproducibility in relation to size of specimen. *Scand J Gastroenterol* 1983; 18:27–32.
7. Scheuer PJ: Changing views on chronic hepatitis. *Histopathology* 1986; 10:1–4.
8. Cooksley WGE, Bradbear RA, Robinson W, et al: The prognosis of chronic active hepatitis without cirrhosis in relation to bridging necrosis. *Hepatology* 1986; 6:345–348.
9. Sherlock S, Thomas HC: Treatment of chronic hepatitis due to hepatitis B virus. *Lancet* 1985; 2:1343–1346.
10. Davis GL, Hoofnagle JH: Interferon in viral hepatitis: Role in pathogenesis and treatment. *Hepatology* 1986; 6:1038–1041.
11. Nair PV, Tong MJ, Stevenson D, et al: A pilot study on the effects of prednisolone withdrawal on serum HBV DNA and HBeAg in chronic active hepatitis B. *Hepatology* 1986; 6:1319–1324.
12. Perrillo RP. The use of corticosteroids in conjunction with antiviral therapy in chronic hepatitis B with ongoing viral replication. *J Hepatol* 1987, in press.
13. Hoofnagle JH, Mullen KD, Jones DB, et al: Treatment of chronic non-A, non-B hepatitis with recombinant human alpha infeteron. A preliminary report. *N Engl J Med* 1986; 315:1575–1578.
14. Czaja AJ, Beaver SJ, Shiels MT: Sustained remission after corticosteroid therapy of severe hepatitis B surface antigen-negative chronic active hepatitis. *Gastroenterology* 1987; 92:215–219.
15. Hegarty JE, Nouriaria KT, Portmann B, et al: Relapse following treatment withdrawal in patients with autoimmune active hepatitis. *Hepatology* 1983; 3:685–691.
16. Walshe JM, Dixon AK: Dangers of non-compliance in Wilson's disease. *Lancet* 1986; 1:845.
17. Van Caillie-Bertrand M, Degenhard HJ, Visser HKA, et al: Oral zinc sulphate for Wilson's disease. *Arch Dis Child* 1985; 60:656.
18. Sherlock S: Hepatic transplantation. *Southern Med J* 1987; 80:357–361.

21

Hepatorenal Syndrome: What are the new concepts?

MURRAY EPSTEIN, M.D., F.A.C.P.

Several acute azotemic syndromes occur with increased frequency in patients with hepatic and biliary disease. Although acute azotemia often represents classic acute renal failure (acute tubular necrosis [ATN]), cirrhotic patients may also develop a unique form of renal failure for which a specific cause cannot be elucidated—hepatorenal syndrome (HRS). This chapter will review the management of the hepatorenal syndrome.

Progressive oliguric renal failure commonly complicates the course of patients with advanced hepatic disease.[1-4] This condition has been designated by many names including "functional renal failure" and "the renal failure of cirrhosis," but the more appealing albeit less specific term to describe this syndrome is "hepatorenal syndrome." For the purpose of this discussion, the hepatorenal syndrome may be defined as unexplained renal failure occurring in patients with liver disease in the absence of clinical, laboratory, or anatomical evidence of other known causes of renal failure.

It should be emphasized that when confronted with a patient who has concomitant renal and hepatic disease, the clinician should consider not only HRS, but a number of potentially treatable disorders that simultaneously involve the liver and the kidney. These disorders,

termed "pseudo" hepatorenal syndromes, include toxic, hematologic, neoplastic, genetic, hemodynamic, and infectious processes. The importance of recognizing these disorders lies in the fact that they may be reversible if detected early and treated appropriately.

CLINICAL FEATURES

HRS occurs usually in cirrhotic patients who are alcoholic, although cirrhosis is not a *sine qua non* for the development of HRS. HRS may complicate other liver diseases including acute hepatitis and hepatic malignancy.[5,6] Renal failure may develop with great rapidity, often occurring in patients in whom normal serum creatinine levels have been previously documented within a few days of onset of HRS. Papadakis and Arieff[7] have suggested that the serum creatinine may be a poor index of renal function in patients with chronic liver disease, often masking markedly reduced glomerular filtration rates (GFR). Implicit in such a formulation is the concept that HRS represents a progression in patients who already have markedly impaired renal function.

Numerous reports have emphasized the development of renal failure following events that reduce effective blood volume including abdominal paracentesis, vigorous diuretic therapy, and gastrointestinal bleeding, although it can occur in the absence of an apparent precipitating event. In this context, several careful observers

---

Portions of this chapter are adapted from Epstein M: Hepatorenel syndrome, in Epstein M, (ed): *The Kidney in Liver Disease*, ed 3. Baltimore, Williams & Wilkins, 1988, pp 89–117.

have recently noted that HRS patients seldom arrive in the hospital with preexisting azotemia. Rather, HRS seems to develop in the hospital, suggesting that iatrogenic events might precipitate this syndrome.[1,4]

Virtually all HRS patients have ascites, which is often tense; other clinical stigmata of chronic liver disease and portal hypertension are usually present. The degree of jaundice is extremely variable, and occasionally renal failure may develop at a time when the serum bilirubin concentration is decreasing. Thus, although the majority of reports suggest that HRS occurs in patients who manifest evidence of severe hepatocellular disease, it is quite apparent that HRS can occur with minimal jaundice and with little evidence of severe hepatic dysfunction.[8] There are no apparent clinical, functional, renal, or hepatic laboratory characteristics to identify patients with cirrhosis who will ultimately develop renal failure.

The overwhelming majority of patients with HRS die, and recoveries are sufficiently rare to be considered worthy of reporting.[9] On the other hand, some investigators have reported a higher incidence of spontaneous recovery.[10,11] It should be noted that the mortality of this syndrome may be exaggerated by the very concept holding that survival of an episode of acute azotemia, per se, constitutes evidence that the patient did not have hepatorenal syndrome.

DIAGNOSTIC CONSIDERATIONS

Although measurement of serum creatinine concentration is in general the best of the widely available clinical means of assessing GFR, there is a diagnostic pitfall in the setting of liver disease (i.e., spurious interference of creatinine measurements by a variety of endogenous and exogenous metabolites). Although the interference by bilirubin in the measurement of serum creatinine levels has been recognized in the technical literature for several years,[12,13] most clinicians are unfamiliar with this phenomenon. The magnitude of the error varies with the autoanalyzer used, but the spurious depression can be as much as 57% with some commonly used instruments.[12] Recognition of this laboratory artifact is important because, depending on the instrument used for bilirubin measurement, an increase in serum creatinine could be masked. Conversely, a decrease in serum creatinine could be interpreted as improvement in renal function. It has been suggested, however, that the end point Jaffé method can overcome the interference of bilirubin.[14] In summary, it is clear that changes in serum creatinine concentrations should be interpreted with caution in the presence of extreme hyperbilirubinemia.

HRS patients manifest a rather characteristic urine excretory pattern, voiding urine that is practically sodium-free and retaining the capacity to concentrate urine

TABLE 21–1.
Differential Diagnosis of Acute Azotemia in the Patient with Liver Disease: Important Differential Urinary Findings*

	Prerenal Azotemia	Hepatorenal Syndrome	Acute Renal Failure (ATN)
Urine sodium concentration (mEq/L)	< 10	<10	> 30†
Urine-to-plasma-creatinine ratio	< 30:1	> 30:1	< 20:1
Urine osmolality	At least 100 mOsm > plasma osmolality	At least 100 mOsm > plasma osmolality	Equal to plasma osmolality
Urine sediment	Normal	Unremarkable	Casts, cellular debris

*From Epstein M (ed): *The Kidney in Liver Disease*, ed 3. Baltimore, Williams & Wilkins, 1988, p. 92.
†It has recently been appreciated that radiocontrast agents and sepsis may lower urinary sodium concentration in the patient with ATN.

to a modest degree. As seen in Table 21–1, the biochemical characteristics of the urine in such patients are indistinguishable from those seen in the setting of hypovolemia, which emphasizes the importance of considering hypovolemia in any diagnostic evaluation of azotemia in the setting of liver disease.

PATHOGENESIS

A substantial body of evidence lends strong support to the concept that the renal failure in HRS is functional in nature. Despite the severe derangement of renal function, pathologic abnormalities are minimal and inconsistent.[1, 4] Furthermore, tubular functional integrity is maintained during the renal failure, as manifested by a relatively unimpaired sodium reabsorptive capacity and concentrating ability. Finally, more direct evidence is derived from the demonstration that kidneys transplanted from patients with HRS are capable of resuming normal function in the recipient, and that renal function returns when the patient with HRS successfully receives a liver transplant.[1]

Despite extensive study, the precise pathogenesis of HRS remains obscure. Many studies using diverse hemodynamic techniques have documented a significant reduction in renal perfusion.[15] Because a similar decrement of renal perfusion is compatible with urine volumes exceeding 1 L in many patients with chronic renal failure, it is unlikely that a decrease in mean blood flow per se is responsible for the encountered oliguria.[16]

My laboratory applied the ^{133}Xe washout technique and selective renal arteriography to the study of HRS and demonstrated a significant reduction in calculated mean blood flow and a preferential reduction in cortical perfusion.[15] In addition, cirrhotic patients manifested marked vasomotor instability characterized not only by variability between serial xenon washout studies but also by instability within a single curve.[15] This phenomenon has not been encountered in renal failure of other etiologies. As detailed in a recent review,[1] the mediators of this intense renal vasoconstriction have not been fully defined.

TREATMENT

The initial step in management is not to equate decreased renal function with HRS, but rather to search diligently for and treat correctable causes of azotemia, such as volume contraction, cardiac decompensation, and urinary tract obstruction. The diagnosis of ATN should clearly be considered because ATN occurs commonly in the cirrhotic patient. Furthermore, cirrhotic patients with ATN may be more apt to recover if supported with dialytic therapy than HRS patients.

Although I commonly invoke the caveat of *primum non nocere*, it takes on greater meaning than it had in earlier times. Increasing knowledge of the effects of numerous drugs in the setting of liver disease has now amplified the myriad ways in which such agents may actually induce acute renal failure in the cirrhotic patient (Table 21–2). Thus, it is well established that nonsteroidal anti-inflammatory drugs (NSAID) that inhibit prostaglandin synthetase activity are capable of inducing detrimental effects on renal function in the patient with liver disease and ascites.[17, 18] Similarly, the broad-spectrum antibiotic, demeclocycline, has been shown to be capable of inducing acute azotemia in the patient with cirrhosis and ascites.[19, 20] Finally, we should be cognizant of the fact that drugs that may be indicated for the management of complications of liver disease (e.g., lactulose for

TABLE 21–2.
Drugs and Procedures that Adversely Affect the Patient with Liver Disease and Ascites

Drugs
    Nonsteroidal anti-inflammatory drugs
    Demeclocycline
    Lactulose
Procedures
    Overly vigorous or inordinately rapid diuresis
    Nonjudicious abdominal paracentesis

the treatment of hepatic encephalopathy) are capable of inducing profound hypovolemia with resultant azotemia. Clearly, we are encountering ever-increasing "diseases of medical progress" in the management of the patient with advanced liver disease.

The next step in management is to exclude reversible prerenal azotemia (Table 21–3). Because HRS and prerenal azotemia have similar urinary diagnostic indices, one must often use a functional maneuver (i.e., administration of volume expanders) to differentiate between these two entities. In this regard, it should be underscored that the frame of reference for the cirrhotic patient may be quite different from that of other disease states. The degree of volume expansion necessary to replete the cirrhotic patient may at times be marked, occasionally requiring the infusion of massive amounts of colloids.

It should be pointed out that there is no defined regimen that allows one to approximate the amount of volume expanders necessary to replete the cirrhotic patient suspected of being hypovolemic. Rather, I believe that the expanders should be infused in a setting in which alteration of clinical status (blood pressure, urine flow rate, creatinine clearance) as well as central hemodynamics (central venous pressure [CVP], Swan-Ganz catheter) can be monitored. Furthermore, it should be stressed that the changes in CVP often are important rather than the absolute level (i.e., a CVP reading may not necessarily be extremely low and yet may not change [increase] until large amounts of expanders are administered). Such guidelines do not presuppose that there is a correlation between central hemodynamics and the volume deficit. Rather, I use such manometric determinations as a safety guideline to determine when to discontinue volume expansion to avoid overt fluid overload.

Once the correctable causes of renal functional impairment are excluded, the mainstay of therapy is careful restriction of sodium and fluid intake. A number of specific therapeutic measures have been attempted, but none has proved to be of practical value. Attempts at volume expansion with different exogenous expanders have resulted in only transient improvement in renal hemodynamics and function without significant improvement in the outcome.[1] Similarly, attempts at reinfusion of ascites using peritoneal fluid which has been concentrated have not provided any lasting improvement.

The role of paracentesis in the treatment of HRS, with or without simultaneous plasma volume expansion, remains controversial. The potential renal benefit of a reduction of ascitic fluid volume includes diminished intra-abdominal pressure with possible relief of inferior vena caval obstruction and augmentation of cardiac output. Improvement in renal function, when it occurs, is transient, and because the abnormal hydraulic pressures that sustain ascites formation are not altered by paracentesis, continued fluid removal is necessary and may result in progressive depletion of intravascular volume with subsequent deterioration in cardiac

TABLE 21–3.
Principles of Management of the Patient with Hepatorenal Syndrome*

I. General measures
  A. Try not to make the diagnosis
    1. Attempt to rule out other likely diagnoses
      a) Acute renal failure
      b) Prerenal azotemia
        Use of CVP or Swan-Ganz catheter
        Volume challenge
  B. *Primum non nocere*
II. Specific therapeutic considerations
  A. General
    1. Sodium and fluid restriction
    2. Correct acid–base disturbances
    3. Correct severe anemia
    4. Treat encephalopathy
  B. Ascites reinfusion
  C. Infusion of vasodilators
    1. Acetylcholine
    2. Phentolamine
    3. Prostaglandins A_1 and E
    4. Dopamine
  D. Portacaval shunting
  E. Dialysis
  F. Continuous arteriovenous ultrafiltration (CAVU)
  G. LeVeen (peritoneovenous) shunt
  H. Hepatic transplantation

*From Epstein M (ed): *The Kidney in Liver Disease*, ed 3. Baltimore, Williams & Wilkins, 1988, p. 108.

function and renal perfusion. Nevertheless, a recent report by Arroyo and coworkers[21] suggests that paracentesis may induce a more favorable response than previously thought.

In view of the prominent role assigned to renal cortical ischemia in the pathogenesis of HRS, it is not altogether surprising that there have been numerous attempts to treat HRS with vasodilators.[1] Intrarenal infusion of nonspecific vasodilators, such as acetylcholine and papaverine, improves renal blood flow but does not augment GFR. Similarly, blockade of vasoconstrictor alpha-adrenergic nerves by intrarenal infusion of phentolamine or phenoxybenzamine or stimulation of vasodilator beta-adrenergic nerves with isoproterenol has no significant effect on GFR. Direct stimulation of renal dopaminergic receptors by infusion of nonpressor doses of dopamine produces renal vasodilatation, but again, GFR and urine flow are virtually unaffected despite infusions for as long as 24 hours. A report suggests that dopamine infusion for longer periods provides some increase in urine flow and sodium excretion, but these effects are modest, and the studies were uncontrolled. Infusion of vasodilator prostaglandins to correct a possible renal prostaglandin deficiency has been unrewarding. In summary, although such therapeutic manipulations with vasodilators have occasionally resulted in salutary effects on renal function, the benefits have not been sustained.

Treatment of HRS with Invasive Procedures

Dialytic Techniques

Although dialysis has previously been reported to be ineffective in the management of HRS,[22] it is presently apparent that it may be helpful and is warranted in certain patients[23] (see below).

Peritoneal Dialysis. There are few published data concerning the treatment of HRS with peritoneal dialysis.[24-26] Of a total of 47 patients with fulminant hepatic failure and HRS treated with peritoneal dialysis, there were only four survivors. In patients with cirrhosis, only one of 35 patients survived. Ring-Larsen and coworkers[24] reported 12 patients with cirrhosis and 5 with acute hepatic insufficiency and HRS who were treated with peritoneal dialysis to correct hyponatremia. Several patients had hepatic encephalopathy. Despite correction of the electrolyte abnormalities, all of the patients died within a few days.

Included among the difficulties in instituting peritoneal dialysis in the HRS are (1) coagulopathy requiring surgical rather than percutaneous placement of the catheter, (2) ascites rendering the exchanges less efficient and augmenting protein losses, and (3) insufficient rates of solute clearance.

Hemodialysis and Ultrafiltration. Several investigators have reported that hemodialysis is ineffective in the management of HRS.[23-29] My recent experience, however, suggests that such a condemnation should be qualified. Although most of the published literature indeed suggests a dismal prognosis for patients who are dialyzed, such reports have dealt almost exclusively with patients with chronic end-stage liver disease. My experience and that of others[26] (Table 21-4) suggests that in carefully selected patients (i.e., patients with acute hepatic dysfunction) in whom there is reason to believe that the underlying liver disease may reverse (making long-term survival and even spontaneous recovery of renal function possible), dialytic therapy is indicated. Thus, sporadic case reports describe prolonged survival and improvement in renal function in selected patients with acute, or acute superimposed on chronic, liver disease treated by dialysis alone[30, 31] or combined with other modalities.[32, 33]

Recently, various continuous extracorporeal therapeutic modalities have been applied to select patients.[23] These methods permit an enhanced level of fluid and solute removal in association with hemodynamic stability and have been applied to the sicker, unstable patient with multiple-organ failure. In addition, fluid balance is improved, permitting a higher in-

TABLE 21-4.
Hemodialysis in the Hepatorenal Syndrome
Associated with Chronic Liver Disease*

Author/year	No. patients	Survival
Topchiashuili and Sergienko (1971)	8	2
Klinger and Cronin (1972)	5	2
Wilkinson et al (1977)	5	0
Coratelli et al (1985)	8	0
Ellis and Avner (1986)[†]	12	4

*From Epstein M (ed): *The Kidney in Liver Disease,* ed 3. Baltimore, Williams & Wilkins, 1988, p. 619.
[†]In patients undergoing hepatic transplantation.

take with much less risk of fluid overload. Increased experience with these therapies, as well as greater awareness of their capabilities, has prompted several groups to apply them to the treatment of renal complications associated with liver disease.

Dialysis may also have a role in the treatment of acute renal failure in patients with severe end-stage liver disease awaiting hepatic transplantation.[29] Aside from complicating the medical management, the development of acute renal failure in this setting is associated with considerable morbidity and mortality not improved by dialysis. Nevertheless, in one study, dialytic therapy was helpful in the life support of patients awaiting liver transplantation, and four of seven patients with HRS experienced recovery of renal function 1 to 5 weeks after successful hepatic replacement.[29]

In addition to stabilizing renal function, it is often necessary to mobilize fluid, either to prevent life-threatening emergencies such as acute pulmonary edema or to facilitate administration of requisite fluids such as bicarbonate solutions or hyperalimentation. Although hemodialysis often constitutes the therapeutic modality of choice in effecting such interventions, it is not feasible in many patients with severe liver disease who have associated hemodynamic instability. Unfortunately, patients with decompensated cirrhosis frequently become hypotensive in response to institution of hemodialysis. To circumvent this problem, I have used continuous arteriovenous ultrafiltration (CAVU) as an alternative maneuver in a few patients with hepatorenal syndrome and have been successful in mobilizing fluid without concomitant hemodynamic instability.[34] Additional experience will be required to clarify the role of this approach to managing patients with hepatorenal syndrome.

Role of Dialysis in Patients with Hepatic Coma. Because many patients with HRS are in hepatic coma, dialysis with a large-pore polyacrilonitrile membrane may have a beneficial effect.[35-37] The available studies suggest that removal of toxic middle-sized molecules with this membrane may be responsible for the improvement in mental status and possibly survival noted in some patients. Unfortunately the number of patients with a clearly established diagnosis of HRS was not specified in most reports.

Opolon has summarized his clinical experience with polyacrylonitrile hemodialysis in the treatment of 39 patients with coma due to fulminant hepatic failure.[37] Although there was an overall improvement in neurologic status in 61% of cases, survival was not different from that of untreated patients.

An adjunctive modality for treatment of hepatic coma consists of hemoperfusion through an extracorporeal device filled with activated charcoal or ion-exchange resins.[38-40] Although the initial results appeared to be encouraging, numerous problems were encountered, especially charcoal embolism, thrombocytopenia, and damage to red blood cells. The introduction of polymeric noncoated charcoal with spherical granules and the concomitant use of prostacyclin infusions appear to obviate many of these complications.

Potential Advantages and Disadvantages of Dialysis in Patients with Decompensated Liver Disease (Table 21–5). The possible beneficial effects of dialysis in the setting of hepatorenal syndrome include correction of fluid, electrolyte, and acid–base abnormalities; correction of the platelet defect of uremia; and removal of toxic metabolites that may contribute to hepatic (such as ammonia, mercaptans, amino acids, and octopamine) and/or uremic encephalopathy. Potential disadvantages include dialysis-induced hypotension, increased risk of infection, worsening of coagulopathy, and changes in drug–protein binding.

Dialysis may correct pulmonary edema in patients requiring fluids for the treatment of shock or coagulopathy. In addition, the removal of excess fluid may permit the daily administration of adequate amounts of parenteral nutrition.

It is unlikely that dialysis per se improves the renal perfusion defect associated wtih end-stage liver disease (HRS). A recent study has shown that hemodialysis with a large-pore membrane is capable of removing endotoxin fragments from the bloodstream. Because the etiologic role of endotoxemia in the pathogenesis of the HRS remains controversial and because all the treated patients in the series of Coratelli et al had a fatal outcome (28) we do not anticipate that the benefits of dialytic intervention operate through such a mechanism.

Peritoneovenous Shunts (PVS)

In 1974, LeVeen and associates introduced PVS for the treatment of refractory ascites.[41] Subsequently, these authors reported five long-term survivals in nine patients with HRS treated with PVS. Other reports that followed[42–50] claimed long-term survival rates approaching 40%. Nevertheless, careful scrutiny of the reported cases reveals that the diagnosis of HRS was frequently inadequately documented, and that many of the original cases were included in subsequent series.[51,52] The only clear-cut beneficial results in patients with carefully established HRS were those of Schroeder and co-workers.[45] Four of their five cases treated in this manner experienced long-term survival; nevertheless, all of their patients exhibited creatinine clearances greater than 50 ml/min prior to shunting, suggesting that they were treated at a very early stage of HRS. Of interest, there was no long-term survival in 10 patients with well-established criteria for HRS reported by Smith and co-workers.[50]

Only two prospective randomized studies of the role of the PVS in the treatment of HRS have been performed.[53,54] Linas and co-workers[53] prospectively compared the effects of PVS ($n = 10$) and medical

TABLE 21–5.
Theoretical Advantages and Disadvantages of Dialysis in Combined Renal and Hepatic Failure*

Advantages	Disadvantages
Correction of fluid and electrolyte disturbances	Dialysis-induced hypotension
Improvement in platelet function	Increased risk of infection
Improvement in hepatic coma	Worsening of coagulopathy
Normalization of plasma amino acid levels	Lack of correction of ascites
Facilitated administration of nutritional supplements	Changes in drug–protein binding
Removal of endotoxin fragments	

*From Epstein M (ed): *The Kidney in Liver Disease*, ed 3. Baltimore, Williams & Wilkins, 1988, p. 621.

therapy ($n = 10$) on renal function and mortality in 20 patients with HRS associated with alcoholic liver disease. After 48 to 72 hours, body weight and serum creatinine were increased with medical therapy and decreased (from 3.6 ± 0.4 to 3.0 ± 0.5, $p < 0.05$) in patients with the shunt. Despite improvement of renal function, only one patient with the PVS had a prolonged survival (210 days). In the remainder, survival was 13.0 ± 2.2 days compared to 4.1 ± 0.6 days with medical therapy.

The preliminary results of the VA Cooperative study are also available in abstract form.[54] Although there were seven long-term survivals in a group of 14 patients treated with PVS, the results were not statistically significantly different when compared to those of a group of 19 patients undergoing medical therapy. The mean half-life of patients treated with the shunt did not differ significantly from that of controls. Of note, the group of patients with HRS was carefully selected, and patients with severe complications of chronic liver disease were excluded. From the above information, it can be concluded that the role of PVS in the treatment of HRS has not been established. Although some patients exhibit an improvement in renal function, further controlled studies, with larger numbers of patients, are necessary to assess the effect of PVS on long-term survival, quality of life, and incidence of complications.

Portacaval Shunt

Schroeder and co-workers reported encouraging results in patients with HRS treated with side-to-side portacaval shunts.[45] Unfortunately the results have not been confirmed by others. In addition, the procedure itself is attended by substantial morbidity and mortality. This procedure should be regarded as experimental and not established therapy.[54a]

Hepatic Transplantation

This is the ultimate modality of therapy, which results in correction not only of HRS[55] but also many of the metabolic complications of advanced liver disease. Obviously the procedure is complicated, expensive, and performed in only a few centers around the world. Thus, transplantation does not currently constitute a practical cost-effective approach to managing these patients.

Water Immersion

I am often asked in consultation if water immersion might be tried as a therapeutic maneuver for a patient who has been diagnosed as having HRS. There has been an increasing awareness that the underlying abnormality in patients with decompensated cirrhosis is not solely an excess of total body fluid, but to a greater extent a maldistribution of extracellular fluid. Consequently, much attention has been focused on developing procedures to redistribute body fluids—not only between compartments, as with PVS, but also within the vascular compartment.

Studies from my laboratory have provided substantial evidence that head-out water immersion markedly augments central blood volume.[56-58] To the extent that diminished effective blood volume constitutes a major determinant of renal sodium retention in established liver disease, one might justifiably speculate on the use of water immersion as a means of replenishing the contracted effective volume. Although at first glance such a proposal appear attractive, repeated use of water immersion would be a time-consuming and costly procedure requiring the continuous attendance of paramedical personnel. These clinically fragile patients exposed to the marked hemodynamic alterations that attend immersion require close medical monitoring. Finally, a patient could only reasonably be immersed for a small percentage of the day, and it is unknown if this confers a lasting beneficial effect.

The "chronic" effect of water immersion on central blood volume is unknown. Certainly, water immersion constitutes a powerful and highly productive means of investigating deranged volume homeostasis in many edematous disorders, including cirrhosis. I believe, however, that at

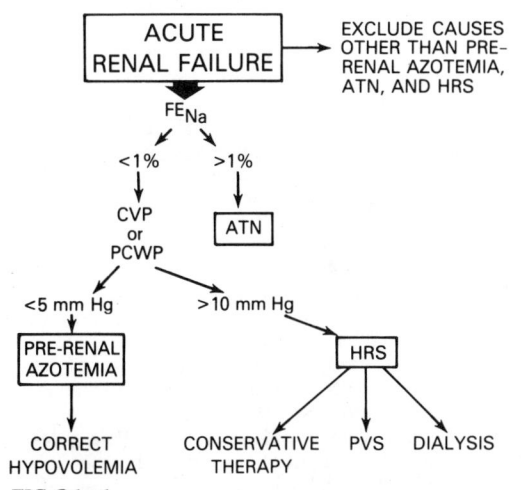

FIG 21–1.
Algorithm for the evaluation and management of a cirrhotic patient with acute renal failure. (From Epstein M (ed): *The Kidney in Liver Disease*, ed 3. Baltimore, Williams & Wilkins, in press.

the present time, pending carefully controlled investigative studies, its application as therapy in managing those patients with decompensated cirrhosis is inappropriate.

In summary, I recommend the following schema for the evaluation and management of acute renal failure in cirrhosis (Fig 21–1). The three important diagnostic considerations are prerenal azotemia, acute tubular necrosis, and HRS. The fractional excretion of sodium (FE_{Na}) or the urinary sodium concentration in a spot urine and the pulmonary capillary wedge pressure (PCWP) or the central venous pressure (CVP) may help to distinguish among these diagnostic possibilities. There is, however, considerable overlap among the three categories, and often patients present with more than one diagnosis. For example, patients with HRS often exhibit acute tubular necrosis, and HRS and prerenal failure often coexist. In fact, the response to colloid infusion is the only feature that helps differentiate the latter two conditions. Of note, because of the low peripheral resistance associated with cirrhosis, volume expansion frequently does not result in a marked increase in CVP or PCWP. Intensive hemodialysis or hemoperfusion is indicated for the management of HRS complicating acute (reversible) liver injury. To avoid systemic hypotension, which often complicates traditional hemodialysis, the clinician might consider continuous extracorporeal therapeutic modalities, which tend to circumvent this problem. In patients with chronic cirrhosis, dialysis may maintain the patient until a suitable liver donor is found. Otherwise, good-risk patients may be treated by PVS.

SUMMARY

In summary, despite considerable progress in the past three decades, there is no comprehensive understanding of the factors that produce the hepatorenal syndrome. Although there has been some progress in characterizing the pathogenesis of this condition, therapy remains largely empirical. The numerous attempts at treating HRS empirically with vasodilators have not resulted in important therapeutic innovations. The failure of many HRS patients to survive despite partial correction of their renal hemodynamic abnormality is a reflection of the precarious state of the patient with liver failure.

It is apparent that any future breakthroughs providing definitive treatment of HRS must be predicated on greater clarification of mechanisms and delineation of mediators. The role of hemodialysis has recently undergone reappraisal, and it is apparent that dialysis may be warranted as a supportive measure in some patients with apparently reversible hepatic failure.

Dialytic techniques have a defined role in the management of renal complications of liver disease. In patients with intractable ascites, ascites reinfusion, dialytic ultrafiltration of ascites, or CAVU may be helpful and may obviate the use of surgical procedures such as PVS. Hemodialysis, preferably with polycrylonitrile membranes, may be warranted in patients with acute, potentially reversible liver disease and hepatic coma or HRS, and in patients with severe chronic liver disease awaiting hepatic transplantation. Particular attention should be given to the dialysis prescription and drug usage in these seriously ill patients.

Acknowledgment

I am indebted to Maria I. Martinez for her expert preparation of this manuscript.

References

1. Epstein M: Hepatorenal syndrome, in Epstein M (ed): *The Kidney in Liver Disease*, ed 3. Baltimore, Williams & Wilkins, 1988, pp. 89–117.
2. Epstein M: Renal functional abnormalities in cirrhosis: Pathophysiology and management, in Zakim D, Boyer TD (eds): *Hepatology. A Textbook of Liver Disease*. Philadelphia, WB Saunders, 1982, pp 446–464.
3. Epstein M: Liver disease, in Massry SG, Glassock RJ (eds): *Textbook of Nephrology*. Baltimore, Williams & Wilkins, 1983, pp 6.304–6.313.
4. Epstein M: Hepatorenal syndrome, in Berk JE (ed): *Bockus Gastroenterology*, ed 4. Philadelphia, WB Saunders, 1985, pp 3138–3149.
5. Ritt DJ, Whelan G, Werner DJ, et al: Acute hepatic necrosis with stupor or coma. *Medicine* 1969; 48:151–172.
6. Vesin P, Roberti A, Viguie RR: Defaillance renale fonctionnelle terminale chez des malades atteints de cancer du foie, primitif ou secondaire. *Sem Hop Paris* 1965; 26:1216–1220.
7. Papadakis M, Arieff AI: Unpredictability of clinical evaluation of renal function in cirrhosis: A prospective study. *Am J Med* 1987; 82:945–952.
8. Epstein M, Oster JR, DeVelasco RE: Hepatorenal syndrome following hemihepatectomy. *Clin Nephrol* 1976; 5:128–133.
9. Goldstein H, Boyle JD: Spontaneous recovery from the hepatorenal syndrome. Report of four cases. *N Engl J Med* 1965; 272:895–898.
10. Reynolds TB: The hepatorenal syndrome, in Schaffner F, Sherlock S, Leevy CM (eds): *The Liver and Its Diseases*. New York, Intercontinental Medical Book Corp, 1974, pp 307–313.
11. Gordon JA, Anderson RJ: Hepatorenal syndrome. *Seminars in Nephrology* 1981; 1:37–41.
12. Halstead AC, Nanji AA: Artefactual lowering of serum creatinine in the presence of hyperbilirubinemia—a method dependent artefact. *JAMA* 1984; 251:38–39.
13. Nanji AA, Halstead AC: Spurious decrease in serum creatinine in patients with hyperbilirubinemia. *Dig Dis Sci* 1982; 27:1051.
14. Daugherty NA, Hammond KB, Osberg IM: Bilirubin interference with the kinetic Jaffé method for serum creatinine. *Clin Chem* 1978; 24:392–393.
15. Epstein M, Berk DP, Hollenberg NK, et al: Renal failure in the patient with cirrhosis. The role of active vasoconstriction. *Am J Med* 1970; 49:175–185.
16. Hollenberg NK, Epstein M, Basch RI, et al: Acute oliguric renal failure in man: Evidence for preferential renal cortical ischemia. *Medicine* 1968; 47:455–474.
17. Boyer TD, Zia P, Reynolds TB: Effect of indomethacin and prostaglandin A_1 on renal function and plasma renin activity in alcoholic liver disease. *Gastroenterology* 1979; 77:215–222.
18. Epstein M: Renal prostaglandins and the control of renal function in liver disease. *Am J Med* 1986; 80 (Suppl 1A):46–55.
19. Oster JR, Epstein M, Ulano HB: Deterioration of renal function with demeclocycline administration. *Curr Ther Res* 1976; 20:794–801.
20. Carrilho F, Bosch J, Arroyo V, et al: Renal failure associated with demeclocycline in cirrhosis. *Ann Intern Med* 1977; 87:195–197.
21. Arroyo V, Gines P, Planas R, et al: Paracentesis in the management of cirrhotics with ascites, in Epstein M (ed): *The Kidney in Liver Disease*, ed 3. Baltimore, Wilkins & Wilkins, 1988, pp. 578–592.
22. Perez GO, Oster JR: A critical review of the role of dialysis in the treatment of liver disease, in Epstein M (ed): *The Kidney in Liver Disease*, ed 1. New York, Elsevier, 1978, pp 325–336.
23. Perez GO, Oster JR, and Epstein M: Role of dialysis and ultrafiltration in the treatment of the renal complications of liver disease, in Epstein M (ed): *The Kidney in Liver Disease*, ed 3. Baltimore, Williams & Wilkins, 1988, pp. 613–624.
24. Ring-Larsen H, Clausen E, Ranek L: Peritoneal dialysis in hyponatremia due to liver failure. *Scand J Gastroenterol* 1973; 8:33–40.
25. Jacobson S, Bell B: Recognition and management of acute and chronic hepatic encephalopathy. *Med Clin North Am* 1973; 57:1569–1577.
26. Wilkinson SP, Weston MJ, Parsons V, et al: Dialysis in the treatment of renal failure in patients with liver disease. *Clin Nephrol* 1977; 8:287–292.
26a. Topchiashuili ZA, Sergienko VS: Hemodialysis in hepatorenal insufficiency. *Khirurgila* 1971; 47:14–16.
27. Klingler EL Jr, Cronin RJ: Renal failure in cirrhosis of the liver: Observations during intermittent hemodialysis (abstract). *Am Soc Artif Intern Organs* 1972; 26.
28. Coratelli P, Passavanti G, Munno I, et al: New trends in hepatorenal syndrome. *Kidney Int* 1985; 17:S143–S147.
29. Ellis D, Avner ED: Renal failure and dialysis therapy in children with hepatic failure in the perioperative period of orthotopic liver transplantation. *Clin Nephrol* 1986; 25:295–303.
30. Strand V, Mayor G, Ristow G, et al: Concomitant renal and hepatic failure treated by polyacrylonitrile membrane hemodialysis. *Int J Artif Organs* 1981; 4:136–139.
31. Keller F, Wagner K, Lenz T, et al: Hemodialysis in "hepatorenal syndrome": Report on two cases. *Gut* 1985; 26:208–211.
32. Kearns PJ, Polhemus RJ, Oakes D, et al: Hepatorenal syndrome managed with hemodialysis then reversed by peritoneovenous shunting. *J Clin Gastroenterol* 1985; 7:341–343.
33. Landini S, Coli U, Lucatello S, et al: Plasma-ex-

change and dialysis. Combined treatment in acute renal insufficiency secondary to severe hepatopathies. *Minerva Nefrol* 1981; 28:179–186.
34. Epstein M, Perez GO, Bedoya LA, et al: Continuous arteriovenous ultrafiltration in cirrhotic patients with ascites or renal failure. *Int J Artif Organs* 1986; 9:253–256.
35. Opolon P, Rapin JR, Huguet C, et al: Hepatic failure coma (HFC) treated by polyacrylonitrile membrane (PAN) and hemodialysis (HD). *Trans Am Soc Artif Intern Organs* 1976; 22:701–710.
36. Silk DBA, Williams R: Experiences in the treatment of fulminant hepatic failure by conservative therapy, charcoal hemoperfusion and polyacrylonitrile hemodialysis. *Int J Artif Organs* 1978; 1:29–33.
37. Opolon P: Large pore hemodialysis in fulminant hepatic failure, in Brunner G, Schmidt FW (eds): *Artificial Liver Support*. Berlin, Springer Verlag, 1981, pp 141–146.
38. Gazzard BG, Weston MJ, Murray-Lyon IM, et al: Charcoal hemoperfusion in the treatment of fulminant hepatic failure. *Lancet* 1974; i:1301–1307.
39. Gelfand MC, Knepshield JM, Cohan S, et al: Treatment of hepatic coma with hemoperfusion through polyacrilamide hydrogen-coated charcoal. *Kidney Int* 1976; (suppl 7):S239–S243.
40. Chang T, Ming S: Hemoperfusion alone and in series with ultrafiltration or dialysis for uremia, poisoning, and liver failure. *Kidney Int* 1976; 10:305–311.
41. LeVeen HH, Christoudias G, Luft R, et al: Peritoneovenous shunting for ascites. *Ann Surg* 1974; 180:580–590.
42. LeVeen HH, Wapnick S, Grosberg S: Further experience with peritoneovenous shunt for ascites. *Am Surg* 1976; 184:574–581.
43. Grosberg SJ, Wapnick S: A retrospective comparison of functional renal failure in cirrhosis treated by conventional therapy or the peritoneovenous shunt (LeVeen). *Am J Med Sci* 1978; 276:287–291.
44. Fullen WD: Hepatorenal syndrome: Reversal by peritoneovenous shunt. *Surgery* 1977; 82:337–341.
45. Schroeder ET, Anderson GH, Smulyan H: Effects of a portacaval or peritoneovenous shunt on renin in the hepatorenal syndrome. *Kidney Int* 1979; 15:54–61.
46. Kinney MJ, Schneider A, Wapnick S, et al: The hepatorenal syndrome and refractory ascites: Successful therapy with the LeVeen-type peritoneal-venous shunt and valve. *Nephron* 1979; 23:228–232.
47. Greig PD, Blendis LM, Langer B: Renal and hemodynamic effects of the peritoneovenous shunt. II. Long-term effects. *Gastroenterology* 1981; 80:119–125.
48. Schwartz ML, Vogel SB: Treatment of hepatorenal syndrome. *Am J Surg* 1980; 139:370–373.
49. Bernhoft RA, Pellegrini CA, Way LW: Peritoneovenous shunting for refractory ascites. *Arch Surg* 1982; 117:631–635.
50. Smith RE, Nostrant TT, Eckhauser FE, et al: Patient selection and survival after peritoneovenous shunting for nonmalignant ascites. *Am J Gastroenterol* 1984; 79:659–662.
51. Epstein M: The peritoneovenous shunt in the management of ascites and the hepatorenal syndrome. *Gastroenterology* 1982; 82:790–799.
52. Epstein M: The LeVeen shunt for ascites and hepatorenal syndrome. *N Engl J Med* 1980; 302:628–630.
53. Linas SL, Schaefer JW, Moore EE, et al: Peritoneovenous shunt in the management of the hepatorenal syndrome. *Kidney Int* 1986; 30:736–740.
54. Stanley MM and Members of VA Cooperative Study #142: Peritoneovenous shunting vs medical treatment of alcoholic cirrhotic ascites. *Hepatology* 1985; 5:980.
54a. Epstein M: Role of the peritoneovenous shunt in the management of ascites and the hepatorenal syndrome, in Epstein M (ed): *The Kidney in Liver Disease*, ed 3. Baltimore, Williams & Wilkins, 1988.
55. Iwatsuki S, Popovtzer MM, Corman JL, et al: Recovery from "hepatorenal syndrome" after orthotopic liver transplantation. *N Engl J Med* 1973; 289:1155–1159.
56. Epstein M: Renal effects of head-out water immersion in man: Implications for an understanding of volume homeostasis. *Physiol Rev* 1978; 58:529–581.
57. Levinson R, Epstein M, Sackner MA, et al: Comparison of the effects of water immersion and saline infusion on central hemodynamics in man. *Clin Sci Mol Med* 1977; 52:343–350.
58. Epstein M, Larios O, and Johnson G: Effects of water immersion on plasma datecholamines in decompensated cirrhosis. *Mineral Electrolyte Metab* 11:25–34, 1985.

22

Hepatitis Immunization: Who? When?

RICHARD S. PHILLIPS, M.D., F.A.C.P., F.A.C.G.
K. RAJENDER REDDY, M.D., F.A.C.P.

The commonly known viruses that cause hepatitis are type A, type B, non-A, non-B, and Delta agent. Infrequently other viruses, mainly cytomegalovirus and Epstein-Barr virus, can cause hepatitis. The clinical spectrum associated with viral hepatitis includes the anicteric presentation, carrier state (particularly with hepatitis B virus), chronic hepatitis, fulminant or subfulminant hepatic failure, and finally cirrhosis. The treatment of these conditions is often limited and frustrating. Type A hepatitis often has a benign course, and prophylactic measures using immune serum globulin are highly successful; vaccines at this time are not commercially available. Hepatitis B viral infection continues to be a major public health problem worldwide with a high prevalence rate in the Far East and among Alaskan Eskimos, Pacific Islanders, sub-Saharan Africans, and among the population of intravenous drug users, hemodialysis patients, homosexuals, and hemophiliacs in the United States. This disease is associated with serious consequences such as chronic hepatitis, cirrhosis, and hepatocellular carcinoma. Currently, although several antiviral and immunomodulatory drugs are being evaluated, there is none that has unequivocally proven beneficial in controlling or clearing the viral infection. Immunoprophylactic measures against hepatitis B infection can be effective. Postexposure prophylaxis with hepatitis B immunoglobulin is protective and highly immunogenic, and safe hepatitis B vaccines have been marketed and offer the best chance of interrupting the transmission of this infection. Our knowledge of non-A, non-B hepatitis is limited because of the failure to identify the causative agent and specific serologic markers. This has impaired the development of any definitive form of immunoprophylaxis.

VIRAL HEPATITIS A

Viral hepatitis A is not new to mankind. Reports of outbreaks of epidemic jaundice, which we presume to be hepatitis A, have been ascribed to Hippocrates in ancient Greece and to writing from B.C. Babylonia. There have been numerous accounts of epidemic jaundice during the American Civil War, the Franco-Prussian War, World War I, and World War II. Yet the agent responsible for this illness was not successfully identified until 1973 when Feinstone and associates first visualized hepatitis A viral particles by immune electron microscopy in the feces of patients acutely infected with hepatitis A.[1] More recently, propagation of hepatitis A virus in cell cultures and molecular cloning of hepatitis A viral genome have further enhanced our understanding of the nature and character of this virus.[2,3]

The hepatitis A virus is a 27-mm RNA agent with characteristics of the picornavirus family.[4] Most hepatitis A viral infections are self-limited and less than 1 month in duration.[5-7] Complications are exceedingly rare and include fulminant disease (1 to 8 per 1,000), cholestasis, and relapsing infections.[7-11] Fortunately, chronic carriage of virus and chronic hepatic disease is not believed to be a sequela of this illness, nor is it thought to have any association with hepatocellular carcinoma.[12,13]

The diagnosis of hepatitis A is now easily made by detecting circulating antibody to hepatitis A virus (anti-HAV) in the bloodstream of infected individuals. The initial antibody response is composed of IgM anti-HAV and confirms the diagnosis of acute hepatitis A. The IgM anti-HAV response, which is typically short-lived, reaches peak titer levels within the first 3 weeks and declines progressively thereafter.[14] By 4 to 5 months, fewer than 50% will have detectable titer levels.[15] During the recovery phase of the illness, IgG anti-HAV becomes the predominant antibody, reaching peak levels within 3 to 12 months.[13] The detection of IgG anti-HAV denotes previous hepatitis A virus infection as well as immunity to reinfections with the virus. The detection of IgG anti-HAV has also been quite helpful in studying the prevalence of past infections in various subpopulations.[16,17] Surveys in major U.S. cities have demonstrated that approximately 40% to 70% of the adult population have antibodies to hepatitis A.[17] Contact transmission by the fecal–oral route represents the major mode of spread of hepatitis A.[13,18,19] Studies have demonstrated that the virus is shedded in large numbers in the stool for approximately 2 weeks before and 1 to 2 weeks after the onset of clinical hepatitis and jaundice.[20] Thus, the likelihood of transmission from an infected individual is before a diagnosis of hepatitis has been established. Person-to-person transmission most often is limited to close contacts within the household. This is particularly true in areas of poor sanitation and crowding. Young children (not toilet-trained) in preschool day-care centers are frequently implicated as transmitters of this enteric infection, not only among themselves but among staff and family as well.[21-23] Sexual transmission of hepatitis A virus is another important mode of spread among homosexual men engaging in oral–anal contact.[24,25] A recent study showed a 22% annual seroconversion rate for hepatitis A virus among its homosexual male population.[25] Contamination of food or water by an infected person is occasionally a source of transmission. Neither perinatal nor transplacental transmission has been reported,[26] and percutaneous or transfusion-related transmission is believed to be quite rare.[27]

Immune Serum Globulin (ISG)

Immune serum globulins (ISG) are sterile, colorless, slightly opalescent solutions of antibodies from human plasma, obtained from outdated donor blood and from fresh plasma collected from commercial donors who undergo plasmapheresis. Each production pool usuallly includes plasma from thousands of donors, the majority of which consists of the immunoglobulin of the IgG class. Although there are no specific federal requirements for ISG to contain a minimum titer of antibody against hepatitis A virus, studies indicate their presence in most ISG preparations. Recently, Hoofnagle and Waggoner investigated the hepatitis A antibody status of ISG preparations.[28] They measured hepatitis A viral antibody titers in 62 lots of ISG prepared by four different U.S. manufacturers between 1962 and 1977. Their results showed that the hepatitis A viral titers in immune serum globulin were quite stable and had not changed over the 15-year period studied. The geometric mean titer was approximately 1 to 1,000 with a range of 1 to 500 and 1 to 4,000. Although the minimum effective titer of anti-HAV needed for prophylaxis still needs to be better defined, titers reported from this study were found to be quite comparable to those lots of ISG that were effective in previous clinical trials in the prevention of hepatitis A.[28,29]

Adverse reactions to ISG are uncommon and generally consist of pain or tenderness at the injection site.[30,31] Although anaphylactic shock and angioneurotic edema have been reported, these are generally limited to intravenous administration and not intramuscular injections.[32] ISG has not been demonstrated to be contaminated with antibody to the human immunodeficiency virus (HIV), and there have been no reported cases of AIDS in recipients of ISG.[33]

Passive Immunization—Postexposure (Table 22–1)

The first efforts at prevention of viral hepatitis A date back to the summer of 1944 when Stokes and Neefe first evaluated the efficacy of immune serum globulin.[34] Their study was conducted at a summer camp in the Pocono Mountains of Pennsylvania during an extensive outbreak of "infectious" viral hepatitis. ISG was administered to 53 campers and counselors. The remainder of the camp was not innoculated. Follow-up showed that those individuals who had received the globulin innoculation had a significantly lower incidence of contracting icteric hepatitis. The positive protective effect of ISG was also supported in two other clinical trials conducted that same year involving military personnel and institutionalized children.[35,36] Additional studies from the United States, England, and New Zealand have confirmed immune serum globulin to be 80% to 90% effective in reducing clinically recognizable hepatitis A.[37–39]

Rates of icteric hepatitis among children contacts within the infected household have been reported as high as 45%, while among adults somewhat less at 5% to 20%.[13] Comparable secondary attack rates are found within institutional settings, such as prisons, army camps, psychiatric wards, homes for the mentally retarded, and foster homes of refugee children. Day-care centers also represent an important source of hepatitis A in many communities. Hadler and associates reported that 40% of over a thousand reported cases of hepatitis A in Phoenix occurred in persons closely associated with day-care centers.[21] Williams and co-workers, summarizing ten outbreaks reported to the Centers for Disease Control (CDC) over a 10-year period, noted that hepatitis A spread among day-care children was usually asymptomatic, while the household contacts of these preschool children accounted for the majority of icteric

TABLE 22–1.
Recommendations for Immune Serum Globulin Prophylaxis for Hepatitis A*

Circumstance	Dose	Frequency
Pre-exposure		
Travel or residence in underdeveloped areas		
Residence for 3 months or less	0.02 ml/kg	Once
Residence for 4 months or more	0.06 ml/kg	Once every 4–6 months
Workers with nonhuman primates	0.06 ml/kg	Once every 4–6 months
Travel to or residence in highly developed countries	Not recommended	
Positive screening IgG anti-HAV	Not recommended	
Postexposure		
Close personal contacts (household, prisons, day-care centers, institutions)	0.02 ml/kg	Once within 2 weeks of episode
Common vehicle exposure		
Co-foodhandlers	0.02 ml/kg	Once
Patrons	0.02 ml/kg	Once within 2 weeks of direct exposure
Casual contacts (school, office, hospital, factory)	Not recommended unless overt epidemic	

*From Recommendations for protection against viral hepatitis. MMWR 1985; 34:313–316.

cases.[40] Similar observations were also reported by Storch and associates while investigating eleven outbreaks occurring over 1 year in the New Orleans area.[22] It is in these three circumstances that the U.S. Public Health Service recommends administration of ISG prophylactically.[41] For the more casual contacts occurring in such places as the classroom, offices, or factories where hepatitis A is frequently transmitted, routine prophylaxis is not generally recommended.[41]

The doses of immune serum globulin used during the three initial investigations in 1944 were arbitrarily chosen and were quite large (0.16 to 0.3 ml/kg).[34-36] Because of the high cost, limited national supply and the discomfort when such doses were given intramuscularly, a series of investigations were undertaken to define a lower effective dose. Over the ensuing years, progressively lower doses were found to be effective. Stokes and associates showed that a dose of 0.02 ml/kg was equally effective in reducing the incidence of overt hepatitis.[42] Subsequent trials showed that even a lower dose of 0.01 ml/kg could provide adequate protection.[43, 44] Only one study found low-dose immune serum globulin to be less effective than higher doses in prevention of overt hepatitis.[45] However, in retrospect, it is recognized that many of the cases of overt hepatitis in this series were types B and non-A, non-B hepatitis. The U.S. Public Health Service currently recommends a single intramuscular dose of 0.02 ml/kg of immune serum globulin for postexposure prophylaxis.[41]

The timing of immune serum globulin administration also plays an important role in evaluating the efficacy of passive immunization. It has been generally regarded that the closer in time the ISG is given to the initial exposure, the greater its protective ability. Mosley and associates showed that ISG administered to household contacts within 2 weeks of exposure was able to prevent clinical hepatitis in 87% of those innoculated.[46] Variability of the incubation period among infected individuals makes 100% protection an unrealistic goal. It is the present view of the Advisory Committee on Immunization Practices that immune serum globulin be given as soon as possible after exposure, and not be recommended more than 2 weeks after exposure.[41]

Passive Immunization—Pre-Exposure (Table 22-1)

Once postexposure immunoprophylaxis with ISG became firmly established, systematic administration of ISG soon became advocated for pre-exposure use as well. This has been specifically directed toward two high-risk groups: travelers to developing countries where, as a result of substandard sanitation, viral hepatitis A exists in endemic proportions; and personnel who care for nonhuman primates in whom high secondary attack rates of hepatitis A have been reported.[47, 48]

Data collected from the U.S. Armed Forces, Peace Corps, and American missionaries have provided the core of experience with ISG prophylaxis for persons living in endemic regions of the world.[35, 49-52] These studies clearly demonstrated significantly lower attack rates among innoculated individuals. Woodson and Clinton observed that most cases of icteric hepatitis in Peace Corp volunteers occurred following the sixteenth week after administration of ISG.[49] Furthermore, Krugman observed cases of icteric hepatitis in institutionalized retarded children 6 months after receiving ISG.[6] These studies illustrated that the protective effect of ISG is limited to 4 to 6 months, and to achieve more effective prophylaxis, ISG needs to be administered at shorter intervals. Two studies have demonstrated a relatively low risk for viral hepatitis A in short-term travelers.[53, 54] The U.S. Public Health Service currently recommends 0.02 ml/kg of ISG be given to those who stay abroad for less than 3 months, while larger doses of 0.06 ml/kg be administered every 4 to 6 months to anyone who remains in an endemic region for longer periods.[41] Travelers to developed countries and those individuals detected to have IgG anti-HAV require no immunoprophylaxis.

Active Immunization

Currently, there is no vaccine available to prevent type A hepatitis. However, research efforts are underway to develop live attenuated, inactivated vaccines using recombinant techniques and synthetic peptide sequences. The role for such vaccines would be limited for several reasons. Motivation for mass vaccination may not be high because the disease is often of a benign nature, with no progression to chronicity. Additionally, type A hepatitis is mainly a problem of the developing countries where the cost of the vaccine is a serious consideration.

VIRAL HEPATITIS B

Since the discovery, approximately two decades ago, of the "Australia antigen," now called the hepatitis B surface antigen (HbsAg), considerable progress has been made in the fields of molecular biology, virology, immunology, and epidemiology to help us better understand the multiple ramifications of this common infection. It is estimated that there are approximately 215 million hepatitis B virus carriers worldwide and over 75% of these live in Asian countries.[55] Considering that the world population is approximately 4 billion, the carrier rate of hepatitis B virus can be estimated at around 5% or more, which would clearly qualify it as a major public health problem.

The carrier rate in the United States is 0.1% to 0.3% among the general population; however, in high-risk populations such as hemophiliacs, dialysis patients, homosexuals, and intravenous drug abusers, the prevalence has been reported to vary from 5% to 7%.[56] The CDC has estimated the incidence of HBV infection in the United States at over 300,000 cases per year.[57]

Hepatitis B virus is a double-shelled DNA virus belonging to the hepadnavirus class of animal viruses. The infectious complete virus (Dane particle) is 42 nm in diameter and has an outer coating of hepatitis B surface antigen (HbsAg) and an inner component of hepatitis B core antigen (HbcAg). The inner core has a single molecule of circular, partially double-stranded DNA and an endogenous DNA polymerase. In addition to the Dane particle, the serum of an HBV-infected patient has an abundance of immunogenic but non-infectious 16 to 25-nm HbsAg particles circulating in the form of spheres and tubules. The sequelae of HBV infection are multiple and include an acute infection often leading to complete recovery, a chronic carrier state, chronic hepatitis, cirrhosis, and hepatocellular carcinoma. The serologic markers that are detected following hepatitis B infection are dependent on the duration (acute or chronic), and the clearance of the infection (immunity). A full discussion of the entire serologic patterns along with the significance of their titers in acute, chronic, and resolved infection is beyond the scope of this chapter. In simpler terms, the serologic markers of acute B infection are hepatitis B surface antigen (HbsAg) and antibody to hepatitis B core antigen of the IgM type (anti-HbcIgM). A chronically infected patient has a positive HbsAg and anti-Hbc which is often not of the IgM type. Hepatitis B viral DNA (HBV DNA), DNA polymerase and HbeAg, a protein fraction of hepatitis B core antigen, are markers of active viral replication and denote high infectivity. A person who has recovered from hepatitis B infection has a negative hepatitis B surface antigen (HbsAg) and one or both antibodies to HbsAg (anti-Hbs) and HbcAg (anti-Hbc).

The modes of transmission of hepatitis B are by perinatal, parenteral, and sexual routes. The most significant route is maternal–infant transmission. This is a major occurrence in endemic areas in Asia and Africa. The likelihood of infection is high if the mother develops acute hepatitis during pregnancy or was HbeAg positive. Tong and associates have noted a 71% chance of the infant becoming HbsAg positive if the mother developed acute hepatitis in the third trimester of pregnancy.[58] In Japan, maternal–infant transmission of the HbsAg has been observed to range from 60% to 100% in HbeAg-positive mothers as compared to 0% to 8% in

TABLE 22–2.
Persons at Increased Risk for Hepatitis B*

Health-care workers with frequent contact with blood
Clients and staff of institutions for the mentally retarded—biting and scratching prevalent
Hemodialysis patients
Homosexually active men
Abusers of illicit injected drugs
Recipients of certain blood products. Clotting factor concentrate
Household and sexual contacts of carriers
Other contacts of carriers. Contacts of deinstitutionalized mentally retarded carriers who behave aggressively
Special high risk populations: Alaskan Eskimos, Pacific Islanders, immigrants and refugees from eastern Asia, Haiti,[61] and Sub-Sahara Africa
Inmates of long-term correctional facilities
Heterosexually active persons with multiple sexual contacts
International travelers planning to reside in areas with high levels of endemic viral B hepatitis

*From Recommendations for protection against viral hepatitis. MMWR 1985; 34:313–316.

HbeAg-negative mothers.[59] Over 90% of infections occur perinatally and in utero transmission is noted in the minority of cases. Presently the Centers for Disease Control recommends only prenatal screening for mothers who are considered to be at high risk for hepatitis B[41, 60] (Table 22–2). However when these criteria were evaluated at a large county hospital, approximately half the hepatitis B surface antigen-positive mothers did not fulfill them and therefore would have escaped screening.[61]

In 1977, Mario Rizzetto identified delta virus (HDV agent) in Italian carriers of HbsAg.[62] The delta virus is a defective RNA virus that is smaller than most conventional viruses and requires hepatitis B virus to replicate and express itself. Therefore, delta infection is seen only in patients with hepatitis B infection because the viral encapsidation is with hepatitis B surface antigen. HDV is highly infectious and has a worldwide distribution. Groups at risk for HBV infection are also susceptible to HDV infection. However it has been noted predominantly in intravenous drug abusers,[63] and perinatal transmission of HDV has not been observed to occur as readily as HBV infection alone. Three types of clinical presentation can be seen in HBV/HDV infection: simultaneous acute B and acute delta infection, acute delta superimposed on chronic hepatitis B infection, and chronic delta infection in a patient with chronic hepatitis B infection. A simultaneous acute B and acute delta infection, as compared to HBV infection alone, is more likely to lead to fulminant hepatic failure; the mortality, among age-matched patients, does not appear to be different from fulminant hepatic failure due to hepatitis B virus alone.[64] A superinfection in carriers of HBV is ominous and has a propensity to progress onto chronic HDV.[65] Furthermore, chronic delta infection is more likely to aggravate the underlying histologic lesion of chronic hepatitis and accelerate the clinical course of underlying HBV-related liver disease.[65, 66] Presently, the only serologic marker of HDV available commercially is anti-HDV. A definitive diagnosis of HDV infection and a distinction between an acute and chronic HDV infection can be made by immunohistochemical identification of delta antigen in the liver, IgM and IgG anti-HD in serum by RIA or EIA, delta antigen and HDV RNA in the serum which at the present time are only available in research centers.

Pre-exposure Prophylaxis (Table 22–3)

Currently two types of hepatitis B vaccines proven to be highly immuno-

TABLE 22–3.
Recommendations for Passive–Active Immunoprophylaxis of Hepatitis B*

Circumstance	Previously Vaccinated Individual	Unvaccinated Individual

HbsAg(+) source
Percutaneous needle stick, transmucosal entry, splash into mouth, eye
	• Test exposed individual for anti-Hbs
	• If titer > 10 mIU/ml—no treatment
	• If titer > 10 mIU/ml and vaccination is incomplete—complete vaccine series
	• If titer < 10 mIU/ml, give HBIG 0.06 ml/kg and
	  a. Booster dose of vaccine
	  b. Incomplete vaccination—complete series
	• Known nonresponder: HBIG 0.06 ml/kg once, repeat vaccine series
		• Test exposed individual for anti-Hbs
		• HBIG 0.06 ml/kg immediately
		• Initiate and complete vaccine series if protective antibody is negative
		• If anti-Hbs < 10 mIU/ml on tested sera and if individual refuses vaccine, repeat HBIG 0.06 ml/kg 1 month from first dose

HbsAg status of source unknown
High risk
	• Test source for HbsAg if exposed individual is known vaccine nonresponder.
	• If source HbsAg(+) give exposed person
	  a. HBIG 0.06 ml/kg once
	  b. Vaccine booster dose
		• Initiate hepatitis B vaccine series
		• Test source for HbsAg and individual for anti HBS
		• If source HbsAg(+) and individual has anti-Hbs < 10, give HBIG 0.06 ml/kg

Low risk	As above	As above
Sexual exposure to acute hepatitis B	• 0.06 ml/kg HBIG along with vaccine series if protective antibody is negative	
Perinatal	• 0.5 ml HBIG along with vaccine series Test child for HbsAg and anti-Hbs 1 year later to determine if prophylaxis is effective	

*Data from Recommendations for protection against viral hepatitis. *MMWR* 1985; 34:313–316; and Koff RS, Galambos JT: Viral hepatitis, in Schiff L, Schiff ER (eds): *Diseases of the Liver*, ed 6. Philadelphia, JB Lippincott, 1987.

genic, safe, and protective are commercially available. After extensive clinical trials,[67, 68] a plasma-derived vaccine was licensed in 1982 and a recombinant DNA vaccine[69] was licensed in 1986. Several groups of individuals (Table 22-2) are at risk of contracting hepatitis B and should be recommended for active immunization with the hepatitis B vaccine.

Since the introduction of the plasma-derived vaccine in 1982, several issues, such as its safety, immunogenicity and efficacy among various populations, duration of protection, appropriate screening tests, reason for nonresponsiveness, and costs and strategies, have been raised. The plasma-derived vaccine is treated with pepsin, 8M urea, and formalin which inactivate all viruses including non-A, non-B hepatitis agent(s), parvoviruses, slow viruses, and retroviruses, including HIV. The yeast-produced recombinant vaccine has a plasmid containing the gene for the hepatitis B surface antigen. It undergoes steps of sterile filtration and formalin treatment and is in a nonglycosylated form, unlike the plasma-derived HbsAg which is 25% glycosylated.[57] The recombinant DNA vaccine has more than 95% HbsAg protein.[57] Both hepatitis B vaccines are highly immunogenic and protective in immunocompetent individuals, and this has been repeatedly demonstrated by several studies.[67-69] In immunoincompetent patients, such as those on hemodialysis, an immunogenic response has been poor even with higher than normal doses of the vaccine.[70] The responsiveness to hepatitis B vaccine is lowered further in renal transplant and oncology patients.[71] The duration of protection from a single series of hepatitis B vaccine is unclear. Currently available studies indicate that the majority of individuals have detectable anti-Hbs beyond 36 months,[72] and these individuals, along with the minority who have lost their anti-Hbs, have an anamnestic response to a single booster dose of 20 µg of the hepatitis B vaccine.[73] Based on current observations, there is general agreement that revaccination should be done every 5 years in individuals with a good initial immunogenic response.[57] Genetic factors have been implicated in nonresponsiveness; a higher frequency of DR alleles DR7 and DR3 has been observed in these individuals.[74] Freezing is ill-advised because it destroys the immunogenicity of the vaccine.[57] Furthermore, gluteal muscle injection is linked to a poor response, and therefore it is recommended that the vaccine be given in the deltoid muscle in adults and anterolateral thigh muscle in neonates or infants.[57] Combined passive-active immunization with HBIG and hepatitis B vaccine has been observed neither to limit the immune response to the vaccine nor to cause immune-complex phenomenon and injury.[58, 75, 76] Controversy exists regarding the appropriate screening tests and the populations to be screened. In high-risk groups, such as homosexuals, with an HbsAg carrier rate of 5% to 7%, anti-Hbc would be the appropriate test because this would eliminate the large number of HbsAg carriers and individuals with acquired immunity from previous exposure to HBV and thereby spare vaccination. In populations with a lower carrier rate, such as health-care workers, anti-Hbs is a reasonable screening test to determine previous exposure. An antibody level greater than 10 mIU/ml of anti-Hbs (approximately equal to ten sample ratio units) is necessary to be protective.[57] Postvaccination testing for anti-Hbs at 6 months after completion of the series is recommended to document seroconversion and also to estimate the titer because the duration of persistence of antibody is directly related to the peak response after the vaccine series.[77]

Unfortunately, despite evidence for the high safety of the vaccines, the use of the plasma-derived hepatitis B vaccine has only been modest. The reasons for the less than expected use of plasma-derived vaccine are: slow implementation of vaccine programs by the hospitals, mainly smaller ones of fewer than 100 beds[57]; high cost of the vaccination; and poor compliance partly related to the unfounded fear of HIV infection.[78] Furthermore, the focus of its use is mainly in health-care personnel, hemodialysis patients, and staff and residents of institutions for the mentally retarded who constitute less than 10% of cases of hepatitis B. The majority of cases of hepatitis occur in homosexual men, intravenous drug abusers, and by heterosexual exposure, and vaccination programs have not effectively reached these groups. Furthermore, up to 30% of individuals with hepatitis B infection offer no history identifying them in any high-risk group.[57] The cost of the vaccination has been a major concern, particularly in the highly endemic developing countries. A low-dose (2 µg) intradermal vaccine regimen has been evaluated and noted to have similar immunogenic response as standard vaccination.[79] This study involved a small group of health workers; further larger studies are necessary to clarify issues such as frequency and rapidity of seroconversion and degree and persistence of antibody response, especially among high-risk immunoincompetent patients. Until vaccination strategies are devised to reach all high-risk group populations, the vaccine is made more affordable, and the compliance rate improves in areas where programs are established, the incidence of hepatitis B will continue to be high and probably will rise.

Postexposure Prophylaxis (Table 22–3)

There is little argument that antibody to HbsAg (anti-Hbs) is the neutralizing antibody and offers protection against hepatitis B infection. These antibodies can be acquired after recovery from hepatitis B infection, passively transmitted with injection of immune serum globulin (ISG) or hyperimmune hepatitis B immune globulin (HBIG), or develop as a response to active vaccination. The titer of anti-HBs in HBIG, however, is often in excess of 1:100,000 as compared to ISG which, on an average among various lots, has a titer of 1:500.[80] The three major clinical situations in which postexposure prophylaxis is used are perinatal exposure, needlestick or permucosal exposure, and sexual exposure to an index case of acute hepatitis B. Passive–active immunization with HBIG and hepatitis B vaccine is highly effective in interrupting maternal–fetal transmission with reported efficacy of greater than 85%.[75, 76] Although at the present time the CDC does not recommend that all pregnant mothers be screened for HBsAg, based on our observations and those of others, it would be cost-effective to screen all pregnant mothers and institute appropriate immunoprophylaxis.[61,81] Recommendations for postexposure prophylaxis in cases of needle exposure and sexual contacts are less well established and somewhat controversial. Controlled clinical studies have shown that passive immunization with HBIG to needle stick exposure and sexual contact of a HbsAg-positive case offers protection in approximately 75% of cases.[82–84]

Currently no passive and active immunoprophylactic measures are available to prevent delta infection. However, it can be prevented by immunoprophylaxis directed against hepatitis B infection.

The recommendations of the Immunization Practices Advisory Committee are summarized in Table 22–3. (Other modifications are also indicated.)

NON-A, NON-B VIRAL HEPATITIS

Non-A, non-B viral hepatitis first became accepted as a possible third etiologic cause of viral hepatitis in humans more than 10 years ago. This was accomplished only after highly sensitive and specific techniques for serologic identification of hepatitis A and B virus were developed.

Although much has been learned about non-A, non-B hepatitis, extensive investigative efforts have failed to identify and characterize this agent. Seto and co-workers suggested that the non-A, non-B hepatitis agent could be related to a retrovirus when they detected reverse transcriptase activity in human non-A, non-B sera.[85] Unfortunately, these results have not been confirmed by other laboratories. Further doubt has been cast by filtration studies which show this virus to be too small to be consistent with the larger retroviruses.[86] Not only the characterization of the non-A, non-B agent is unsettled, but also the actual number of potential viruses associated with non-A, non-B hepatitis. What once was thought to be only a single virus transmitted solely by blood transfusions has now been expanded to include at least two viruses with many epidemiologic similarities to the hepatitis B virus. To add to the frustration of investigators, endemic and enterically transmitted non-A, non-B hepatitis has been reported in India, Pakistan, South East Asia, the Soviet Union, and Mexico.[87-91]

Therefore, it is clear that our overall knowledge of non-A, non-B hepatitis is still quite limited and evolving. Unfortunately, until specific serologic markers for this disease are developed or until the causative agent is identified, much of our information will continue to be derived by inference. This has retarded the development for any definitive form of immunoprophylaxis, including the development of a vaccine. Nevertheless, efforts are being made toward prevention of non-A, non-B hepatitis. Most interest in prophylaxis of hepatitis non-A, non-B has focused on transfusion-associated hepatitis.

TRANSFUSION-ASSOCIATED HEPATITIS

Hepatitis following blood transfusions was first described in 1943.[92,93] Since that time, viral hepatitis has become recognized as the most serious post-transfusion complication and is considered a major public health problem in the United States.[94] With the advent of highly sensitive third generation immunoassays for screening hepatitis B surface antigen in potential blood donors, it has become apparent that the principal agent in transfusion-associated hepatitis is a non-A, non-B virus.[95,96] In fact, multiple studies have shown that non-A, non-B virus attributes to over 90% of the cases of transfusion-associated hepatitis.[97] With attacks occurring in up to 10% of multitransfused patients with volunteer blood, it is estimated that 200,000 to 300,000 cases occur in the United States each year.

Overall, the clinical features are quite similar to those of hepatitis B. However, acute non-A, non-B hepatitis tends to be a somewhat milder disease.[97-101] Patients are generally less symptomatic, have lower peak serum transaminase activity, and are more often anicteric as jaundice develops in only 25% of cases. Less often, the hepatitis will be severe enough to require acute hospitalization. Fulminant disease, although reported, is considered a rare occurrence.[100]

The most significant consequence of non-A, non-B hepatitis is the high percentage of chronic sequelae that occur with this disease. In a review of 17 studies of transfusion-associated hepatitis, Dienstag noted alanine aminotransferase (ALT) elevations in 10% to 70% of patients who were followed for 6 months or more.[100] In ten of these studies, chronic transaminase elevations were appreciated in over 50% of the patients.[100] Approximately 40% of chronic non-A, non-B hepatitis patients had chronic active hepatitis, and as many as 20% had cirrhosis either on initial or repeat biopsy.[101-103] To further illustrate the significant long-term consequences of this disease, Alter and Dienstag have presented the following scenario. Assuming that 5% to 10% of multitransfused individuals will develop an acute non-A, non-B hepatitis, and that approximately 50% will progress into chronic hepatitis, of whom 20% will ultimately develop cirrhosis, it can be estimated that as many as 1% of all multitransfused patients will eventually develop cirrhosis.[104] Based on these calculations, because approximately 3 million patients are transfused each year in the United States, cirrhosis could be anticipated in up to 30,000 of these individuals. These figures, in fact, may even underestimate the actual incidence of ensuing cirrhosis. Many recipients of multitransfusions may die from the morbidity of the underlying situation or, in the case of the elderly, from natural causes before liver involvement can progress into a cirrhotic state.

Thus it is clear that non-A, non-B transfusion-associated hepatitis is more than just a benign transaminasemia. The chronic sequela of this disease is appreciable and can be associated with significant morbidity and mortality. What should be done to prevent and treat this disease is a problem facing all physicians and transfusion recipients. There is no effective therapy[104-106] except for recent encouraging results noted with the use of alpha$_2$ interferon.[107] Therefore, prevention is very important. Unfortunately, our abilities to prevent this disease are limited by the unavailability of specific viral markers which could identify infected blood products prior to transfusion. Nevertheless, surrogate markers have been proposed to detect potential non-A, non-B carriers, and a number of studies and clinical reports using immune globulin[108-119] or hepatitis B immune globulin[120, 121] in the prevention of transfusion-associated hepatitis have been published.

Immune Serum Globulin (ISG)

ISG was first evaluated for prevention of transfusion-associated hepatitis (possibly B and non-A, non-B) by Grossman and his associates in 1945.[108] Their patients were U.S. Army soldiers who had received multiple blood transfusions after battle casualties. Grossman administered two 10-ml injections of ISG to alternate soldiers and demonstrated a significant reduction in the incidence of hepatitis in the ISG-treated group.

This study set the stage for other trials investigating ISG in the prophylaxis of transfusion-associated hepatitis. Of the 12 subsequent large-scale trials conducted,[108-119] significant discrepancies in the results have created much controversy. Seven studies have noted a positive effect of ISG,[108, 110, 111, 113-115, 119] while five studies have shown no beneficial effects.[109, 112, 116-118] A positive response to ISG was either a reduction in the incidence of transfusion-associated hepatitis or a decrease in severity of the disease.

It is not entirely clear why results of these studies differed, but it is perhaps related to the multitude of differences in study designs as well as the criteria used to diagnose hepatitis. The different investigators used different routes, amounts, and timing of administration of ISG. Furthermore, different ISG products, which may have varied in antibody titer levels, were used. The average volume of blood transfused to each of the patients varied, as did the type of blood units and even tests to screen potential blood donors. Many of the trials involved cardiac surgical patients who had received large quantities of blood. It has been suggested by Seeff and Hoofnagle that in many of these patients, passively transferred antibody may have been washed out.[122] Finally, and importantly, all but three trials were conducted before serologic tests for hepatitis A and B were available.[110, 118, 119]

The first of these trials was conducted in 11 Veterans Administration hospitals during a 49-month period, beginning in early 1969.[110] In this double-blind, randomized study, 1094 out of a total of 2204 patients received ISG given in 10-ml injections within 96 hours of the initial transfusion and approximately 1 month later. Greater than 50% of these patients received at least one unit of blood from commercial blood banks. Although there was a significantly reduced incidence of icteric non-B hepatitis among recipients of ISG, no difference was appreciated in the overall incidence of hepatitis. ISG did not significantly alter the incubation period, duration, and severity of the disease. Perhaps their most important observation was the extraordinarily high risk factor accompanying the use of commercial blood products.

Shortly after the Veterans Administration Cooperative trials were begun, Kuhns and his associates began their own controlled trial of passive immunization for prevention of post-transfusion hepatitis.[118] One hundred and ninety-five patients who had cardiovascular surgery and had received large quantities of blood in the perioperative period were randomly assigned to a control group or were administered two 10-ml vials of ISG, which did not appear to reduce the incidence of post-transfusion hepatitis. However, Kuhns did note the severity of the disease among the ISG recipients to be somewhat less severe, although the differences were not felt to be statistically significant.

The most recent large-scale study of the

effect of ISG on the incidence of post-transfusion hepatitis was conducted by Knodell and his associates from the Walter Reed and Letterman Army Medical Centers.[119] Their patients all had received multiple units of blood during cardiac surgery. Preoperatively, each patient was randomized to receive either 10 ml of ISG, hepatitis B immune globulin (HBIG), or albumin placebo, and was followed periodically for 9 months. Both gamma globulin preparations were equally effective and were significantly better than the albumin placebo in reducing the frequency of hepatitis. Furthermore, preoperative gamma globulin prophylaxis significantly reduced the progression to chronic liver disease in those who had acquired acute non-A, non-B post-transfusion hepatitis.[123]

Despite the favorable evidence from Knodell's trial in reducing the incidence of non-A, non-B hepatitis, and thereby its progression to chronic hepatitis, the use of ISG is not routinely recommended for prophylaxis of transfusion-associated non-A, non-B hepatitis. Further trials confirming these observations are needed prior to recommending it for routine use.

Hepatitis B Immune Globulin (HBIG)

HBIG has been used as well as ISG in attempts to prevent non-A, non-B transfusion-associated hepatitis. This was first assessed on hemodialysis patients by Nicole Simon in the late 1970s and early 1980s.[120] In the 3-year study, patients were randomly allocated to either a control group or to a treatment group which received injections of 5 ml of the HBIG intramuscularly. Non-A, non-B hepatitis was noted to occur in only 3% of 67 patients who received HBIG, compared to 37% of the 83 in the control group. Unfortunately, this prophylactic effect was a transient one, as the attack rate among the treated patients once off HBIG became similar to controls.

In contrast to this study was a randomly controlled trial of intravenous HBIG administered preoperatively and immediately postoperatively involving over 400 cardiac surgery patients.[121] Although a trend toward lower frequency of non-A, non-B hepatitis in the HBIG-treated patient group was noted, these differences were statistically insignificant. Therefore, from the limited studies available at the present time, HBIG cannot be recommended for routine prophylaxis against post-transfusion, non-A, non-B hepatitis.

Use of Surrogate Markers

Because ISG and HBIG cannot be recommended for routine prophylaxis of non-A, non-B transfusion-associated hepatitis, we have begun to depend on the use of surrogate markers to help identify viral carriers among blood donors. Two major studies—a multicenter transfusion-transmitted virus study and a National Institutes of Health (NIH) study—have proposed two surrogate markers to detect non-A, non-B virus carriers—SGPT (ALT) and hepatitis-B core antibody.[124, 125] These two independent studies, which together provided data on more than 8000 donors and 1500 recipients, showed a significant correlation between donor ALT levels and the incidence of non-A, non-B hepatitis in transfusion recipients. Both studies predict that routine screening of donor blood for elevated ALT levels could prevent almost 30% of the transfusion-related hepatitis at the expense of losing 1.5% to 3% of the donor population.

More recently, the data from these two original studies have been further analyzed to access the potential use of testing hepatitis-B core antibody in blood donors.[126, 127] Both showed a significant association between hepatitis B core antibody-positive donor blood units and recipient non-A, non-B hepatitis. Calculation of the maximal corrected efficacy predicted that exclusion of hepatitis B core antibody-positive donors may have prevented as many as 43% of non-A, non-B hepatitis in the NIH trial, while possibly preventing 33% of cases in the Transfusion-Transmitted Viruses Study (TTVS) multicenter study. The most plausible explanation for this association, between donor hepatitis B core antibody and recipient non-A, non-B hepatitis, is probably related to the strong epidemiologic similarities of the two viruses (i.e., if a person is exposed to one, the likelihood is that there has been some exposure to the other virus as well).[126] A major disadvantage of hepatitis B core antibody screening to prevent transmission of non-A, non-B hepatitis is the high prevalence of this marker in the donor population. If hepatitis B core antibody screening were instituted, as many as 4% to 6% of donor units would have to be eliminated.[126, 127] This represents almost twice as many donor units discarded from screening ALT elevations. Combined screening with hepatitis B core antibody and ALT would certainly increase the sensitivity for detecting potential carriers of non-A, non-B hepatitis but would further increase the number of donor units discarded to around 7.5%.[126]

Debate continues as to whether blood banks should routinely screen all potential donors for one or both of these surrogate markers. The New York City blood bank was the first major facility to begin routine screening of ALT. Several other blood banks have also begun routine screening.

At the present time, no specific guidelines can be recommended for the prevention of non-A, non-B transfusion-associated hepatitis. Nevertheless, we still advocate administration of ISG to certain patient populations with an unequivocal strong likelihood of receiving multiple transfusions. This is particularly true in coronary bypass patients. In these people, we give 10 ml of ISG prior to surgery and then 1 month later. Although this measure may help some, this is certainly not the answer to this difficult problem. Unfortunately, until a specific non-A, non-B agent is identified, we must depend, in the interim, on non-specific measures, such as using autologous blood for elective surgery, avoiding single unit transfusions, using blood products only when absolutely necessary, minimizing the volume of blood transfusions or blood products, identifying donors with known infection, and using surrogate markers for screening.

References

1. Feinstone SM, Kapikian AZ, Purcell RH: Hepatitis A: Detection by immune electron microscopy of a viruslike antigen associated with acute illness. Science 1973; 182:1026–1028.
2. Provost PJ, Hilleman MR: Propagation of human hepatitis A virus in cell culture in vitro. Proc Soc Exp Biol Med 1979; 160:213–221.
3. Ticehurst JR, Racaniello VR, Baroudy BM, et al: Molecular cloning and characterization of hepatitis A virus CDNA. Proc Natl Acad Sci USA 1983; 80:5885–5889.
4. Provost PJ: Biophysical and biochemical properties of CR 326 human hepatitis A virus. Am J Med Sci 1975; 287:87.
5. Routenberg JA, Dienstag JL, Harrison WO, et al: Foodborne outbreak of hepatitis A: Clinical and laboratory features of acute and protracted illness. Am J Med Sci 1979; 278:123–137.
6. Krugman S, Ward R, Giles JP: The natural history of infectious hepatitis. Am J Med 1962; 32:717–728.
7. Misch AM, Gust ID: Clinical, serologic and epidemiologic aspects of hepatitis A viral infection. Semin Liver Dis 1986; 6:42–45.
8. Gust ID: The epidemiology of viral hepatitis, in Vyos GN, Dienstag JH, Hoofnagle JH (eds): Viral Hepatitis and Liver Disease. Orlando FL, Grune & Stratton, 1984, p 415.
9. Gust ID: Viral hepatitis, in Warren KS, Mahmoud AAF (eds): Tropical and Geographical Medicine. New York, McGraw Hill, 1984, pp 572–588.
10. Gordon SC, Reddy KR, Schiff L, et al: Prolonged intrahepatic cholestasis secondary to acute hepatitis A. Ann Intern Med 1984; 101:635–637.
11. Jacobson IM, Nath BJ, Dienstag JL: Relapsing viral hepatitis type A. J Med Virol 1985; 16:163.
12. Lemon SM: Type A viral hepatitis—new developments in an old disease. N Engl J Med 1985; 313:1059–1067.
13. Koff RS, Galambos JT: Viral hepatitis, in Schiff L, Schiff ER (eds): Diseases of the Liver. Philadelphia, JB Lippincott, 1986, pp 457–581.
14. Flehmig B: A solid-phase radioimmunoassay for detection of IgM antibodies to hepatitis A virus. J Infect Dis 1979; 140:169.
15. Hatzakis A, et al: Sex-related differences in immunoglobulin and in total antibody response to hepatitis A virus observed in two epidemics of hepatitis A. Am J Epidemiology 1984; 120:936.
16. Maynard JE, et al: Preliminary serologic studies of antibody to hepatitis A virus in populations in the U.S. J Infect Dis 1976; 134:528–530.
17. Szmuness W, et al: Distribution of antibody to

hepatitis A antigen in urban adult populations. N Engl J Med 1976; 295:755–759.
18. Mosley JW, Speers JF, Chin TDY: Epidemiologic studies of a large urban outbreak of infectious hepatitis. Am J Public Health 1963; 53:1603.
19. Capps RB, Bennett AM, Stokes J Jr: Endemic infectious hepatitis in an infants' orphanage. Epidemiologic studies in student nurses. Arch Intern Med 1952; 89:6.
20. Dienstag JL, et al: Fecal shedding of hepatitis A antigen. Lancet 1975; 1:765.
21. Hadler SC, Webster HM, Erben JJ, et al: Hepatitis A in day-care centers: A community-wide assessment. N Engl J Med 1980; 302:1222–1227.
22. Storch G, McFarland LM, Kelso K, et al: Viral hepatitis associated with day-care centers. JAMA 1979; 242:1514–1518.
23. Benenson MW, Takafuji ET, Bancroft WH, et al: A military community outbreak of hepatitis type A related to transmission in a child care facility. Am J Epidemiol 1980; 112:471–481.
24. Christenson B, Brostrom C, Bottiger M, et al: An epidemic outbreak of hepatitis A among homosexual men in Stockholm: Hepatitis A, a special hazard for the male homosexual subpopulation in Sweden. Am J Epidemiol 1982; 116:599–607.
25. Corey L, Holmes KK: Sexual transmission of hepatitis A in homosexual men: Incidence and mechanism. N Engl J Med 1980; 302:435–438.
26. Tong MJ, Thursby M, Rakela J, et al: Studies on the maternal–infant transmission of viruses which cause acute hepatitis. Gastroenterology 1981; 80:999–1004.
27. Hollinger FB, Kahn NC, Oefinger PE, et al: Post-transfusion hepatitis type A. JAMA 1983; 250:2313–2317.
28. Hoofnagle JH, Waggoner JG: Hepatitis A and B virus markers in immune serum globulin. Gastroenterology 1980; 78:259.
29. Hall WT, et al: Protective effect of immune serum globulin against hepatitis A infection in a national epidemic. Am J Epidemiol 1977; 106:72.
30. Seiff LB, Hoofnagle JH: Immunoprophylaxis of viral hepatitis. Gastroenterology 1979; 77:161–182.
31. Risk of post-transfusion hepatitis in the United States. A prospective cooperative study. JAMA 1972; 220:692–701.
32. Baybutt JE: Hypersensitivity to gamma globulin. JAMA 1959; 171:415–416.
33. Centers for Disease Control: Provisional public health service inter-agency recommendations for screening donated blood and plasma for antibody to the virus causing acquired immunodeficiency syndrome. MMWR 1985; 34:1.
34. Stokes J Jr, Neefe, J: The prevention and attenuation of infectious hepatitis by gamma globulin. JAMA 1945; 127:144–145.
35. Gellis SS, Stokes J Jr, Brother GM, et al: The use of human immune serum globulin in infectious hepatitis in the Mediterranean Theater of Operations. JAMA 1945; 128:1062–1063.
36. Havens WP Jr, Paul JR: Prevention of infectious hepatitis with gamma globulin. JAMA 1945; 129:270–272.
37. Landrigan PJ, et al: The protective efficacy of immune serum globulin in hepatitis A: A statistical approach. JAMA 1971; 223:74.
38. Andrews DA: Immunoglobulin prophylaxis of infectious hepatitis. NZ Med J 1971; 73:199.
39. Assessment of British gamma globulin in preventing infectious hepatitis: A report to the Director of the Public Health Laboratory Service. Br Med J 1968; 3:451.
40. Williams SU, Huff JC, Bryan JA: Hepatitis A and facilities for preschool children. J Infect Dis 1975; 131:491–494.
41. Recommendations for protection against viral hepatitis. MMWR 1985; 34:313–316.
42. Stokes J Jr, Farquhar JA, Drake ME, et al: Infectious hepatitis: Length of protection by immune serum globulin during epidemics. JAMA 1951; 147:714.
43. Drake ME, Ming C: Gamma globulin in epidemic hepatitis: Comparative value of two dosage levels approximately near minimum effective level. JAMA 1954; 155:1302.
44. Arch RD, Elsea WR, Lyerly J, et al: Efficacy of varied doses of gamma globulin during an epidemic of infectious hepatitis, Hoonah, Alaska, 1961. Am J Public Health 1963; 53:1623.
45. Krugman S, Ward R, Giles JP, et al: Infectious hepatitis. Studies on the effect of gamma globulin and on the incidence of inapparent infection. JAMA 1960; 174:823–830.
46. Mosely JW, Reisler DM, Brachott D, et al: Comparison of two lots of immune serum globulin for prophylaxis of infectious hepatitis. Am J Epidemiol 1968; 87:539.
47. Pattison CP, Maynard JE, Bryan JS: Subhuman primate hepatitis. J Infect Dis 1975; 132:478–480.
48. Hepatitis A in humans associated with non-human primates—Ohio. MMWR 1973; 22(49):407–408.
49. Woodson RD, Clinton JS: Hepatitis prophylaxis abroad. Effectiveness of immune serum globulin in protecting Peace Corps volunteers. JAMA 1969; 209:1053–1058.
50. Cline AL, et al: Viral hepatitis among American missionaries abroad: A preliminary study. JAMA 1967; 199:551.
51. Frome JD: Hepatitis among missionaries in Ethiopia and Sudan. Susceptibles at high risk. JAMA 1967; 203:389–392.
52. Woodson RD, Cahill KM: Viral hepatitis abroad. Incidence in Catholic missionaries. JAMA 1972; 219:1191–1193.
53. Kendrick MA: Study of illness among Americans returning from international travel, July 11–August 24, 1971. J Infect Dis 1972; 126:684.
54. Kendrick MA: Summary of study on illness among Americans visiting Europe, March 31, 1969–March 30, 1970. J Infect Dis 1972; 126:685.
55. Scientific group on viral hepatitis B and its related liver disease. Report to the Manila, World Health Organization Regional Office for the Western Pacific, 1982.
56. Hoofnagle JH, Alter HJ: Chronic viral hepatitis

and liver disease, in Vyas GN, Dienstag JL, Hoofnagle JH (Eds): *Viral Hepatitis and Liver Disease*. Orlando, FL, Grune & Stratton, 1984.
57. Update on hepatitis B prevention. Recommendations of the Immunization Practices Advisory Committee. Centers for Disease Control, Department of Health and Human Services, Atlanta, Georgia. *Ann Intern Med* 1987; 107:353–357.
58. Tong MJ, Nair PB, Thursby M, et al: Prevention of hepatitis B infection by hepatitis B immune globulin in infants born to mothers with acute hepatitis during pregnancy. *Gastroenterology* 1985; 89:160–164.
59. Nishioka K: Predominant mode of transmission of hepatitis B virus: Perinatal transmission in Asia, in Vyas GN, Dienstag JL, Hoofnagle JH (eds): *Viral Hepatitis and Liver Disease*. Orlando, FL, Grune & Stratton, 1984.
60. Schiff E: Immunoprophylaxis of viral hepatitis. A practical guide. *Am J Gastroenterol* 1987; 82:287–291.
61. Jonas MM, Schiff ER, O'Sullivan MJ: Failure of Centers for Disease Control criteria to identify hepatitis B infection in a large municipal obstetrical population. *Ann Intern Med* 1987; 107:335–337.
62. Rizzetto M, Canese MG, Arico S, et al: Immunofluoresence detection of a new antigen–antibody system (delta/anti-delta) associated with hepatitis B virus in liver and serum of HbsAg carriers. *Gut* 1977; 18:997–1003.
63. DeCock KM, Govindarajan S, Chin KP, et al: Delta hepatitis in the Los Angeles area: A report of 126 cases. *Ann Intern Med* 1986; 105:108–114.
64. Govindarajan S, Chin KP, Redeker AG, et al: Fulminant B viral hepatitis: Role of delta agent. *Gastroenterology* 1984; 86:1417–1420.
65. Smedile A, Dentico P, Zaretti A, et al: Infection with the HBV-associated delta (d) agent in HbsAg carriers. *Gastroenterology* 1981; 81:992–997.
66. Rizzetto M, Verme G, Recchia S, et al: Chronic HbsAg hepatitis with intrahepatic expression of delta antigen. An active and progressive disease unresponsive to immunosuppressive treatment. *Ann Intern Med* 1983; 98:437–441.
67. Szmuness W, Stevens CE, Howley ES, et al: Hepatitis B vaccine: Demonstration of efficacy in a controlled clinical trial in a high-risk population in the United States. *N Engl J Med* 1980; 303:834.
68. Szmuness W, Stevens CE, Zang EA, et al: A controlled clinical trial of the efficacy of the hepatitis B vaccine (Hepatovax B): A final report. *Hepatology* 1981; 1:377.
69. Emini EA, Ellis RW, Miller WJ, et al: Production and immunological analysis of recombinant hepatitis B vaccine. *J Infect* 1986; 13(Suppl. A):3–9.
70. Stevens CE, Alter JH, Taylor PE, et al: Hepatitis B vaccine in patients receiving hemodialysis: Immunogenicity and efficacy. *N Engl J Med* 1984; 311:496–501.
71. Dienstag JL: Hepatitis B vaccines. AASLD postgraduate course. Hepatology uptake-portal hypertension; viral hepatitis, pp. 256–269, 1986.
72. Stevens CE, Taylor PE, Tong MJ, et al: Hepatitis B vaccine: An overview, in Vyas GN, Dienstag JL, Hoofnagle JH (eds): *Viral Hepatitis and Liver Disease*. Orlando, FL, Grune & Stratton, 1986, pp 275–291.
73. McLean AA, Buynack EB, Kuter BJ, et al: Clinical experience with hepatitis B vaccine, in Millman I, Eisenstein TK, Blumberg BS (eds): *Hepatitis B: The Virus, the Disease and the Vaccine*. New York, Plenum, 1984, pp 149–159.
74. Craven DE, Anden ZL, Kunches LM, et al: Nonresponsiveness to hepatitis B vaccine in health care workers. Results of revaccination and genetic typings. *Ann Intern Med* 1986; 105:356–360.
75. Beasley RP, Hwang LY, Lee GCY, et al: Prevention of perinatally transmitted hepatitis B virus infections with hepatitis B immune globulin and hepatitis B vaccine. *Lancet* 1983; ii:2099–2102.
76. Stevens CE, Toy P, Tong MJ, et al: Perinatal hepatitis B virus transmission in the United States: Prevention by passive–active immunization. *JAMA* 1985; 253:1740–1745.
77. Jilg W, Schmidt M, Dienhardt F, et al: Hepatitis B vaccination: How long does protection last? (letter). *Lancet* 1984; 2:458.
78. Poiesz B, Tomar R, Lehr B, et al: Hepatitis B vaccine: Evidence confirming lack of AIDS transmission. *MMWR* 1984; 33:685–687.
79. Redfield RR, Innis BL, Scoff RM, et al: Clinical evaluation of low-dose intradermally administered hepatitis B virus vaccine. *JAMA* 1985; 254:3202–3206.
80. Koff RS, Galambos JT: Viral hepatitis, in Schiff L, Schiff ER (eds): *Diseases of the Liver*, ed 6, Philadelphia, JB Lippincott, 1987.
81. Arevalo JA, Washington AE: Cost-effectiveness of prenatal screening and immunization for hepatitis B virus. *JAMA* 1988; 259:365–369.
82. Grady GF, Lee VA, Prince AM, et al: Hepatitis B immune globulin for accidental exposure among medical personnel: Final report of a multicenter controlled trial. *J Infect Dis*, 1978; 138:625.
83. Seeff LB, Wright EC, Zimmerman HJ, et al: Type B hepatitis after needle-stick exposure: Prevention with hepatitis B immune globulin. *Ann Intern Med* 1978; 88:285.
84. Redeker AG, Mosley JW, Gocke DJ, et al: Hepatitis B immune globulin as a prophylactic measure for spouses exposed to acute type B hepatitis. *N Engl J Med* 1976; 294:728.
85. Seto B, Coleman WG Jr, Iwarson S, et al: Detection of revese transcriptase activity in association with non-A, non-B hepatitis agent(s). *Lancet* 1984; 2:941–943.
86. Bradley DW, Maynard JE: Etiology and natural history of post-transfusion and enterically transmitted non-A, non-B hepatitis. *Semin Liver Dis* 1986; 6:56–63.
87. Wong DC, Purcell RH, Screenivasan MA, et al:

Epidemic and endemic hepatitis in India: Evidence for a non-A, non-B hepatitis virus etiology. *Lancet* 1980; 2:876–879.
88. Khuroo MS: Study of an epidemic of non-A, non-B hepatitis: Possibility of another human hepatitis virus distinct from post-transfusion non-A, non-B type. *Am J Med* 1980; 68:818–824.
89. Balayan MS, Andjaparidze AG, Savinskaya SS, et al: Evidence of a virus in non-A, non-B hepatitis transmitted via the fecal–oral route. *Intervirology* 1983; 20:23–31.
90. Maynard JE: Epidemic non-A, non-B hepatitis. *Semin Liver Dis* 1984; 4:336–339.
91. Enterically transmitted non-A, non-B hepatitis—Mexico. *MMWR* 1987; 36:597–602.
92. Morgan HV, Williamson DAJ: Jaundice following administration of human blood products. *Br Med J* 1943; 1:750–753.
93. Beeson PB: Jaundice occurring one to four months after transfusion of blood or plasma: Report of seven cases. *JAMA* 1943; 121:1332–1334.
94. Chalmers TC, Koff RS, Grady GF: A note on fatality in serum hepatitis. *Gastroenterology* 1965; 49:22–26.
95. Feinstone SM, Kapikian AZ, Purcell RH, et al: Transfusion associated hepatitis not due to viral hepatitis type A or B. *N Engl J Med* 1975; 292:767–770.
96. Dienstag JL, Feinstone SM, Purcell RH, et al: Non-A, non-B post-transfusion hepatitis. *Lancet* 1977; 1:560–567.
97. Alter HJ, Purcell RH, Holland PV, et al: Clinical and serological analysis of transfusion-associated hepatitis. *Lancet* 1975; 2:838–841.
98. Aach RD, Kahn RA: Post-transfusion hepatitis: Current perspectives. *Ann Intern Med* 1980; 92:539–546.
99. Aach RD, Londer JJ, Sherman LA, et al: Transfusion-transmitted viruses: Interim analysis of hepatitis among transfused and non-transfused patients, in Vyas GN, Cohen SN, Sepmed R (eds): *Viral Hepatitis*. Philadelphia, Franklin Institute Press, 1978; pp 383–396.
100. Dienstag JL: Non-A, non-B hepatitis I. Recognition, epidemiology, and clinical features. *Gastroenterology* 1983; 85:439–452.
101. Koretz RL, Stone O, Gitnick G: The long-term course of non-A, non-B post-transfusion hepatitis. *Gastroenterology* 1980; 79:893–898.
102. Alter HJ, Hoofnagle JH: Non-A, non-B: Observations on the first decade, in Vyas GN, Dienstag JL, Hoofnagle HJ (eds): *Viral Hepatitis and Liver Disease*. Orlando, FL, Grune & Stratton, 1984; pp 345–354.
103. Realdi G, Alberti A, Rugge M, et al: Long-term follow-up of acute and chronic non-A, non-B post-transfusion hepatitis: Evidence of progression to liver cirrhosis. *Gut* 1982; 23: 270–275.
104. Dienstag JL, Alter HJ: Non-A, non-B hepatitis: Evolving epidemiologic and clinical perspective. *Semin Liver Dis* 1986; 6:67–81.
105. Hoofnagle JH: Chronic hepatitis: The role of corticosteroids, in Szmuness W, Alter HJ, Maynard JE (eds): *Viral Hepatitis: 1981 International Symposium*. Philadelphia, Franklin Institute Press, 1982, pp 573–583.
106. Pappas SC, Hoofnagle JH, Young N, et al: Treatment of chronic non-A, non-B hepatitis with acyclovir: Pilot study. *J Med Virol* 1985; 15:1–9.
107. Hoofnagle JH, Mullen KD, Jones DB, et al: Treatment of chronic non-A, non-B hepatitis with recombinant human alpha-interferon. *N Engl J Med* 1986; 315:1575–1578.
108. Grossman EB, Stewart SG, Stokes J Jr: Post-transfusion hepatitis in battle casualties. *JAMA* 1945; 129:991–994.
109. Risk of post-transfusion hepatitis in the United States. A prospective cooperative study. *JAMA* 1972; 220:692–701.
110. Seeff LB, Zimmerman HJ, Wright EL, et al: A randomized double-blind, controlled trial of the efficacy of immune serum globulin for the prevention of post-transfusion hepatitis. A VA Co-op study. *Gastroenterology* 1977; 72:111–121.
111. Katz R, Rodriguez R, Ward R: Post-transfusion hepatitis—Effect of modified gamma globulin added to blood in vitro. *N Engl J Med* 1971; 285:925–932.
112. Duncan GG, Christian HA, Stokes J Jr, et al: An evaluation of immune serum globulin as a prophylactic agent against homologous serum hepatitis. *Am J Med Sci* 1947; 213:53–57.
113. Csapo J, Budai J, Bartos A, et al: Prevention of transfusion hepatitis. *Acta Paedriatr Med Sci Hubg Y* 1963; 4:195–198.
114. Mirick GS, Ward R, McCallum RW: Modification of post-transfusion hepatitis by gamma globulin. *N Engl J Med* 1965; 273:59–65.
115. Creutzfeldt W, Severldt HJ, Brachmann H, et al: Untersuchungen zur prophylaxe der transfusion hepatitis durch gamma globulin. *Dtsch Med Wochenschr* 1966; 91:1905–1908.
116. Holland PV, Rubinson RM, Morrow AG, et al: Gammaglobulin in the prophylaxis post-transfusion hepatitis. *JAMA* 1966; 196:471–474.
117. Spellberg MA, Berman PM: The incidence of post-transfusion hepatitis and the lack of efficacy of gamma globulin in its prevention. *Am J Gastroenterol* 1971; 55:564–574.
118. Kuhns WJ, Prince AM, Brotman B, et al: A clinical and laboratory evaluation of immune serum globulin from donors with a history of hepatitis: Attempted prevention of post-transfusion hepatitis. *Am J Med Sci* 1976; 272:255–261.
119. Knodell RG, Conrad ME, Gingsberg AL, et al: Efficacy of prophylactic gammaglobulin in preventing non-A, non-B post-transfusion hepatitis. *Lancet* 1976; 1:557–561.
120. Simon N: Prevention of non-A, non-B hepatitis in haemodialysis patients by hepatitis B immunoglobulin. *Lancet* 1984; 2:1047.
121. Sugg V, Schneider W, Hoffmaster HE, et al: Hepatitis B immune globulin to prevent non-A, non-B post-transfusion hepatitis. *Lancet* 1985; 1:405–406.
122. Seef LB, Hoofnagle JH: Immunoprophylaxis of viral hepatitis. *Gastroenterology* 1979; 77:161–182.

123. Knodell RG, Conrad ME, Ishak KG: Development of chronic liver disease after acute non-A, non-B post-transfusion hepatitis. Role of gamma globulin prophylaxis in its prevention. *Gastroenterology* 1977; 72:902–909.
124. Aach RO, Szmuness W, Mosley JW, et al: Serum alanine aminotransferase of donors in relation to the risk of non-A, non-B hepatitis in recipients. The transfusion transmitted virus study. *New Engl J Med* 1981; 304:889–993.
125. Alter HJ, Purcell RH, Holland PV, et al: Donor transaminase and recipient hepatitis. *JAMA* 1981; 246:630–634.
126. Stevens CE, Aach RO, Hollinger B, et al: Hepatitis B virus antibody in blood donors and the occurrence of non-A, non-B hepatitis in transfusion recipients. An analysis of the transfusion-transmitted viruses study. *Ann Intern Med* 1984; 101:733–738.
127. Koziol DE, Holland PV, Alling DW et al: Antibody to hepatitis B core antigen. A paradoxical marker for non-A, non-B hepatitis agents in donated blood. *Ann Intern Med* 1986; 104:488–495.

V
Biliary Tract

23

Gallstones:
Dissolution? Fracture? Removal?

HANS FROMM, M.D.
MAURO MALAVOLTI, M.D.

BACKGROUND

Prevalence and Epidemiology

Gallstones are very common. Various epidemiologic and clinical studies suggest that approximately 10% of the general population in North America and Europe is afflicted by this condition.[1,2] Gallstones are about twice as common in females as in males. Their prevalence increases with age. While only approximately 2.1% of men and 2.9% of women have gallstones at the age of 25, these figures increase to about 11% and 27%, respectively at the age of 55.[1]

Two major classes of gallstones can be distinguished, namely cholesterol and pigment stones. The former variety can be found in about 85% of the cases; pigment stones are present in the remaining 15%. For therapeutic reasons, it is important to subdivide the so-called cholesterol stones into several types. As will be described in more detail later in this chapter, only those stones that consist predominantly of cholesterol and do not contain significant admixtures of calcium salts, mucin, or pigment can be treated by medical means. Although no exact data are available, it can be estimated that only the minority of gallstones, probably not more than 20% to 30%, is free of significant contaminations by these three substances. Recent data indicate that the response to medical dissolution therapy is poor if the cholesterol content of the stones drops below 70%.[3] Stone age and, associated with this, stone size bear a relation to stone composition. With increasing age and size, the stone is more likely to be calcified and contain layers enriched in mucin and pigment. Young and small stones are more prone to have a very high cholesterol content, especially if they are of the floating variety, as defined by oral cholecystogram.[4] It appears likely that the latter type of stones will become more prevalent in clinical practice, as more gallstone carriers are identified at an earlier age by ultrasonographic screening. However, in most published series of patients selected for gallstone dissolution therapy, only 10% to 20% of the cases had floating stones.[5-8]

The prevalence of gallstones differs considerably among different ethnic groups in the United States. Particularly noteworthy is the very high prevalence in many Indian tribes, in which the majority of women above the age of 30 have cholesterol gallstones.[9]

Etiology, Pathogenesis, Physical Chemistry, and Clinical Presentations of Gallstones

The etiology, pathogenesis, and physical chemistry of cholesterol gallbladder stones are obviously different from those of pigment stones. The etiology of cholesterol stones is not entirely known. However, presently available information points toward a strong role of dietary factors, in particular an increased intake of both calories and cholesterol. Part of the absorbed cholesterol is excreted in bile.[10, 11] In addition, overweight is associated with increased hepatic synthesis and biliary secretion of cholesterol.[12] Normally, cholesterol is fully solubilized by bile acids and lecithin. At low rates of bile acid secretion, cholesterol appears to be transported mainly in lecithin vesicles.[13–15] At higher rates of bile acid secretion, cholesterol in bile is solubilized in mixed micelles, consisting of bile acids and lecithin.[13–15] Above certain concentrations, cholesterol precipitation may occur. Experimental evidence is growing that vesicles are an essential stage in the events that may lead to formation of gallstones. Precipitation of cholesterol crystals appears to be consistently preceded by the conglomeration of cholesterol-rich vesicles. The levels at which cholesterol is saturated and supersaturated in bile have been defined.[16–18] It is now well accepted that, in the majority of cases, cholesterol-supersaturated bile is the result of enhanced cholesterol secretion.[19, 20] However, in some cases, the major defect underlying cholesterol saturation appears to be a decrease in bile acid secretion.[21]

Although cholesterol supersaturation constitutes a prerequisite for the formation of cholesterol gallstones, it can be present without stones being formed. Recently, researchers have identified in human bile nucleating as well as antinucleating proteins that promote and counteract, respectively, the crystallization of cholesterol.[22, 23] Rapid crystal formation is now understood to be due to the presence of nucleating proteins in the gallbladder.[22] In contrast, the absence of nucleation in some subjects who show supersaturation for prolonged periods of time can be explained by an increased secretion of antinucleating proteins.[23] The factors responsible for the secretion of either protein are not known.

Finally, gallstone formation can be promoted by the secretion of mucin in the gallbladder as well as by decreased gallbladder contractility.[24, 25] Current information suggests that these two cholelithogenic factors develop as a consequence or complication of cholesterol-supersaturated bile.

The pathogenesis of pigment stones is less well defined than that of cholesterol gallstones. Principally, there are two types of pigment stones, black and brown.[26] The former type of stone is usually formed in the gallbladder in sterile bile. In contrast, the development of brown pigment stones occurs in bile ducts and is frequently associated with bacterial infection.[27] The exact mechanism of pigment stone formation is not known. It has been hypothesized that brown stones form as the result of the hydrolysis of conjugated bilirubin by bacterial β-glucuronidase.[27] Unconjugated bilirubin is much less soluble than the bilirubin conjugate. It may, therefore, precipitate and serve as a nidus for the growth of bilirubinate stones. However, bacterial deconjugation of bilirubin has not been proven to be the primary event in the genesis of pigment stones.[28] A more likely possibility is, perhaps, that motility disorders of the biliary tree lead to stasis and the subsequent accumulation and activation of hydrolytic enzymes secreted by the liver, pancreas, or the mucosa of the bile ducts and gallbladder.[29] Both lecithin and bilirubin could then be hydrolysed, leading to a reduction of the capacity of bile acid–lecithin micelles to solubilize cholesterol as well as an increased risk of the precipitation of calcium bilirubinate and of calcium salts of fatty acids.

Considerable progress has been made in the understanding of the natural history of gallstones. Several carefully conducted studies in the United States and Italy have shown that, in the majority of cases, gallstones are silent (i.e., cause no symptoms).[30–32] The risk of a subject with silent gallstones to develop biliary pain is only about 2% per year. The annual risk of a complication from gallstones is even lower (i.e., approximately 0.1%). Symptom-free gallstones carriers, are, therefore, managed conservatively.[30] Prophylactic cholecystectomy is not recommended anymore for silent gallstones. Contrary to earlier claims, recent studies also indicate that the mortality of diabetic patients undergoing surgery for acute biliary tract disease is not significantly increased in comparison to nondiabetic patients.[33] Therefore, nonsurgical management appears to be also the treatment of choice for asymptomatic gallstone carriers who have diabetes.

Prospective studies of the natural history have also shown that complications from gallstones are virtually always preceded by several episodes of biliary pain.[30] In other words, there is usually plenty of time for a gallstone patient and his physician to choose among the various available treatment options before he is seriously threatened by a complication.

Current Treatment Methods for Gallstones

Subjects with silent stones can either be managed expectantly without any therapeutic intervention (since, at an average, their risk to develop biliary pain during their life time is only about 20%) or, in selected cases, undergo oral cholelitholytic treatment with ursodeoxycholic acid (UDCA, 3 alpha, 7 beta-dihydroxy-5-cholanoic acid) or a combination of this bile acid with chenodeoxycholic acid (CDCA, 3 alpha, 7 beta-dihydroxy-5-cholanoic acid). For symptomatic gallstones, several therapeutic modalities are now available. The most commonly used mode of therapy is still the time-honored cholecystectomy, used successfully for more than a century.[34] Although considered to be a very safe procedure, it carries a mortality of about 0.4% and is associated with a significant morbidity, as well as with the costs of the operation and postoperative in-hospital care. Furthermore, in spite of the surgical removal of the gallbladder as a locus of gallstone formation, stones either can be left behind during the operation or they can recur in the bile ducts. The frequency at which this occurs is difficult to assess. However, figures found in the literature ranging from 5% to 15% are probably representative of the average risk of a patient to develop bile duct stones after a cholecystectomy. For these reasons, major efforts are underway to develop nonsurgical methods for the treatment of symptomatic gallstones. Considerable and clinically applicable progress toward this goal has recently been evident. Two new methods will probably move rapidly out of the experimental stage into clinical practice. One is invasive and involves the instillation of methyl tert-butyl ether (MTBE) into the gallbladder through a transhepatically placed catheter.[35] The other method is noninvasive and employs extracorporeally induced shock waves.[36] Shock wave fragmentation has become the treatment of choice for most renal stones. Recently, increasing evidence is accumulating, primarily from studies in Munich, Germany, that this new treatment can also be used for gallstones with a high degree of efficacy and safety.[36] The patient selection criteria for both the MTBE and shock wave treatments are similar to those of oral cholelitholytic treatment with UDCA or a UDCA–CDCA combination (see below), except for the fact that the oral systemic dissolution treatment is reserved for patients who have either no or only minor biliary symptoms. Both the MTBE and shock wave treatments can be combined with oral bile acid therapy.

Mechanisms for Drug Treatment of Gallstones

As discussed above, pharmacologic intervention is possible in both a local and systemic manner. The first mode of gallstone dissolution treatment which has become clinically feasible involves the systemic use of UDCA or a UDCA–CDCA combination.[6-8, 37-44] The therapeutic effect of the two bile acids is principally based on a dual mechanism of action, namely the suppression of both the hepatic synthesis and biliary secretion of cholesterol. Most studies show that CDCA as well as UDCA inhibit (1) the activity of the rate-limiting enzyme of cholesterol synthesis, the hydroxy methyl glutaryl-CoA reductase (HMG-CoAR) and (2) the biliary secretion of cholesterol.[41] The latter effect of the two bile acids is understood to be a result of their relatively hydrophilic nature. An increase in hydrophilicity (and consequent decrease in hydrophobicity) is associated with a fall in the micellar solubilizing power for cholesterol. Hydrophilic compounds, such as UDCA, solubilize cholesterol mainly by a nonmicellar, liquid crystalline mechanism.[43, 44] It appears that at the hepatocellular membrane level the shift from micellar to liquid-crystalline solubilization leads to a decrease in the biliary secretion of cholesterol. Although less hydrophilic than UDCA, CDCA is more hydrophilic that cholic acid, which constitutes a major bile acid in human bile. Enrichment of the bile in UDCA or UDCA–CDCA leads, therefore, to a decrease in the hepatocellular and biliary capacity for micellar transport of cholesterol. In view of the fact that cholesterol secretion is markedly suppressed, the overall solubility of cholesterol in bile during UDCA or UDCA–CDCA treatment is significantly improved. As a result of changing a cholesterol-supersaturated bile to one which is undersaturated, cholesterol stones slowly dissolve.

Theoretically, there are a number of additional possibilities for systemic pharmacologic intervention to improve the efficacy of UDCA and UDCA–CDCA. They consist of the development of pharmaca which have the following features: (1) suppress the hepatic synthesis, as well as biliary secretion of cholesterol; (2) increase the hepatic synthesis and biliary secretion of bile acids; (3) induce a major enhancement in the biliary solubility for cholesterol; and (4) have no adverse effects. Attempts have been made to synthesize bile acid analogues that fulfill these demanding requirements. However, it has been proven to be very difficult to develop a compound which, in the overall balance, offers advantages over UDCA.

The second method of gallstone dissolution treatment involves the local application of solvents. Two compounds have been introduced into clinical practice. One of the two, MTBE, is used mainly to dissolve gallbladder stones,[35] whereas the other, monooctanoin, is infused into the common bile duct to dissolve bile duct stones.[45–48] The local MTBE therapy can be supplemented by systemic UDCA or UDCA–CDCA treatment in order to facilitate clearing of incompletely dissolved stone particles from the gallbladder.

To improve local cholelitholytic therapy, current research efforts focus on the development of solvents able to safely dissolve calcified stones, which constitute a major proportion of gallstones resistant to both local and systemic dissolution treatment.

GALLSTONE DISSOLUTION THERAPY

Historical Perspective

Attempts have been made for centuries to dissolve gallstones by either natural compounds or drugs.[7] In spite of many claims, few of these treatments have stood the test of time. The two bile acids, CDCA and UDCA, which represent the only compounds known to be effective for systemic gallstone dissolution therapy, have only recently been introduced.[5–8, 37–41, 49–52] The feasibility of in vivo cholelitholytic therapy was probably first recognized when gallstones implanted into the dog gallbladder were found to dissolve. The physical–chemical basis for gallstone dissolution therapy was provided by studies which showed that ingestion of CDCA resulted in the desaturation of bile which was previously supersaturated in cholesterol.[53] Gallstone dissolution was then observed to occur when CDCA treatment was continued for several months.[49] The ability of UDCA to dissolve gallstones was recognized later.[51, 52] This bile acid had been used for several decades in Japan for the treatment of chronic liver diseases. Because CDCA and UDCA are structurally closely related compounds, it was natural that UDCA's cholelitholytic potential was tested after CDCA became known to dissolve gallstones.

The history of local cholelitholytic therapy is relatively short. Only recently, appropriate nonoperative techniques and devices have been developed to allow the safe instillation of gallstone-dissolving solutions into the bile ducts and gallbladder. Together with these developments, the search for litholytic agents has resulted in the successful introduction of monooctanoin and MTBE for the treatment of common bile duct stones and gallbladder stones, respectively.[35, 45–48]

Dissolution Treatment with Bile Acids

Mode of Action and Pharmacology

As described elsewhere in this chapter, the main pharmacologic action of both bile acids consists of their decreasing biliary cholesterol secretion. While the pharmacodynamics and kinetics of CDCA have been extensively studied, those of UDCA are less well defined.[53, 54] Free CDCA is, as the sodium salt, completely absorbed in the upper small intestine by nonionic diffusion, in contrast to the glycine or taurine-amidated compounds, which are mainly absorbed in the terminal ileum. Following absorption, CDCA is transported in the portal blood to the liver where it is amidated with glycine or taurine. It is then reexcreted with the endogenous bile acids in bile and stored in the gallbladder at night and between meals. When a meal enters the small intestine, cholecystokinin is released from the intestinal mucosa and stimulates both the contraction of the gallbladder and relaxation of the sphincter of Oddi, facilitating the secretion of bile into the duodenum. In the small intestine, the bile acids form micelles with the products of fat digestion and are then reabsorbed by active transport in the terminal ileum. The CDCA-enriched bile acid pool undergoes approximately two enterohepatic cycles during each meal.

Following the ingestion of therapeutic doses of CDCA, this compound constitutes 70% to 90% of the total bile acids in bile.[55, 56] This high enrichment of the bile with CDCA is a result of the suppression of bile acid synthesis. In some cases, there can be considerable biotransformation of CDCA to UDCA, mainly via 7-ketolithocholic acid as an intermediate.[55, 57, 58] Following its formation by bacteria in the intestine, the intermediate is either directly reduced by bacterial enzymes or first absorbed and then reduced in the liver.[58, 59] The principal product of the enzymatic reduction of 7-ketolithocholic acid by intestinal bacteria is UDCA.[59] In contrast, the liver converts the intermediate mainly to CDCA.[59]

The site and rate of absorption of UDCA are similar to those of CDCA. However, in contrast to CDCA, UDCA does not suppress bile acid synthesis.[60–62] Therefore, the enrichment of bile with UDCA is lower than that with CDCA during the respective bile acid treatments. The biliary UDCA content during UDCA treatment usually does not exceed 50% to 60%.[6, 7] UDCA is biotransformed by intestinal bacteria. The principal metabolite of CDCA and UDCA is lithocholic acid, the product of 7-dehydroxylation. Small fractions of lithocholic acid, which are mainly formed in the proximal colon, are reabsorbed and enter the enterohepatic circulation. Lithocholic acid is both in its free form and as the glycine amidate very insoluble and thus rapidly excreted in stool.[63] In contrast, the sulfate of lithocholic acid, which is formed in the liver, is water soluble and consequently excreted in the urine.[64] Another important bacterial biotransformation of UDCA is represented by its epimerization to CDCA, mainly via the intermediate, 7-ketolithocholic acid.[59] The rates of the 7-dehydroxylation as well as oxido-reduction reactions of UDCA appear to be slower than those of CDCA.[65, 66]

Efficacy and Safety

CDCA and UDCA are similarly effective in dissolving gallstones.[6, 37] However, there are differences between these two bile acids as far as their safety is concerned. CDCA treatment is often associated with adverse effects consisting of diarrhea, moderate serum transaminase elevations, and minor increases in serum LDL cholesterol.[5-8, 67] In contrast, UDCA has proven to be very safe.[6-8, 36-41] Indeed, recent observations indicate that UDCA may have hepatoprotective properties[41, 68] and may stimulate hepatic LDL catabolism through an up-regulation of the LDL receptor.[69] If, for example, CDCA is combined with UDCA, the liver test abnormalities observed with the single use of CDCA disappear.[41] UDCA also does not cause any increases in serum cholesterol.

Clinical Application

CDCA and UDCA find their main application in oral gallstone dissolution therapy. In Japan, UDCA is also being used for the treatment of chronic hepatitis. Recently, investigators in Europe have not only corroborated the experience of Japanese clinicians concerning the beneficial effect of UDCA in chronic hepatitis[70] but also have provided preliminary evidence that this bile acid may arrest the progression of primary biliary cirrhosis.[68]

Thus far, only CDCA has been approved by the FDA and is marketed in the United States. However, in view of the described adverse effects CDCA has if used as a single agent, it is likely that it will be supplanted by UDCA as the drug of choice once the latter has received FDA approval.

Both CDCA and UDCA are only effective in radiolucent gallstones. The gallbladder has to be functioning as evidenced by its visualization during an oral cholecystogram. The efficacy of the cholelitholytic treatment is mainly dependant on stone size and composition. The best results in terms of rate and completeness of gallstone dissolution are seen in patients with floating stones.[5, 6] The floating quality signifies a relatively pure cholesterol stone. Stones which are smaller than 0.5 cm in diameter dissolve in approximately 70% of the cases. However, the average efficacy of the treatment drops to less than 40% if the stone diameter increases to more than 1.5 cm. Massive obesity is another factor which is known to lower the prospect of treatment success.

Doses

Both CDCA and UDCA are taken per os in capsules or coated tablets. The drugs appear to have optimal effect if taken at bedtime.[71] This allows the overnight enrichment of gallbladder bile with CDCA and UDCA. Maximal nocturnal levels of the cholelitholytic compounds in the bile are desirable because cholesterol supersaturation is most pronounced at night. It is recommended to ingest the bedtime dose of UDCA with a snack to allow mixing of the drug with bile which is secreted into the intestine following food-stimulated contraction of the gallbladder. This recommendation is based on the concern that UDCA may not be absorbed completely if it is not solubilized by endogenous bile acids in the intestine. The solubility of UDCA is lower than that of CDCA. However, as previously mentioned, published data concerning bioavailability of UDCA preparations are incomplete.

The optimal dose of CDCA is approximately 15 mg/kg/day.[72] In many patients, this dose is not tolerated because it may cause diarrhea. Tolerance of the drug is improved by increasing the drug slowly to the optimal level over a period of several days or weeks. The optimal dose of UDCA has not been reliably determined. The dose range at which UDCA does not show any significant change in cholelitholytic efficacy appears to be considerably wider than that of CDCA.[6-8, 36-40] Most studies indicate doses between approximately 5 and 13 mg/kg/day to be equally effective. There does not seem to be any gain in increasing the dose above 13 mg/

kg/day. If the two bile acids are combined, a CDCA dose of approximately 7.5 mg/kg/day and a UDCA dose of 6.5 mg/kg/day have been used successfully without side effects.[41]

Adverse Effects

The adverse effects of CDCA, namely diarrhea, liver test abnormalities, and elevations of serum LDL cholesterol, are relatively minor and dose dependent.[5-8] The increases of liver-associated enzymes, in particular of L-alanine aminotransferase in serum, are almost invariably transient and disappear, in spite of continued CDCA treatment, usually within 3 to 6 months.[5-7] The increase in serum LDL cholesterol occurs gradually. The total cholesterol rises by about 15 mg/dL over a period of 2 years.[5,67] This relatively small cholesterol change is difficult to document in the individual case and has only become apparent in the study of large numbers of patients in the National Cooperative Gallstone Study.[5,67] UDCA has no known adverse effects. To the contrary, it may favorably affect both cholesterol metabolism and certain liver diseases.[68,70,73] There is experimental evidence that UDCA not only lowers intestinal cholesterol absorption, but also directly stimulates hepatic LDL receptor activity.[69] As mentioned previously in this chapter, there is also preliminary evidence that UDCA exerts a therapeutically favorable effect in primary biliary cirrhosis and chronic active hepatitis.[68,70]

The authors are not aware of any significant untoward interactions between CDCA or UDCA and any drugs.

Contraindications

The treatment should not be conducted during pregnancy, although there are no known teratogenic or other harmful effects associated with the use of either CDCA or UDCA in pregnant women. There are few other contraindications, especially if UDCA or a UDCA–CDCA combination is used, and if the previously described selection criteria are observed. In contrast to UDCA, CDCA, if used alone, may be toxic in preexistent liver disease and may worsen diarrhea and malabsorption.

Monooctanoin

Mode of Action and Pharmacology

Monooctanoin, a medium chain monoglyceride, is a locally applied solvent of cholesterol gallstones.[45-47] The compound is infused through a catheter into the gallstone-containing bile duct. Monooctanoin, similar to other organic solvents, floats and thus has the tendency to separate from bile and the stone.[74] Proper catheter placement, which facilitates intimate contact of the solvent with the stone, is, therefore, important. Monooctanoin does not dissolve pigment or calcified stones.

Once it passes into the small intestine, monooctanoin is hydrolysed by pancreatic lipase to octanoic acid and glycerol.[75] Octanoic acid is absorbed and oxidized mainly in the liver.

Efficacy and Safety

Monooctanoin is more effective than the amidates of CDCA or UDCA in dissolving gallstones. It also dissolves gallstones faster than does taurocholate, which has been used in the past for the treatment of stones in the common bile duct.[45-47] However, the solubilization power of monooctanoin is lower than that of MTBE (see below). Although the efficacy of monooctanoin reported in the literature varies considerably, a relatively recently published survey by other investigators indicates it to be quite low.[47] Complete disappearance of stones was observed in 26% of the cases. Partial dissolution with subsequent ability to extract the stones by mechanical means was reported in another 29%. The authors are not aware of reports of serious adverse effects of monooctanoin treatment which can be attributed to the compound itself. Cases of pancreatitis and other complications, which have been observed, are probably sequelae of extrahepatic bile duct obstruction rather than the drug. Overall, the safety of monooctanoin appears to compare favorably to that of other locally infused agents, such as bile salts or MTBE.

Clinical Application

Monooctanoin (Capmul(R), consisting of approximately 70% glyceryl monooctanoate and 30% glyceryl dioctanoate) finds its main application in the dissolution treatment of retained common bile duct stones which cannot be removed by papillotomy or mechanical extraction. The number of cases in which monooctanoin is being used is likely to decline with the increasing application of new technologies of shock wave, ultrasonic, and laser lithotripsy to the treatment of gallstones. In addition, the refinement of mechanical extraction techniques will further decrease the need for monooctanoin. For detailed description of the techniques of the infusion of the solvent, the reader is referred to the literature.[45-47, 76] The infusion pressure can be monitored with a manometer broken off at the 30-cm mark.[76] A stopcock is positioned in such a manner that the infusion pump, bile duct, and manometer are in communication. It usually takes several days, often more than a week, before the stones are either dissolved or small enough to be amenable to mechanical extraction or to pass spontaneously.

Because Capmul has a freezing point of 20° C, the compound is often solid. The viscosity of the solution is decreased by the addition of small amounts of water (10 parts water to 90 parts Capmul(R).[77] Water also lowers the freezing point of Capmul, which makes it easier to infuse the material.

Doses

Capmul usually is infused at a rate of 3 to 5 ml/hr, using an infusion pump. The infusion is interrupted during mealtime and for brief periods of ambulation, when the patient is disconnected from the infusion pump.[76] No dietary restrictions are necessary.

Adverse Effects

One possible adverse reaction can occur in response to increased pressure in the common bile duct during the infusion. In that case, patients may experience right upper-quadrant abdominal pain, chills, fever, and nausea.[45-47, 76] A second untoward effect is related to the use of higher rates of monooctanoin infusion, which can be associated with abdominal cramps and diarrhea. As far as other adverse effects and complications are concerned, which have been observed during the infusion of monooctanoin, it is difficult to determine whether they were due to the drug or severe biliary disease.

Contraindications

There do not seem to be any distinct contraindications to monooctanoin infusion treatment if the proper selection criteria are observed. Only patients with noncalcified cholesterol stones can be expected to benefit from the treatment.

Other Compounds for Dissolution Treatment for Bile Duct Stones

A number of other agents being studied have potential to be useful for the dissolution of bile duct stones. Among these are limonene and various monooctanoin-based mixtures. D-limonene (p-metha-1, 8-diene) is a monoterpene which has been used by Igimi and co-workers with excellent results in the treatment of bile duct stones.[78] A summary of the current experience with this compound can be found in a recent review article by Neoptolemos and co-workers.[79]

Because monooctanoin has the tendency to separate from the aqueous medium of the bile, attempts have been made to improve the ability of the solvent to form an emulsion.[80] However, it is presently not proven that the addition of bile salts and nonionic detergents, such as Pluronic F-68 (polyoxyethylenepolyoxypropylene polymer), improves the clinical dissolution efficacy.[80, 81]

Methyl Tertiary Butyl Ether (MTBE)

MTBE ($C_2H_5OC_2H_5$) is mainly used for local dissolution of cholesterol gallstones in the gallbladder. Is it also being used for the treatment of common bile duct stones, although the propriety of the latter is being debated.[74] The rationale for the use of MTBE is primarily based on both its lipid solubilizing power and relative safety. The boiling point of MTBE is 52.2 C—higher than that of other ethers previously tried for gallstone dissolution. It remains, therefore, liquid at body temperature. MTBE is used with the aim to restrict its action to the site of the gallstones, namely, the gallbladder or bile ducts. While is is obviously easier, by proper catheter placement, to impair the outflow of MTBE from the gallbladder into the cystic duct, special balloon devices and manipulations are required to prevent excessive flow of the solvent from the common bile duct into the intestine. Significant absorption occurs once MBTE passes into the intestine. The patient may fall asleep as a result of the narcotic effect of the compound.[34, 82] The majority of the absorbed MTBE is exhaled in unaltered form. The small remaining portion is metabolized to methane and formate.[34] Concentrations of MTBE in breath have been found to range below those associated with danger of explosion.[34]

An important point to be considered regarding the pharmacodynamics of organic solvents, such as MTBE and monooctanoin, relates to their floating quality and tendency to separate from the bile and gallstones.[74] Proper positioning of the patient and placement of the catheter tip in proximity of the stones are, therefore, necessary to achieve the maximal possible efficacy of the solvent.

Efficacy and Safety

In spite of being the strongest gallstone-dissolving agent currently available, MTBE does not dissolve pigment or calcified stones.[34, 74, 82] It is presently the only solvent that can be used for local dissolution of gallstones in the gallbladder. Monooctanoin is not strong enough for this purpose because it has to be infused for several days, before the gallstones are dissolved.

In the hands of a physician who is experienced in the transhepatic or endoscopic placement of catheters into the gallbladder, the cholelitholytic treatment with MTBE should be quite safe. However, greater precautions are necessary with the use of MTBE than they are with that of monooctanoin or bile acids. The patient has to be monitored very closely for narcotic effects of MTBE. In addition, nausea, vomiting, and diarrhea appear to be more pronounced during treatment with MTBE than during that with the other dissolving agents.

Clinical Application

For dissolution of stones in the gallbladder, MTBE is instilled through a catheter (7 F polyethylene) which is placed either transhepatically or endoscopically in a retrograde manner into the gallbadder.[82] A similar catheter, which can also be introduced endoscopically, is used for MTBE treatment of common bile duct stones.[82] It should be noticed that some catethers not made of polyethylene may be eroded by MTBE.[83] Every attempt should be made to limit the passage of ether into the intestine by both placing the catheter correctly and adjusting the instilled volume of ether in such a manner that overflow is avoided. In the future, MTBE therapy will probably be combined with lithotripsy. Lithotripsy is likely to speed up the dissolution by MTBE. In the treatment of common bile duct stones, it is often necessary to complement the MTBE infusion by endoscopic papillotomy and instrumental extraction of undissolved stone fragments.

Presently, MTBE treatment of gallbladder stones is reserved to patients with biliary pain who either object to a cholecystectomy or for whom abdominal surgery and general anesthesia pose a high risk. Similar to the other dissolution methods, the gallbladder has to be functioning and the gallstones have to be radiolucent and free of calcifications.

Doses

For dissolution of gallbladder stones, 2 to 5 ml of MTBE are instilled through the catheter into the gallbladder. The gallbladder content is then withdrawn after 30 minutes. This cycle of infusion and aspiration is repeated until the stones are dissolved. Depending on the size and composition of the stones, several hours are usually required until dissolution has been accomplished.[45–47, 82] For treatment of common bile duct stones, 5 to 10 ml of MTBE are injected. After 1 to 3 minutes, the contents of the common duct are withdrawn. Injection and aspiration are then repeated until the stones are dissolved.

Adverse Effects

Sedation or general anesthesia constitutes probably the most important untoward effect of MTBE, if significant amounts of the ether pass into the intestine and are absorbed. The foul-smelling odor of MTBE, which is noted in the patient's breath, requires adequate ventilation of the procedure room. In addition, smoking and other fire-hazardous activities must be prohibited because of the volatile and flammable nature of the ether. The narcotic effect of MTBE needs to be considered if the patient is sedated for the procedure. The tolerance for MTBE may be especially low in the presence of significant liver or lung disease and the ensuing decrease in the metabolization and exhalation of the ether. A second potential adverse effect of MTBE relates to its powerful lipid-solubilizing capacity. If, due to improper catheter placement, the compound is injected into blood vessels or the liver, hemolysis and tissue necrosis, respectively, can occur. Most patients experience upper abdominal pain at the beginning of the infusion.[82] Nausea, vomiting, and duodenitis are additional untoward effects which can be seen in MTBE-treated patients. The frequency and severity of undesirable reactions to the treatment are very much related to the expertness and carefulness with which the procedure is carried out.

Contraindications

MTBE treatment is contraindicated both in patients with silent gallstones and in those who present with jaundice, cholangitis, or pancreatitis. A low tolerance of narcotics, as it may be present in patients with severe pulmonary, liver, or heart disease, has to be carefully weighed against both the expected benefit of MTBE treatment and the comparative risk of alternative procedures.

LITHOTRIPSY

Various lithotriptic technologies currently being developed are likely to revolutionize the treatment of gallstones. They include the use of extracorporeally generated shock waves and of laser. The former technology appears to hold the most promise as far as fragmentation of both gallbladder and bile duct stones is concerned.[36, 84] The principle and technique of crushing gallstones by extracorporeal shock waves are essentially the same as those for kidney stone fragmentation.[85] There is currently no published experience with shock wave therapy of gallstones in the United States. However, an increasing data from two centers in Germany suggest that the treatment may be both effective and safe in selected patients with cholesterol gallstones.[36, 84]

Efficacy and Safety

Although it is presently difficult to evaluate efficacy and safety of extracorporeal shock wave therapy of gallstones, the results emerging mainly from two medical centers in Germany are encouraging. They encompass experience with more than 300 patients. The efficacy is very dependent on proper patient selection. If carefully selected (see below), and if shock wave lithotripsy is combined with UDCA or a combination of UDCA and

CDCA, complete disappearance or dissolution of gallbladder stones has been reported to occur in 70% to 80% of the cases.[84] The contribution of UDCA or UDCA–CDCA to the disappearance of the gallstone fragments from the gallbladder after lithotripsy is not known. However, according to the reports by investigators from Germany, the success rate (complete stone disappearance) increases from 20% to 30% 2 to 3 months after shock wave treatment to 70% to 80% after longer periods of continued dissolution therapy with UDCA or UDCA–CDCA.[84] While complete evacuation of the stone fragments from the gallbladder may occur spontaneously, this may not often be the case. Because cholesterol supersaturation of bile is likely to continue after lithotripsy in most patients, the stone fragments may act as nidus for renewed gallstone growth. Furthermore, a continuing motility disorder may impair complete emptying of the gallbladder. However, placebo-controlled studies of the therapeutic role of or need for UDCA or UDCA–CDCA after shock wave fragmentation of the gallstones have not yet been conducted.

The published experience thus far indicates the safety of shock wave lithotripsy to be acceptable.[36,84] Biliary pain has been reported to occur in approximately 25% of the patients after lithotripsy. The majority of the cases was managed medically. However, pancreatitis was observed in 2% to 3% of the patients. The interval between shock wave treatment and pancreatitis varied from a few days to several weeks. While the pancreatitis responded to conservative measures in most instances, an endoscopic papillotomy was found to be necessary in several patients.[36,84] The papillotomy was considered to be well tolerated and effective in all of them. Cystic duct obstruction and cholecystitis were observed after lithotripsy in 3 of 157 patients in one recently reported study. In two of the three the cystic duct opened up after conservative treatment. The third patient, who showed unsatisfactory fragmentation of the stones, underwent elective cholecystectomy. In appears, therefore, that patients require careful monitoring after shock wave treatment. Both gastroenterologists and surgeons versed in the proper management of biliary tract disease need to be intimately involved in the postlithotripsy follow-up of the patients. Expertise in the performance of ERCP and endoscopic papillotomy is required, and good radiology is essential.

Clinical Application

Currently, shock wave lithotripsy is combined with oral bile acid dissolution therapy, using UDCA either alone or in combination with CDCA.[36,84] Lithotripsy may also prove to be useful in conjunction with the topical application of MTBE, allowing complete dissolution of the stones within a few hours in one single treatment. The technology and clinical application of shock wave lithotripsy are in a process of rapid improvement and refinement. A detailed review of this subject is beyond the scope of this chapter. The new generations of lithotriptors, which are manufactured by several companies in Europe and the United States (1) no longer require the positioning of the patient in a water bath, (2) are equipped with sophisticated ultrasound devices for locating the gallstones, (3) emit shock waves in a manner and at energy levels that either reduce or eliminate the need for anesthesia or analgesics, and (4) are multipurpose devices which can be used for the fragmentation of kidney and bile duct, as well as gallbladder stones.

Adverse Effects

Air-containing structures such as lungs or air-filled colon loops have to be shielded from or removed out of the shock wave path. The shock wave is transmitted through water and tissue mainly composed of water. Significant change in the acoustic impedance of a structure from that of water to that of air or stones leads to the development of tear and shear forces. Because the right kidney is in the proximity of the shock wave path directed at the biliary system, gallstone lithotripsy is frequently followed by transient microhematuria. In a small percentage of cases, macrohematuria may be present for 1 to 2 days.

Indications and Contraindications

Shock wave lithotripsy is presently used only in symptomatic gallstones. It is contraindicated in silent gallstones. Presently, the selection criteria are otherwise similar to those of systemic dissolution treatment with UDCA or UDCA–CDCA. The gallbladder has to be functioning, as evidenced by its visualization by oral cholecystography, and the stones have to be radiolucent (i.e., composed mainly of cholesterol). Diffusely calcified stones are usually not amenable to lithotripsy. The success rate is highest in patients with single stones not exceeding a diameter of 2.0 to 2.5 cm. If the stones are larger than 2.5 cm or if the number of stones is higher than three, the efficacy of shock wave fragmentation is limited.

SUMMARY

During the last decade, the concepts concerning the pathogenesis, natural history, and treatment of gallstones have been advanced considerably. Silent gallstones can either be managed expectantly or, in selected cases, be dissolved by systemic bile acid therapy, using UDCA or a combination of UDCA and CDCA. A number of new medical treatment modalities, including MTBE treatment and extracorporeal shock wave lithotripsy, may prove to offer effective and safe alternatives to cholecystectomy in selected patients with radiolucent cholesterol stones. However, cholecystectomy will continue to be the treatment of choice in the majority of patients with symptomatic gallstones, in particular in those in whom gallstones are diffusely calcified. The selection of the proper treatment for gallstone patients, therefore, has to be based on a careful evaluation of (1) the clinical symptoms and signs, (2) the characteristics of the gallstones, and (3) gallbladder function.

References

1. Barbara L for the "Progetto Sirmione": Epidemiology of gallstone disease: The "Sirmione Study," in Capocaccia L, Ricci G, Angelico F, et al (eds): *Epidemiology and Prevention of Gallstone Disease*. Lancaster, MTP Press Limited, 1984; pp 23–25.
2. Ricci G and the GREPCO Group: The GREPCO research programmes: Aims and prevalence data, in Capocaccia L, Ricci G, Angelico F, et al (eds): *Epidemiology and Prevention of Gallstone Disease*. Lancaster, MTP Press Limited, 1984; pp 9–14.
3. Smith BF: Dissolution of cholesterol gallstones in vitro. Gallstone matrix content and diameter, not cholesterol content, predict gallstone dissolution in monooctanoin. *Gastroenterology* 1987; 93:98–105.
4. Dolgin SM, Schwartz JS, Kressel HY, et al: Identification of patients with cholesterol or pigment gallstones by discriminant analysis of radiographic features. *N Engl J Med* 1981; 304:808–811.
5. Schoenfield LJ, Lachin JM, and the Steering Committee and The National Cooperative Gallstone Study Group: Chenodiol (chenodeoxycholic acid) for dissolution of gallstones: The National Cooperative Gallstone Study. *Ann Intern Med* 1981; 95:257–282.
6. Fromm H, Roat JW, Gonzalez V, et al: Comparative efficacy and side effects of ursodeoxycholic and chenodeoxycholic acids in dissolving gallstones: A double blind controlled study. *Gastroenterology* 1983; 85:1257–1264.
7. Bachrach WH, Hofmann AF: Ursodeoxycholic acid in the treatment of cholesterol cholelithiasis. *Dig Dis Sci* 1982; 27:737–856.
8. Fromm H: Gallstone dissolution therapy. Current status and future prospects. *Gastroenterology* 1986; 91:1560–1567.
9. Samplinear RE, Bennett PH, Comess LJ, et al: Gallbladder disease in Pima Indians: Demonstration of high prevalence and early onset by cholecystography. *N Engl J Med* 1970; 283:1358–1364.
10. Long TT, Jakoi L, Stevens R, et al: The sources of rat biliary cholesterol and bile acid. *J Lipid Res* 1978; 19:872–878.
11. DenBesten L, Connor WE, Bell S: The effect of dietary cholesterol on the composition of human bile surgery. *Surgery* 1973; 73:266–273.
12. Bennion LJ, Grundy SM: Effects of obesity and caloric intake on biliary lipid metabolism in man. *J Clin Invest* 1975; 56:966–1011.
13. Somjen GJ, Gilat T: A nonmicellar mode of cholesterol transport in human bile. *FEBS Lett* 1983; 156:265–268.
14. Pattison NR, Chapman BA: Distribution of biliary cholesterol between mixed micelles and nonmicelles in relation to fasting and feeding in humans. *Gastroenterology* 1986; 91:697–702.
15. Kibe A, Breuer AC, Holzbach RT: Cholesterol nucleation in human bile by video-enhanced control differential interference microscopy

(VEM). The role of vesicles in metastable saturation (abstract). *Gastroenterology* 1984; 86:1326.
16. Hegardt FG, Dam H: The solubility of cholesterol in aqueous solutions of bile salts and lecithin. *Z Ernahrungswiss* 1971; 10:228–233.
17. Holzbach RT, Marsh M, Olszewski M, et al: Cholesterol solubility in bile: Evidence that supersaturated bile is frequent in healthy man. *J Clin Invest* 1973; 52:1467–1479.
18. Carey MC, Small DM: The physical chemistry of cholesterol solubility in bile. Relationship to gallstone formation and dissolution in man. *J Clin Invest* 1978; 61:998–1026.
19. Northfield TC, Hofmann AF: Biliary lipid output during three meals and an overnight fast. I. Relationship to bile acid pool and cholesterol saturation of bile in gallstone and control subjects. *Gut* 1975; 16:1–11.
20. Shaffer EA, Small DM: Biliary lipid secretion in cholesterol gallstone disease. The effect of cholecystectomy and obesity. *J Clin Invest* 1977; 59:828–840.
21. Grundy SM, Metzger AL, Adler RD: Mechanisms of lithogenic bile formation in American Indian women with cholesterol gallstones. *J Clin Invest* 1972; 51:3026–3043.
22. Gallinger S, Harvey PRC, Petrunka CN, et al: Biliary proteins and the nucleation defect in cholesterol cholelithiasis. *Gastroenterology* 1987; 92:867–875.
23. Holzbach RT, Kibe A, Thiel E, et al: Biliary proteins: Unique inhibitors of cholesterol crystal nucleation in human gallbladder bile. *J Clin Invest* 1984; 73:35–45.
24. Smith BF, LaMont JT: Identification of gallbladder mucin bilirubin complex in human cholesterol gallstone matrix. Effects of reducing agents on in vitro dissolution of matrix and intact gallstones. *J Clin Invest* 1985; 76:439–445.
25. La Morte WW, Schoetz DJ, Birkett DH, et al: The role of the gallbladder in the pathogenesis of cholesterol gallstones. *Gastroenterology* 1979; 77:580–592.
26. Trotman BW: Formation of pigment gallstones, in Cohen S, Soloway RD (eds): *Gallstones. Contemporary Issues in Gastroenterology*. New York, Churchill Livingstone, 1985; pp 299–307.
27. Maki T: Pathogenesis of calcium bilirubinate gallstone. *Ann Surg* 1966; 164:90–100.
28. Trotman BW: Insights into pigment gallstone disease. *J Lab Clin Med* 1979; 93:349–352.
29. Robins SJ, Fajulo JM, Patton GM: Lipids of pigment gallstones. *Biochim Biophys Acta* 1982; 712:21–25.
30. Gracie WA, Ransohoff DF: The natural history of silent gallstones: The innocent gallstone is not a myth. *N Engl J Med* 1982; 307:798–800.
31. Ransohoff DF, Gracie WA, Wolfenson LB, et al: Prophylactic cholecystectomy or expectant management for silent gallstones. *Ann Intern Med* 1983; 99:199–204.
32. Capocaccia L and the GREPCO Group: Clinical symptoms and gallstone disease: Lessons from a population study, in Capocaccia L, Ricci G, Angelico F, et al (eds): *Epidemiology and Prevention of Gallstone Disease*. Lancaster, MTP Press Limited, 1984, pp 153–157.
33. Ransohoff DF, Miller GL, Forsythe SB, et al: Outcome of acute cholecystitis in patients with diabetes mellitus. *Ann Intern Med* 1987; 106:829–832.
34. Langenbuch C: Ein Fall von Extirpation der Gallenblase wegen chronischer Cholelithiasis. Heilung. *Berliner Klinische Wochenschrift* 1882; 48:725–727.
35. Allen MJ, Borody TJ, Bugliosi TF, et al: Rapid dissolution of gallstones by methyl tert-butyl ether. Preliminary observations. *N Engl J Med* 1985; 312:217–220.
36. Sauerbruch T, Delius M, Paumgartner G, et al: Fragmentation of gallstones by extracorporeal shock waves. *N Engl J Med* 1986; 314:818–822.
37. Tokyo Cooperative Gallstone Study Group: Efficacy and indications of ursodeoxycholic acid treatment for dissolving gallstones. A multicenter double-blind trial. *Gastroenterology* 1980; 78:542–548.
38. Roda E, Bazzoli F, Morselli Labate AM, et al: Ursodeoxycholic acid vs. chenodeoxycholic acid as cholesterol gallstone-dissolving agents: A comparative randomized study. *Hepatology* 1982; 2:804–810.
39. Tint GS, Salen G, Colalillo A, et al: Ursodeoxycholic acid: A safe and effective agent for dissolving cholesterol gallstones. *Ann Intern Med* 1982; 97:351–356.
40. Fromm H: Dissolving gallstones. *Adv Intern Med*, In Stollerman GH, LaMont JT (eds): *Advances In Internal Medicine*, Chicago, Year Book Medical Publishers, 1988, pp. 409–30.
41. Fromm H: Gallstone dissolution and the cholesterol-bile acid-lipoprotein axis: Propitious effects of ursodeoxycholic acid (editorial). *Gastroenterology* 1984; 87:229–233.
42. Roehrkasse R, Fromm H, Malavolti M, et al: Gallstone dissolution treatment with combination of chenodeoxycholic and ursodeoxycholic acids. Studies of safety, efficacy and effects on bile lithogenicity, bile acid pool and serum lipids. *Dig Dis Sci* 1986; 31:1032–1040.
43. Corrigan OI, Su CC, Higuchi WI, et al: Mesophase formation during cholesterol dissolution in ursodeoxycholate-lecithin solutions: A new mechanism for gallstone dissolution in man. *J Pharm Sci* 1980; 69: 869–871.
44. Salvioli G, Igimi H, Carey MC: Cholesterol gallstone dissolution in bile. Dissolution kinetics of crystalline cholesterol monohydrate by conjugated chenodeoxycholate-lecithin mixtures: Dissimilar phase equilibria and dissolution mechanisms. *J Lipid Res* 1983; 24:701–720.
45. Leuschner U, Wurbs D, Landgraf H: Dissolution of biliary duct stones with mono-octanoin. *Lancet* 1979; ii:103–104.
46. Leuschner U, Wurbs D, Baumgartel H, et al: Alternating treatment of common bile duct stones with a modified glyceryl-l-monooctanoate preparation and a bile acid–EDTA solution by nasobiliary tube. *Scand J Gastroenterol* 1981; 16:497–503.

47. Thistle JL, Carlson GL, Hofmann AF, et al: Monooctanoin, a dissolution agent for retained cholesterol bile duct stones; Physical properties and clinical application. *Gastroenterology* 1981; 78:1016–1022.
48. Palmer KR, Hofmann AF: Intraductal mono-octanoin for the direct dissolution of bile duct stones: Experience in 343 patients. *Gut* 1986; 27:196–202.
49. Danzinger RG, Hofmann AF, Schoenfield LJ, et al: Dissolution of cholesterol gallstones by chenodeoxycholic acid. *N Engl J Med* 1972; 286:1–8.
50. Fromm H, Eschler A, Tollner D, et al: In vivo dissolving of gallstones: The effect of chenodeoxycholic acid. *Dtsch Med Wochenschr* 1975; 100:1619–1624.
51. Nakagawa S, Makino I, Ishizaki T, et al: Dissolution of cholesterol gallstones by ursodeoxycholic acid. *Lancet* 1977; II:367–369.
52. Fromm H: Ursodeoxycholic acid for gallstone dissolution: The emergence of a new therapeutic application for an old bile acid, in Fisher MM, Goresky CA, Shaffer EA, et al (eds): *Gallstones*. New York, Plenum, 1979; pp 363–370.
53. Thistle JL, Schoenfield LJ: Lithogenic bile among young Indian women. Lithogenic potential decreased with chenodeoxycholic acid. *N Engl J Med* 1971; 284:177–181.
54. Berge-Henegouwen GP Van, Hoffman AF: Pharmacology of chenodeoxycholic acid. II. Absorption and metabolism. *Gastroenterology* 1977; 73:300–309.
55. Fromm H, Erbler HC, Eschler A, et al: Alterations of bile acid metabolism during treatment with chenodeoxycholic acid. Studies of the role of the appearance of ursodeoxycholic acid in the dissolution of gallstones. *Klin Wschr* 1976; 54:1125–1131.
56. Thistle JL, Hofmann AF, Yu PYS, et al: Effect of varying doses of chenodeoxycholic acid on bile lipid and biliary bile acid composition in gallstone patients: A dose-response study. *Am J Dig Dis* 1977; 22:1–6.
57. Fromm H, Sarva RP, Bazzoli F, et al: Formation of ursodeoxycholic acid from chenodeoxycholic acid in the human colon: Studies of the role of 7-ketolithocholic acid as an intermediate. *J Lipid Res* 1983; 24:841–853.
58. Salen G, Tint GS, Eliav B, et al: Increased formation of ursodeoxycholic acid in patients treated with chenodeoxycholic acid. *J Clin Invest* 1974; 53:612–621.
59. Fromm H, Carlson GL, Hofmann AF, et al: Metabolism in man of 7-ketolithocholic acid: A precursor of chenodeoxycholic and ursodeoxycholic acids. *Am J Physiol* 1980; 239:G161–G166.
60. Nilsell K, Angelin B, Leijd B, et al: Comparative effects of ursodeoxycholic acid and chenodeoxycholic acid on bile acid kinetics and biliary lipid secretion in man. Evidence for different modes of action on bile synthesis. *Gastroenterology* 1983; 85:1248–1256.
61. Hardison WGM, Grundy SM: The effect of ursodeoxycholate and its taurine conjugate on bile acid synthesis and cholesterol absorption. *Gastroenterology* 1984; 87:130–135.
62. Von Bergmann K, Epple-Gutsfeld M, Leiss O: Differences in the effects of chenodeoxycholic and ursodeoxycholic acids on biliary lipid secretion and bile acid synthesis in patients with gallstones. *Gastroenterology* 1984; 87:136–143.
63. Carey MC, Wu SJ, Watkins JB: Solution properties of sulfated monohydroxy bile salts. Relative insolubility of the disodium salt of glycolithocholate sulfate. *Biochim Biophys Acta* 1979; 575:16–26.
64. Palmer RH: The formation of bile acid sulfates: A new pathway of bile acid metabolism in humans. *Proc Natl Acad Sci USA* 1967; 58:1047–1050.
65. Fedorowski T, Salen G, Tint GS, et al: Transformation of chenodeoxycholic acid and ursodeoxycholic acid by human intestinal bacteria. *Gastroenterology* 1979; 77:1068–1073.
66. Bazzoli F, Fromm H, Sarva RP, et al: Comparative formation of lithocholic acid from chenodeoxycholic and ursodeoxycholic acids in the colon. *Gastroenterology* 1982; 83:753–760.
67. Albers JJ, Grundy SM, Cleary PA, et al and the National Cooperative Gallstone Study Group: National Cooperative Gallstone Study: The effect of chenodeoxycholic acid on lipoproteins and apolipoproteins. *Gastroenterology* 1982; 82:638–646.
68. Poupon R, Chretien Y, Poupon RE, et al: Is ursodeoxycholic acid an effective treatment for primary biliary cirrhosis? *Lancet* 1987; i:834–836.
69. Malavolti M, Fromm H, Ceryak S, et al: Modulation of low density lipoprotein receptor activity by bile acids: Differential effects on chenodeoxycholic and ursodeoxycholic acids in the hamster. *J Lipid Res* 1987; 28:1281–1295.
70. Leuschner U, Leuschner M, Sieratzki J, et al: Gallstone dissolution with ursodeoxycholic acid in patients with chronic active hepatitis and two years follow-up. A pilot study. *Dig Dis Sci* 1985; 30:642–649.
71. Kupfer RM, Maudgal DP, Northfield TC: Gallstone dissolution rate during chenic acid therapy: Effect of bedtime administration plus low cholesterol diet. *Dig Dis Sci* 1982; 27:1025–1029.
72. Iser JH, Dowling HR, Mok HYI, et al: Chenodeoxycholic acid treatment of gallstones—A follow-up report analysis of factors influencing response to therapy. *N Engl J Med* 1975; 293:378–383.
73. Fromm H: Serum lipid and lipoprotein analysis in patients treated with chenodeoxycholic and ursodeoxycholic acids, in Barbara L, Dowling RH, Hofmann AF, et al (eds): *Recent Advances in Bile Acid Research*. New York, Raven Press, 1985; p 225.
74. Thistle JL: Monooctanoin in the dissolution of gallstones in bile ducts: Limitations and precautions. *Hepatology* 1987; 7:192–194.
75. Schwabe AD, Cozzetto F, Bennett LR, et al: Estimation of fat absorption by monitoring of expired radioactive carbon dioxide after feeding a radioactive fat. *Gastroenterology* 1962; 42:285–291.
76. Gadacz TR: The effect of monooctanoin on retained common duct stones. *Surgery* 1981; 89:527–531.
77. Bogardus JB: Importance of viscosity in the dis-

solution rate of cholesterol in monooctanoin solutions. *J Pharm Sci* 1984; 73:906–910.
78. Igimi H, Hisatsugu T, Nishimura M: The use of d-Limonene preparation as a dissolving agent of gallstones. *Dig Dis Sci* 1976; 21:926–939.
79. Neoptolemos JP, Hofmann AF, Moossa AR: Chemical treatment of stones in the biliary tree. *Br J Surg* 1986; 73:515–524.
80. Leuschner U, Baumgartel H, Wurbs D: Auflosung von Cholesterin-Gallengangssteinen mit einer modifizierten Capmul 8210-Emulsion and einer EDTA-Gallensalzlosung. *Leber Magen Darm* 1980; 10:284–287.
81. Allen MJ, Borody TJ, LaRusso NF, et al: Gallstone dissolution—A comparison of solvents for direct biliary perfusion (abstract). *Hepatology* 1983; 3:871.
82. Teplick SK, Haskin PH, Goldstein RC, et al: Common bile duct stone dissolution with methyl tertiary butyl ether: Experience with three patients. *AJR* 1987; 148:372–374.
83. Van Sonnenberg E, Hofmann AF, Neoptolemus J, et al: Gallstone dissolution with methyl tert-butyl ether via percutaneous cholecystostomy: Success and caveats. *AJR* 1986; 146:865–867.
84. Greiner L, Wenzel H, Jakobeit CH: Biliary shock-wave lithotripsy: Fragmentation and lysis—A new method. *Dtsch Med Wschr* 1987; 49:1893–1896.
85. Chaussy CH, Brendel W, Schmiedt E: Extracorporeally induced destruction of kidney stones by shock waves. *Lancet* 1980; 1265–1268.

24

Sclerosing Cholangitis: Treatment or Transplant?

NICHOLAS F. LARUSSO, M.D.
RUSSELL H. WIESNER, M.D.

Primary sclerosing cholangitis (PSC) is a chronic, cholestatic syndrome of unknown etiology characterized by diffuse inflammation and fibrosis of the biliary system. The pathologic process leads to obliteration of intrahepatic and extrahepatic bile ducts and to cirrhosis. The course is variable but often is one of slow progression, perhaps over decades, to portal hypertension and death from liver failure. In a subset of asymptomatic patients with PSC, the disease may remain stable for years. PSC may occur alone but is commonly (> 50%) associated with inflammatory bowel disease, usually chronic ulcerative colitis (CUC).

SYMPTOMS AND SIGNS

PSC usually begins insidiously; this makes it difficult to determine the onset of the disease accurately. Nevertheless, most patients have had symptoms for an average of 24 months before diagnosis. The gradual onset of progressive fatigue and pruritus followed by jaundice is the most frequent symptom complex that leads to the diagnosis of PSC. Clinical evidence of cholangitis (recurrent right upper-quadrant pain, fever, and jaundice) is uncommon unless previous bile duct reconstructive surgery has been done. More recently, totally asymptomatic patients with PSC are being diagnosed because of abnormalities on routine blood tests which prompt further work-up, including cholangiography. Although some patients with PSC may have a normal physical examination, most patients have some abnormality, most commonly hepatomegaly, jaundice, and splenomegaly.

BIOCHEMICAL TESTS

Virtually all patients with PSC have a cholestatic biochemical profile. The serum alkaline phosphatase is almost always abnormal, although it may fluctuate. The vast majority of patients have an increase in serum aspartate transaminase level, usually to a mild degree. Approximately one-half of the patients will have a modest increase in their total serum bilirubin; however, these values may be normal or sometimes very high.

Tests related to copper metabolism are virtually always abnormal in patients with PSC. For example, hepatic copper levels are elevated in approximately 90% of patients while urine levels are increased in up to two-thirds; in both cases, the levels are increased to the degree seen in primary biliary cirrhosis (PBC), Wilson's disease, and Indian childhood cirrhosis. Similarly, serum copper and ceruloplasmin levels are usually increased in patients with PSC as they commonly are in patients with primary biliary cirrhosis.

RADIOLOGIC FEATURES

Early articles, based largely on findings at surgery, emphasized the extrahepatic location of the ductal changes in PSC. Recently, however, use of improved cholangiographic techniques indicates that the intrahepatic ducts are almost always involved radiographically in this syndrome, often to a greater degree than the extrahepatic ducts. Endoscopic or transhepatic cholangiography show diffusely distributed strictures of the intrahepatic and extrahepatic bile ducts in virtually all patients. Most commonly, the strictures are short (1 to 2 cm long) and annular with intervening segments of apparently normal or slightly dilated ducts which produce the characteristic "beaded" appearance. Focal dilatation of bile ducts between strictures is also a common finding, but diffuse nonsegmental dilatation is unusual.

LIVER HISTOLOGY

In virtually all patients with PSC, histologic abnormalities are evident on liver biopsy specimens. The characteristic features on liver biopsy specimens are bile duct proliferation, periductal fibrosis, periductal inflammation, ductal obliteration, and loss of bile ducts. Most commonly, the disease begins with enlargement of portal tracts (stage I), characterized by some edema, connective tissue and proliferation of interlobular bile ducts; inflammatory infiltrates are not prominent. With progression, tongues of connective tissue grow into the periportal parenchyma (stage II), again with only mild cellular inflammation. This process leads to the formation of fibrous septa (stage III) and biliary cirrhosis (stage IV). The pathognomonic histologic changes on liver biopsy specimens occur in the early stages; these changes are characterized by fibrous-obliterative cholangitis leading to replacement of duct segments by solid cords of connective tissue and to complete loss of interlobular and adjacent septal bile ducts with time.

PATHOGENESIS

The cause of PSC is unknown; genetic factors, acquired factors, or both, could be involved. Several recent observations are consistent with an important role for genetic factors in PSC. For example, the frequency of HLA-B8 is significantly higher in patients with PSC (60%) than in control subjects (25%). Also, recent reports have described the familial occurrence of both PSC and CUC, further evidence suggesting a genetic component to the disease.

Important acquired factors could theoretically include toxins, infectious agents, or altered immunity. Although elevated hepatic copper levels were initially thought to be an important potential toxin in the initiation or perpetuation of the disease, recent negative results from a controlled trial with D-penicillamine (see below) make it unlikely that elevated hepatic copper levels are pathogenetically important. Recently, extrahepatic biliary tract disease closely mimicking PSC has been described following infusions with the chemotherapeutic agent, 5-fluorodeoxyuridine. This drug apparently causes small vessel arteriopathy which likely leads to bile duct fibrosis and destruction. This syndrome, however, represents a type of secondary sclerosing cholangitis rather than PSC. Only few data are available concerning the possible role of infectious agents in the etiopathogenesis of PSC. Results of several studies have excluded the hepatitis B virus as a causative agent. Cytomegalovirus may affect intrahepatic bile ducts, but the histologic picture differs from that seen in PSC. Reovirus type 3 has been associated with neonatal biliary atresia which, like PSC, is characterized by obliterative cholangitis. However, reovirus infections have not so far been directly linked to the development of PSC, and a preliminary report indicates that elevated titers of antibody to reovirus type 3 are not more prevalent in patients with PSC than in the general population.

Currently, the pathogenesis of PSC is most closely linked with alterations in the immune mechanisms. Although serologic markers (e.g., mitochondrial or smooth muscle antibodies) are generally absent, other data strongly support disturbed alterations in immunity. For example, PSC is associated with HLA-B8 and HLA-DR3, two haplotypes frequently noted to be present in autoimmune diseases. Other more direct lines of evidence supporting an immunologic basis include the inhibition of leukocyte migration by biliary antigens, elevated IgM levels, the presence of circulating immune complexes, decreased clearance of immune complexes, and increased complement metabolism. Also, cells involved in the destruction of bile ducts in PSC have recently been shown to be T lymphocytes and abnormalities in lymphocyte subsets in peripheral blood have also been demonstrated. Finally, enhanced autoreactivity of suppressor/cytotoxic T lymphocytes from peripheral blood of patients with PSC has been reported. All these studies support alterations in the immune system as pathogenetically related to the development or perpetuation of PSC, although the exact mechanisms are still not understood.

MANAGEMENT

General Guidelines

The management of PSC provides a real challenge to the clinician, given the array of symptoms and complications that can develop and the absence of any effective specific therapy. The first decision regarding management relates to whether or not any therapeutic intervention is necessary in a patient with newly diagnosed PSC. In the asymptomatic patient with mild liver test abnormalities and early histologic disease by liver biopsy, because the prognosis is probably quite good and no specific therapy is available, observation would be reasonable. Alternatively, therapy might be considered in the context of a randomized trial. If a decision is made to intervene therapeutically, one needs to identify the goal of treatment. Specifically, therapy should be directed toward either symptoms, complications, or the underlying hepatobiliary disease. For example, pruritus and fat-soluble vitamin deficiencies are common problems in patients with PSC; conventional approaches to management of these problems, which will not be reviewed here, are reasonable. Also, when complications such as varicele bleeding develop, appropriate intervention (such as varicele sclerosis) should be considered.

Treatment of Complications

There are, however, complications relatively specific for PSC, including recurrent cholangitis and bacteremia, dominant strictures, and cholangiocarcinoma. Patients with recurrent episodes of cholangitis without dominant stricture formation should be treated with broad-spectrum antibiotics as needed. Prophylactic antibiotics are favored by some in patients with frequent episodes of cholangitis, but the efficacy of this approach has not been established. Also, patients may develop dominant strictures in the biliary tract that can lead to rapid increases in serum bilirubin levels, recurrent episodes of cholangitis, or pruritus. Consideration of dilation of these strictures in the symptomatic patient is reasonable; depending on their location, a transhepatic or endoscopic approach with or without stent placement may be useful. Indeed, our experience with the transhepatic approach in symptomatic patients with PSC and dominant strictures suggests that balloon dilation is very effective in alleviating pruritus and in diminishing the frequency of cholangitic episodes secondary to dominant strictures. Our experience also suggests that cholangiocarcinoma develops in probably 10% to 15% of patients with PCS. The management of a suspected or established cholangiocarcinoma superimposed on PSC is complicated and is currently in evolution. If the cholangiocarcinoma is surgically resectable and the patient is not currently a candidate for liver transplantation, an attempt at surgical resection would seem reasonable. Alternatively, if the cholangiocarcinoma is not surgically resectable, or if it is resectable but the patient has advanced parenchymal liver disease, the physician should consider orthotopic liver transplantation.

Surgical Treatment of the Underlying Hepatobiliary Disease

Currently, there is no specific treatment for the underlying hepatobiliary disease in PSC. This reflects, in part, our lack of knowledge about the exact pathogenesis of the disease. Nevertheless, therapeutic approaches for the underlying hepatobiliary disease can be categorized as mechanical, medical, and surgical. Advocates have suggested that balloon dilation of dominant strictures may be beneficial to the natural history of the underlying hepatobiliary disease. There are no studies to support this position and intuitively, given the diffuse nature of the disease and the fact that patients die from parenchymal dysfunction and liver failure, it is not attractive. Thus, we recommend balloon dilation of dominant strictures only for symptomatic relief of jaundice or pruritus and not for treatment of the underlying hepatobiliary disease.

Three surgical procedures have been considered of potential benefit in the treatment of PSC: biliary tract reconstructive procedures, protocolectomy in a patient with PSC and CUC, and orthotopic liver transplantation.

Biliary Tract Reconstructive Procedures

We consider biliary tract reconstructive procedures in the same category as balloon dilation of dominant strictures (i.e., as palliative procedures to alleviate symptoms and ones that are unlikely to affect the natural history of the disease). However, no good published data are currently available to allow one to confidently evaluate the role of biliary tract reconstructive procedures in treatment of the underlying liver disease. Our own data, currently being evaluated, suggest no beneficial effect of these types of procedures on the natural history of the disease.

Proctocolectomy

Some have suggested that proctocolectomy in a patient with PSC and CUC may favorably affect the hepatobiliary disease. This is not only because beneficial treatment for PSC is needed, but because proctocolectomy in patients with PSC and CUC may be associated with considerable morbidity. Recently, we have prospectively studied the effects of proctocolectomy on the progression of clincial, biochemical, cholangiographic, and hepatic histologic features in 53 patients with PSC and CUC. Patients with both diseases who had undergone proctocolectomy ($n = 23$) were compared to those who had not ($n = 30$) over 4 years. New onset of complications, serial changes in biochemical tests, histologic progression on liver biopsy, and survival did not differ in the two groups. We concluded that proctocolectomy for chronic ulcerative colitis is not beneficial for primary sclerosing cholangitis in patients with both diseases.

Liver Transplantation

Finally, liver transplantation is a serious consideration for patients with any form of advanced liver disease, including PSC. Indeed, at many major transplant centers, including our own, PSC is one of the most frequent indications for liver transplantation in adults. Although data are still evolving, recent preliminary results suggest that the outcome of liver transplantation in patients with PSC is no different from that in patients with other forms of noninfectious, chronic liver disease, with 5-year survivals of approximately 60%. Our own preliminary experience supports this conclusion. Indeed, in a recent comparison of patients with PSC and PBC transplanted at Mayo, the 2-year estimated survival was 83% in both diseases, even though the operating time, number of reoperations, and frequency of chronic rejection and retransplantation were greater in PSC.

Medical Treatment of the Underlying Hepatobiliary Disease

Medical approaches for the treatment of the underlying hepatobiliary disease in

PSC have centered primarily on the use of cupruretic, antifibrogenic, and immunosuppressive agents. To date, however, no controlled trials of any form of medical therapy in PSC have been published in manuscript form.

Cupruretic Agents

The finding of elevated hepatic copper levels in PSC and early reports showing apparent biochemical improvement induced by D-penicillamine in PBC, another chronic cholestatic liver disease with many similarities to PSC, prompted a therapeutic trial of D-penicillamine in PSC in 1980. In a randomized prospective double-blind trial, 39 patients received penicillamine (250 mg three times a day) and 31 received a placebo. The two groups were highly comparable at entry with regard to clinical, biochemical, radiologic, and hepatic histologic features. Although a predictable cupruresis and a decrease in levels of hepatic copper were achieved in patients taking penicillamine, there was no beneficial effect on disease progression within 36 months or on overall survival. Progressive symptoms, deterioration in serial hepatic laboratory values, and histologic progression on sequential liver biopsy specimens were similar in both groups. The development of major side effects led to the permanent discontinuation of penicillamine in 21% of the patients taking the drug. We concluded from this study that the use of penicillamine in PSC is not associated with a beneficial effect on disease progression or survival and has considerable toxicity.

Immunosuppressive Agents

Corticosteroids have been used both topically and systemically in several small studies in PSC. A small controlled trial of nasobiliary lavage with corticosteroids versus placebo has recently been reported; the results were negative. Uncontrolled observations in a small number of patients with a marked inflammatory component to their PSC have shown impressive responses to orally administered corticosteroids. In one study, seven of ten patients with PSC showed objective biochemical improvement and some beneficial effect on liver histology while receiving long-term corticosteroid therapy. Previous smaller uncontrolled studies have not shown any beneficial effect of corticosteroids. Azathioprine has been used in at least two instances without apparent benefit. Also, use of low-dose methotrexate has recently been reported in two patients with PSC. In this small study, methotrexate caused improvement in biochemical studies, apparently stabilized bile duct scarring, and led to improvement in liver histology. The potential hepatotoxicity of methotrexate and the very small number of patients in this report necessitate that this drug not be used until results from controlled trials are available. Cyclosporine, a new immunosuppressive drug which inhibits the production of interleukin-2 by T lymphocytes resulting in decreased T lymphocyte activation and proliferation, is currently under investigation at Mayo in a double-blind, controlled trial. Preliminary results are not yet available.

Antifibrogenic Agents

Recently, interest has developed in the use of antifibrogenic agents, specifically colchicine, in PSC, given the promising but preliminary results of colchicine in PBC. We recently reported preliminary experience with combined prednisone and colchicine in 12 patients with PSC compared to 12 untreated patients matched for age, sex, initial biochemical levels, and liver histology. We observed impressive improvement in bilirubin, alkaline phosphatase, and aspartate aminotransferase levels when patients were reevaluated at 6 and 12 months after entry. A prospective, controlled, randomized trial employing this combination is currently underway at Mayo.

SUMMARY AND CONCLUSIONS

Primary sclerosing cholangitis is a generally progressive, sometimes fatal, chronic hepatobiliary disorder for which no effective medical or surgical therapy now exists. The syndrome occurs most frequently in young men and is characterized by chronic cholestasis, frequent association with CUC, a paucity of serologic markers, hepatic copper overload, and characteristic abnormalities in some liver biopsy specimens and in virtually all cholangiograms. The natural history of the syndrome is unclear; the disease likely progresses slowly and relentlessly over a decade or longer from a asymptomatic stage to a condition characterized by symptoms of cholestasis and complicated by cirrhosis and portal hypertension and carcinoma of the bile ducts. A subset of asymptomatic patients appears to have a more benign course. Management should first involve a thoughtful decision to observe, which is reasonable in the asymptomatic patient with early disease, or to intervene, particularly in patients with symptoms. Therapeutic goals should be defined and should concentrate on either alleviating symptoms, dealing with complications, or attempting to affect the underlying hepatobiliary disease. Symptomatic treatment and therapy for complications are similar to treatment employed in other chronic liver diseases, but also involve balloon dilation of dominant strictures in appropriately selected symptomatic patients. Biliary tract reconstructive surgery may alleviate symptoms in selected patients with PSC, but its effect on the natural history of the syndrome has not been determined. Proctocolectomy for CUC in a patient with CUC and PSC does not beneficially affect the progression of the underlying hepatobiliary disease. In contrast, orthotopic liver transplantation may be life-saving for patients with advanced disease. Medical therapy directed at arresting the progression of the underlying hepatobiliary disease is currently experimental and includes cupruretic, immunosuppressive, and antifibrogenic agents. Although a single recently completed controlled trial makes it unlikely that cupruretic agents will be helpful in this syndrome, antifibrogenic and immunosuppressive agents alone or in combination are currently undergoing evaluation in randomized trials.

Bibliography

Reviews

1. Wiesner RH, LaRusso NF: Clinicopathologic features of the syndrome of primary sclerosing cholangitis. *Gastroenterology* 1980; 79:200–206.
2. LaRusso NF, Wiesner RH, Ludwig J, et al: Primary sclerosing cholangitis. *N Engl J Med* 1984; 310:899–903.
3. Chapman RWG, Orborgh BAM, Rhodes JM, et al: Primary sclerosing cholangitis: A review of its clinical features, cholangiography and hepatic histology. *Gut* 1980; 21:870–877.

Complications of PSC

4. Wee A, Ludwig J, Coffey RJ, et al: Hepatobiliary carcinoma associated with primary sclerosing cholangitis and chronic ulcerative colitis. *Hum Pathol* 1985; 16(7):719–726.
5. MacCarty RL, LaRusso NF, May GR, et al: Cholangiocarcinoma complicating primary sclerosing cholangitis: Cholangiographic features. *Radiology* 1985; 156:43–46.
6. Gluskin LE, Payne JA: Cystic dilatation as a radiographic sign of cholangiocarcinoma complicating sclerosing cholangitis. *Am J Gastroenterol* 1983; 78:661–664.
7. Wiesner RH, LaRusso NF, Dozois RR, et al: Peristomal varices after proctocolectomy in patients with primary sclerosing cholangitis. *Gastroenterology* 1986; 90:316–322.

PSC and Radiology

8. MacCarty RL, LaRusso NF, Wiesner RH, et al: Primary sclerosing cholangitis: Findings on cholangiography and pancreatography. *Radiology* 1983; 149:39–44.
9. Li-Yeng C, Goldberg HI: Sclerosing cholangitis: Broad spectrum of radiographic features. *Gastrointest Radiol* 1984; 9:39–47.

PSC and Hepatobiliary Histology

10. Ludwig J, Barham SS, LaRusso NF, et al: Morphologic features of chronic hepatitis associated with primary sclerosing cholangitis or chronic ulcerative colitis. *Hepatology* 1981; 1:632–640.
11. Ludwig J, MacCarty RL, LaRusso NF, et al: Intrahepatic cholangiectases and large-duct obliteration in primary sclerosing cholangitis. *Hepatology* 1986; 6:560–568.

Etiopathogenesis of PSC

12. Bodenheimer HC Jr, LaRusso NF, Thayer WR Jr, et al: Elevated circulating immune complexes in primary sclerosing cholangitis. *Hepatology* 1983; 3:150–154.
13. Quigley EMM, LaRusso NF, Ludwig J, et al: Familial occurrence of primary sclerosing cholangitis and chronic ulcerative colitis. *Gastroenterology* 1983; 85:1160–1165.
14. MacFarlane IG, Wojeica BM, Tsantoulas DC, et

al: Leukocyte migration inhibition in response to biliary antigens in primary biliary cirrhosis, sclerosing cholangitis, and other chronic liver diseases. *Gastroenterology* 1979; 76:1333–1340.

Management of PSC

15. May GR, Bender CE, LaRusso NF, et al: Nonoperative dilatation of dominant strictures in primary sclerosing cholangitis. *Am J Radiol* 1985; 145:1061–1064.
16. LaRusso NF, Wiesner RH, Ludwig J: Recent advances in the diagnosis and management of primary sclerosing cholangitis. *Current Concepts in Gastroenterology* 1983; 8:6–9.
17. Wiesner RH, Ludwig J, LaRusso NF, et al: Diagnosis and treatment of primary sclerosing cholangitis, in Schaffner F (ed): *Seminars in Liver Disease*. New York, Thieme Inc., 1985, pp 241–253.
18. Pitt HA, Thompson HH, Tompkins RL, et al: Primary sclerosing cholangitis: Results of an aggressive surgical approach. *Ann Surg* 1984; 199:637–647.

VI
Small Intestine

# 25

Chronic Diarrhea:
How should we approach the diagnosis?

NORTON J. GREENBERGER, M.D.

Chronic diarrhea is a common problem facing the practitioner of medicine. Despite impressive advances in diagnostic technology, many patients continue to have chronic diarrhea without a firm diagnosis being established. Importantly, the history obtained and the physical examination performed are often perfunctory and the patient often undergoes a number of contrast and imaging studies, endoscopic procedures, and laboratory investigations, which may still be nondiagnostic. In all patients with chronic diarrhea, which I will arbitrarily define as diarrhea that has persisted over at least a 2-month period, there is need for a careful orderly approach to the differential diagnosis. In this chapter I will detail a method that I have employed in approaching such patients. The method emphasizes a careful history and physical examination; judicious and sequential use of laboratory investigations, contrast studies, and endoscopic procedures; and special situations in which more detailed investigations are required. I have found that unless I go through the detailed differential diagnostic approach to the patient with chronic diarrhea I will miss disorders that can be readily diagnosed, and, more importantly, such patients can be given inappropriate treatment.

HISTORY TAKING AND PHYSICAL EXAMINATION

The important diagnostic considerations in the patient with chronic diarrheal disorder are listed in Table 25-1. A careful history and physical examination will often provide the important clues in establishing diagnosis of several disorders listed in Table 25-1. This is now presented in more detail.

Iatrogenic Dietary Factors

A careful dietary history often is not obtained in patients with chronic diarrheal disorders. Several important questions that need to be asked, include the following: (1) How much coffee, tea, and other caffeine-containing beverages are ingested each day? (2) How much cola beverage is ingested each day? In this regard, it should be recalled that a 16-oz bottle of soda pop contains 40 gm of fructose as the sweetener, and approximately 15% of normal subjects will not absorb this amount of fructose completely.[1] (3) How much sorbitol-containing food does the patient ingest? Sorbitol is a potent laxative and is found in gum, mints, apples, peaches, pears, prunes, fortified fruit juices, and dietetic foods.[2] Importantly, many dietetic foods for diabetics are erroneously labeled "sugarless" when in fact such foods contain significant amounts of sorbitol. (4) How much pastry, candy, cookies, and chocolate does the patient ingest? (5) Does the patient have an eating disorder such as bulimia? A classic triad of physical findings—loss of enamel on the teeth, parotid enlargement, and roughening of the skin on the dorsum of the hand[3]—should alert the physician to

TABLE 25–1.
Differential Diagnosis of Chronic Diarrhea

1. Iatrogenic dietary factors
   A. Excess colas, coffee, fructose- and sorbitol-containing foods
   B. Bulimia and other eating disorders
2. Infections
   A. Amebiasis, giardiasis, Campylobacter
   B. Special considerations in immunocompromised and homosexual patients (AIDS)
3. Inflammatory bowel disease
   A. Idiopathic ulcerative colitis/regional enteritis
4. Idiopathic secretory diarrhea
   A. Microscopic colitis/collagenous colitis
   B. Idiopathic bile salt catharsis and variants
   C. Large-volume secretory diarrhea of uncertain cause
5. Incontinence
   A. Diabetes, anorectal surgery, errant episiotomy, and so forth
6. Irritable bowel syndrome
7. Drugs
8. Diverticular disease of the colon
9. Lactose intolerance
10. Laxative use and abuse
    A. NaOH test for phenolphthalein-containing laxatives
11. Metabolic
    A. Diabetes, hyperthyroidism, hypoadrenalism
12. Malabsorption
    A. Pancreatic exocrine insufficiency, regional enteritis, short bowel syndrome, bacterial overgrowth
13. Mechanical
    A. Fecal impaction (anticholinergics, tricyclics)
14. Neoplasms
    A. Carcinoma pancreas
    B. Endocrine tumors: Gastrinoma, VIP-oma, carcinoid, medullary cancer thyroid

the possibility that a patient has bulimia nervosa. In addition, it should be emphasized that many patients with bulimia nervosa have attempted to control their weight by other measures including the use of diuretics, use of laxatives, and alternating periods of starvation and binge eating.

Infections

A careful travel history should be obtained on all patients who have chronic diarrhea. Patients may have traveled to areas of the world where infections such as giardiasis, amebiasis, and Campylobacter enteritis are endemic. Immunocompromised patients and patients with AIDS are particularly prone to chronic gastrointestinal infections (see Table 25–2). Accordingly, a careful sexual history should be obtained on all patients with a chronic diarrheal disorder. Further, the finding of proctitis in a homosexual male should prompt consideration of several of the disorders listed in Table 25–2.

Inflammatory Bowel Disease

The inflammatory bowel diseases, idiopathic ulcerative colitis and regional enteritis, are usually diagnosed by employing composite criteria that include the history, physical examination, abnormalities identified in x-ray contrast studies, abnormalities identified on endoscopic examination, and histologic abnormalities noted in biopsy specimens. Several extraintestinal manifestations point to the diagnosis of inflammatory bowel disease, and these include aphthous ulcers of the mouth, uveitis, skin lesions, arthritis, arthralgia, fever, weight loss, and anemia. Physical examination may reveal a palpa-

TABLE 25–2.
Chronic Diarrheal Disorders in AIDS Patients and HIV-Positive Patients with Constitutional Symptoms

Amebiasis
Giardiasis
Histoplasmosis
Chlamydia trachomatis
Campylobacter
Cytomegalovirus*
Cryptosporidiosis
Candidiasis*
Isosporiasis
Mycobacterium avium intracellulare*
Clostridium difficile
AIDS enteropathy*

*Most frequent

ble mass in the right lower quadrant and evidence of perirectal disease (fissure-in-ano, rectal fissure), and both of these findings point toward a diagnosis of regional enteritis. Crohn's disease can also affect the vulva.

Idiopathic Secretory Diarrhea

A history of painless watery diarrhea should point away from the diagnosis of irritable bowel syndrome and toward several other diagnostic considerations. For example, painless watery diarrhea may be a manifestation of idiopathic bile salt catharsis or one of its variants. In this regard, approximately 5% of patients who undergo cholecystectomy develop diarrhea postoperatively and 5% to 10% of patients undergoing truncal vagotomy and a drainage procedure develop similar diarrhea. In both of these settings, diarrhea often responds to a bile salt-sequestering agent such as cholestyramine. Patients with microscopic colitis/collagenous colitis may also present with painless watery diarrhea that has failed to respond to symptomatic measures such as anticholinergic drugs.[4,5] Patients with painless watery diarrhea may also have an underlying secretory diarrhea due to endocrine neoplasm such as a gastrinoma or vasoactive intestinal peptide-secreting tumor (VIP-oma). Patients with the pseudo-VIP-oma syndrome (clinical features simulating a VIP-oma but without biochemical confirmation) have also been termed patients with large-volume secretory diarrhea of uncertain cause. It is possible, however, that as yet unidentified diarrheagenic factors or mediators may be present in such patients causing a large-volume secretory diarrhea. Some of the clinical features employed to differentiate between secretory and osmotic (alimentary) diarrhea are listed in Table 25–3. Patients with a secretory diarrhea usually have 24-hour stool volumes greater than 1.0 L, exhibit no change or only a modest decrease in stool volume after fasting, and frequently show a minimal stool osmolality gap. The latter criterion is the most controversial because several authorities have cited values for an appropriate stool osmolality gap as being less than 40, less than 50, and even less than 100 mmole. Other examples of secretory diarrhea include cholera, toxin-producing *Escherichia coli* infections, villous adenoma, and medullary carcinoma of the thyroid.

Incontinence

I am amazed at how often physicians neglect to ask patients with diarrhea whether they ever lose their stool (i.e., are incontinent). Patients are often embarrassed to tell their physicians that they are, in fact, occasionally incontinent of stool. If a patient is incontinent, it should prompt consideration of several disorders including diabetes mellitus, prior anorectal surgery, or errant episiotomy with resultant anal sphincter damage.[6] It is important for incontinence to be recognized because such patients can often be benefited by retraining exercises to enhance basal and squeeze and rectal pressures as well as anorectal volumes.

Irritable Bowel Syndrome

Important considerations in the diagnosis of irritable bowel syndrome and clinical criteria frequently employed in establishing this diagnosis are listed in Ta-

TABLE 25–3.
Features of Secretory and Osmotic (Alimentary) Diarrhea

Feature	Secretory Diarrhea	Osmotic Diarrhea
24-hr stool volume	Usually > 1.0 L	usually < 1.0 liter
Effect of fasting on stool volume	No change or modest ↓ (< 50% basal volume)	↓ > 50% of basal volume
Stool osmolality gap* (total osmolality minus 2 × measured Na$^+$ + K$^+$)	< 40*	> 40*
Examples	• Cholera • Toxin-producing *Escherichia coli* • Gastrinoma • VIP-oma • Villous adenoma • Medullary cancer thyroid	• Lactose intolerance • Laxative abuse • Diabetes mellitus • Short bowel syndrome • Ileal resection • Post gastric surgery

*Controversial test with values cited ranging from 40 and 50 to 100 mmole.

TABLE 25–4.
Diagnosis of Irritable Bowel Syndrome

1. Important clues from the history
   A. Absence of nocturnal diarrhea
   B. Absence of systemic symptoms or signs
      1. Anorexia, weight loss, fever, anemia
   C. Feeling of incomplete evacuation
   D. Bowel motions primarily in the morning
   E. Relief of discomfort after evacuation
   F. Female preponderance
   G. Long history frequent—unusual for onset to occur after age 50
2. Clinical criteria frequently employed
   A. Presence of abdominal pain with diarrhea or alternating diarrhea and constipation
      1. Presence of *painless* watery diarrhea should prompt other diagnostic considerations (see below)
   B. No hematochezia, melena, occult blood in stool
   C. Normal sigmoidoscopic examination
   D. Normal barium enema
   E. Exclusion of the disorders listed in Table 25–1
3. Differential diagnosis of irritable bowel syndrome
   A. Inadvertent dietary indiscretion/intolerance
   B. Subclinical carbohydrate malabsorption
   C. Lactose intolerance
   D. Laxative/diuretic abuse/eating disorder
   E. Colonic diverticular disease, usually with myochosis
   F. Drug associated
   G. Bile salt catharsis syndromes
      1. Idiopathic postcholecystectomy, postvagotomy, and gastric surgical procedure
   H. Incompletely understood motility disorders of colon or small bowel

ble 25-4. It can be seen that there are several important clues from the history. The differential diagnosis of irritable bowel syndrome will be commented on in detail below.

Drugs

A careful drug history must be obtained on all patients with chronic diarrhea. Several medications can cause diarrhea including antacids (which the patient may not regard as a drug), diuretics, antibiotics (which may or may not be related to *Clostridium difficile* infection), promotility drugs such as Reglan, and antigout medications such as colchicine.

Diverticular Disease of the Colon

Patients with diverticular disease of the colon, especially if myochosis is also present, often develop diarrhea. However, it is unusual for patients with diverticular disease of the colon to have persistent unremitting diarrhea for several months at a time. Accordingly, in a patient with diverticular disease of the colon and persistent diarrhea, the presence of diverticular disease does not obviate the need for a more detailed evaluation of the patient.

Lactose Intolerance

Primary lactose intolerance not associated with any underlying disease is a common clinical problem. All patients with diarrhea should be asked specifically about their ingestion of milk or milk products to determine whether there is temporal relationship between ingestion of milk products and the subsequent development of crampy abdominal pain and diarrhea. In addition, patients who are lactose intolerant often develop gas, bloating, and abdominal distention. The amount of lactose that may cause such symptoms is highly variable and may range from as little as 3 gm to as much as 60 gm of lactose. Diagnosis of primary lactose intolerance is usually established by the history of intolerance to lactose-containing foods and amelioration of such symptoms with a lactose-restricted diet. In equivocal cases, a lactose tolerance test with measurement of breath hydrogen can be used to confirm the diagnosis. It is not generally appreciated that approximately one-third of patients with proven lactose intolerance will not experience amelioration of abdominal pain and diarrhea with a lactose-restricted diet. Such patients may have either an underlying irritable bowel syndrome or secondary lactose intolerance (i.e., lactose intolerance associated with disorders such as regional enteritis, nontropical sprue, postgastric surgery syndrome and so forth).

Laxative Use and Abuse

A careful history of laxative use should be obtained with all patients with chronic diarrhea. However, some patients who abuse laxatives deny doing so. Accordingly, it is necessary to check the stool for presence of laxatives. Phenolphthalein-containing laxatives can be detected in the stool by addition of small amounts of sodium hydroxide: Phenolphthalein is an acid-base marker and the development of a red color indicates the presence of phenolphthalein.[7] The addition of hydrochloric acid will reverse the color change. Only a few currently available laxatives, however, contain phenolphthalein and thus, the diagnosis of chronic laxative abuse can be easily missed. Another clue to the presence of laxative abuse is the presence of hypokalemia. Such patients may or may not exhibit inappropriate potassium losses in the urine (i.e., so-called kaliopenic neuropathy due to laxative abuse).

Metabolic

Patients with diabetes, hyperthyroidism, and hypoadrenalism may have diarrhea as a primary symptom of their underlying endocrine disorder. Accordingly, a blood glucose determination and a T_4 should be obtained on all patients with unexplained diarrhea. Patients with unexplained weight loss, nausea and vomiting, eosinophilia, or salt craving, especially if this constellation of clinical features occurs in the presence of hyponatremia and hyperkalemia, should have appropriate plasma cortisol determinations and more definitive tests to diagnose hypoadrenalism. It should be emphasized, however, that if such patients receive intravenous fluids, especially saline, the above noted electrolyte abnormalities may not be evident, and the diagnosis may be masked.

Malabsorption

The most frequent disorders causing malabsorption include pancreatic exocrine insufficiency, regional enteritis with extensive ileal disease or following ileal resection, short bowel syndrome, and bacterial overgrowth of the proximal small bowel. A history of chronic ethanol abuse coupled with weight loss and diarrhea should raise the question of pancreatic exocrine insufficiency. The clues to the diagnosis of regional enteritis have been noted above. The diagnosis of short bowel syndrome would be evident from the history. Several conditions that predispose to abnormal bacterial proliferation of the proximal small bowel include hypomotility disorders (scleroderma), diabetes mellitus, after subtotal gastrectomy, strictures, fistulas, immunoglobulin deficiency, and pernicious anemia. Tests used for assessing intestinal absorptive function are detailed in Table 25–5.

Mechanical

It is not generally appreciated that patients with fecal impaction can present with diarrhea as the predominant symptom. Thus, in elderly patients who reside in nursing homes and who present with diarrhea, a fecal impaction must be excluded. Use of anticholinergic drugs and tricyclic antidepressants, which have anticholinergic properties, often predispose to the development of fecal impaction, and this diagnosis should be excluded in such patients.

Neoplasms

Several neoplasms associated with the development of diarrhea are carcinoma of the pancreas, endocrine tumors such as gastrinoma, VIP-oma, carcinoid tumor, medullary carcinoma of the thyroid, and villous adenoma. In any patient who is past the age of 50 and who develops diarrhea accompanied by any of the symptoms (weight loss, anorexia, abdominal pain, fever, back pain, and flushing) or signs of diabetes, *neoplasm* must be excluded. Carcinoma of the pancreas is the most frequent neoplasm encountered, and approximately 20% of patients with carcinoma of the pancreas present with diarrhea.

SUGGESTED WORK-UP FOR PATIENTS WITH CHRONIC DIARRHEA

The suggested work-up for patients with chronic diarrhea is detailed in Table 25–5. For purposes of this discussion, chronic diarrhea has been arbitrarily defined as diarrhea that has persisted for at least 2 months. Several patients at the time of presentation will have had many of the tests listed under category I (i.e., tests usually done on all patients before they are seen by a consultant). All too often, however, the tests carried out may not have been of the requisite quality. Accordingly, it is often necessary to repeat the tests listed under category I. It should also be emphasized that not all the tests in this category need be done if a diagnosis becomes evident from a careful history, physical examination, and carefully selected tests within category I. However, to be sure that treatable disorders are not missed, it is often necessary to proceed in an orderly fashion and carry most of the tests listed in category I. These tests are now discussed in detail.

Stool Examinations

Stool specimens should be obtained for analysis of occult blood, culture for en-

Table 25-5.
Suggested Work-up for Patients with Chronic Diarrhea*

I. Usually done on all patients
   A. Stool examinations
      1. Occult blood
      2. Culture for enteric pathogens (*Campylobacter, Chlamydia, Yersinia* and so forth)
      3. White blood cells
      4. Ova and parasites
      5. Qualitative/quantitative fat determination, especially if weight loss and/or abnormal chemistry profile is present
      6. Test for phenolpthalein-containing laxative (NaOH test)
   B. Sigmoidoscopy (rigid or flexible)
      1. With biopsy
      2. With cultures
   C. Contrast studies
      1. Barium enema
      2. Upper GI and small bowel series
   D. Blood tests
      1. Glucose, T_4, immunoglobulin, eosinophils
      2. Gastrin, VIP, calcitonin (if secretory diarrhea is present)
   E. Tests of intestinal absorptive function
      1. Chemistry profile: serum calcium, albumin, K^+, cholesterol, protime
      2. Qualitative/quantitative fat determinations
      3. D-xylose, Schilling test for B_{12} absorption
      4. Breath test if bacterial overgrowth suspected (lactulose), etc.
      5. Small bowel biopsy, aspirate, and culture, especially if malabsorption suspected
II. Frequently done tests/procedures
      1. Lactose tolerance test with measurement breath H_2
      2. UGI endoscopy and colonoscopy with biopsies
      3. CT scan abdomen
      4. Urine for 5-hydroxyindoleacetic acid (5-HIAA) (rarely helpful)
III. Carried out if indicated
      1. Endoscopic retrograde cholangiopancreatography (ERCP)
      2. Pancreatic function tests (chymex-bentiromide)
      3. Celiac/mesenteric angiography
IV. Therapeutic trials
      1. Restricted diets:
         a. Lactose, sugar, fat
      2. Medications—Cholestyramine, anticholinergics, antibiotics, corticosteroids, phenothiazines, pancreatic enzymes, histamine-H_2-receptor blockers, nonsteroidal anti-inflammatory drugs (NSAID), lithium, somatostatin analogues

*Most important

teric pathogens such as *Campylobacter, Chlamydia,* and *Yersinia*, white blood cells, ova, and parasites. Examination of the stool for leukocytes is particularly important because the presence of fecal leukocytes indicates a disease process that has caused damage to the colonic mucosa—is most frequently an infectious or inflammatory disease process.[8] If the patient has lost weight or if the chemistry profile is abnormal (especially if the serum calcium, albumin, cholesterol, and prothrombin time are abnormal), then it is important to determine whether malabsorption is present. A properly performed qualitative stool fat, if abnormal, will be a reliable indicator that the patient has steatorrhea. However, the gold standard remains the quantitative fecal fat determination. If this is abnormal, then a detailed search must be made to establish the correct diagnosis. Finally, in any patient with chronic diarrhea, the stool should be tested for the presence of phenolphthalein-containing laxatives with the sodium hydroxide test.

Endoscopic Procedures

Usually, patients with diarrhea that has persisted for over 2 months will have had a sigmoidoscopic examination. If this has not been obtained, then it is reasonable to carry out a flexible sigmoidoscopic examination and obtain biopsy specimens even if the colonic mucosa appears normal. It has been shown, for example, that patients with microscopic colitis/collagenous colitis may have a perfectly normal appearing colonic mucosa but may have clearly abnormal biopsy specimen suggestive of this disorder. If ulcerations are encountered, then it is also important to obtain appropriate cultures. In patients in whom Crohn's disease is a diagnostic possibility, it is important to carry out full colonoscopy to better assess the entire colon and to determine whether skip lesions are present.

Contrast Studies

If total colonoscopy has been performed, it will obviate the need for barium studies of the colon. If flexible sigmoidoscopy examination with biopsy and a good quality barium enema examination have been performed, then this will usually obviate the need for additional procedures such as total colonoscopy. If there is evidence of malabsorption, especially if steatorrhea is present and the cause is not evident, then a good quality small bowel series should be obtained. A small bowel enema or enteroclysis is a superior examination, but it is not cost effective to start with this procedure.

Blood Tests

As noted above, it is important to obtain routine blood tests (fasting and/or 2-hr postprandial blood glucose, T_4, immunoglobulins) and to check for eosinophilia. If watery diarrhea is present or if secretory diarrhea is suspected, then it is also reasonable to check serum gastrin and VIP levels. If there is a family history of medullary carcinoma of the thyroid or if there is an abnormal neck examination, it is also reasonable to determine serum calcitonin levels.

Tests of Intestinal Absorptive Function

The routine chemistry profile provides clues that the patient may have impaired intestinal absorptive function. Thus, the serum calcium, albumin, cholesterol, prothrombin time, iron, and potassium should be checked. In the presence of diarrhea and weight loss, qualitative stool fat determination is also an important test to do. If that is abnormal, then the full gamut of intestinal absorptive studies should be carried out including the d-xylose test, Schilling test for vitamin B_{12} absorption (see Table 25-6), small bowel biopsy aspirate and culture, and breath test(s) if bacterial overgrowth is suspected.

Frequently Done Tests and Procedures

The lactose tolerance test with measurement of breath hydrogen will confirm that a patient has either primary or secondary lactose intolerance. However, as noted above, patients with lactose intolerance may have an underlying disorder. If lactose intolerance is suspected, it is reasonable to place the patient on a lactose-free diet and observe whether amelioration of symptoms occurs. If the patient continues to have symptoms, this usually indicates the need for additional studies. Upper gastrointestinal endoscopy is frequently performed if a small bowel biopsy is needed because it is reasonable to obtain a biopsy by this method. If Zollinger-Ellison syndrome (gastrinoma) is suspected, a very careful examination of the duodenum is needed because 6% to 8% of

TABLE 25–6.
Schilling Test in Malabsorption Disorders

Part	Without Intrinsic Factor	With Intrinsic Factor	After Antibiotic	After Specific Rx for Ileal Disease	After Pancreatic Enzyme	Interpretation and Comment
I	+	–	–	–		An abnormal part I test is nonspecific and consistent with gastric disorders, intraluminal disorders, ileal disease, and pancreatic insufficiency.
II		+				The Schilling test will normalize in > 90% of patients with pernicious anemia or postgastrectomy B_{12} malabsorption. An abnormal part II test is consistent with intraluminal factors (bacterial overgrowth, Zollinger-Ellison syndrome), ileal disease (regional enteritis), and pancreatic insufficiency.
III			+			Correction of B_{12} malabsorption after antibiotics directed against aerobic and anaerobic bacteria supports a diagnosis of bacterial overgrowth of the small bowel.
IV				+		Normalization of Schilling test after corticosteroid therapy implies improvement in ileal function in patients with regional enteritis.
V					+	Approximately 40% of patients with pancreatic insufficiency have B_{12} malabsorption which is corrected with pancreatic enzymes.

gastrinomas are located in the duodenum. CT scan of the abdomen is useful in diagnosing carcinoma of the pancreas, carcinoma of the stomach, and intra-abdominal lymphoma/Hodgkin's disease. CT scan of the abdomen will be abnormal in approximately 75% to 80% of the patients with carcinoma of the pancreas. In one quarter of the abnormal tests, the only finding will be an enlarged pancreas.

Tests Carried Out If Indicated

Endoscopic retrograde cholangiopancreatography (ERCP) is often employed to confirm the presence of a pancreatic ductal lesion (i.e., most likely carcinoma). Invasive pancreatic function tests, such as the secretin-CCK-PZ test, are not widely available. Accordingly, if chronic pancreatic disease is suspected a screening test such as the Chymex (bentiromide) test may be carried out. If this test is abnormal, it would indicate the need for more detailed tests of the pancreas (i.e., CT scan of the abdomen or ERCP). It is important to emphasize, however, that whenever the bentiromide test is employed the d-xylose test should also be performed. If both of these tests are performed, and the bentiromide test is abnormal and the xylose test is normal, an abnormal value has a sensitivity of approximately 65% and a specificity of approximately 90% indicating that a pancreatic disease process is present. Celiac and mesenteric angiography are often employed if a pancreatic endocrine tumor is suspected; such angiographic studies will detect a few such tumors not identified by CT scan, and this is a useful procedure to consider if pancreatic endocrine tumor is strongly suspected. Angiography is also occasionally useful for patients with carcinoma of the pancreas, but use in this setting has largely been superceded by the advent of CT scanning and ERCP.

Therapeutic Trials

In occasional patients, even after the performance of all the tests listed in Table 25–5, a diagnosis is not evident. Such patients may have idiopathic secretory diarrhea of uncertain cause or very small endocrine tumors which have eluded identification by CT scanning, angiography, and even laparotomy. It is often necessary, therefore, to use therapeutic trials to see if improvement in diarrhea can be effected. Diets restricted in lactose, simple sugars, and fat have been employed with variable success. A number of medications are available for treating diarrhea. Cholestyramine and other bile salt-sequestering agents should be considered in patients with painless watery diarrhea of uncertain cause. Anticholinergics are rarely effective in controlling chronic diarrhea. If bacterial overgrowth is suspected but cannot be verified, a trial with antibiotics active toward both anaerobic and aerobic gram-negative microorganisms (Bactrim) might be considered. If pancreatic insufficiency is suspected, a trial of pancreatic enzymes is reasonable. In patients with idiopathic secretory diarrhea, there have been variable responses to corticosteroids, nonsteroidal anti-inflammatory drugs (NSAID), lithium, and somatostatin analogues.

References

1. Ravich WJ, Bayless TM, Thomas M: Fructose: Incomplete intestinal absorption in humans. *Gastroenterology* 1983; 84:26–29.
2. Hyams JS: Sorbitol intolerance: An unappreciated cause of functional gastrointestinal complaints. *Gastroenterology* 1983; 84:30–33.
3. Mitchell JE, Seim HC, Colon E, et al: Medical complications and medical management of bulimia. *Ann Intern Med* 1987; 107:71–77.
4. Bo-Lin GW, Vendrell D, Lee E, et al: An evaluation of the significance of microscopic colitis in patients with chronic diarrhea. *J Clin Invest* 1985; 75:1559–1569.
5. Jessuruh Y, Yardley JH, Lee EL, et al: Microscopic and collagenous colitis: Different names for the same condition. *Gastroenterology* 1986; 91:1583–1584.
6. Read NW, Harford WV, Schmuler AC, et al: Clinical study of patients with fecal incontinence and diarrhea. *Gastroenterology* 1979; 76:747–756.
7. Kramer P, Pope CE: Fractitious diarrhea induced by phenolphthalein. *Arch Intern Med* 1964; 114:634–636.
8. Harris JC, DuPont HL, Harnick RB: Fecal leukocytes in diarrheal illness. *Ann Intern Med* 1972; 76:697–703.

26

Work-up of the Patient with Recurrent Right Upper-Quadrant Pain

JOHN E. STONE, M.D.
WALTER J. HOGAN, M.D.
JOSEPH E. GEENEN, M.D.

Evaluation of patients with recurrent upper abdominal pain frequently discloses the presence of gallstones and often leads to cholecystectomy. Following cholecystectomy, it is estimated that 5% to 15% of patients continue to have similar complaints of pain.[1] Considering the fact that 475,000 cholecystectomies were performed in the United States in 1985, it follows that at least 50,000 patients each year continue to have symptoms of upper abdominal pain despite removal of their gallbladder.[2] This pain problem is identified clinically as the "postcholecystectomy syndrome."

The pivotal point to successful management of patients with the postcholecystectomy syndrome is to maintain an "open-minded" approach to the differential diagnosis. Often, there is difficulty determining whether the pain truly originates from the biliary tract or whether it originates from another organ system. Secondly, one needs to distinguish between organic (structural) lesions and functional (motor) abnormalities.

In this chapter, we define the postcholecystectomy syndrome and review the clinical features of typical and atypical biliary pain symptoms. We outline disorders, both organic and functional, associated with the postcholecystectomy syndrome and discuss our current approach to the diagnosis and management of this clinical syndrome.

POSTCHOLECYSTECTOMY SYNDROME

Definition

The postcholecystectomy syndrome is a complex of pain symptoms which persist or occur de novo shortly after cholecystectomy. Classically, biliary-like pain is usually epigastric or very often right upper quadrant in location, and it is often precipitated by food intake. Commonly, there are associated dyspeptic symptoms. Objective findings associated with pancreaticobiliary disease are often lacking. The postcholecystectomy syndrome may be the result of (1) error in diagnosis prior to the removal of the gallbladder, or (2) a problem that develops or continues despite the appropriate operative removal of the gallbladder. Postcholecystectomy pain symptoms may not relate to biliary tract disease at all. Other upper abdominal organs can cause pain symptoms that imitate, very closely, typical biliary type symptoms.

Incidence and Experience

Glenn and McSherry[1] reviewed their series of 6,366 patients following biliary tract surgery and found that 253 patients, or 4.5%, required a second operation because of persistent postcholecystectomy pain. Eighty-three of these patients had common bile duct stones, 57 patients had "cystic duct disorders," and 19 patients had papillary stenosis. Eighty-seven patients (34%) required "nonbiliary tract" surgery to alleviate their pain.

Several years ago, we reviewed our experience of 97 patients referred to our diagnostic unit with pain and the presumptive diagnosis of the postcholecystectomy syndrome. All of these patients had severe recurrent typical biliary-like pain and had undergone extensive, albeit unrewarding, diagnostic evaluations.

Of these 97 patients, a diagnostic ERCP was successful in 97% of the patients and sphincter of Oddi manometry was obtained in 78% of the patients. A definitive cause for pain was determined for 72 of the 94 patients (77%). Papillary stenosis was present in 31 patients, common bile duct (CBD) stones were found in 30 patients, and chronic pancreatitis was detected in 5 patients. Cystic duct stones, peptic ulcer disease, and carcinoma were found in two patients each. Of particular note, 23% of our patients had no definitive structural or motor abnormality that could be identified as the cause of their pain symptoms.

Blumgart[3] reviewed his series of 52 patients with postcholecystectomy pain and found that 21 patients presented with only colicky pain, while 18 patients presented with jaundice, 8 patients presented with pancreatitis, and 5 patients presented with cholangitis. Although all the patients in this series had diagnostic ERCP as part of their work-up, 13 of the "colic-only" patients (64%) had a normal study, and the cause of the recurrent abdominal pain remained unexplained. This study reinforces the fact that those patients presenting with pain alone can be quite difficult to assess, and many of these patients will be found to have normal biliary and pancreatic anatomy.

Burnett and Shields[4] reported that 20 of 141 of their postcholecystectomy patients indicated that the gallbladder operation did not cure their pain symptoms. Eighteen of these 20 patients had "extra pancreaticobiliary" causes of their distress, which included such disparingly diffuse etiologies as peptic ulcer disease, "adhesions," hiatal hernia, migraine headache, or psychogenic vomiting! There remains a significant number of patients who are labeled as having postcholecystectomy pain syndrome, who have no explanation for their pain symptoms. In this group, the pain may likely be arising from a source other than the biliary tract or pancreas.

THE CHARACTER OF BILIARY TRACT PAIN: A REVIEW OF THE LITERATURE

In point of fact, how accurately can abdominal pain be identified as originating from a specific site such as the biliary tract? Does biliary tract pain possess unique features (e.g., an exclusive right upper-quadrant location or colicky nature)?

Classically, biliary tract pain is described as an intermittent, colicky pain which persists from one to several hours; it usually can be related to meals. Zollinger[5] awakened six patients during cholecystectomy operation and induced gallbladder distention to observe patterns of pain response. In this study, all six subjects experienced severe penetrating epigastric pain. Likewise, CBD distention caused intense epigastric pain and vomiting. Intraoperative electrical stimulation of the CBD induced right upper-quadrant pain or epigastric pain in five of eight patients; however, three patients had periumbilical pain.[6] Four patients in this group experienced radiation of pain into the interscapular area.

Doran[7] induced pain in 45 of 56 postcholecystectomy patients using a balloon catheter placed into the CBD through an indwelling T-tube catheter. Twenty-five of the 45 patients experienced epigastric pain, and 6 of these patients noted radiation of pain into the interscapular region. Only ten patients had right upper-quadrant pain, while nine patients had predominantly back pain (interscapular or right subscapular location). One patient had periumbilical pain.

Layne and Bergh[8] studied pain patterns in 30 postcholecystectomy patients by infusing saline under pressure into the common bile duct through a T-tube catheter.

Twenty-nine of 30 patients developed pain in the epigastrium or right upper quadrant, and 11 patients experienced pain radiating into the interscapular or right subscapular region.

Gallbladder and CBD pain induced by balloon distention or electrical stimulation seems to be sensed as a deep epigastric pain and less often as a right upper-quadrant pain. In the majority of occasions, the distress is experienced as a steady, penetrating pain which does not vary in colicky nature during the study. Approximately one-third of patients experienced pain radiation to the back; a small number of patients presented predominantly with back pain only. While typical biliary tract pain may be sensed predominantly in certain locations of the body, these areas of pain referral, unfortunately, are not specific nor exclusive for pancreaticobiliary disease.

For instance, investigators have studied pain patterns in patients with irritable bowel syndrome using balloon distention of the colon to induce pain. Swarbrick[9] found that balloon inflation in the ascending and transverse colon caused right upper-quadrant pain in 17 of 35 patients and epigastric pain in 12 of 43 patients. However, the same balloon inflation in healthy controls did not cause any right upper-quadrant pain and caused epigastric pain symptoms in only one of nine control subjects.

Kingham and Dawson[10] evaluated 22 patients with chronic right upper-quadrant pain and normal clinical investigation including ERCP examination. Balloon distention of the small intestine and/or right colon reproduced right upper-quadrant pain in 21 of these 22 patients.

Therefore, the dilemma persists for the clinician concerned about the patient's right upper-quadrant pain distress. Although typical biliary tract pain is predominantly epigastric, and to a lesser extent right upper quadrant in location, these anatomical sites are also frequently areas of referred, nonbiliary pain. Unfortunately, the human right upper quadrant is a cosmopolitan location for pain perception from a number of diverse structural and functional GI tract problems. With this realization, the work-up of the patient with recurrent right upper-quadrant pain becomes more complex, time consuming, and often frustrating.

POSTCHOLECYSTECTOMY PAIN VS. IRRITABLE BOWEL SYNDROME

The postcholecystectomy patient who presents clinically with biliary-type pain, yet thorough diagnostic evaluation fails to show pancreaticobiliary disease, presents a most difficult clinical challenge. A significant number of patients in this group have additional dyspeptic problems often seen in the irritable bowel syndrome (IBS).

IBS patients often have upper-quadrant abdominal pains of intestinal origin that may imitate biliary colic. Reviews of the postcholecystectomy pain problems frequently ignore this possibility in many patients. Classically, IBS patients present with bouts of painless diarrhea or episodes of abdominal pain associated with irregularity of bowel habits. Bloating, excessive flatus, and relief of pain following defecation are suggestive of IBS.

Chaudhary[11] reviewed 130 IBS patients and found that 106 patients had abdominal pain. The quality of pain was described as "colicky" by 45 patients, as constant by 37 patients, and as having a mixed character by 15 patients. Of note, 50 of the 106 patients had no relief of pain with defecation, and 52 patients had no exacerbation of pain following meals. It behooves the clinician to determine whether or not the patient's pain symptom profile fits that of IBS. This may deter an exhaustive work-up of the pancreaticobiliary system and may, thereby, allow better definition of treatment objectives and avoidance of needlessly invasive and potentially dangerous procedures.

EVALUATION OF THE PATIENT WITH POSTCHOLECYSTECTOMY SYNDROME

There are a number of disorders which may be responsible for the pain symptoms following cholecystectomy. Some of these disorders are related to biliary tract disease, while some are unrelated. A list includes the following:

A. Postcholecystectomy syndrome; pancreaticobiliary pain source
  1. Common bile duct (CBD) disease
     a. Recurrent or residual ductal calculi
     b. Strictures of the biliary tract
     c. Choledochocele
  2. Cystic duct remnant
     a. Cystic duct calculi
     b. Cystic duct neuroma
  3. Sphincter of Oddi (SO) disorders
     a. Papillary stenosis
     b. SO dyskinesia
  4. Pancreatitis
     a. Acute, recurrent
     b. Chronic
     c. Pancreas divisum
B. Postcholecystectomy syndrome; extra pancreaticobiliary pain source
     a. Gastroesophageal reflux disease (GERD)
     b. Peptic ulcer disease
     c. Primary hepatic disorders
     d. Primary/metastatic carcinoma
     e. Irritable bowel syndrome (IBS)
     f. Abdominal adhesions
     g. Musculoskeletal inflammation

Work-up of a postcholecystectomy patient with pain involves consideration of all of the disorders listed above. The physician needs to focus on a number of clinical points. Chief among these items are a detailed comparison of the patient's precholecystectomy vs. postcholecystectomy symptoms, and an exact description of his or her pain profile. Does the pain occur in discrete episodes? Has the patient ever experienced a similar type pain? How incapacitating is the pain? What is the quality of the pain, its location, or radiation points? How does the patient obtain relief of the pain? Is there a relationship between the intake of food and the pain? (More specifically, are certain food types or groups implicated in the pain?) Is there any relationship of the pain to fecal elimination or flatus? Does fever, nausea, or vomiting occur during the painful episodes? Objective features to pursue include: determination as to whether there has been an elevation of the white blood count, liver chemistry tests, or serum amylase at the time of the pain. If the amylase was mildly elevated, was there an associated increase in the serum lipase? Has a spot urine amylase excluded macroamylasemia? If liver function tests have been abnormal, was the blood obtained before or after an intramuscular injection of analgesic? And, finally, what was found at cholecystectomy, and what features were documented at the time of operation?

At the time of physical examination, the patient is carefully evaluated for signs suggestive of organic disease (e.g., fever, peritoneal irritation, enlarged visceral organs, abdominal masses, acholic stool, hyper-responsiveness to light palpation of the abdomen, and Hemoccult status of the stools).

The radiologic evaluation of the patient with postcholecystectomy pain includes: an abdominal ultrasound and/or CT scan of the abdomen, which are useful in identifying unsuspected organomegaly, abdominal mass lesions, lymphadenopathy, biliary and pancreatic ductal dilatation, pancreatic pseudocysts, and calcifications. Very occasionally, CBD calculi may be identified on CT or ultrasound, but this is unusual. The decision to proceed to ERCP in patients who present with postcholecystectomy pain and objective evidence of organic abnormalities such as jaundice, cholangitis, or pancreatitis, is quite easy. However, the decision to proceed to ERCP in those postcholecystectomy patients who present with only pain complaints and no objective findings is not so easy.

ERCP and SO Manometric Study

The diagnostic ERCP study of the patient with postcholecystectomy pain includes the following: complete contrast definition of both the biliary tree and pancreatic ductal systems noting luminal contour, ductal diameter, and time required for drainage of injected contrast. The latter is an important observation, but its usefulness is obviated by premedication with narcotics, anticholinergics, or the presence of a gallbladder.

Normal CBD drainage time for contrast injected during ERCP in patients without a gallbladder is less than 45 minutes (i.e., the distal CBD should be clear of contrast residue in that time with the patient in a supine position on the radiology table). Normal contrast drainage time from the pancreatic ductal system is less than 10 minutes in our experience. CBD diameter is considered to be abnormal when it is more than 12 mm in the postcholecystectomy state. The dorsal pancreatic duct is considered abnormal if the midportion is more than 5 mm in diameter. Multiple spot-compression films of the gallbladder should be obtained by the radiologist during repositioning maneuvers of the patient if the gallbladder is intact. We have found this maneuver extremely helpful in detecting sludge and gravel which go undetected by other imaging modalities. Additionally, the right hepatic ductal system may not completely fill with the patient in a prone position during routine diagnostic ERCP. In this situation, we turn the patient to a full prone position with both arms over the head to allow the right hepatic lobe to come into a more dependent position. We have seen instances in which it was unclear (on PA imaging) whether or not both the right and left hepatic ductal systems were filled with contrast. It is helpful in this situation to obtain a true lateral view to differentiate between right and left hepatic lobes.

Failure to successfully cannulate a normal appearing papilla does not infer a disease or disorder of the papilla or SO per se. It may not be the endoscopist's day! Furthermore, reproduction of the patient's pain immediately following injection of only 3 to 5 ml of contrast at ERCP is not a specific provocative test, even though it is certain to gain the endoscopist's (and the patient's) attention. A recent study in our laboratory indicates that this phenomenon happens just as often in normal patients as in patients with SO dysfunction.

ERCP manometry has been useful in assessing the possibility of SO dysfunction (SO dyskinesia or papillary stenosis) in our postcholecystectomy patients with pain. Following diagnostic ERCP and evaluation of contrast drainage time, a triple-lumen pressure recording catheter is inserted through the biopsy channel of the endoscope into the papillary orifice and advanced into the biliary ductal system. The manometry catheter must be within the duct in a "free" position and not impacted or sharply angulated within the duct. With our newly developed guidewire-assisted SO manometry catheter, successful placement of the catheter within the ductal system can be achieved more frequently. The guidewire should be removed prior to SO recording because its presence can result in recording artifact. After the SO pressure profile is obtained during catheter pull-through from the duct into the duodenum, (a method previously described),[12] the catheter is then stationed within the zone of the SO during a 5 to 10-minute recording period to evaluate both basal and phasic SO pressures. During this recording period, amyl nitrite inhalant and/or cholecystokinin–octapeptide (CCK-OP; 20 µg/kg/IV) is administered and SO basal pressure is observed for a paradoxical pressure rise. Both of these agents are potent inhibitors of basal SO tone as well as phasic SO activity. Demonstration of this effect indicates that the recorded pressure is generated by SO smooth muscle contraction and is not caused by structural narrowing (stenosis). At the present time, injection of CCK-OP has prompted a paradoxical basal SO contraction in 12 patients with suspected SO motor dysfunction. This phenomenon suggests the possibility of a "denervated" sphincteric mechanism.

SO manometric studies in patients with normal anatomy and those with papillary stenosis or SO dyskinesia have provided us with a range of "normal" manometric values. We have found in the control population that the basal SO pressure is usually detectable over a 4 to 6-mm-long segment in the distal CBD; the basal pressure averages 19 ± 7 (SD) mm Hg.[13] Phasic wave activity has an average frequency of 3 to 5 waves per minute with a duration of 4 to 5 seconds. Phasic waves have an average amplitude of 140 mm Hg ± 15 mm Hg. In the normal population, phasic wave propagation is antegrade 60% of the time, retrograde in 14%, and simultaneous in 26% of sequences. During the SO manometric study of 32 patients with suspected SO dysfunction, we found that 12 of the patients had greater than 50% retrograde phasic waves.[14] Six additional patients were found to have rapid phasic SO wave activity, which has been labeled as "tachyoddia" (8 to 12 waves per minute). Tachyoddia usually occurs in "bursts" of 20 to 30 seconds.[15] Eight of the 32 patients were found to have an elevated basal SO pressure between 50 and 160 mm Hg above duodenal pressure. In these patients, there was no alteration of SO pressure with injection of CCK-OP. However, six other patients were found to have an abnormal SO wave contraction response to CCK-OP, while three other patients responded to CCK-OP with an increase in basal SO pressure. In these latter patients, CCK-OP caused a rise in the mean SO basal pressure from 31 mm Hg to 82 mm Hg and abolished phasic wave activity.

Postcholecystectomy Syndrome and SO Dysfunction

SO dysfunction may result in biliary tract pain secondary to either delayed drainage of bile and/or pancreatic juice. SO dysfunction may be categorized into SO stenosis or SO dyskinesia. SO stenosis is a structural alteration of the SO zone caused by inflammatory stricturing or adenomatosis of the papilla. SO dyskinesia, on the other hand, is a functional disturbance—an SO dysmotility—which is much more rare. Clinically, it may be extremely difficult, if not impossible, to separate these problems. In an effort to help identify symptomatic patients with SO dysfunction and to better define the mechanism of involvement, we have categorized patients with "normal" ERCP ductograms and suspected SO dysfunction into three groups: Biliary I, II, and III. Characterization of these three groups depends on the presence or absence of a number of clinical features, which are discussed below.

Biliary Group I

Patients in this category have the following features:
1. Severe biliary-type pain
2. Elevated LFTs (AST and alkaline-phosphatase > 2 × normal) documented during or immediately after pain attacks on two or more occasions
3. Evidence of a dilated common bile duct (> 12 mm Hg)
4. Evidence of a delayed contrast drainage from the common duct (> 45 minutes)

SO manometric studies are desirable but not necessary for diagnosis in this group.

Biliary Group II

Patients in this category have severe biliary-type upper abdominal pain with one or two of the previously noted objective findings (elevated liver functions, dilated duct, or delayed drainage). These patients require SO manometric study for the diagnosis of papillary stenosis or SO dyskinesia. We now have a 4-year follow-up on 40 patients in this group who were randomized to endoscopic sphincterotomy or sham sphincterotomy prior to SO manometry. In the patient group with basal SO pressure greater than 40 mm Hg, endoscopic spincterotomy significantly relieved symptoms in the great majority of these patients compared to the sham procedure.[16] In the patients of group II who had normal basal SO pressure, there was no difference in the clinical outcome between the group that underwent endoscopic sphincterotomy and the group who had the sham procedure. In summary, SO manometry is helpful in identifying group II patients who will benefit from endoscopic sphincterotomy.

Biliary Group III

Patients in this category have severe biliary-type pain and no other objective features associated with pancreaticobiliary disease. SO manometry is an essential diagnostic study to determine whether papillary stenosis or SO dynkinesia is present. Sphincterotomy may benefit those patients with an elevated basal SO pressure who do not respond to appropriate medical therapy. It is yet uncertain whether sphincterotomy will relieve pain symptoms in group III patients who have evidence of SO dyskinesia, but in whom basal SO pressure is normal. Balloon dilation of the SO in group III patients with normal basal SO pressure has not been useful in alleviating pain symptoms and has been associated with a 20% incidence of complications.[17]

Provocative Testing

Provocative testing has been used to reproduce pain symptoms in those patients with suspected postcholecystectomy pain. The morphine-Prostigmin test (Nardi test), in our experience, has caused pain, abnormal LFTs, or pancreatic enzyme elevation in a significant number of healthy controls, as well as patients with partial common duct obstruction. It, therefore, lacks specificity, and is not useful for management of postcholecystectomy pain.[18]

Reproduction of pain symptoms by injection of contrast into the common duct can be observed in patients without disease and has not been useful in distinguishing patients with SO dyskinesia from patients with papillary stenosis. Reproduction of pain symptoms by CCK-OP injection has also been claimed as a possible provocative test. In our experience, however, this is not specific because it can cause pain in patients with normal SO manometric studies.

Noninvasive Testing

Dodds and co-workers[19] studied a group of 56 patients with postcholecystectomy pain and suspected partial common duct obstruction. These patients were evaluated by fatty meal biliary ultrasound, quantitative hepatobiliary scanning, ERCP, and SO manometry studies. The sensitivities of fatty meal ultrasound and biliary scanning were 67% when used as individual tests and 80% when used together. Biliary scanning resulted in two false-positive studies. These results are encouraging, but additional studies are needed to improve the sensitivity of these tests before they should be considered for routine clinical use.

Diagnostic Approach

Our approach to right upper-quadrant pain in the postcholecystectomy patient is centered on a thorough history taking and complete exam. If the abdominal pain is "typical" in location for biliary distress, colicky in nature and episodic rather than constant, we may proceed with ERCP despite lack of objective findings (group III). When the history and examination do not portray a typical picture of biliary colic, we do not proceed with ERCP unless (1) there is objective radiologic (CT scan or ultrasound) or laboratory evidence to support a pancreaticobiliary etiology, or (2) the patient continues to have severe pain and a thorough diagnostic search for other causes has been unsuccessful (Fig. 26–1). Most patients in group III who have a normal SO manometric study have a symptom complex consistent with IBS.

We use biliary ultrasound to evaluate the liver for focal parenchymal lesions and ductal dilatation, as well as to evaluate the extrahepatic ductal diameter and pancreatic parenchymal. Most patients referred for evaluation of postcholecystectomy pain have previously had upper and lower barium studies and often have had upper GI endoscopy and intravenous pyelogram (IVP) studies.

In summary, the direction of the diagnostic evaluation is heavily dependent on the initial review of the history, surgical records, and exam findings. Laboratory and radiologic studies are often helpful in grouping these patients into high-probability and low-probability groups as to whether their pain originates from the biliary or pancreatic system. ERCP and SO

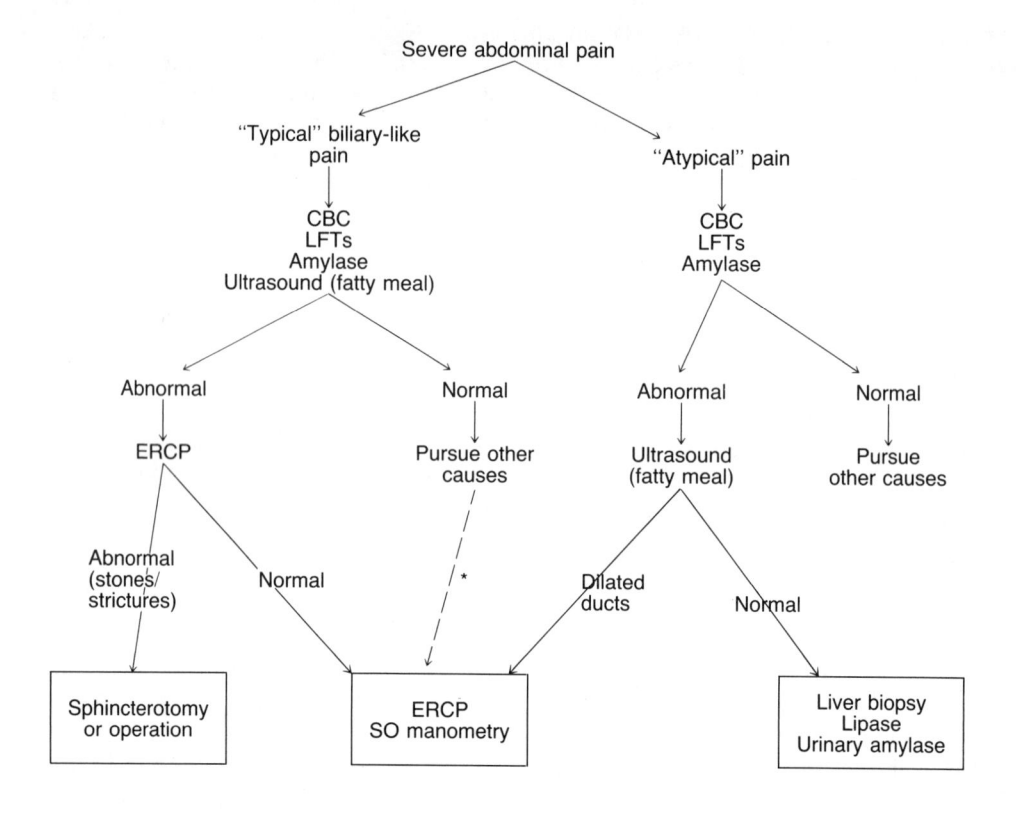

```
                    Severe abdominal pain
                    /                    \
        "Typical" biliary-like        "Atypical" pain
              pain                           |
                |                           CBC
               CBC                          LFTs
               LFTs                        Amylase
              Amylase
         Ultrasound (fatty meal)
          /           \                  /           \
    Abnormal        Normal          Abnormal        Normal
        |             |                |               |
      ERCP      Pursue other       Ultrasound       Pursue
                  causes          (fatty meal)    other causes
      /    \         /              /    \
 Abnormal  Normal   *          Dilated   Normal
 (stones/                       ducts
 strictures)
     |            |                |              |
┌──────────┐ ┌──────────┐    ┌──────────┐
│Sphincterotomy│ │  ERCP    │    │Liver biopsy│
│or operation │ │SO manometry│  │  Lipase    │
└──────────┘ └──────────┘    │Urinary amylase│
                              └──────────┘
```

*If evaluation of other etiologies is negative and severe pain persists, then reconsider ERCP and SO manometry.

FIG 26–1.
An approach to the patient with postcholecystectomy pain syndrome.

manometry studies are quite essential in assessing group II and group III patients, and in identifying patients who are likely to benefit from sphincterotomy.

References

1. Glenn F, McSherry CK: Secondary abdominal operations following biliary tract surgery. *Surg Gynecol Obstet* 1965; 121(5):979–988.
2. Vital and Health Statistics. Detailed Diagnoses and Procedures for Patients Discharged from Short-stay Hospitals—1985. Hyattsville, MD. Department of Health and Human Services, Public Health Service, National Center for Health Statistics. April 1987.
3. Blumgart, LH, Carachi, R, Imrie, CW, et al: Diagnosis and management of post-cholecystectomy symptoms: The place of endoscopy and retrograde choledochopancreatography. *Br J Surg* 1977; 64:809–816.
4. Burnett W, Shields R: Symptoms after cholecystectomy. *Lancet* 1958; 1:923–925.
5. Zollinger R: Observations following distention of the gallbladder and common duct in man. *Proc Soc Exp Biol Med* 1933; 30:1260–1261.
6. Zollinger R, Walter CW: Localization of pain following faradic stimulation of the common bile duct. *Proc Soc Exp Biol Med* 1936; 35:267–268.
7. Doran FSA: The sites to which pain is referred from the common bile duct in man and its implication for the theory of referred pain. *Br J Surg* 1967; 54(7):599–606.
8. Layne JA, Bergh GS: An experimental study of pain in the human biliary tract induced by spasm of the sphincter of Oddi. *Am J Physiol* 1940; 128:18–24.
9. Swarbrick ET, Bat L, Hegarty JE, et al: Site of pain from the irritable bowel. *Lancet* 1980; 2:443–446.
10. Kingham JGC, Dawson AM: Origin of chronic right upper quadrant pain. *Gut* 1985; 26:783–788.
11. Chaudhary NA, Truelove SC: The irritable colon syndrome. A study of the clinical features, predisposing causes, and prognosis in 130 cases. *Q J Med* 1962; 123:307–322.

12. Geenen JE, Hogan WJ, Dodds WJ, et al: Intraluminal pressure recording from the human sphincter of Oddi. *Gastroenterology* 1980; 78:317–324.
13. Toouli J, Hogan WJ, Geenen JE, et al: Action of cholecystokinin–octapeptide on sphincter of Oddi basal pressure and phasic wave activity in humans. *Surgery* 1982; 92(3):497–503.
14. Toouli J, Roberts-Thomson IC, Dent J, et Manometric disorders in patients with suspecte sphincter of Oddi dysfunction. *Gastroenterology* 1985; 88:1243–1250.
15. Hogan WJ, Geenen JE, Venu R, et al: Abnormally rapid phasic contractions of the human sphincter of Oddi (tachyoddia). *Gastroenterology* 1983; 84(5 pt. 2):1189.
16. Geenen JE, Hogan WJ, Dodds WJ, et al: Long-term results of endoscopic sphincterotomy (ES) for treating patients with sphincter-of-Oddi (SO) dysfunction: A prospective study. *Gastroenterology* 1987; 92(5 pt. 2):1401.
17. Bader M, Geenen JE, Hogan WJ, et al: Endoscopic balloon dilatation of the sphincter of Oddi in patients with suspected biliary dyskinesia; Results of a prospective randomized trial. *Gastrointest Endosc* 1986; 32(2):158.

LoGuidice JA, Geenen JE, Hogan WJ, et al: Efficacy of the morphine—Prostigmin test for evaluating patients with suspected papillary stenosis. *Dig Dis Sci* 1979; 24:455–458.
19. Darweesh R, Dodds WJ, Hogan WJ, et al: Efficiency of quantitative hepatobiliary scintigraphy and fatty-meal sonography for detecting partial common duct obstruction. *Gastroenterology* 1987; 92(5 pt. 2):1363.

27

Small Intestinal Biopsy:
Who?
How?
What are the findings?

ROBERT H. RIDDELL

In the last few years there has been a variety of changes in how small bowel biopsies are carried out, the clinical reasons for their being done, and the range of diseases visualized on biopsy. These have raised the following questions:
1. Is endoscopic biopsy an adequate substitute for suction capsule biopsy of the small bowel?
2. What terminology should be used to describe abnormal biopsies?
3. When should small bowel biopsy be considered and what can be expected from the biopsies?
4. Is low-power dissecting microscopy of jejunal biopsies still necessary?

IS ENDOSCOPIC BIOPSY AN ADEQUATE SUBSTITUTE FOR SUCTION CAPSULE BIOPSY OF THE SMALL BOWEL?

Over the last few years capsule biopsies of the jejunum have become less common and have been replaced by biopsies taken through the endoscope under direct vision. Does this trend have a sound pathologic basis? The variables that need to be considered are whether endoscopes can reach the jejunum, and if they cannot, whether duodenal biopsies are an adequate substitute, and whether endoscopic biopsies are adequate to answer the clinical problem posed.

Can Endoscopes Reach the Proximal Jejunum, and If Not Is Duodenal Biopsy an Adequate Substitute?

It has become increasingly apparent that upper gastrointestinal endoscopes can certainly reach the distal (third part) of the duodenum and sometimes proximal jejunum to allow both visualization of disease in this part of the bowel and also to obtain multiple biopsies. One of the major advantages is that focal lesions can be both seen and biopsied. Some diseases such as lymphangiectasia or Whipple's disease, while distinctly uncommon, do tend to have a marked focal tendency; when employing capsule biopsies, random hits of focal lesions are required to make the diagnosis. Endoscopic visualization and biopsy of such lesions facilitates making the diagnosis.

The final part of this question relates to whether distal duodenal biopsies are an adequate substitute for proximal jejunal biopsies. It should be stated at the outset that there is nothing magical about the ligament of Treitz, and the pathology that primarily affects the proximal small bowel affects the duodenum as well as the jejunum. The disadvantages of duodenal biopsies are that villi tend to be smaller, particularly in the first and second parts where Brunner's glands are most pronounced, and that peptic disease occurs primarily in the first part, and to a much lesser extent in the second part of the duodenum. Beyond this, peptic-related diseases are rare unless the patient has had the distal part of the stomach removed, or there is marked hyperchlorhydria such as may be seen in Zollinger-Ellison syndrome. Brunner's glands are much less prominent in the third and fourth parts of the duodenum, while the length of villi in this part of the bowel approximates that seen in the proximal jejunum. Artifacts from biopsies that can be induced by tangential sectioning are therefore much less of a problem in the distal duodenum. In theory, then, biopsy of the distal duodenum is acceptable for making the diagnosis of primary small bowel disease, but the closer the biopsies are taken to (or distal to) the ligament of Treitz, the less the likelihood that they will be subject to the vagaries of peptic ulcer disease or problems caused by the shorter villi and prominent Brunner's glands of the duodenum.

Are Endoscopic Biopsies Adequate in Size for Diagnostic Purposes?

Adequacy of biopsies is a function of size, adequacy of orientation, and the number of biopsies obtained.

The size of biopsies obtained varies tremendously depending on the instrument used and the force with which the biopsy forceps are thrust into the mucosa. At one extreme, endoscopes capable of obtaining jumbo (8 mm open span) biopsies provide tissue that is comparable in size to suction biopsies. They can be properly oriented and sectioned histologically to obtain the best orientation. As the size of the biopsy forceps decreases, the size of biopsies obtained and the ease with which they can be oriented and therefore interpreted are reduced. Well-oriented biopsies become less frequent, nevertheless this defect can be compensated to a large extent by simply increasing the number of biopsies. Even using pediatric endoscopes in infants, it is quite easy to take four to six small biopsies to answer questions such as whether the patient has celiac sprue, for example.

The answer to this question then is that conventional endoscopic biopsies have largely replaced suction biopsies. They are quite adequate, particularly if larger endoscopes are used or if smaller tissue forceps are used when the number of biopsies is increased. However, it is worthwhile remembering that if the primary objective of the endoscopy is to obtain tissue for diagnostic purposes then real consideration should be given to using endoscopes capable of transmitting jumbo biopsy forceps. Arguments that "patients prefer smaller endoscopes" reflect gastroenterologists' preferences rather than those of the patients.

WHAT TERMINOLOGY SHOULD BE USED TO DESCRIBE ABNORMAL BIOPSIES?

The problem of terminology has bedeviled the study of small bowel biopsies since they have been carried out on a regular diagnostic basis. Initially, terminology included terms such as "atrophy," so that biopsies were called, for instance, partial villous atrophy and either total or subtotal villous atrophy, both of the latter terms referring to an identical appearance with a flat villous-less mucosa. In practice, this change was almost completely explained by a marked increase in the length of the crypts that reached the surface as a result of the markedly shortened turnover time, which in celiac sprue may be as short as 6 hours. These terms inevitably were abbreviated to PVA and SVA. Others preferred "flat biopsy" to "subtotal villous atrophy." To my mind the simplest classification is to refer to these lesions as mild, moderate, or severe villous lesions, a severe lesion corresponding to a flat mucosa.[1] This terminology gets around all of the difficulties associated with the use of the term "atrophy," and also problems associated with nonflat biopsies if that classification is preferred.

WHEN SHOULD SMALL BOWEL BIOPSY BE CONSIDERED, AND WHAT CAN BE EXPECTED FROM THE BIOPSIES?

Small bowel biopsy should be considered when
1. The patient has symptoms of malabsorption and the obvious clinical question is whether the patient has a primary small bowel disease such as celiac sprue
2. An immunodeficient patient has diarrhea in which stool cultures and examination are negative
3. A patient has diarrhea and colonoscopic biopsies are normal so that attention is now focused on the small bowel as a potential source of the patient's symptoms
4. The patient is known to have celiac sprue but is doing poorly and the reason for this is unknown
5. The patient has possible or probable Crohn's disease and the question of possible upper gastrointestinal tract involvement is being raised.

What biopsy appearances might the gastroenterologist expect to see under these clinical circumstances?

To understand these questions it is important to appreciate a simple classification for small bowel biopsies and the most usual causes. Table 27–1 shows such a simple classification.

Nonspecific causes of a severe (flat) villous lesion are shown in Table 27–2 while nonspecific causes of inflammation where there is at least partial preservation of the villi are shown in Table 27–3. Tables 27–4 through 27–6 show specific causes of disease.

Investigation of Nonimmunosuppressed Patients with Symptoms Referrable to Small Bowel

In practice, the number of possible underlying diseases is relatively small. In nonimmunosuppressed individuals, the most frequent question regards the poten-

TABLE 27–1.
Classification of Small Bowel Biopsy*

Severe villous lesion (= flat biopsy)
  Nonspecific changes
  Diagnostic changes
Mild/moderate villous lesion
  Nonspecific changes
  Diagnostic changes
Normal villi
  Diagnostic disease

*Modified from Lewin K, Riddell RH, Weinstein WM: Gastrointestinal Pathology with Clinical Implications. New York, Igaku-Shoin, in press.

TABLE 27–2.
Severe (Flat) Villous Lesion—Nonspecific (Nondiagnostic)*

Symptomatic celiac sprue
Dermatitis herpetiformis (some patients)
Other protein injury
Tropical sprue (uncommonly)
Zollinger-Ellison syndrome
Refractory sprue
Familial enteropathy (very rare)

*Modified from Lewin K, Riddell RH, Weinstein WM: Gastrointestinal Pathology with Clinical Implications. New York, Igaku-Shoin, in press.

TABLE 27–3.
Mild/Moderate Villous Lesion—Nonspecific*

Subclinical celiac sprue
  (and some patients with dermatitis herpetiformis)
Infectious gastroenteritis
Crohn's disease
Some tropical sprue
Stasis syndromes
AIDS enteropathy
Geographic variation
Zollinger-Ellison (gastrinoma)
Graft vs. host

*Modified from Lewin K, Riddell RH, Weinstein WM: Gastrointestinal Pathology with Clinical Implications. New York, Igaku-Shoin, in press.

TABLE 27-4.
Severe (Flat) Villous Lesion—Diagnostic

Collagenous sprue
Late onset immunodeficiency
  (common variable hypogammaglobulinemia)

TABLE 27-6.
Normal Villi—Diagnostic*

Giardia lamblia
Hypo- and abetalipoproteinemia
Amyloidosis
X-linked immunodeficiency
Lipid storage diseases
Cytomegalovirus infection
Chronic granulomatous disease
Pigments

*Modified from Lewin K, Riddell RH, Weinstein WM: Gastrointestinal Pathology with Clinical Implications. New York, Igaku-Shoin, in press.

tial possibility of underlying celiac sprue. In *symptomatic* patients, all biopsies should be completely flat to sustain this diagnosis. Some preservation of villi is very rare in symptomatic patients and should cause this diagnosis to be seriously reconsidered.

Investigation of Immunosuppressed Patients with Symptoms Referrable to Small Bowel

In patients with known or suspected acquired immunodeficiency syndrome (AIDS) or hypergammaglobulinemia, a variety of specific infections can be documented on small bowel biopsy: these include *Mycobacterium avium-intracellulare*, *Cryptosporidiosis*, *Isospora*, and, rarely, *Giardia lamblia*. Some patients with AIDS

TABLE 27-5.
Mild/Moderate Villous Lesion—Diagnostic*

Giardia lamblia
Whipple's disease
Mycobacterium avium-intracellulare
Cryptosporidiosis
Isospora belli
Eosinophilic gastroenteritis
Primary intestinal lymphoma
Other parasitic diseases
Fungal diseases
Viral diseases
Macroglobulinemia
Lymphangiectasia (1° or 2°)
Late onset immunodeficiency
  (common variable hypogammaglobulinemia)
Severe B_{12} on folate deficiency

*Modified from Lewin K, Riddell RH, Weinstein WM: Gastrointestinal Pathology with Clinical Implications. New York, Igaku-Shoin, in press.

also have a severe enteropathy in the absence of an obvious infection,[2] the so-called enteropathy of AIDS. Cytomegalovirus may be present in endothelial cells in the submucosa and may not be visible on mucosal biopsy.

Patients with Diarrhea in Whom Colonoscopy with Multiple Biopsies Has Been Negative

In most patients presenting with diarrhea, unless there are good reasons to suspect the upper gastrointestinal tract as the source of symptoms, the investigation begins in the lower gastrointestinal tract. This usually includes not only sigmoidoscopy but also multiple biopsies even if the large bowel appears normal endoscopically. The reason that biopsies must be taken is that a variety of diseases that can cause diarrhea may appear normal endoscopically, including collagenous colitis, "microscopic" (nonspecific) colitis, pseudomelanosis resulting from anthroquinone ingestion, and amyloid. These diseases can all be "missed" if biopsies are omitted.

Virtually all of the diseases listed in Tables 27-2 through 27-6 may be found when investigations continue to the upper small bowel. Crohn's disease may also be found, primarily involving the small bowel, so that small bowel enema is likely to complement upper and lower gastrointestinal endoscopy.

Biopsy Findings in Patients with Documented Celiac Sprue Who Are Not Responding to Therapy

If the patient is either inadvertently or deliberately not adhering to a gluten-free diet, the typical appearances seen in untreated celiac sprue are likely to be present, although lesser degrees of change may be found. Rare complications which may be detected on endoscopy and biopsy include collagenous sprue, the supervention of lymphoma or carcinoma, or the development of ulcerative jejunitis. In patients with lymphoma, the lamina propria may contain a predominantly lymphocytic rather than plasma cell infiltrate. Frank lymphoma or carcinoma may be seen and biopsied. The final complication is ulceration, possibly part of nonspecific, chronic jejunoileitis. However, most of these complications are much more likely to be demonstrated with enteroclysis unless within endoscopic range.

Changes in Patients with Diarrhea Who Have Normal Colonoscopic Biopsies

The list of potential diseases here is large and may include a variety of specific diseases and nonspecific morphologic appearances, as outlined in Tables 27–2 through 27–6. However, in practice, a nonspecific inflammatory infiltrate (mild/moderate villous lesion) is the most common; the vast majority of these lesions are the result of infection or bacterial overgrowth. More recently, specific problems of biopsy interpretation have arisen. An obvious example is the distinction between Whipple's disease and *Mycobacterium avium-intracellulare*. Although at first glance these diseases appear very similar, each being characterized by the presence of an excess of granular macrophages in the lamina propria, both of which are positive with diastase-PAS stain, in practice, a variety of differences between these two disorders are apparent. Perhaps the most obvious is that dilated lymphatics are part of Whipple's disease but are not seen in *Mycobacterium avium-intracellulare*; neutrophils are not infrequent in Whipple's disease but also are not usually seen in *Mycobacterium avium-intracellulare*. However, the simplest general rule is that where either of these two diseases are an issue, a stain for acid-fast organisms should be carried out routinely. In *M. avium* each of the macrophages is stuffed with red staining bacilli while the stain is completely negative in Whipple's disease. In practice then, routine acid-fast stains are mandatory whenever the diagnosis of Whipple's disease is being considered.

Patients with Crohn's Disease in Whom Upper Gastrointestinal Involvement is Suspected

The diagnosis of gastroduodenal Crohn's disease is beyond the scope of this chapter. In particular, the distinction between peptic ulcer disease involving the stomach or proximal duodenum and NSAID in the stomach can be difficult. However, in the third or fourth part of the duodenum or proximal jejunum where peptic ulcer disease is rare, criteria for the diagnosis are essentially similar to those employed in the large bowel, including the combination of endoscopic and histologic appearances. Granulomas are uncommon, but very useful if detected; the combination of marked focality of inflammation within or between biopsies is particularly helpful. In young patients, the combination of gastric and duodenal disease, particularly if it extends into or beyond the second part of the duodenum, is highly suggestive of underlying Crohn's disease rather than peptic ulcer disease.

IS LOW-POWER DISSECTING MICROSCOPY OF JEJUNAL BIOPSIES STILL NECESSARY?

In the early days of jejunal biopsy it became clear that the use of the dissecting microscope could be of value to ensure that the biopsy had been mounted correctly on the mounting medium with the submucosal surface down, and to get an initial impression as to the likely histology. It has been increasingly apparent that the time invested in this procedure is out of proportion to the advantages unless it is done for esthetic or academic reasons.

SUMMARY

In the last few years our approach to small bowel biopsies has changed. There has been a major trend from suction biopsy to multiple endoscopic biopsies of either distal duodenum or proximal jejunum; in children the diagnosis of celiac sprue is often made on multiple biopsies of the first or second part of the duodenum. Dissecting microscopy has largely disappeared. There has been an increasing awareness of Crohn's disease involving the upper gastrointestinal tract down to the proximal jejunum which can be documented in many patients by endoscopy and biopsy. Finally, there has been increasing use of distal duodenal or proximal jejunal biopsies in AIDS patients to detect infections such as *Mycobacterium avium-intracellulare* or *Isospora*, which are not easy to find by examination of the stool; the enteropathy of AIDS in the absence of detectable infection may also be found. Unfortunately, terminologic problems remain, but many traditional terms are now sufficiently ground into our vocabulary that they cease being a problem.

References

1. Lewin K, Riddell RH, Weinstein WM: *Gastrointestinal Pathology with Clinical Implications*. New York, Igaku-Shoin, in press.
2. Gillin JS, Shike M, Alcock C, et al: Malabsorption and mucosal abnormalities of the small intestine in the acquired immunodeficiency syndrome. *Ann Intern Med* 1985; 102:619–622.

28

Short Bowel Syndrome: How do we prolong life?

GARY M. LEVINE, M.D.

The short bowel syndrome usually has been defined as a severe maldigestion/malabsorption state induced by resection of approximately 200 cm or more of small intestine. The definition of the short bowel syndrome can be broadened to include patients who develop severe nutritional disability from diseases such as extensive Crohn's disease, severe radiation enteritis, or idiopathic intestinal psuedoobstruction because these patients present many of the same challenges as patients with massive resection. Patients with the short bowel syndrome present a difficult long-term management problem. The focus of this chapter will be to provide insight into a rational approach to the management of these patients rather than the causes, pathophysiology, and mechanisms of intestinal adaptation which have been discussed in more detail in recent reviews.[1,2]

The degree of *functional* loss and resulting nutritional disability depends on a number of factors in addition to the loss of a significant length of small intestine (Table 28–1). Resection of jejunum, even in excess of 200 cm, is well tolerated; whereas, resection of the ileum, particularly including the ileocecal valve, is not. An intact ileocecal valve has prognostic value because it mitigates against bacterial overgrowth. The presence of distal ileum may allow sufficient reabsorption of bile salts to maintain pool size and allows the "ileal brake" to function in slowing gastric emptying and intestinal motility.[3,4] If the resection is coupled with loss of the colon, the degree of colonic resection also has prognostic value.[5] The presence of an intact colon not only provides additional surface area for the absorption of food and electrolytes, but also allows colonic conservation of carbohydrate by absorption of short chain fatty acids, products of bacterial metabolism.[6,7]

The underlying etiology of short bowel syndrome significantly affects the patient's prognosis. A young patient who suffers a massive loss of intestine from a mechanical problem, such as a strangulation obstruction or malrotation, will probably do better than an elderly patient who has lost an equivalent amount of intestine because of mesenteric vascular disease.

In the past two decades, management of patients with the short bowel syndrome has been revolutionized by advancements in parenteral and enteral nutritional support. Total parenteral nutrition (TPN) has been life saving to pa-

TABLE 28–1.
Prognostic Features in the Short Bowel Syndrome

Favorable	Unfavorable
Age < 50 years	Age > 50 years
Jejunal resection	Ileal resection
Residual bowel > 150 cm	Residual bowel < 50 cm
Presence of ileocecal valve	Loss of ileocecal valve
Presence of colon	Colectomy

tients recovering from an acute, massive intestinal resection. TPN also has allowed us to maintain good nutrition of patients while the process of intestinal adaptation occurs. A better understanding of the factors controlling intestinal adaptation has allowed for more rational diet therapy. The development of specialized enteral diets as well as sophisticated means for delivery of enteral nutrition has also helped patients with the short bowel syndrome.

The clinical management of the short bowel syndrome can be divided into two phases. The first phase involves the immediate care of the patient following bowel resection and the second phase involves long-term care directed at restoring and maintaining performance status.

ACUTE (PERIOPERATIVE) CARE OF THE SHORT BOWEL SYNDROME PATIENT

Most patients develop the short bowel syndrome following an acute catastrophic vascular event such as mesenteric thrombosis or embolus or vascular obstruction as a result of a volvulus, internal hernia, or acute trauma. A lesser number of patients develop the short bowel syndrome following repeated resections for Crohn's disease, abdominal malignancy, or radiation enteritis. In the past, greater than 90% of short bowel patients died in the immediate postoperative period.[8] Today, with advances in critical care techniques, short-term survival has markedly improved. In addition to modern cardiorespiratory support, rational use of antibiotics, and fluid and electrolyte replacement, we are able to provide adequate caloric and nitrogen intake to allow the patient to overcome sepsis, major organ failure (acute respiratory distress syndrome, acute renal failure, and so forth) and ensure wound healing. Almost without exception, all patients should be given TPN during this period of time.[9]

TPN must be administered through a dedicated central venous line. Calories can be provided in the form of dextrose and lipid emulsions. Patients with respiratory failure may benefit from receiving up to 40% to 50% of their calories in the form of lipid.[10] Protein requirements of 1.5 to 2 gm/kg/day are met with a complete amino acid solution. Nitrogen intake may have to be decreased in patients with concomitant renal failure. To date there is no firm evidence that specialized essential amino acid solutions ("renal failure fluid," "hepatic failure fluid") improve survival. In fact, because these specialized amino acids solutions omit nonessential amino acids that may not be synthesized effectively in critically ill patients, they should be avoided. Adequate doses of trace elements (zinc, copper, chromium, iodide, manganese, and selenium) must be provided to these patients because trace mineral deficiencies can occur as early as 2 to 3 weeks after resection.[11]

Another aspect of management particular to patients in the acute phase of the short bowel syndrome is the presence of gastric hypersecretion.[12, 13] Increased acid secretion results from hypergastrinemia as well as from the absence of normal inhibitory gastrointestinal hormones usually secreted by endocrine cells present in the resected small intestine. The lack of these "enterogastrones" may cause the uninhibited release of gastrin as well as a lack of direct inhibition of parietal cells. Adequate doses of H_2 inhibitors must be administered to prevent development of gastroduodenal ulceration as well as to minimize fluid and electrolyte losses. Gastric hypersecretion continues for several months and then spontaneously abates.

Patients in the acute phase of the short bowel syndrome tend to lose large quantities of fluid and electrolytes even while fasted. In patients with high jejunostomies, it is not unusual to lose 2 to 3 L of output per day.[14, 15] With time, in response to volume contraction caused by gastrointestinal losses, compensatory mechanisms lead to reduction in basal intestinal secretion. These mechanisms include the effects of the renin-angiotensin system, increased secretion of antidiuretic hormone, and stimulation of sodium chloride absorption by the systemic acidosis resulting from excessive bicarbonate loss.[16–18]

NUTRITIONAL STABILIZATION AND ADAPTATION

Once the short bowel syndrome patient has surmounted the immediate life-threatening complications in the postoperative period, long-term nutritional planning must begin. Several important issues must be dealt with:

Will the patient require temporary or long-term TPN?

Can enteral or oral intake stimulate adequate intestinal adaptation?

What enteral or oral diet is optimum?

Use of TPN

TPN has revolutionized and vastly improved both the quality and length of life in patients with the short bowel syndrome.[9] Before the availability of TPN, short bowel syndrome patients followed an inexorable downhill course of progressive malnutrition, dehydration, infection, and death. The question is not whether the patient should receive TPN, but for how long will TPN be required? In almost all patients, it is preferable to insert a subcutaneous tunneled long-term Silastic catheter.[19] These catheters reduce the incidence of sepsis and minimize the incidence of venous thrombosis at the site of the catheter. The decision to place a long-term TPN catheter must include determination that the patient and family members or custodial care personnel will be able to succeed with out-of-hospital TPN.[20] A motivated patient can be trained to care for the catheter, connect and disconnect tubing, and operate an infusion perfusion pump within a week to 10 days.

In the past several years, there has been a proliferation in the number of private agencies that provide home nutritional support. It is recommended that each hospital assess the quality of the providers and choose one such agency to administer home TPN to its patients. Ideally, the nutritional support company should provide 24 hours a day/7 days a week nursing and pharmacy coverage as well as routine visits to the patient. A schedule for laboratory testing should be established, and the results of home visits and laboratory tests should be provided regularly to the patient's physician. Before discharge from the hospital, the patient's calorie and nitrogen needs should be established. A program of cyclic TPN should be instituted by gradually shortening the number of hours and increasing the infusion rate. Most TPN patients prefer to receive their infusions during the evening hours so that they may "unplug" themselves in the morning and carry out a normal day's activities.

With meticulous catheter care and support services, home TPN can be provided almost indefinitely. However, the physician should be alert for certain well-known complications of home TPN. Sepsis is the most serious complication of long-term TPN. The incidence of catheter sepsis in well-managed programs is one episode every 2 to 3 patient-years.[19, 20] Other catheter-related problems include venous thrombosis, tubing leaks, and cracked hubs which occur with a frequency of less than one episode every 5 patient-years.[21, 22]

There are several serious metabolic complications of home TPN, which should be recognized and may occur despite our best efforts. Bone disease manifested by bone pain and pathologic fractures has been noted with increasing frequency in patients on long-term parenteral nutrition.[23] The cause of bone disease is unclear and probably is multifactorial. It has been noted that many patients beginning TPN after suffering a catastrophic illness have a state of relative hyperparathroidism secondary to low 25(OH) vitamin D levels.[24] With long-term TPN, additional factors that can cause bone disease include aluminum toxicity and TPN-induced hypercalciuria.[25, 26] In some patients, improvement has been noted after withdrawal of vitamin D from parenteral infusates[23] or increasing parenteral phosphate intake.[27] In other patients, decreasing the amino acid load and lengthening the infusion period may improve symptoms and allow fractures to heal.[26]

The trace metal deficiencies are a sec-

TABLE 28–2.
Trace Metals

	Deficiency State	Daily Requirements
Zinc[11, 29]	Acrodermatitis enteropathica Alopecia Delayed wound healing Dysgeusia	2–5 mg basal plus 10–15 mg/L GI losses
Copper[11, 30]	Anemia Neutropenia	0.2–1.0 mg
Chromium[31]	Glucose intolerance	5–20 µg
Molybdenum[32]	Irritability, confusion Coma	20–30 µg
Selenium[33]	Cardiomyopathy	50–150 µg
Manganese	Not reported	0.2–3.0 mg

ond major metabolic complication of home TPN. These syndromes have been recognized more and more frequently in patients on long-term home TPN. Many short bowel syndrome patients have increased gastrointestinal losses of these minerals in excess of their parenteral intake.[28] As the need for an increasing number of trace metals has been identified, these metals have been added to trace metal mixtures used for parenteral nutrition. Table 28–2 outlines the deficiency states and daily requirements for the trace metals.

Nephrolithiasis frequently occurs in short bowel syndrome patients.[34] Patients develop uric acid stone as a result of oliguria and aciduria induced by excessive gastrointestinal losses of fluid and bicarbonate. Treatment for this type of kidney stone includes increasing fluid intake, oral sodium bircarbonate, and, if necessary, allopurinol. Short bowel syndrome patients who have retained all or part of their colon are susceptible to development of oxalate stone.[35] Measures to prevent oxalate stone formation include increasing fluid intake, a low oxalate diet, and oral supplementation with calcium salts or citric acid.[36]

As more and more patients spend longer and longer on home TPN, other unusual complications have been recognized. Hepatic abnormalities occur, ranging from minor transient elevations of liver function tests to severe cholestasis.[37] The more severe forms of liver disease tend to occur in patients with extensive resections. Recently, an unusual type of liver disease resembling alcoholic hepatitis which can progress to a micronodular cirrhosis has been identified.[37, 38] Gallstones occur with high frequency in short bowel syndrome patients and occasionally may become symptomatic. Factors responsible for stone formation include ileal bile salt malabsorption and lack of enteral feeding which leads to chronic stasis within the gallbladder.[39, 40] Another unusual complication is the occurrence of d-lactic acidosis. This condition results from bacterial metabolism of nonabsorbed carbohydrate, particularly in the residual colon of patients with the short bowel syndrome.[41] This condition tends to occur in patients who are eating in addition to receiving TPN.

For some patients with the short bowel syndrome, home TPN is continued indefinitely and no plans are made for instituting oral intake. However, the vast majority of patients with the short bowel syndrome wish to eat and, unless eating brings on severe symptoms such as abdominal pain and uncontrollable diarrhea, a diet plan needs to be developed. With the current pressures to discharge patients from the hospital as soon as possible, there may be insufficient time to completely tailor a diet program for each patient. The next section will deal with the process of instituting oral intake. Each patient must be treated as an individual because of differences in the amount of remaining gut, presence or absence of a colon, and the presence or absence of an ostomy.

Oral Intake and Intestinal Adaptation

The process by which the residual intestine undergoes hyperplasia is termed intestinal adaptation.[1] The most important mechanism responsible for this process is luminal nutrition.[42] Although it is believed that local and systemic hormones, as well as neurovascular factors, play a role, they are a secondary cascade brought about by the presence of nutrients in the gut.[43] For further discussion of this process the reader is referred to several excellent reviews.[1, 44]

In planning an enteral diet regimen, it should be noted that changes in gastrointestinal transit in the short bowel syndrome are not completely understood. In many studies using an nonabsorbable marker, it has been noted that oral to ostomy transit time is complete in under 3 hours.[14, 15] A single study concerning gastrointestinal motor activity in the short bowel syndrome revealed that interdigestive motor complexes were shorter in duration and higher in frequency than in controls. No differences in gastric emptying activity or postprandial motor activity were seen. The administration of loperamide led to an increase in motor activity characterized by a decrease in the amount of time from taking a meal to the appearance of the interdigestive motor complex. It was suggested that the increase in motility resulted in decrease in net transit because the more frequent contractions decreased the rate at which the meal moved down the gastrointestinal tract.[45]

Enteral feeding should be instituted in patients after establishing a TPN regimen which fills the patient's nutritional needs. There is no one right way to reinstitute enteral feeding. Feeding should not be attempted unless the basal ostomy or stool output is less than 2000 ml/day because patients with large fluid losses will develop worsening dehydration and electrolyte imbalance. With the use of H_2 antagonists and antimotility drugs such as loperamide, diphenoxylate, or paregoric, basal gastrointestinal losses can be reduced to a level that allows enteral nutrition.[45, 46] In patients who have not eaten for several weeks following intestinal resection, the physician should be aware that the small intestine has undergone a marked degree of atrophy.[42] Refeeding should be started slowly and cautiously. If possible, a small bore nasoduodenal tube should be placed, and enteral alimentation should be begun with continuous infusion of an isotonic diet at a relatively low rate (25 ml/hour). The slow infusion of a diet around the clock may minimize GI losses and maximize intestinal adaptation. Whether a suitably diluted chemically defined diet (such as Criticare, Vital, or Vivonex) or a complete, lactose-free isotonic diet (such as Osmolite, Isocal, or Precision) should be used is debatable. Chemically defined diets are potentially advantageous because they do not require digestion by pancreatic enzymes and a critical micellar concentration of bile salts.[47, 48] Chemically defined diets are made up of oligo-, di- and monosaccharides, oligopeptides, and amino acids and usually are fat-free. However, these diets may cause net secretion into the lumen and worsen ostomy output.[49] On the other hand, complete diets, made up of complex carbohydrates, proteins, and fat, may be better tolerated because of their lower osmotic load.[15] Because each patient responds differently, it is my preference to start with a chemically defined diet and switch to a complete diet, if necessary. The rate of infusion is governed by the amount of ostomy or fecal output. The infusion rate may be increased by 25 ml/hour every 3 to 5 days as long as total losses do not exceed 2 to 3 L per day. Losses of fluid and electrolytes will have to be compensated for by augmenting TPN intake.

Ostomy or fecal losses depend on several factors related to diet composition and may be idiosyncratic for each patient. After 1 to 3 weeks, the short bowel syndrome patient should be able to receive a significant fraction of their daily caloric needs enterally. Tube feedings should be discontinued, and the patient should be begun on oral intake. The amount of calories and protein provided by TPN can gradually be decreased, remembering to provide adequate parenteral fluid and electrolytes to prevent dehydration.

In some short bowel syndrome patients, it may be reasonable to avoid the use of the feeding tube and begin with oral feedings from the start. While there are many studies concerning the optimal diet composition in patients with the short bowel syndrome, they have been carried out in chronically adapted patients. There is little information available on what diet is preferred early in the adaptation phase. If the physician chooses to provide an oral diet, several principles should be kept in mind.

Because it may take several months for adaptation to be complete, it is important that the physician and patient not become impatient with the results of a feeding regimen. It is important that diet orders not be changed with such frequency that there is no intelligible information gathered. In many patients, the amount of oral intake is increased too quickly, resulting in excessive gastrointestinal losses making the patient worse rather than better. It is important to provide psychologic support to the patient during the refeeding regimen because initially, increased gastrointestinal losses will occur. Obviously, enteral adaptation will occur more quickly and more efficiently in patients with longer segments of remaining gut. Patients with more than 150 cm of intact jejunum, even without a colon, can successfully return to oral intake alone, whereas patients with less than 40 or 50 cm of jejunum are usually destined to require home TPN for a good part of their nutritional needs.[5]

As patients progress with their enteral/ oral regimen, gastrointestinal losses should be repeatedly quantified. Most patients can collect an adequate 24-hour quantitative stool specimen, which can be analyzed for total weight, fat content, and, electrolyte content.

Long-Term Enteral Feeding

The dietary approach to patients with the short bowel syndrome has come full circle in the past 20 years. In the 1960s, there was renewed interest in the management of these patients with the advent of medium-chain triglycerides (MCT).[48, 50] These early studies indicated that an MCT-enriched diet resulted in decreased steatorrhea. However, careful analysis of these papers does not provide strong evidence that a low-fat, MCT-substituted diet dramatically improved caloric retention or decreased gastrointestinal fluid and electrolyte losses. But, following publication of these studies, it was recommended that patients with the short bowel syndrome be maintained on a high-carbohydrate, low-fat, MCT diet. In the past several years, several studies have indicated that patients with the short bowel syndrome do equally well on a high-carbohydrate, low-fat diet as on a low-carbohydrate, high-fat diet.[14, 15, 51-53] There is uniform agreement that steatorrhea worsens as fat intake increases, but the relative percentage of dietary fat absorbed remains fairly constant over a wide range of dietary intake. Even in patients with less than 150 cm of residual bowel, at least 50% of dietary triglycerides are absorbed.[15, 52] In fact, in some studies the deleterious effects of a high-carbohydrate diet because of the resulting high osmotic load have been demonstrated.[45, 49]

In two recent studies, chronically adapted short bowel syndrome patients were extensively studied.[14, 52] No difference was seen in the assimilation of calories, protein, calcium, and magnesium in patients on either a high-carbohydrate, low-fat diet or a moderate-carbohydrate, high-fat diet. In fact, the authors concluded that there was no role for dietary restriction in short bowel syndrome patients. Some patients may be able to tolerate a high-carbohydrate diet because of excellent digestion whereas others will develop an osmotic diarrhea from the presence of carbohydrate. In some patients, malabsorbed carbohydrate is efficiently converted to short-chain fatty acids by intestinal bacteria and may enhance absorption[7, 54] but in others excessive production of short fatty acids may worsen diarrhea.[47] In contrast, the presence of malabsorbed fat may have no deleterious effect on ostomy output because fat has low osmotic activity. But, in patients with an intact colon, free fatty acids and bacterial conversion of these fatty acids to hydroxy fatty acids may worsen intestinal absorption and cause increased losses.[55] Bile salt malabsorption is usually not a factor causing diarrhea in these patients because the fecal pH is sufficiently low as to keep the colonic aqueous bowel salt concentration very low.[56]

Studies advising high fat intake should be taken with caution because massive steatorrhea may cause fat-soluble vitamin malabsorption. If a high-fat diet is well tolerated by the patient, two to three times the recommended daily allowances of these vitamins may be needed. In some instances, a high-fat diet may increase the losses of divalent cations (calcium, magnesium, zinc, and copper) and produce a negative balance.[14, 28] These minerals will have to be provided in increased quantities in patients with short bowel syndrome. The needs for adequate vitamin D and calcium intake in order to prevent metabolic bone disease are obvious. In addition, vitamin B_{12} should be administered regularly by injection to these patients.

The patient with the short bowel syndrome is a real challenge to the physician. In addition to providing for the patient's medical care and supervision of their nutritional support, the physician must be alert to the serious psychologic and social problems of the patient. In many patients, the concomitant input of psychiatrists, psychologists, and social workers is needed to help the patients adjust to their life after intestinal resection. Additional help can be obtained from organizations such as the National Foundation for Ileitis and Colitis, the Oley Foundation for home nutritional support, and the Ostomy Society. These three organizations provide excellent patient-to-patient support. In addition, they publish newsletters and other material to help inform patients with the short bowel syndrome.

References

1. Weser E: Nutritional aspects of malabsorption. Short gut adaptation. *Am J Med* 1979; 67:1014.
2. Tilson MD: Pathophysiology and treatment of short bowel syndrome. *Surg Clin North Am* 1980; 60:1272–1284.
3. Hofmann AF, Poley JR: Role of bile acid malabsorption in pathogenesis of diarrhea and steatorrhea in patients with ileal resection. *Gastroenterology* 1972; 62:918–934.
4. Spiller RC, Trotman OF, Higgins BF, et al: The ileal brake-inhibition of jejunal motility after ileal fat perfusion in man. *Gut* 1984; 25:365–374.
5. Gouttebel MC, Saint-Aubert B, Astre C, et al: Total parenteral nutrition needs in different types of short bowel syndrome. *Dig Dis Sci* 1986; 31:718–723.
6. Bond JH, Currier BE, Buchwald H, et al: Colonic conservation of malabsorbed carbohydrate. *Gastroenterology* 1980; 78:444–447.
7. Ruppin H, Bar-Mier S, Soergel KH, et al: Absorption of short chain fatty acids by the colon. *Gastroenterology* 1980; 78:1500–1507.
8. Haymond HE: Massive resection of the small intestine. Analysis of 257 collected cases. *Surg Gynecol Obstet* 1935; 61:693–705.
9. Sheldon GF: Role of parenteral nutrition in patients with short bowel syndrome. *Am J Med* 1979; 67:1021–1029.
10. Covelli HD, Black JW, Olsen MS, et al: Respiratory failure precipitated by high carbohydrate loads. *Ann Intern Med* 1981; 95:579–581.
11. Fleming CR, Hodges RE, Hurley LS: A prospective study of serum copper and zinc levels in patients receiving total parenteral nutrition. *Am J Clin Nutr* 1976; 29:70–77.
12. Windsor CWO, Fejfar J, Woodward DAK: Gastric secretion after massive small bowel resection. *Gut* 1969; 10:779–786.
13. Straus E, Gerson CD, Yalow RS: Hypersecretion of gastrin associated with the short bowel syndrome. *Gastroenterology* 1974; 66:175–180.
14. Woolf GM, Miller C, Kurian R, et al: Nutritional absorption in short bowel syndrome. Evaluation of fluid, calorie, and divalent cation requirements. *Dig Dis Sci* 1987; 32:8–15.
15. McIntyre PB, Fitchew M, Lennard-Jones JE: Patients with a high jejunostomy do not need a special diet. *Gastroenterology* 1986; 91:25–33.
16. Kramer P, Levitan R: Effect of 9-fluorohydrocortisone on the ileal excreta of ileostomized subjects. *Gastroenterology* 1972; 62:235–241.
17. Ladefoged K, Olgaard K: Fluid and electrolyte absorption and renin–angiotensin–aldosterone axis in patients with severe short bowel syndrome. *Scand Gastroenterol* 1979; 14:729–735.
18. Charney AN, Haskell LP: Relative effects of systemic pH, PCO_2, and bicarbonate concentration

on ileal ion transport. *Am J Physiol*: 1983; 245:G230–G235.
19. Broviac JW, Scribner GH: Prolonged parenteral nutrition in the home. *Surg Gynecol Obstet* 1974; 139:24–28.
20. Detsky AS, McLaughlin JR, Abrams HB, et al: A cost-utility analysis of the home parenteral nutrition program at Toronto General Hospital: 1970–1982. *JPEN* 1986; 10:49–57.
21. Fleming CR, Beart RW, Berkner S, et al: Home parenteral nutrition for management of the severely malnourished adult patient. *Gastroenterology* 1980; 79:11–18.
22. Howard L, Heaphey LL, Timchalk M: A review of the current national status of the home parenteral and enteral nutrition from the provider and consumer perspective. *JPEN* 1986; 10:416–424.
23. Shike M, Harrison JE, Sturtridge WS, et al: Metabolic bone disease in patients receiving long term parenteral nutrition. *Ann Intern Med* 1980; 92:343–350.
24. Epstein S, Traberg H, Levine G, et al: Bone and mineral status of patients beginning total parenteral nutrition. *JPEN* 1986; 10:263–264.
25. Ott SM, Maloney NA, Klein GL, et al: Aluminum is associated with low bone formation in patients receiving chronic parenteral nutrition. *Ann Intern Med* 1983; 98:910–914.
26. Wood RJ, Bengoa JM, Sitrin MD, et al: Calciuretic effect of cyclic versus continuous total parenteral nutrition. *Am J Clin Nutr* 1985; 41:614–619.
27. Wood RJ, Sitrin MD, Cusson GJ, et al: Reduction of total parenteral nutrition-induced urinary calcium loss by increasing the phosphorus in the total parenteral nutrition prescription. *JPEN* 1986; 10:188–190.
28. Ladefoged K, Nicolaidou P, Jarnum S: Calcium, phosphorus, magnesium, zinc, and nitrogen balance in patients with severe short bowel syndrome. *Am J Clin Nutr* 1980; 33:2137–2144.
29. Wolman SL, Anderson GH, Marliss EB, et al: Zinc in total parenteral nutrition: Requirements and metabolic effects. *Gastroenterology* 1979; 73:458–467.
30. Shike M, Roulet M, Kurian R, et al: Copper metabolism and requirements in total parenteral nutrition. *Gastroenterology* 1981; 81:290–297.
31. Jeejeebhoy KN, Chu RC, Marless EB, et al: Chromium deficiency, glucose intolerance and neuropathy reversed by chromium supplementation in a patient receiving long term total parenteral nutrition. *Am J Clin Nutr* 1977; 30:531–538.
32. Abamrad NN, Schneider AJ, Steel D, et al: Amino acid intolerance during prolonged total parenteral nutrition reversed by molybdate therapy. *Am J Clin Nutr* 1981; 34:2551–2559.
33. Lane HW, Lotspeich CA, Moore CE, et al: The effect of selenium supplementation on selenium status of patients receiving chronic total parenteral nutrition. *JPEN* 1987; 11:177–182.
34. Deren JJ, Porush JG, Levitt MF, et al: Nephrolithiasis as a complication of ulcerative colitis and regional enteritis. *Ann Intern Med* 1962; 56:843–853.
35. Dobbins JW, Binder HJ: Importance of the colon in enteric hyperoxaluria. *N Engl J Med* 1977; 296:298–301.
36. Rudman D, Dedonis JL, Fountain MT, et al: Hypocitraturia in patients with gastrointestinal malabsorption. *N Engl J Med* 1980; 303:657–661.
37. Stanko RT, Nathan G, Mendelow H, et al: Development of hepatic cholestasis and fibrosis in patients with massive loss of intestine supported by prolonged parenteral nutrition. *Gastroenterology* 1987; 92:197–202.
38. Bower GA, Fleming CR, Ludwig J, et al: Does long term home parenteral nutrition in adult patients cause chronic liver disease? *JPEN* 1985; 9:11–17.
39. Roslyn JJ, Pitt HA, Mann LL, et al: Gallbladder disease in patients on long term parenteral nutrition. *Gastroenterology* 1983; 84:148–154.
40. Cano N, Cicero F, Ramieri F, et al: Ultrasonographic study of gallbladder motility during total parenteral nutrition. *Gastroenterology* 1986; 91:313–317.
41. Ramakrishnan T, Stokes P: Beneficial effects of fasting and low carbohydrate diet in d-lactic acidosis associated with short-bowel syndrome. *JPEN* 1985; 9:361–363.
42. Levine GM, Deren JJ, Yezdimir EA: Small bowel resection: Oral intake is the stimulus for hyperplasia. *Dig Dis Sci* 1976; 21:542–546.
43. Dworkin LD, Levine GM, Farber NJ, et al: Small intestinal mass of the rat is partially determined by indirect effects of intraluminal nutrition. *Gastroenterology* 1976; 71:626–630.
44. Williamson RC: Intestinal Adaptation. *N Engl J Med* 1978; 298:1292–1302, 1444–1450.
45. Remington M, Malagelada JR, Zinmeister A, et al: Abnormalities in gastrointestinal motor activity in patients with short bowels: Effect of a synthetic opiate. *Gastroenterology* 1983; 85:629–636.
46. Remington M, Fleming CR, Malagelada JR: Inhibition of postprandial pancreatic and biliary secretion by loperamide in patients with short bowel syndrome. *Gut* 1982; 23:98–101.
47. Ameen VZ, Powell GK, Jones LA: Quantitation of fecal carbohydrate excretion in patients with short bowel syndrome. *Gastroenterology* 1987; 92:493–500.
48. Winawer SJ, Broitman SA, Wolochow DA, et al: Successful management of massive small bowel resection based on assessment of absorption defects and nutritional needs. *N Engl J Med* 1966; 274:72–78.
49. Smith JL, Arteaga C, Heymsfield SB: Increased ureagenesis and impaired nitrogen use during infusion of a synthetic amino acid formula. *N Engl J Med* 1982; 506:1013–1018.
50. Zurier RB, Campbell RG, Hashim SA, et al: Use of medium chain triglyceride in management of patients with massive resection of the small intestine. *N Engl J Med* 1966; 274:450–493.
51. Simko V, McCarroll AM, Goodman S, et al: High-fat diet in a short bowel syndrome. Intestinal absorption and gastroenteropancreatic hor-

mone responses. *Dig Dis Sci* 1980; 25:333–339.
52. Woolf G, Miller C, Kurian R, et al: Diet for patients with a short bowel: High fat or high carbohydrate? *Gastroenterology* 1983; 84:823–828.
53. Ovesen L, Chu R, Howard L: The influence of dietary fat on jejunostomy output in patients with severe short bowel syndrome. *Am J Clin Nutr* 1983; 38:270–277.
54. Schmitt MG, Soergel KH, Wood CM, et al: Absorption of short chain fatty acids from the human ileum. *Dig Dis Sci* 1977; 22:340–347.
55. Ammon HV, Phillips SF: Inhibition of colonic water and electrolyte absorption by fatty acids in man. *Gastroenterology* 1973; 65:744–749.
56. McJunkin B, Fromm H, Sarva RP, et al: Factors in the mechanism of diarrhea in bile acid malabsorption: Fecal pH—a key determinant. *Gastroenterology* 1981: 80:1454–1464.

Intestinal Gas:
What do we offer the patient?

MICHAEL D. LEVITT, M.D.

Because I have performed research on intestinal gas for the past 20 years, I am frequently asked by other gastroenterologists to consult on their difficult patients with gas problems. I usually try to avoid seeing these patients because I seldom have anything to offer that has not been previously tried, and found wanting, by the referring gastroenterologist. Thus, I would like to stress at the outset of this chapter that I make no claims that I can handle gaseous problems more effectively than can the average, knowledgeable physician.

The first thing I do when a patient tells me that they have a gas problem is to clarify the nature of the complaint. Is the patient referring to belching, bloating and distention, or the excessive passage of flatus? I believe these three problems have different origins and require different evaluations and treatment.

CHRONIC ERUCTATION

Chronic eructation is a nervous habit in which the patient repeatedly aspirates air into the esophagus and then immediately regurgitates most of this air. Fluoroscopy clearly demonstrates that in chronic eructation the esophagus fills from above and then empties. Some of the gas may be propelled into the stomach, and belchers often have a large gastric air bubble. However, the physician should realize that the excess gastric air is a result, not a cause, of the eructation. When questioned, some patients claim that they perform this seemingly pointless maneuver in an attempt to relieve some sort of thoracic or abdominal distress. In fact, many patients claim that for a few moments, the eructation actually does produce very transitory relief of the discomfort. Thus, it is useful to question the patient concerning various organic or functional causes of chest and abdominal discomfort. Frequently chronic belchers have associated irritable bowel syndrome. In other patients, chronic eructation appears to be nothing more than a nervous habit driven by some sort of irresistible urge.

If the patient has symptoms suggestive of some thoracic or abdominal problem, an appropriate work-up is indicated. However, I don't believe that the isolated complaint of chronic eructation requires evaluation.

If an underlying organic lesion is uncovered, this condition should, of course, be treated. The patient almost always is wedded to the idea that certain foods cause the belching. However, a careful history usually shows no logical pattern to the foods that allegedly cause belching, and I don't believe any form of dietary manipulation is useful in these patients. I am convinced that education is the most important form of therapy. It must be explained to the patient, in no uncertain terms, that the gas being eructated is not coming from the stomach or intestines but is being aspirated by the mouth. Often, this does not square with the patient's longstanding belief that the stomach or intestines are the source of the problem. To demonstrate the voluntary nature of eructation, I like to aspirate air and belch at the patient several times. I'm not sure if this cures the patient, but they seldom ever complain to me again of belching. It is also useful to explain that belching is not helping the real or perceived abdominal or thoracic problem. In fact, in many patients there appears to be a vicious cycle in which abdominal discomfort (usually functional) leads to chronic eructation. Some of the aspirated air may enter the gut and aggravate the irritable bowel syndrome, which leads to more eructation. If the patient can control the eructation, the vicious cycle is interrupted and the abdominal discomfort may actually improve.

Despite my best efforts, many patients are not able to suppress the urge to eructate. I believe it is totally irrational to treat these patients with medication directed at the stomach and intestine, and age-old remedies such as clenching a pencil between the teeth are totally impractical. All one can do is to tell the patient to live with their chronic eructation.

BLOATING AND DISTENTION

By far the most common gaseous complaint is bloating and distention, which the patient attributes to excessive bowel gas. Most of what I think I know about this problem I learned from a study we carried out to measure the volume of intestinal gas.[1] To this end, we rapidly perfused argon into the gut by a tube at the ligament of Treitz and quantitatively collected all gas washed out at the rectum. This study showed that bloating patients had the same volume of bowel gas as did normal controls—about 200 ml. This observation is supported by x-ray studies, which seldom show excessive intestinal gas in patients who complain of bloating. However, bloating patients had much more discomfort during the argon infusion than did the controls. Many of these patients developed such severe pain that the gas infusion had to be discontinued. There also was a tendency for more of the infused argon to reflux back into the stomach in the bloating patients as compared to controls.

Thus, I believe the basic problem of bloating patients has nothing to do with excessive bowel gas: rather, these subjects are suffering from a variation of the irritable bowel syndrome that affects primarily the small bowel. The intestine of these subjects does not seem to propel gas (or liquids) in a well-coordinated fashion and, as a result, the patient senses that the gut is overdistended. It seems likely that this irritability of the bowel causes the patient to sense overdistention when the gut is actually distended to a degree that would not be perceived as painful by healthy controls. It is also possible that isolated loops of gut actually are overdistended with gas (or liquid) even though the total volume of gas in the gut is normal.

The evaluation required for the patient with bloating and distention is dependent on a number of factors including age and duration of the problem. Organic disease of the gut—particularly carcinoma of the colon and Crohn's disease—can present with bloating and distention. Thus, colon cancer must be ruled out in patients over 50 years of age, particularly when there is a short history of symptoms and no previous colonic evaluation. In younger patients, little if any diagnostic evaluation is indicated in the otherwise healthy patient. The presence of unexplained weight loss, diarrhea, or occult blood in the stools requires evaluation of the gastrointestinal tract.

There are exceptions to the general rule that patients who complain of excessive gas have normal volumes of bowel gas. An occasional patient will demonstrate gaseous distention on an abdominal x-ray. These patients usually have some sort of severe motility disorder (such as intestinal pseudo-obstruction) that causes huge volumes of gas to collect in the gut.

Treatment of the bloating patient usually is not curative. In my opinion, the most important component of therapy is psychological rather than physical. Often these patients are concerned that their abdominal discomfort represents some severe disease, usually cancer. This worry causes the patient to concentrate on their abdominal distress, and that, in time, tends to aggravate the problem. The physician first must convince the patient that there is not life-threatening disease in the abdomen. To this end, I will sometimes carry out more diagnostic tests than are truly indicated—but I consider such testing to be therapeutic rather than diagnostic.

Improvement in these patients is dependent on a logical and sympathetic explanation of their problem, avoiding even the slightest suggestion that it is all "in the head." Thus, I carefully explain that the gut is a long muscular tube that normally propels liquid and gas in an orderly fashion. However, the patient has a irritable gut that does not move things along in such an orderly fashion, and this disordered motility gives him or her the sensation of distention. In many patients such simple reassurance and explanation lead to dramatic improvement. If the patient does not improve with reassurance, in my experience it is very unlikely that any therapy will be dramatically effective.

Is there any point in attempting to reduce the volume of gas in the gut? It seems possible that normal volumes of gas cause discomfort in these subjects. In particular, I have the impression that repeated attempts to eructate gas lead to air swallowing, which aggravates the problem. Thus if the bloating patient is a chronic eructator, I try to have the patient suppress the urge to eructate, as described previously. Dietary manipulation to reduce gas production, such as the elimination of legumes or lactose restriction in lactase-deficient subjects, seems to be helpful in a few patients, but I suspect that the benefit represents a placebo response to dietary manipulation. Nevertheless, I always suggest lactose restriction in the lactase-deficient patient. I am not a believer in taking a careful dietary history in bloating subjects. Most of these subjects have developed a list of foods they believe they cannot tolerate. Ordinarily there seem to be no features by which one could logically link these foods to distention. In addition, careful questioning usually indicates that all foods (even water, on occasion) cause a problem, but, for some reason, the patient has decided to implicate only certain dietary items. Despite published evidence to the contrary,[2] I am not convinced that patients can actually identify specific foods that cause functional abdominal distress.

My impression is that increasing dietary intake of fiber does not help these patients, and there are no data in the literature to indicate that fiber is useful for complaints of bloating or abdominal pain. In fact, fiber increases gas production in the gut, and many subjects complain of increased bloating with fiber.

There are few well-controlled trials of drugs in bloating patients. These subjects are very susceptible to the placebo effect, and improvement in poorly controlled trials may merely reflect a placebo response. What follows is a brief summary of my anecdotal experience in treating bloating patients. This information may have no true basis in fact. Anticholinergic drugs are of little benefit and may actually increase bloating and distention. Antacids are of no benefit and may aggravate symptoms. Thus, I commonly take patients off antacids. Simethicone and pancreatic supplements are ineffective, and there are no well-controlled studies to convince me that I am mistaken. However, I will sometimes use such compounds more as a harmless placebo than with any confidence in their true effectiveness. Some patients seemingly respond favorably to metaclopramide, and there is a controlled study to support this idea.[3] Because of the central nervous system side effects of metaclopramide, I do not use this drug routinely in bloating subjects. But during periods of great discomfort, it seems to be helpful. Lastly, I believe that various antidepressants may be helpful in patients who have no evidence of depression. The compound I have the most experience with is doxepin, and I prescribe this drug in very small doses, frequently just 10 mg at bedtime.

The degree of improvement noted by the patient with any form of therapy for bloating and distention (as is the case with irritable bowel) is very strongly dependent on the words that go with the medicine. If a convincing and enthusiastic rationale is provided along with the drug, the chances of improvement are markedly enhanced. For example, a much better response will result if the prescription of a high-fiber diet is associated with a description of how fiber holds water in the gut and distends the gut preventing the bowel from the "overcontraction" that causes discomfort. Such a beneficial response that is dependent on words rather than medication is no doubt a placebo effect. However with chronic, otherwise untreatable conditions such as bloating and distention, I am more than willing to accept any type of beneficial response, including a placebo response.

FLATUS

The third type of gaseous problem is the complaint of passage through the rectum of excessively voluminous or odiferous gas. A surprisingly difficult problem in these patients is the determination as to whether the patient truly is abnormal or merely perceives himself or herself to be abnormal with regard to flatus excretion. We found that healthy 25- to 35-year-old males passed gas about 14 ± 4.5 (1SD) per day.[4] While only a small group of subjects was studied, it appears that the upper limit of normal for passages per day is about 23. Very unsatisfactory attempts to measure flatus volume using a rectal tube have convinced me that the measurement of flatus frequency (as opposed to volume) are the only data that can be obtained on flatus excretion in the clinical situation. Thus my first action with patients complaining of excessive flatus is to have them count the number of times they pass gas each day. At least 50% of these patients will be well within normal limits. I explain to these subjects that they are suffering from a misperception of normality as opposed to being truly abnormal. This reassures some patients, while others would like to be even more normal.

The patient who truly passes gas with excessive frequency (which I equate with excessive volume) presumably has some abnormality. The flatus of such individuals virtually always contains large percentages of H_2 and CO_2, two gases produced in the lumen during bacterial fermentation of carbohydrate. Thus the abnormality of such subjects presumably consists of some combination of excessive carbohydrate malabsorption and a fecal flora that is unusually adept at producing gas from a given amount of carbohydrate.

I do not carry out any investigative procedures on the otherwise healthy, but flatulent, patient. I recommend a trial diet free of sorbitol, lactose, and legumes for several weeks while the patient continues to count the number of gas passages to provide a semiobjective record of response. If sufficient benefit is not obtained, the patient is unlikely to respond to any form of therapy. However, in the willing patient I recommend a diet totally carbohydrate free with the exception of rice. (Studies with the commonly ingested starches showed that all are malabsorbed by normal subjects with the exception of rice.[5]) Almost without exception, flatulence will decrease markedly on this diet. However, the diet is intolerable to most subjects. The addition of one complex carbohydrate every week or two until flatulence reoccurs (which it always does) shows the limit of carbohydrate that can be ingested. Patients are then left with the choice of a markedly restricted carbohydrate diet or flatulence, and they nearly always choose flatulence.

Drugs that I have not found to be of value in flatulence include simethicone, pancreatic supplement, charcoal, and antibiotics. With regard to charcoal, there are studies in the literature both supporting[6,7] and refuting[8] its value. We found that charcoal did not decrease flatulence or breath H_2 excretion following ingestion of baked beans. There are few objective tests of the value of antibiotics in flatulence. Of the few patients I treated, most thought their flatulence was increased while on antibiotics. Rats clearly excrete more H_2 while on a variety of antibiotics than in the control state.[9] This enhancement of H_2 excretion appears to represent a dimunition in H_2-consuming bacteria such that a greater fraction of the H_2 liberated is available for excretion.

The complaint of malodorus flatus is not uncommon. The lack of objective tests of odor makes it impossible to rationally assess this complaint. My only therapeutic suggestion is dietary manipulation to reduce the volume of flatus, presumably allowing more of the odiferous gas to be absorbed and less to be excreted per rectum. Activated charcoal will effectively absorb odors when dry but is much less effective when wet. I do believe (without solid evidence) that ingestion of activated charcoal may reduce flatus odor. I have had no success with dietary manipulations designed to alter the delivery of substrates that are metabolized to odiferous compounds or antibiotics that alter the colonic flora.

References

1. Lasser RB, Bond JH, Levitt MD: The role of intestinal gas in functional abdominal pain. *N Engl J Med* 1975; 293:524–526.
2. Jones VA, McLaughlan P, Shorthouse M, et al: Food intolerance: A major factor in the pathogenesis of irritable bowel syndrome. *Lancet* 1982; 2:1115–1117.
3. Johnson AG: Controlled trial of metoclopramide in the treatment of flatulent dyspepsia. *Br Med J* 1971; 2:25–26.
4. Sutalf LO, Levitt MD: Follow-up of a flatulent patient. *Dig Dis Sci* 1979; 24:652–654.
5. Levitt MD, Hirsh P, Fetzer CA, et al: H_2 excretion to detect carbohydrate malabsorption. *Gastroenterology* 1987; 92:383–389.
6. Jain NK, Patel VP, Pitchumoni CS: Activated charcoal, simethicone, and intestinal gas: A double-blind study. *Ann Intern Med* 1986; 105:61–62.
7. Hall GH Jr, Thompson H, Strother A: Effects of orally administered activated charcoal on intestinal gas. *Am J Gastroenterol* 1981; 75:192–196.
8. Potter T, Ellis C, Levitt M: Activated charcoal: In vivo and in vitro studies of effect on gas formation. *Gastroenterology* 1985; 88:620–624.
9. Levitt MD, Berggren T, Hastings J, et al: Hydrogen (H_2) catabolism in the colon of the rat. *J Lab Clin Med* 1974; 84:163–167.

VII
Large Intestine

30

Fecal Incontinence:
How should it be contained?

ARNOLD WALD, M.D.

Fecal incontinence is a physically and emotionally distressing condition with potentially grave consequences in terms of social disruption and damage to self-esteem. Patients are often embarrassed to mention their soiling problem even to their physicians and often will not volunteer information unless directly questioned. Unfortunately, many physicians (including gastroenterologists) are inadequately trained to evaluate and treat fecal soiling and may be unaware that effective therapy is available. This situation was exemplified by a recent inquiry from an elderly patient. For many years, she had suffered from fetal incontinence and had been told by her physician that she "had to live with her problem" because there was nothing to be done.

Appropriate management of fecal soiling begins with an understanding of anorectal physiology and continence mechanisms because a number of abnormalities of anorectal function may contribute to incontinence.

ANORECTAL ANATOMY AND CONTINENCE MECHANISMS[1]

The main function of the anorectum is to store and eliminate feces in a socially acceptable manner. To accomplish these tasks, a storage reservoir is provided by the rectum, regulation of defecation and continence is maintained by two anal sphincters and the pelvic floor muscles, and a sensory mechanism exists to make the individual aware of rectal filling and impending defecation.

Rectal Sensation

The rectum is supplied with afferent nerves which allow awareness of rectal distension with volumes as small as 5 ml of air. Indirect evidence suggests that mechanoreceptors that mediate this awareness lie in the perirectal tissues. Rectal sensation can be evaluated by inflating balloons placed in the rectum with different volumes of air and at different rates of inflation.

Anal Sphincters

Approximately 80% of the resting pressure of the anal canal is derived from the tone of the internal anal sphincter (IAS) which arises from the circular smooth muscle of the rectum and is not under voluntary control. Anal canal pressure (and thus resistance to passage of feces) is augmented by the tone of the external anal sphincter (EAS) and can be greatly increased by voluntary contraction of the EAS, a striated muscle which is innervated by the pudendal nerves arising from the sacral plexus. The EAS can be stimulated to transiently contract in response to rectal distension, postural changes, cough, and perianal pinprick.

Anal sphincter tone and strength can be assessed subjectively by digital examination and more objectively using manometric techniques. Indirect assessment of anal sphincter integrity is made using tests of solid sphere continence and (in patients with diarrhea) with saline loading studies.[2]

Anorectal Angle

Anteroposterior angulation of the anorectum is maintained by the puborectalis muscle which inserts anteriorly to the symphysis pubis (Fig 30–1). Contraction of the puborectalis narrows the anorectal angle and enhances resistance to passage of stool through the anal canal.[3] Assessment of puborectalis function can be made during digital examination of the rectum or by obtaining lateral radiographs of the anorectum (chain proctogram) (Fig 30–2).

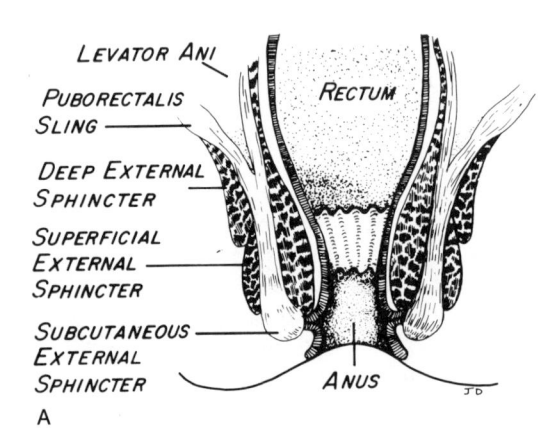

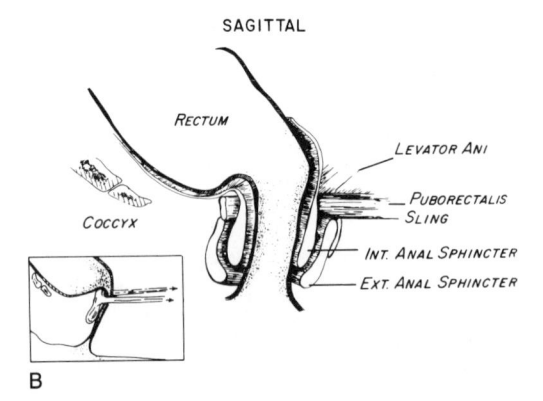

Reservoir Capacity

The rectum acts as a storage reservoir through adaptive compliance and accommodation; thus, rectal pressures increase by relatively small amounts in response to increases in rectal contents.[4] Rectal volume can be assessed through lateral radiographs of the rectum following instillation of barium or can be measured by determining pressure–volume relationships in response to progressive filling of a rectal balloon (rectometrogram).

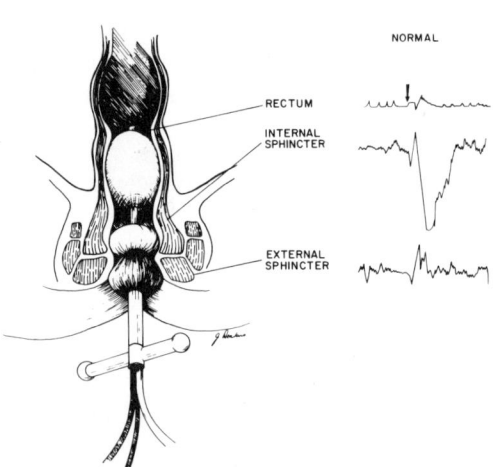

FIG 30–1.
Transverse (**A**) and sagittal (**B**) views of the anorectum indicating important structural components. Inset illustrates anterior pull of anorectum during contraction of the puborectalis muscle. (Modified from Wald A: Fecal incontinence: Effective nonsurgical treatments. *Postgrad Med* 1986; 80:123–130. Used by permission.)

FIG 30–2.
Lateral radiographs of the anorectum (chain proctogram) in a normal subject at rest (**A**) and while straining (**B**). The anorectal angle is defined by a line drawn along the rectum and a beaded chain in the anal canal. The pelvic floor is defined by a line drawn from the symphysis pubis and the tip of the coccyx. (Wald A: Abnormalities of anorectal function, in Cohen S, Soloway RD (eds): *Functional Disorders of the GI Tract.* New York, Churchill Livingstone, 1987, pp 121–138.)

Maintenance of fecal incontinence is achieved by the coordinated actions of the above mechanisms together with motivation to make the appropriate responses. Most patients with fecal incontinence have demonstrable abnormalities of one or more of these mechanisms.

DISORDERS OF CONTINENCE—ADULTS

Iatrogenic Anal Sphincter Damage

Many patients develop fecal incontinence following obstetric trauma to the sphincters or damage occurring from surgical procedures involving the anal canal. These include repeated anal dilation for chronic pain, fissures, or hemorrhoids; surgical division of the EAS to repair anal fistulae; internal anal sphincterotomy; and hemorrhoidectomy.

Idiopathic Fecal Incontinence

This condition occurs predominantly in middle-aged and elderly women who have no history of anorectal disease or trauma. Often, there has been longstanding constipation or excessive straining with defecation. On examination, diminished anal sphincter pressure is noted with little or no increase during voluntary sphincter contraction; similarly puborectalis contraction is often weak.

Manometric studies confirm diminished anal sphincter pressures at rest and following maximal voluntary contraction. Such patients are often unable to retain saline infused into the rectum in volumes that can be retained by normal continent individuals, and less force is required to overcome anal sphincter resistance during the solid sphere continence test. Lateral radiographs of the anorectum frequently show a more obtuse anorectal angle and abnormal descent of the pelvic floor at rest or during strain when compared to continent subjects.[5] These findings suggest weakness of the puborectalis and pelvic floor muscles in addition to impaired anal sphincters.

Recent studies suggest that weakness of these muscles may occur because of repetitive damage to the pudendal nerves associated with excessive descent of the pelvic floor during chronic straining associated with defecation.[5] This condition has been termed the *descending perineum syndrome*. In patients with more severe weakness of the pelvic floor, rectal prolapse of varying degrees may occur. Fecal incontinence in patients with full thickness prolapse is often associated with denervation weakness of the EAS and/or puborectalis muscles due to stretch injury to the pudendal nerves.

Diabetes Mellitus

Fecal incontinence occurs in as many as 20% of diabetic patients,[6] most of whom have diarrhea associated with peripheral and autonomic neuropathy. Several recent studies have demonstrated multiple abnormalities of anorectal function including impaired rectal sensation, decreased resting anal canal pressures, impaired continence of liquids and solids, and frequent absence of EAS contraction in response to rectal distention.[7,8] The pathogenesis of impaired rectal sensation is uncertain but is not related to changes in viscoelasticity of rectal smooth muscle.

Rectal Disorders

A number of disorders may be associated with impaired rectal storage capacity and often are associated with urgency and incontinence. These include rectal carcinomas and large villous adenomas, idiopathic inflammatory bowel diseases involving the rectum, radiation damage to the rectum,[9] subtotal colectomy with ileoanal anastomosis, sphincter-saving procedures for rectal lesions, and chronic rectal ischemia.[10] The diagnosis can be made by history, physical examination, and conventional proctoscopic and radiographic studies. Manometric findings include decreased rectal viscoelasticity and rectal size with correspondingly reduced reservoir capacity. However, excepting patients with anal or perianal involvement, anal sphincter pressures and rectal sensation are normal.

Neurologic Incontinence

Neurogenic disorders associated with fecal incontinence include injury to the sacral cord or plexus, damage to the spinal cord above the sacrum, and diseases of the frontal cortex or subcortical pathways. Rectal sensation is frequently impaired in the first two disorders, and EAS and puborectalis muscle denervation is common, particularly with involvement of the sacral cord or plexus. In contrast, in the last disorder rectal sensation and sphincter tone are retained, but the ability to inhibit reflex emptying of the rectum is lost. Thus, eating results in reflex movement of stool into the rectum with uninhibited defecation. This condition is often found in patients with cerebrovascular disease.

Incontinence Associated with Diarrhea

In many patients, fecal incontinence develops only after diarrhea occurs. Liquid stool may be more difficult to perceive and, particularly when associated with urgency, more difficult to retain. In the absence of massive diarrhea or conditions that render patients unable to reach the commode, incontinence associated with diarrhea is usually associated with underlying abnormalities of anorectal continence mechanisms.[11]

Incontinence Associated with Constipation

Incontinence associated with constipation is frequently found in elderly and physically immobilized people; the two frequently coexist in the institutionalized elderly population.[11] Constipation may lead to fecal impaction; soft, poorly formed stools may seep around the obstructing fecal bolus and may be passed many times per day. This is frequently misinterpreted as diarrhea, which may result in inappropriate treatment. The correct diagnosis can be made on rectal examination or, in the case of impactions more proximally, by abdominal radiographs. The importance of excluding a fecal impaction before treating diarrhea or fecal incontinence in an elderly or debilitated patient is worth reemphasizing.

DISORDERS OF CONTINENCE—CHILDREN

Encopresis

The vast majority of children with encopresis have constipation and overflow soiling, often associated with megarectum and megacolon. Similar to adults with fecal impactions, the correct diagnosis is made by rectal examination, palpation of fecal masses on abdominal examination, or by abdominal radiographs. Although many physicians continue to emphasize psychologic or behavioral determinants, it is my experience and that of others,[12] that behavioral abnormalities are often secondary to the underlying bowel dysfunction and often disappear following successful therapy. Despite the presence of fecal incontinence, sphincter continence mechanisms are normal, and rectal sensory impairment is probably due to megarectum which normalizes with successful treatment. Recent studies[13] have found that up to 40% of encopretic children have abnormal patterns of defecation characterized by inappropriate contractions of the EAS or puborectalis muscle. This may represent an unconscious learned behavior which might contribute to constipation and fecal retention in some children.

Meningomyelocele (Spina Bifida)

Fecal incontinence is often associated with constipation, which can lead to fecal impaction, megarectum, and megacolon if neglected. EAS denervation and decreased anal sphincter tone occur in most children, and rectal sensation is often irreversibly impaired. Not uncommonly, other sensorimotor abnormalties are present, and retardation or behavioral problems may exist. Such individuals often require comprehensive care and extensive evaluation in addition to bowel control programs.

Imperforate Anus

Fecal incontinence may be variously associated with decreased rectal compliance, anal sphincter weakness, dysfunction due to poor surgical correction, and, occasionally, a stricture with fecal impaction and overflow incontinence. Therefore, a complete diagnostic evaluation is necessary to document which abnormalities may be present.

DIAGNOSTIC ASSESSMENT OF ADULTS WITH FECAL INCONTINENCE

Evaluation begins with considerations of possible contributing factors during history taking and when performing the physical examination (Table 30–1). A careful examination of the anorectum, focused neurologic testing and evaluation of mental status, and psychosocial assessment are particularly important at both ends of the age spectrum. Failure of the anal canal to close after digital examination (anal "gaping") indicates EAS denervation, whereas the finding of fecal impaction or anorectal deformity has been previously emphasized. However, in general, digital estimation of anal sphincter tone and strength correlates only moderately well with objective testing in the laboratory.

Initial studies should also include sigmoidoscopy and, in the presence of diarrhea, an appropriate assessment as to possible and potentially treatable causes (Table 30–1). I find it particularly helpful to have the patient keep a calendar for several weeks to assess the frequency, severity, and temporal relationship of defecations and incontinence. In addition to providing recent objective information, an estimate of the patient's reliability and cooperation can be obtained, which may be important in selecting therapeutic modalities. This assessment is appropriate before referral or treatment and can be supplemented by specialized tests to assess

TABLE 30–1.
Evaluation of Fecal Incontinence*

History

Frequency, duration, severity
Pattern (diurnal, nocturnal, both)
Associated symptoms (e.g., urgency, lack of warning, diarrhea, constipation, straining at defecation)
Other relevant factors (e.g., anorectal trauma or surgery, diabetes, laminectomy, urinary incontinence, immobility, dementia, neurologic disease, multiple childbirths, inflammatory bowel disease, medications)

Physical examination

Rectal examination (prolapse, fecal impaction or rectal mass, anal deformity or disease, anal "gaping," atrophy of gluteal muscles)
Neurologic examination (mental status, sacral reflexes, perineal sensation, basic neurologic evaluation)

Initial investigation

Sigmoidoscopy (proctitis, tumor, melanosis coli)
Incontinence calendar
Presence of diarrhea (stool for culture, ova and parasites; 72-hr stool collection for weight, fat, reducing substances; barium enema; small bowel series; medication and diet histories)

*Modified from Wald A: Fecal incontinence: Effective nonsurgical treatments. *Postgrad Med* 1986; 80:123–130. Used by permission.

TABLE 30-2.
Specialized Laboratory Studies for Fecal Incontinence

Test	Information Obtained
Anorectal manometry (pull-through)	Resting anal pressure (IAS and EAS)
	Augmented anal pressure (EAS)
Anorectal manometry (balloon or perfused)	Rectal sensation
	IAS relaxation
	EAS contraction to all stimuli
Rectometrogram	Rectal elasticity and accommodation
Solid sphere continence	Resting and augmented anal continence (IAS and EAS)
Saline continence	Continence for liquids
Chain proctogram	Anorectal angle (puborectalis muscle)
	Pelvic floor muscles (perineal descent)
	Rectal size and distensability

continence mechanisms performed at a center experienced with such techniques (Table 30–2).

TREATMENT OF ADULTS

Anal Sphincteric Abnormalities

Patients in this category include those with iatrogenic sphincter damage and most patients with idiopathic fecal incontinence. Although surgical approaches have been advocated as the treatment of choice,[14] on the basis of personal experience[15,16] and the experience of others,[17] I believe that biofeedback (operant conditioning) should be the initial approach for patients in this category because it is simple, risk-free, and effective in many patients. The classic method as originally described and used in many centers employs an anorectal manometer which is often used for diagnostic studies (Fig 30–3). The principle of the technique is that the recording apparatus provides information about EAS responses (feedback) so that the patient can tell whether sphincteric contractions are appropriate. Essentially, biofeedback is a trial-and-error learning process that uses a visual display to monitor performance. The program that I employ consists of three phases.

1. Patients watch the recording of their sphincteric responses and are asked to contract the EAS. A normal response is illustrated, and patients are praised if they can produce an appropriate (similar) contraction. The ability to make an appropriate contraction is achieved through trial and error; the first phase ends when the subject produces that response repeatedly.
2. The contraction response is synchronized with rectal distention (and, therefore, IAS relaxation). Responses are monitored by watching the recording to ensure appropriate synchronization with IAS relaxation.
3. Patients are weaned from the instrument by having their view of the recording blocked. During this phase, patients are informed by the instructor when sphincteric responses are appropriate. When this occurs consistently, the training session is complete.

Subsequently, patients are instructed to practice contraction exercises three or four times daily and to contract the sphincter whenever they sense rectal distention or urgency. Routine reinforcement sessions are generally not needed for adults and are reserved for those patients in whom initial responses are suboptimal or relapse occurs.

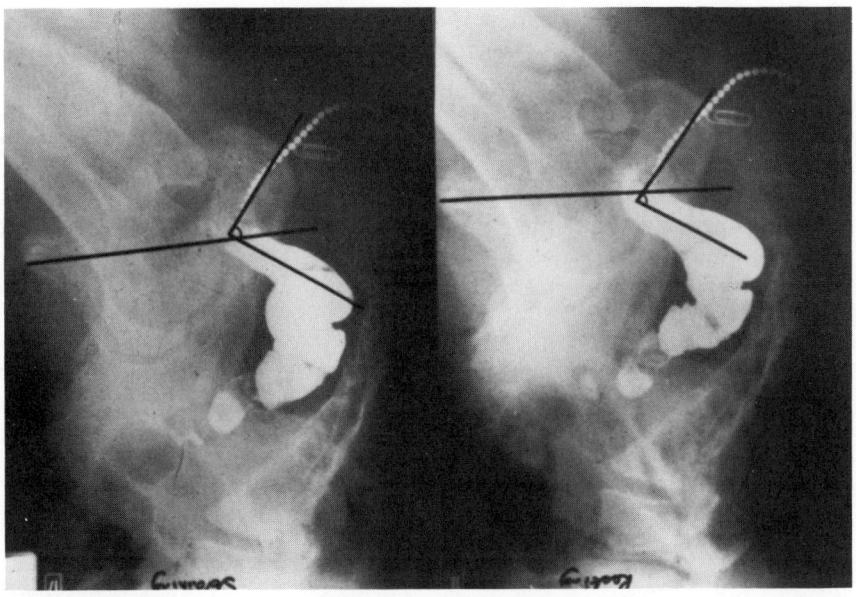

FIG 30–3.
Anorectal manometer composed of three air-filled balloons shown in the anorectum with normal sphincteric responses shown on right. Transient distention of the rectum by inflating the proximal balloon *(arrow)* produces reflex relaxation of the internal anal sphincter and transient contraction of the external anal sphincter. (From Wald A: Fecal incontinence: Effective nonsurgical treatments. *Postgrad Med* 1986; 80:123–130. Used by permission.)

For biofeedback to be successful, the patient must be motivated and able to comprehend and follow directions, sense rectal distention in the normal range, and contract the EAS or gluteal muscles. Success has been achieved in more than 70% of patients who meet these requirements.

Recently, a biofeedback technique directed at EAS contraction only was reported to be equally effective in treating this category of fecal incontinence.[18] In this technique, the electric impulse of EAS contractions is presented in the form of audible and visual signals using an intraanal plug and an electromyometer. No attempt is made to monitor IAS responses or to coordinate EAS contractions with rectal distention. Success rates similar to those treated with classic biofeedback were obtained. The advantages of this approach are the use of less sophisticated and expensive monitoring equipment and its suitability for office use.

If biofeedback or other measures fail to restore satisfactory continence, surgical measures should be considered. Surgical approaches include anal sphincter repair to restore sphincteric competency and techniques such as postanal repair which simply aims to restore the anorectal angle.[14] The choice of surgery thus depends on the clinical picture and diagnostic studies that evaluate the anorectal angle and the integrity of the anal sphincters. Postanal repair has been advised as the procedure of choice for idiopathic fecal incontinence, for patients with incontinence after surgical repair of a rectal prolapse, and soiling after anal dilation. Sphincter repair is preferred for trauma or iatrogenic damage to the anal canal.

Diabetes Mellitus

Because many patients with diabetes and fecal incontinence have diarrhea, it is important to carefully assess potential causes and institute appropriate therapy. Nonetheless, because the majority of diabetics with fecal incontinence have abnormalities of anorectal continence mechanisms, my approach has been similar to that used with nondiabetics with one modification.

In patients with abnormal conscious rectal sensation, I start with a rectal sensory conditioning program in which the threshold of rectal sensation is decreased in the following manner: Once the smallest volume of rectal distention sensed by the patient is determined, progressively smaller distention volumes are administered in decrements of 1 to 5 ml of air. Each time a smaller volume is sensed consistently, the volume is further decreased, and the process is repeated until the patient exhibits no further improvement.

Once sensory conditioning is successful, the biofeedback program proceeds in a manner identical to that for patients with normal rectal sensation. Good to excellent results have been obtained in more than 70% of a relatively small number of diabetic patients.[8] If biofeedback is ineffective, loperamide may be used in an attempt to control diarrhea (see below).

Rectal Disorders

Therapeutic approaches depend on the underlying disease. Rectal urgency and incontinence caused by proctitis often respond to steroid retention enemas, which may be supplemented with loperamide or diphenoxylate to control diarrhea and cramping. Patients with soiling associated with subtotal colectomy and ileoanal anastomosis often lack localizing rectal sensation as well as adequate reservoir capacity. Treatment includes reduction of fecal volume through fiber restriction, use of loperamide or diphenoxylate to prolong transit time and promote intestinal absorption of fluids and electrolytes, and planning defecation after a meal or other known stimulating factor. With time, improved ileal cacpacity with restoration of continence occurs in some patients.

Neurologic Abnormalities

Treatment consists of combining planned regular defecation with use of constipating agents. To take advantage of the "gastrocolic reflex," patients should be seated on a commode after breakfast and encouraged to defecate. In many patients, evacuation can be effected and soiling minimized with this approach alone. If soiling persists, an approach that minimizes the frequency of defecation can be employed. Fecal volume is reduced through fiber restriction, and loperamide or diphenoxylate taken two to four times per day can minimize stool frequency. To prevent fecal impaction in patients who require such an approach, a phosphate enema followed by bisacodyl suppositories can be administred once or twice each week.

Diarrhea

In a disorder such as irritable bowel syndrome that is characterized by low-volume diarrhea, fiber supplements may help to regulate bowel habits and improve continence. In cases where diarrhea is nonspecific, antidiarrheal agents are often effective. On the basis of recent studies, loperamide (up to 4 mg four times daily, as needed) appears to be more effective than diphenoxylate in achieving continence;[19] this may be due to its beneficial effect on continence mechanisms.[20] Codeine probably should not be used for long-term control because of its potentially addictive properties.

Constipation

Treatment begins with administration of hypertonic enemas once or twice daily until there is no fecal return. Neglecting to completely evacuate the colon with repeated enemas is the most frequent reason for treatment failure. If the fecal impaction is hard and cannot be evacuated with simple enemas, a mineral oil enema should be administered to soften the stool. Digital disimpaction is an unpleasant task that is rarely necessary.

Once evacuation is complete, preventive measures should be taken, especially if the patient remains relatively immobile.

Once or twice a week, a phosphate enema followed by bisacodyl suppositories will assure periodic colonic evacuation and prevent recurrence of the problem.

TREATMENT OF CHILDREN

Encopresis[21,22]

Because the vast majority of children with encopresis have constipation and overflow soiling, the key to initial management is colonic evacuation with laxatives or enemas. Enemas (4½ oz of phosphate solution in a disposable plastic squeeze bottle or 1 qt of warm water administered by bag drip) are administered twice daily for at least 3 days; occasionally, children must be hospitalized to accomplish this critical task.

After colonic evacuation, 1 or 2 tablespoons of lactulose (Chronulac) or mineral oil are given twice daily to produce one or two soft, formed stools per day. A bowel training program is also instituted: The child is instructed to sit on the toilet for 20 minutes after a selected meal (preferably breakfast) to take advantage of the gastrocolic reflex. A footstool should be used so that the child's legs are firmly supported. A calendar is kept to record patterns of defecation and soiling. The lactulose or mineral oil can be tapered 6 to 12 months after continence is established and eventually can be discontinued.

Office counseling is generally sufficient if individual or family problems are uncovered, but more formal psychotherapy may be necessary in some cases. Encopresis without constipation or fecal impaction responds poorly to treatment and suggests the presence of severe underlying psychopathic factors.[23]

Spina Bifida

With good bowel programs, megarectum, megacolon, and fecal impactions can be avoided and satisfactory continence can often be achieved. Toilet training should be started at age 2 or 3 years by placing the child on a commode 20 to 30 minutes after a meal. Rectal evacuation can be aided by manually increasing abdominal pressure or by Valsalva's maneuver. Insertion of a glycerin suppository shortly after the child eats may promote defecation. If results from such measures are unsatisfactory, a 2¼ oz disposable phosphate enema can be administered 30 minutes after meals to evacuate the distal colon.

In some patients, successful toilet training cannot be accomplished or diarrhea is a problem. A constipating diet low in fiber and lactose (in lactose-intolerant children), supplemented by loperamide or diphenoxylate to reduce stool frequency, may be helpful. Phosphate or warm water enemas once or twice a week will prevent fecal impaction. Laxatives and cathartics should be avoided, and Colace is not helpful.

Some children with spina bifida have been successfully treated with biofeedback techniques in which gluteal muscle contraction substitutes for the external sphincter.[24] Although only a few children are eligible, a successful outcome can be gratifying in terms of independence and control over a bodily function. Potential candidates should be strongly motivated and able to learn, capable of standing or ambulating without full leg braces, and have normal rectal sensation by objective testing.[25] An average of four to six reinforcement sessions at 2-week intervals is required, unlike biofeedback training in adult patients.

Imperforate Anus

Treatment approaches will differ according to the specific abnormalities present. Biofeedback may be effective for external sphincter dysfunction alone; anal dilation, bowel cleansing, and bowel training as previously detailed are effective if constipation and impaction are present. Decreased rectal compliance or capacity is difficult to correct surgically. Measures to reduce stool volume combined with constipating drugs and weekly or twice weekly enemas may be employed in such patients.

SUMMARY

Management of the patient with fecal soiling begins with a careful evaluation of possible contributing factors, followed by anorectal examination, neurologic and psychosocial testing, and workup for chronic diarrhea, if present. These procedures can be supplemented by radiologic and manometric studies to determine if structural or functional anorectal abnormalities are present. Therapeutic approaches include behavioral, pharmacologic, and surgical methods, which should be carefully considered in relation to the underlying cause of incontinence. Therapy can be gratifyingly effective and can dramatically improve the quality of life of many patients with fecal soiling.

Acknowledgment

The author thanks Pamela Simmons and Virginia Hunt for their expert assistance in the preparation of this manuscript.

References

1. Whitehead WE, Schuster MM: Anorectal physiology and pathophysiology. *Am J Gastroenterol* 1987; 82:487–497.
2. Henriksen FW, Anthonisen B: Measurement of the anal sphincter strength by a simple method suitable for routine use. *Scand J Gastroenterol* 1972; 7:555–558.
3. Dickinson VA: Maintenance of anal continence: A review of pelvic floor physiology. *Gut* 1978; 19:1163–1174.
4. Arhan P, Faverdin C, Persoz B, et al: Relationship between viscoelastic properties of the rectum and anal pressure in man. *J Appl Physiol* 1976; 41:677–682.
5. Henry MM, Parks AG, Swash M: The pelvic floor musculature in the descending perineum syndrome. *Br J Surg* 1982; 69:470–472.
6. Feldman M, Schiller LR: Disorders of gastrointestinal motility associated with diabetes mellitus. *Ann Intern Med* 1983; 98:378–384.
7. Schiller LR, Santa Ana CA, Schmulen AC, et al: Pathogenesis of fecal incontinence in diabetes mellitus: Evidence for internal-anal-sphincter dysfunction. *N Engl J Med* 1982; 307:1666–1671.
8. Wald A, Tunuguntla AK: Anorectal sensorimotor dysfunction in fecal incontinence and diabetes mellitus. *N Engl J Med* 1984; 310:1282–1287.
9. Touchais J-Y, Paillot B, Denis P, et al: Severe rectal urgency and fecal incontinence following pelvic irradiation. *Gastroenterol Clin Biol* 1982; 6:1003–1007.
10. Devroede G, Vobecky S, Masse S, et al: Ischemic fecal incontinence and rectal angina. *Gastroenterology* 1982; 83:970–980.
11. Brocklehurst JC: Management of anal incontinence. *Clin Gastroenterol* 1975; 4:479–487.
12. Wald A, Handen BL: Behavioral aspects of disorders of defecation and fecal continence. *Ann Behavioral Med* 1987; 9:19–23.
13. Wald A, Chandra R, Gabel S, et al: Anorectal function and continence mechanisms in childhood encopresis. *J Pediatr Gastroenterol Nutr* 1986; 5:346–351.
14. Keighley MRB, Fielding JWL: Management of fecal incontinence and results of surgical treatment. *Br J Surg* 1983; 70:463–468.
15. Wald A: Biofeedback therapy for fecal incontinence. *Ann Intern Med* 1981; 95:146–149.
16. Wald A: Fecal incontinence: Effective nonsurgical treatments. *Postgrad Med* 1986; 80:123–130.
17. Cerulli MA, Nikoomanesh P, Schuster MM: Progress in biofeedback conditioning for fecal incontinence. *Gastroenterology* 1979; 76:742–746.
18. MacLeod JH: Management of anal incontinence by biofeedback. *Gastroenterology* 1987; 93:291–294.
19. Palmer KR, Corbett CL, Holdsworth CD: Double-blind cross-over study comparing loperamide, codeine and diphenoxylate in the treatment of chronic diarrhea. *Gastroenterology* 1980; 79:1272–1275.
20. Read M, Read NW, Barber DC, et al: Effects of loperamide on anal sphincter function in patients complaining of chronic diarrhea with fecal incontinence and urgency. *Dig Dis Sci* 1982; 27:807–814.
21. Levine MD, Bakow H: Children with encopresis: A study of treatment outcome. *Pediatrics* 1976; 58:845–852.
22. Lowery SP, Srour JW, Whitehead WE, et al: Habit training as treatment of encopresis secondary to chronic constipation. *J Pediatr Gastroenterol Nutr* 1985; 4:397–401.
23. Wald A: Incontinence, in Bayless TM (ed): *Current Therapy in Gastroenterology and Liver Disease—2*, Toronto, Decker Inc, 1986, pp 307–310.
24. Wald A: Use of biofeedback in the treatment of fecal incontinence in patients with meningomyelocele. *Pediatrics* 1981; 68:45–49.
25. Wald A: Biofeedback for neurogenic fecal incontinence: Rectal sensation is a determinant of outcome. *J Pediatr Gastroenterol Nutr* 1983; 2:302–306.

31

Ischemic Bowel:
How often is it misdiagnosed?

LAWRENCE J. BRANDT, M.D., F.A.C.G.

The term "ischemia," when applied to the gastrointestinal tract, connotes more than just a reduction in blood flow. Ischemia is actually a spectrum of disorders, each with its own presentation and natural history and each requiring its own plan of management—albeit with overlap between types of ischemic injury. Injury may be acute or chronic and involve part or all of the small and/or large bowel. In addition, the clinical presentation of ischemia may be catastrophic, gradual, delayed, or even recurrent. In this section we will concentrate on several frequently asked questions about the diagnosis and management of the spectrum of ischemic disorders; among these questions are:
1. How does one distinguish between patients with ischemia of the small bowel and patients with colonic ischemia? (Table 31–1)
2. What is the role of angiography in the diagnosis of acute mesenteric ischemia and colonic ischemia? (Fig 31–1)
3. How does one make the diagnosis of intestinal angina?

A practical approach to the diagnosis and management of ischemic bowel disorders considers four broad categories of disease; in three there is a single episode of acute ischemia, and in the fourth, chronic mesenteric ischemia, there are multiple recurrent attacks:
1. Acute mesenteric ischemia—acute ischemia of major portions of the small intestine with or without involvement of the colon
2. Focal mesenteric ischemia—acute ischemia of localized segments of small intestine
3. Colonic ischemia—acute ischemia involving only the colon
4. Chronic mesenteric ischemia—ischemia of small and large bowel but without loss of tissue viability

ACUTE MESENTERIC ISCHEMIA

Acute mesenteric ischemia is far more common than is chronic mesenteric ischemia and may be caused by a superior mesenteric artery embolus or thrombus, nonocclusive mesenteric ischemia ("low-flow" syndrome with vasoconstriction), or mesenteric venous thrombosis. Superior mesenteric artery embolus is the most common cause of acute mesenteric ischemia today and accounts for approximately 50% of cases. Nonocclusive mesenteric ischemia, which previously was more common, is being reported less often today. This reduction in frequency is probably because of better monitoring in intensive care units with correction of hemodynamic abnormalities before hypotension occurs and the more widespread use of systemic unloading (vasodilating) agents in the management of congestive heart failure and myocardial ischemia. Regardless of its cause, acute mesenteric

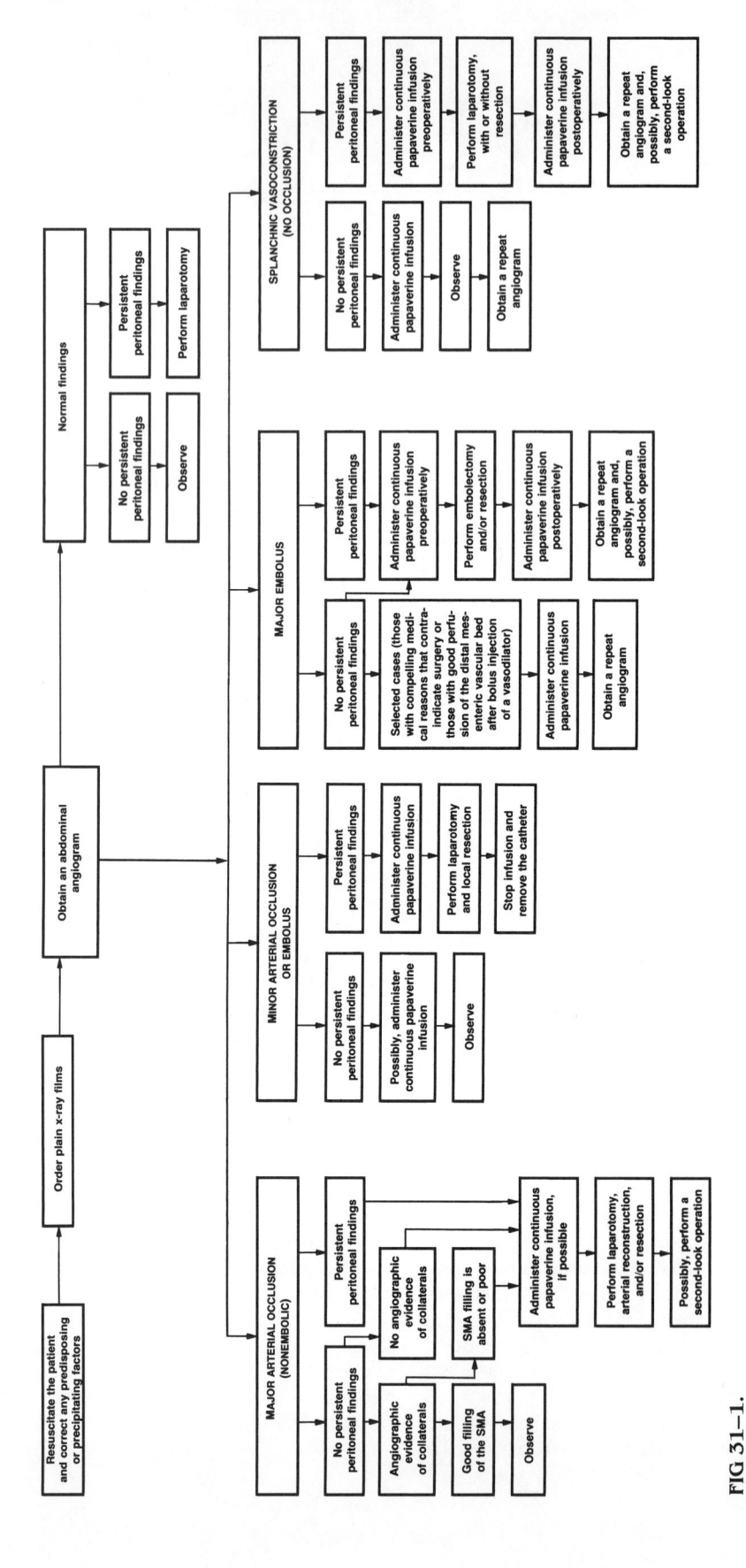

FIG 31–1.
Managing acute mesenteric ischemia based on the angiographic findings.

TABLE 31–1.
Differential Diagnosis of Acute Mesenteric Ischemia and Colonic Ischemia

Acute Mesenteric Ischemia	Colonic Ischemia
Older >> younger patients	90% in patients over 60 years of age
Acute precipitating cause usual (e.g., myocardial infarction, congestive heart failure, cardiac arrhythmias, hypotensive episodes)	Acute precipitating cause rare
Predisposing lesion uncommon (excluding atherosclerosis)	Predisposing associated lesion present in 20% (e.g., colonic carcinoma, stricture, diverticulitis, fecal impaction)
Usually appear ill	Do not appear seriously ill
Pain more severe; abdominal findings are minimal early in course but become pronounced later	Usually have mild abdominal pain with minimal tenderness and guarding
Rectal bleeding and diarrhea uncommon until late in the course	Moderate rectal bleeding or bloody diarrhea
Should have angiography first	Should have barium enema or colonoscopy first

ischemia is an intra-abdominal catastrophe as lethal today as 50 years ago, with an average mortality of 70% to 80%. In 1973, Boley and colleagues[1] proposed an aggressive plan of managment calling for earlier and more extensive use of angiography and the intra-arterial infusion of papaverine to interrupt splanchnic vasoconstriction. This is the only management plan that has resulted in an impressive improvement in survival and salvage of compromised bowel.

Early diagnosis depends on two important points.

1. *Recognition of patients at risk.* Patients at risk are usually older than 50 years of age, with congestive heart failure, cardiac arrhythmias, recent myocardial infarction, hypovolemia, hypotension, or sepsis. Attempts to acutely digitalize these patients may play an adjunctive etiologic role, because digitalis is a potent splanchnic vasoconstrictor.
2. *Recognition that a characteristic of early acute mesenteric ischemia is a disparity between the severity of the abdominal pain and the paucity of significant abdominal findings.* Acute mesenteric ischemia is a painful syndrome although the pain may vary in severity and location. The severity of pain helps to differentiate acute mesenteric ischemia from colonic ischemia in which pain is a much less impressive symptom (Table 31–1). It cannot be overstated how important it is to recognize that the combination of severe abdominal pain and a paucity of significant abdominal findings in a patient "at risk" demands that acute mesenteric ischemia be excluded. Reluctance to undertake early angiography in these often critically ill patients is the primary cause of continuing high mortality. Improved survival will only come when it is recognized that the dangers of waiting for definite physical signs (the "acute abdomen") or roentgenologic signs of ischemia (ileus, thumbprinting, free or intramural air) outweigh the risks of early invasive studies in patients in whom acute mesenteric ischemia is a real possibility.

Abdominal pain may be absent in 15% to 25% of patients; especially those with nonocclusive mesenteric ischemia. Unexplained abdominal distention or gastrointestinal bleeding may be the only indication of acute intestinal ischemia, and distention may be the first sign of impending intestinal infarction. As infarction develops, increasing tenderness, rebound tenderness, and muscle guarding become more prominent. Significant abdominal findings are strong evidence for the presence of nonviable bowel. Nausea, vomiting, fever, rectal bleeding, hematemesis, intestinal obstruction, back pain, shock, and increasing abdominal distention are other late signs.

Leukocytosis above 15,000 cells/mm^3 occurs in approximately 75% of patients with acute mesenteric ischemia, and a metabolic acidosis with increased base deficit is present in about 50%. Elevations in serum and peritoneal fluid amylase, alkaline phosphatase, and inorganic phosphates have been reported, but the consistency and specificity of these findings have not been established. Leukocytosis, especially if out of proportion to the physical findings, an elevated hematocrit, and blood-tinged peritoneal fluid, often with a high amylase content, are signs of advanced intestinal necrosis.

The initial treatment of any patient at risk suspected of having acute mesenteric ischemia is to correct predisposing or precipitating causes. Relief of acute congestive heart failure, correction of cardiac arrhythmias, and replacement of blood volume precede any diagnostic studies. In general, efforts at increasing intestinal blood flow will be futile if low cardiac output, hypotension, or hypovolemia persists. Patients who are hypotensive, hypovolemic, or in shock should *not* have angiography because mesenteric vasoconstriction always will be evident—even without intestinal ischemia. Such patients should *not* receive papaverine intra-arterially because this will increase the size of the vascular bed and aggravate the hypovolemia.

The management of associated congestive heart failure or shock may be especially difficult because digitalis preparations have a direct vasoconstrictor action on superior mesenteric artery smooth muscle and are therefore to be avoided. Vasopressors are also contraindicated in the treatment of shock if mesenteric ischemia is suspected. A helpful development is increased use of systemic vasodilators in the therapy of congestive heart failure and myocardial infarction. These drugs (e.g., hydralazine, prazosin, nitroglycerin, and nitroprusside) reduce arterial impedance by diminishing preload and/or afterload and theoretically are ideal agents to treat low mesenteric flow syndromes associated with congestive failure.

When intestinal ischemia has progressed to the extent that systemic alterations are present, correction of plasma volume deficits, gastrointestinal decompression, and parenteral antibiotics are essential *before* any roentgenologic studies. After these initial measures, roentgenologic studies are undertaken irrespective of the abdominal physical findings or the surgeon's decision whether to operate.

Plain film examination of the abdomen is performed to exclude other diagnosable causes of abdominal pain (e.g., a perforated viscus or intestinal obstruction). Another important axiom for the successful management of these patients is that *a normal plain film does not exclude a diagnosis of acute mesenteric ischemia.* Indeed, in patients suspected of having acute mesenteric ischemia, the combination of severe abdominal pain lasting several hours, an unimpressive abdominal examination, and a normal plain film of the abdomen denotes to our group precisely the kind of patient who is a prime candidate for angiography—for this is the patient with acute mesenteric ischemia who will not have infarcted bowel and who will therefore probably survive! Signs of intestinal ischemia on plain film studies occur late and usually indicate bowel infarction. If the plain films do not reveal another cause for the pain, angiography is performed.

Emergency angiography is the keystone of our aggressive approach (Fig 31–1). Even when the decision to operate has been made, an angiogram must be obtained to manage the patient properly at operation. Emboli, thrombosis, and mesenteric vasoconstriction can be diagnosed, and the adequacy of the splanchnic circulation can be evaluated; the angiographic catheter also provides a route for the administration of intra-arterial vasodilators. Relief of mesenteric vasoconstriction is an integral part of the therapy for emboli and thromboses, as well as for "low flow" states, and can best be achieved by intra-arterial infusion of papaverine through the angiography catheter.

The use of anticoagulants in the management of acute mesenteric ischemia is controversial. We do not use heparin in the perioperative period, except with venous thrombosis, because of the danger of intestinal hemorrhage. Because of the occurrence of thromboses late in the postoperative period, we start anticoagulation 48 hours postoperatively following embolectomy or arterial reconstruction.

Laparotomy is indicated to restore intestinal arterial flow (i.e., after an embolus or thrombosis) or to resect irreparably damaged bowel. There is no proven reliable objective means of determining the viability of ischemic intestine, especially early in the course of ischemia when the mucosa and submucosa are injured and serosal blood flow is preserved. Nonetheless, despite advancing technology, clinical assessments of the color of the bowel and the presence of pulsations, bleeding and peristalsis remain the inexact criteria on which judgment of viability usually is made. If there is any question of the viability of any remaining intestine, a planned reexploration or "second-look" is performed within 12 to 24 hours.

Although mortalities of 70% to 90% have been reported through 1979 using conventional methods, the aggressive approach can reduce these catastrophic figures.[2] Of the first 50 patients so managed, 35 (70%) proved to have acute mesenteric ischemia, and 19 of these (54%) survived. Eighty-five percent of the survivors did not lose any bowel or had excision of less than 3 ft of small intestine, thus enabling relatively normal bowel function. Similar results have been reported by the group at the University of Cincinnati using our aggressive approach.[2a]

In another study of 47 patients with intestinal ischemia resulting from superior mesenteric artery emboli, the survival rate was 55% in patients managed according to an aggressive protocol, whereas only 20% of those treated by traditional methods survived.[3]

Complications of angiographic studies and prolonged infusions of vasodilator drugs have not been excessive. Three of our first 50 patients developed transient acute tubular necrosis. There were several instances of local hematomas at the arterial puncture site. Problems with prolonged papaverine infusions have been minimal.

COLONIC ISCHEMIA

Ischemia of the colon is the most common vascular disorder of the intestines. It presents in one of several fashions including reversible colonic ischemia (33%), transient ischemic colitis (16%), chronic ischemic colitis (21%), colonic stricture (12%), and gangrene (18%).[4]

The most important initial clinical problem in managing a patient with colonic ischemia is to differentiate it from acute mesenteric ischemia. This is mandatory because the approach to management and the prognosis of patients with these two disorders are very different (Table 31–1). As reviewed before, patients with acute mesenteric ischemia usually present with severe abdominal pain associated with certain predisposing clinical situations (e.g., congestive heart failure, cardiac arrhythmias, and hypovolemia). Successful management is based on recognition of the disparity between the severity of the abdominal pain and the paucity of abdominal findings; prompt angiography (with or without intra-arterial papaverine) is indicated—even if surgery is contemplated—if no other cause for the pain is found on plain film study of the abdomen.

In contradistinction to acute mesenteric ischemia, patients with colonic ischemia are usually *not* ill, abdominal pain is typically mild, prognosis is excellent in at least one half of instances, and diagnosis is supported by barium enema or colonoscopy; mesenteric angiography plays *little* role in diagnosis and management.

In most cases of colonic ischemia, no specific etiology or vascular occlusion is identified. The greater frequency of colonic ischemia in the elderly does suggest a relationship to degenerative changes in the vascular tree, although angiography only rarely has demonstrated a significant occlusion or abnormality. What finally triggers the ischemic episode is still conjectural, but the combination of a normally low blood flow and further diminution during functional activity would seem to make the colon uniquely susceptible to ischemic injury. One possible etiologic factor in some cases of colonic ischemia is a distal colonic lesion, which in about half the cases is a carcinoma and in the others is a variety of entities including diverticulitis, stricture, and fecal impaction. Such a potentially obstructing lesion could theoretically decrease the colon circulation in the small mucosal and submucosal vessels of the proximal colon, thus rendering it ischemic.

Typically, colonic ischemia presents with the sudden onset of mild lower abdominal crampy pain, usually localized to the left side. The pain is frequently accompanied by or followed within 24 hours by bloody diarrhea or bright red blood per rectum. With irreversible transmural necrosis or accompanying small bowel involvement, the pain may be quite severe. Characteristically, blood loss is minimal; massive bleeding militates against a diagnosis of colonic ischemia.

Initially, the only physical finding is mild abdominal tenderness of the involved left colon. Signs of peritoneal irritation have been noted with ultimately reversible lesions, but if these persist for more than a few hours, they should be considered evidence of irreparable tissue damage.

If acute mesenteric ischemia is not believed to be present, the elderly patient with sudden abdominal pain and rectal bleeding or bloody diarrhea should have a "gentle" barium enema or colonoscopy within 48 hours. However, distending the colon, either by barium or gas, when it has suffered a vascular insult may theoretically worsen an ischemic injury. This is because increasing intraluminal pressure beyond 30 mm Hg diminishes intestinal blood flow, especially to the mucosa. At pressures greater than 30 mm Hg, which routinely are generated during barium enema examination and colonoscopy, there is a progressive reduction in the arteriovenous oxygen difference and a shunting of blood away from the mucosa to the serosa, thus increasing the risk of ischemia. We have tried to minimize this problem by using carbon dioxide rather than room air to inflate the colon during these diagnostic studies. Carbon dioxide is rapidly absorbed from the colon thus leading to a more comfortable examination with shorter periods of distention. Because distention is less prolonged, colonic blood flow is less compromised. Carbon dioxide, because of its vasodilating effects, actually increases colonic blood flow at the lower range of intracolonic pressures studied and therefore is probably a safer agent with which to insufflate the colon, especially in elderly patients with suspected or proven colonic ischemia.[5]

Conventional or rigid sigmoidoscopy is of value only if the segment of involved bowel is within reach of the sigmoidoscope and the typical submucosal hemorrhages of colonic ischemia are present. Colonic ischemia involves the sigmoid in approximately 50% to 60% of instances and the rectum in less than 10% of cases.[6] Depending on the stage at which sigmoidoscopy or colonoscopy is performed, findings vary greatly. Thus, during a bout of acute colonic ischemia, purplish blebs representing mucosal and submucosal hemorrhage may be seen. As the hemorrhage is resorbed, signaling the healing phase of the process, varying degrees of necrosis, inflammation, ulceration, and mucosal sloughing occur; patients seen in this phase of disease are frequently given an incorrect diagnosis of ulcerative colitis or Crohn's disease. Nonspecific inflammatory changes neither establish nor exclude an antecedent ischemic episode. Characteristic of colonic ischemia is the sequential spontaneous changes which typically evolve over an interval of 10 to 14 days; from submucosal hemorrhage to "colitis" and finally normal mucosa.

The so-called thumbprints, or pseudotumors, which disappear on serial studies, are the major criterion of ischemia on roentgenologic diagnosis. Thumbprints represent submucosal hemorrhage and are present only in the acute stage of colonic ischemia. A barium enema repeated 1 week after the initial study should reflect the evolution of the ischemic injury. Either the hemorrhages are resorbed and the study returns to normal, or the thumbprints are replaced by a segmental colitis pattern as the mucosa ulcerates.

Colonic ischemia is almost always a single event. Only 5% of patients experience recurrent episodes. The usual episode of colonic ischemia resolves spontaneously and completely in about half of the patients. The other half can be divided into three roughly equal groups: patients who present with gangrene and perforation, patients with chronic colitis, and those who present weeks to months later because of a colonic stricture. In mild cases, symptoms and signs usually subside in 24 to 48 hours, and complete clinical and roentgenologic healing occurs within 1 to 2 weeks. In more severe ischemia, areas of mucosa may slough with complete healing over 1 to 6 months. Patients with a prolonged course may be clinically well even in the presence of persistent enema changes.

Irreversible lesions may become obvious in hours when gangrene or perforation occurs or may follow a protracted course when chronic colitis or stricture develops. The diagnosis of colonic infarction is made on the basis of abdominal tenderness, guarding, rebound tenderness, a rising fever, leukocytosis, and evidence of paralytic ileus. These signs, not specific for infarction, dictate the need for emergency laparotomy.

Treatment of acute colonic ischemia is based on early diagnosis and continued monitoring of both the patient and the roentgenologic or colonoscopic appearance of the colon. Systemic antibiotics are administered when indicated, and blood and fluid loss is corrected as necessary. It is best to place the bowel at rest and provide fluids intravenously. Contrary to their efficacy in idiopathic ulcerative colitis, corticosteroids are of no proven value. Serial barium studies or colonoscopies are essential: they establish the diagnosis definitively, verify the reversibility of the colonic damage, or demonstrate progression to an ischemic colitis or stricture. If deterioration in the clinical course is suggested by increasing abdominal signs, fever, and leukocytosis, or if the diarrhea, bleeding, or both persist for more than 2 weeks, irreversible damage almost certainly has occurred and surgical intervention is indicated. Operative treatment consists of local resection with primary anastomosis.

CHRONIC MESENTERIC ISCHEMIA (ABDOMINAL ANGINA, INTESTINAL ANGINA)

Patients with chronic mesenteric ischemia experience recurrent acute episodes of insufficient blood flow during periods of maximal gastrointestinal work. The pain is analogous to that arising in the myocardium with angina pectoris or in the calf muscles with intermittent claudication. Intestinal angina is almost always caused by atherosclerosis of the splanchnic vessels. The consistent feature is abdominal discomfort or pain. Most commonly pain occurs 10 to 15 minutes after eating, gradually increases in severity, reaches a plateau, and then slowly abates in 1 to 3 hours. The pain most often is crampy, located in the upper abdomen, and may radiate from the epigastrium through to the back. Some patients find it can be relieved by squatting or assuming a prone position. Initially, the pain occurs only after a large meal, but characteristically the pain pattern progresses such that the patient will reduce the size of his meals ("small meal syndrome") and become reluctant to eat. Weight loss is characteristic and often severe. Bloating, flatulence, and abnormal motility with constipation or diarrhea are also seen. Intermittent episodes of vomiting occur less commonly. Steatorrheic stools are observed by half of the patients. Physical findings are limited and nonspecific. A systolic bruit is heard in the upper abdomen in approximately one half of the patients, but similar bruits have been reported in up to 15% of healthy patients and are *not* diagnostic.

There is no specific or reliable diagnostic test for abdominal angina. The diagnosis is based on the typical clinical symptoms, the arteriographic demonstration of an occlusive process of the splanchnic arteries, and exclusion of other gastrointestinal disease. Conventional roentgenologic examinations of the gastrointestinal tract usually are unremarkable. Angiographic demonstration of stenoses or occlusions of one, two, or even all of the major vessels does *not* by itself establish the diagnosis of arterial insufficiency or intestinal angina.

Three means of attempting to make a definitive diagnosis of intestinal angina are:

1. The provocative D-xylose test in which the urinary excretion and hence the absorption of orally administered D-xylose is measured before and after a meal. Interference with absorption of the sugar implies a fixed or diminished intestinal blood supply to the intestine and possibly suggests a "steal" syndrome. Clinical experience with this test is needed before its use can be widely recommended.
2. A rather demanding method of assessing the adequacy of splanchnic blood flow has been described by Hansen and co-workers.[7] Splanchnic blood flow is defined as the total blood flow through the three splanchnic arteries and extrasplanchnic collaterals. It is determined by measuring hepatic venous blood flow with indocyanin-green, both in the fasting state and after a standard meal. Oxygen consumption in the splanchnic bed is also measured. In their study of 15 patients with abdominal pain, there was a significant failure of patients with abdominal angina to increase their splanchnic blood flow after the test meal. After arterial reconstruction, the postprandial increase was similar to that in the control group. This technique involves catheterization of the radial artery, an arm vein, and a hepatic vein. In spite of the technical expertise needed to perform these studies, if the observations of Hansen and co-workers are corrobrated, this method will provide objective means for determining the need for operation.
3. Recently, tonometry has been applied to studying the problem of intestinal angina in a canine experimental model.[8] Tonometry is a new technique by which intestinal blood flow can be measured indirectly. By measuring the bicarbonate concentration in a specimen of arterial blood and the partial pressure of carbon dioxide in fluid placed within a semipermeable balloon in the lumen of the bowel, the intramural pH of the bowel can be calculated using the Henderson-Hasselbalch equation. The intramural pH is a metabolic marker of the adequacy of oxygenation and hence blood supply in the bowel. Using this technique, a decrease in the intestinal intramural pH was seen when, in the presence of a partially obstructed celiac and superior mesenteric artery, cream was placed in the stomach of the experimental animal; this suggested that a hemodynamic "steal" of blood from the intestine to the stomach was prompted by the food in the stomach. Much more experience with this technique is needed.

In the past, treatment of intestinal angina was some form of operative arterial reconstruction. Today, transluminal angioplasty may afford an alternative approach of lesser magnitude and risk. A patient with classic abdominal angina and unexplained weight loss whose diagnostic evaluation has excluded other gastrointestinal disease and whose angiogram shows occlusive involvement of at least two of the three major arteries should be treated. The issue has been much less clear if only one major vessel is involved.

References

1. Boley SJ, Sprayregen S, Veith FJ, et al: An aggressive roentgenologic and surgical approach to acute mesenteric ischemia, in Nyhus LM (ed): *Surgery Annual*. New York, Appleton-Century-Crofts, 1973, p 355.
2. Boley SJ, Sprayregen S, Siegleman SS, et al: Initial results from an aggressive roentgenological and

surgical approach to acute mesenteric ischemia. *Surgery* 1977; 82:848–855.
2a. Clark RA and Gallant TE: Acute mesenteric ischemia: Angiographic spectrum. AJR 1984; 3:555–562.
3. Boley SJ, Feinstein FR, Sammartano R, et al: New concepts in the management of emboli of the superior mesenteric artery. *Surg Gynecol Obstet* 1981; 153:561–569.
4. Brandt LJ: *Gastrointestinal Disorders of the Elderly*. New York, Raven Press, 1984.
5. Brandt LJ, Boley SJ, Sammartano R: Carbon dioxide and room air insufflation of the colon: Effects on colonic blood flow and intraluminal pressure in the dog. *Gastrointest Endosc* 1986; 32:324–329.
6. Boley SJ, Brandt LJ, Veith FJ: Ischemic disorders of the intestines. *Curr Probl Surg* 1978; 15:1–85.
7. Hansen HJB, Engell HC, Ring-Larsen H, et al: Splanchnic blood flow in patients with abdominal angina before and after arterial reconstruction. *Ann Surg* 1977; 186:216–220.
8. Poole JW, Sammartano R, Boley SJ: Hemodynamic basis of the pain of chronic mesenteric ischemia. *Am J Surg* 1987; 153:171–176.

32

Ulcerative Proctitis:
Tractable or intractable?

RICHARD G. FARMER, M.D., F.A.C.P.

Ulcerative proctitis is encountered, with relative frequency, by gastroenterologists, digestive disease surgeons, internists, and family practitioners. The major reasons for referral, and thus for consultation by a gastroenterologist or other specialist are (1) accuracy of diagnosis, (2) concern over clinical significance and prognosis, (3) fear of cancer, and (4) by far the most common, failure to respond to medical therapy. However, the "failure to respond" is often relative because patients may have only rectal bleeding (i.e., no diarrhea, abdominal pain, weight loss, fever etc.) and the anxiety caused by this alarming symptom may be a dominant clinical feature. If the physician then implies that it is somehow the "fault" of the patient (usually by invoking some stress-related issue), the effect can be to intensify the symptoms rather than alleviating them. On the other hand, trivializing the symptoms will be viewed as illogical because patients are well aware that rectal bleeding is an abnormal situation. Thus, dealing with a patient who has well-established and recurrent ulcerative proctitis for which much treatment has already been given can be a true dilemma for the consultant. As with most conditions treated by physicians and endured by patients, an understanding of ulcerative proctitis will be of benefit in approaching the clinical problem as intelligently and as objectively as possible.

HISTORICAL PERSPECTIVE

Proctitis, inflammation of the rectal mucosa, is a descriptive term encompassing a group of conditions that may be difficult to categorize. The hallmark symptom of proctitis is rectal bleeding, frequently alarming to the patient, but often unassociated with other symptoms and often self-limited.

The major clinical emphasis over the past 50 years has been the relationship of proctitis to inflammatory bowel disease, particularly ulcerative colitis. Even this, however, has not been universally accepted; although, the statement made by Lennard-Jones and co-workers[1] that "proctitis represents a real form of proctocolitis" generally has been considered true. In one of the first large studies on proctitis by Thaysen,[2] the term "simple" proctitis was used, implying that it was different from ulcerative colitis because of the better prognosis. In 1966 we[3] used the term "ulcerative proctitis" to emphasize the relationship to ulcerative colitis (Lennard-Jones and co-workers had used the term "idiopathic" proctitis"[1]). Subsequent to this, it became recognized that the inflammation could involve the rectosigmoid rather than the rectal mucosa only, and the term proctosigmoiditis became more commonly used.[4,5]

Although ulcerative proctitis represents an idiopathic condition that is treated empirically, "specific" causes of proctitis do exist and the physician must be aware of them. There has been a greatly increasing interest and knowledge in "specific" causes of proctitis in recent years, and, with the marked increase in incidence of Crohn's disease in the past 20 years,[6, 7] the relationship of this disease to proctitis has also attracted considerable attention. The rapid increase in incidence of Crohn's disease now appears to have reached a plateau, and the incidence of ulcerative colitis has remained relatively stable.[6] An important aspect is that the frequency of proctitis or proctosigmoiditis (also called distal colon ulcerative colitis) has proportionately increased among the cases of ulcerative colitis observed. Thus, the clinical observation that among patients with inflammatory bowel disease, those with ulcerative colitis seem to have a "milder" clinical course than those patients with Crohn's disease relates primarily to the increasing number of cases of distal colon ulcerative colitis observed. Recent studies from Sweden,[8] Denmark,[9] and South Africa[10] showed percentages of proctitis among patients with ulcerative colitis to range from about 25% to 50% of the entire group of patients. In the large study by Nordenvall and co-workers,[8] there were 1,274 total cases with 25% of patients having proctitis and 38% having left-sided colitis over a 25-year follow-up period. A study of patients with ulcerative colitis at London's St. Mark's hospital over a 10-year period found that 58%[11] had proctitis or proctosigmoiditis only. Thus, based on the clinical observations of groups from a variety of locations around the world over a 25-year period, these comments can be made: (1) ulcerative proctitis/proctosigmoiditis does not appear to be the "benign end of the spectrum" of ulcerative colitis, and (2) the relative incidence of localized distal form of the disease is increasing in relationship to the number of cases of ulcerative colitis observed in any one center (Table 32–1).

Another observation of clinical significance is that the age of onset of patients with ulcerative proctitis/proctosigmoiditis is generally older than those with inflammatory bowel disease; patients with proctosigmoiditis at the Cleveland Clinic were, on the average, 10 years older than patients with inflammatory bowel disease.[12] Although the disease can occur in children[13] and the peak age of onset is in the third decade of life,[6] there has been an increasing interest in the clinical characteristics of patients with "late onset" ulcerative colitis, typically as manifested by the distal colon form of the disease. Recent studies from England[14] and Israel,[15] while differing in their definition of "late onset," arrived at similar conclusions regarding the relative frequency of distal colon disease in older patients. In both studies, the potential for complications was much more likely in older patients than in younger patients with localized disease.

Other clinical features known to exist among patient groups with ulcerative colitis do not appear to be proportionally different among patients with proctitis or proctosigmoiditis. While the sex incidence is variable, overall there is a slight male preponderance.[6, 11, 12] An increasing fre-

TABLE 32–1.
Follow-up and Extension of Disease in Patients with Proctitis and Proctosigmoiditis

Authors	Year	Number of Patients	Follow-up (years)	Extended (%)
Lennard-Jones et al.[1]	1962	100	2–5	10
Farmer and Brown[3]	1966	51	6.5	10
Sparberg et al.[29]	1966	45	10±	10
Nugent et al.[4]	1970	234	10±	12
Powell-Tuck et al.[28]	1977	219	10	12
Ritchie et al.[11]	1978	76	11	5
Farmer[12]	1979	359	11	10
Mir-Madjlessi et al.[13]	1986	66	14.6	35

quency of observing the disease in more than one member of the same family has occurred,[7, 13] a relative preponderance among white populations has continued,[6, 9, 10] but data concerning the relative incidence among Jews are not entirely clear. In the well-defined racial mix of Cape Town, South Africa, the incidence among the Jewish population there was over three times that of the rest of the white population.[10]

The role of psychologic or psychosomatic factors in initiation and perpetuation of the inflammation has largely been discounted in recent years. In the past, the belief was that "emotional factors" played a role in a significant number of clinical situations. While, undoubtedly, anxiety and depression over persistence or recurrence of rectal bleeding and fear of cancer or complications may exist, the recent emphasis has been on infectious or "specific" causes of proctitis in the differential diagnosis rather than on emotional or psychosomatic aspects.

DIFFERENTIAL DIAGNOSIS: INFECTIOUS CAUSES (TABLE 32-2).

Infectious causes of proctitis have been increasingly recognized in recent years,[16] and much of this renewed interest relates to a marked increase of such infections among homosexual men.[17] Despite the increased awareness and the considerable publicity given to diseases associated with homosexuality, the most commonly encountered infectious causes of proctitis are *Campylobacter*, *Salmonella*, and *Shigella* organisms.[16] The rectum can be involved in cases of amebiasis as well as in *Yersinia* enterocolitis, but these are usually associated with more proximal involvement of the colonic mucosa.[16]

The symptoms of acute infectious proctitis include rectal pain, rectal bleeding, and tenesmus. In addition, there may be a flulike syndrome, although this is more common with viral gastroenteritis in which there is no specific rectal involvement.[16] The rectal mucosa of a patient with *Campylobacter* proctitis may bear a superficial resemblance to the mucosa of ulcerative proctitis, with granularity and friability; however, there is generally not the diffuse and uniform involvement found in ulcerative proctitis.[16] Both shigellosis and amebiasis have a more dramatic endoscopic picture with punched out, discrete lesions in amebiasis and acute ulceration with bleeding in shigellosis.[18] Salmonellosis and *Yersinia* enterocolitis generally friability and ulceration.[16]

There has been a marked increase in infectious proctitis in male homosexuals which is now considered a part of "gay bowel syndrome."[18] In addition to the organisms that can be found generally in patients with proctitis, giardiasis may be present in the enteritis-type of infection, although not usually present with only proctitis. However, the organisms that have created the most interest have been those not commonly found in the usual

TABLE 32-2.
Proctitis: Clinical Diagnosis and Differential Diagnosis

Diagnosis	Acute Onset	Rectal Bleeding	Rectal Pain	Tenesmus	Diarrhea	Mucosal Friability	Lesions
Ulcerative colitis	±	+ +	0	+	±	+ +	0
Crohn's disease	±	±	+	+	+ +	±	+ +
Campylobacter	+ +	+	0	+	+	+	0
Antibiotic associated	+ +	±	0	+	+ +	±	0
Herpes simplex	+ +	±	+ +	+ +	0	0	+ +
Chlamydia	+	+	+ +	+ +	+	0	+ +

0 = usually absent; ± = may be present; + = usually present; + + = prominent.

medical practice, either specifically related to venereal disease or organisms not frequently encountered generally. Included in the former are gonorrhea proctitis and herpes simplex proctitis, and included in the latter are organisms associated with lymphogranuloma venereum. Further, in cases of infectious proctitis associated with male homosexuality, more than one organism may be present.[16, 17]

Herpes simplex virus is associated with severe rectal pain and tenesmus, and the symptoms are more striking than those with proctitis associated with gonorrhea. Primary anorectal syphilis usually causes only mild symptoms. More recently recognized has been proctitis associated with lymphogranuloma venereum, and particularly *Chlamydia trachomatis*. In addition, *Cryptosporidia* have been found to be present in enteric infections but not typically associated with proctitis. In a study by Quinn,[18] the most commonly found organisms in homosexual men with proctitis were *Neisseria gonorrhoeae*, *Entamoeba histolytica*, herpes simplex virus, *Giardia lamblia*, *Chlamydia trachomatis*, and *Campylobacter jejuni*.

Proctitis is also found in antibiotic-associated diarrhea, also known as pseudomembranous colitis.[16] Although this condition has been known for many years, understanding of the syndrome has been greatly enhanced by the recognition that the cause is a toxin-producing strain of *Clostridium difficile*. While it is usually self-limited and responds to withdrawal of the antibiotic agent, at times the proctitis may be severe and may be associated with a pseudomembrane.[16] The visual appearance is more similar to Crohn's disease than ulcerative colitis, without the diffuse uniform granularity and friability associated with the latter.

DIFFERENTIAL DIAGNOSIS: CROHN'S DISEASE

Crohn's disease has been known to affect the distal large bowel only but typically has a different clinical picture than the proctitis associated with ulcerative colitis or with infectious agents. Ritchie and Lennard-Jones[19] reported the most frequent types of anal lesion encountered were external anal tags, perianal fistulae, anal fissures, perirectal abscesses, anal canal stenosis, and rectal mucosal ulceration. The clinical course and long-term prognosis for patients with anorectal Crohn's disease are usually different than for patients with other types of proctitis who may require operation. Crohn's disease of the distal large bowel typically is associated with external manifestations, including perirectal fistulae and abscesses, with relatively less involvement of the rectal mucosa itself. On the other hand, ulcerative proctitis affects the rectal mucosa itself, with diffuse and uniform granularity and friability, and without significant external lesions being present.

DIFFERENTIAL DIAGNOSIS: OTHER CAUSES OF PROCTITIS

As emphasized, proctitis is a descriptive term meaning inflammation of the rectal mucosa and thus can have many causes, including trauma, vasculitis, amyloidosis, and Behçet's syndrome.[16] Diverticulitis typically is not associated with acute proctitis or with mucosal abnormalities similar to that seen in other forms of proctitis. Ischemic proctitis may present with acute rectal bleeding and may mimic inflammatory bowel disease.[14] Radiation proctitis may also mimic idiopathic proctitis, but the typical history is that of pelvic radiation and the typical clinical picture is that of diarrhea and tenesmus. Patients who have undergone colonic diversion, usually a colostomy, and have had the fecal stream diverted may develop a form of acute rectal or colonic inflammation generally known as "diversion colitis."[20] This condition is usually found in patients who have undergone colostomy for a reason other than inflammatory bowel disease, usually cancer, and can generally be differentiated on this basis. The solitary rectal ulcer syndrome (localized colitis cystica profunda)[21] is usually seen in young people with only minor rectal bleeding and an endoscopic picture of a discrete and relatively nodular lesion.

PATHOLOGIC DIFFERENTIATION

While rectal biopsy is an obvious diagnostic tool which should be of great clinical significance, the relative nonspecificity of histologic findings has limited its value. Thus, in the assessment of a patient with proctitis, the clinical correlation with the anticipated histologic findings are important and relate particularly to the timing of the biopsy. While studies have shown value in the ability to differentiate inflammatory bowel disease from other forms of proctitis,[22] the differential diagnosis histologically of various causes of proctitis[21] and the lack of specific histologic characteristics have proved to be a problem for both clinicians and pathologists.

Surawicz and Belic[22] evaluated histologic features and applied statistical methods and predictive probability to their findings. The features with a high predictive probability (over 85%) of diagnosing, inflammatory bowel disease were distorted crypt architecture, increased number of round cells and neutrophils in the lamina propria, and villous changes on the surface, in addition to epithelioid granulomata, crypt atrophy, lymphoid aggregates, and isolated giant cells. They found that biopsy features of acute self-limited colitis were less diagnostic, including presence of edema, surface erosions, preservation of normal crypt architecture, acute inflammation in the lamina propria, and purulent exudate on the surface.

In a recent review by Rickert,[21] the importance of "imposters" was emphasized in the differential diagnosis of inflammatory bowel disease. Ischemia may create histologic findings similar to inflammatory bowel disease. Among the infectious diseases, Campylobacter "has proven to be the most frequently identified cause of acute infectious colitis" recognized in the laboratory. The biopsy appearance is characterized by mucosal edema, variable loss of surface epithelium, a sparse inflammatory infiltrate, and focal changes in the crypts. The lesions of amebiasis may mimic Crohn's disease more than ulcerative colitis, and the same is true of opportunistic infections associated with the acquired immune deficiency syndrome (AIDS). The characteristic lesion of antibiotic-associated colitis is a focal erosion of the surface epithelium covered by an adherent plaque of fibrinopurulent and mucoid exudate. Histologic changes in radiation proctitis are not specific and include patchy mucosal injury. Diversion-related proctitis is associated with focal patchy mucosal inflammation.

In the steadily increasing number of reports of intestinal infections and abnormalities among male homosexuals, a recent report has documented the spectrum of rectal biopsy abnormalities in homosexual men with and without intestinal symptoms.[23] In this study there were 5% who had biopsy features comparable to those seen in inflammatory bowel disease, and these patients were infected with *Treponema pallidum* or *Chlamydia trachomatis*. Although these histologic features were those of acute inflammation, chronic inflammatory changes do not occur and can further mimic inflammatory bowel disease.

DIAGNOSIS

The diagnosis of ulcerative proctitis/proctosigmoiditis relates primarily to the clinical history and the sigmoidoscopy findings. Virtually all patients have a history of bright red rectal bleeding, often without other symptoms and frequently without diarrhea, abdominal pain, tenesmus, weight loss, or other "systemic" features. Typically, the onset is gradual, and the patient (and sometimes the initial physician) ascribes the bleeding to hemorrhoids; however, anoscopic, proctoscopic, or sigmoidoscopic examination demonstrates diffuse and uniform mucosal friability with (usually) touch bleeding, edema, loss of vascular pattern, and a visual appearance usually described as "sandy" or "mossy" as a result of edema. There is usually a mucopurulent discharge and, almost invariably, the examiner can observe bright red blood. Characteristically, for patients with proctitis, the inflammatory lesion begins at the dentate line and extends proximal for about 15 cm or more. Beyond this there is a "clear upper limit" with visibly normal mucosa above. Emphasis has been placed on the importance of the "clear upper limit" in the past.[1,3,24] However, because with the use of the rigid sigmoidoscope it was not always possible to visualize the exact upper extent of inflammation and because the clinical behavior of the patients observed was similar, there has been a merging of the concepts of proctitis and proctosigmoiditis into a more general emphasis on inflammation in the distal colon.[4,5] We[12] observed 359 patients at the Cleveland Clinic from 1960 to 1972, with a 97% follow-up (mean of 11 years). There was male preponderance and mean age at diagnosis of 40 years (37 patients were over the age of 60 years at the time of original diagnosis). All patients had rectal bleeding as the primary symptom; none had significant abdominal pain, although tenesmus was occasionally noted. None had significant weight loss, and few other symptoms were present. None had significant perianal disease. All had typical sigmoidoscopic appearances, and all had normal barium enema examinations. None had significant anemia or hypoalbuminemia. The clinical features described were similar to those reported by Lennard-Jones et al.[1] and Nugent et al.[4]

Prior to the development of colonoscopy, exact definition of the extent of disease was difficult and even controversial. In recent years, with the use of colonoscopy and double contrast barium enema examination, there has been a much greater ability to define the extent of disease. Das and colleagues[25] performed a colonoscopy study in patients with idiopathic proctitis, with multiple mucosal biopsies from area of inflammation as well as from portions of the proximal colon. Although the visual inflammatory changes extended to approximately 18 to 20 cm proximal to the dentate line, mucosal biopsy abnormalities were frequently found in more proximal locations of the large bowel. We evaluated 100 consecutive patients with distal colon ulcerative colitis who underwent colonoscopy; two thirds of the patients were found to have mucosal abnormalities proximal to the rectosigmoid but not extending proximal to the splenic flexure.[26] Twelve patients had histologic abnormalities proximal to the splenic flexure, including three with total colonic involvement despite a clinical diagnosis of proctosigmoiditis. Therefore, we advocated fiberoptic endoscopy (colonoscopy, limited colonoscopy, or fiberoptic sigmoidoscopy) to determine the extent of disease (1) when no upper limit of inflammatory process was visualized on sigmoidoscopy; (2) when there was a questionable mucosal abnormality on barium enema; and (3) for a patient who has multiple recurrences of rectal bleeding and sigmoidoscopic findings of proctitis or proctosigmoiditis. Subsequent and current experience have indicated the value of fiberoptic endoscopic examination in patients with distal colon ulcerative colitis, particularly when following the patient over a long period of time.

The double contrast barium enema has also been effective in detection of mucosal abnormalities and determination of extent of disease. In a study by Williams and co-workers,[27] a comparison between double contrast barium enema examination and proctosigmoidoscopy found that endoscopy was more sensitive than double contrast examination in detection of disease of the distal colon and rectum, and neither examination misclassified a case of Crohn's disease as ulcerative colitis. Double contrast examination demonstrated disease proximal to the range of the proctosigmoidoscope of a greater severity than that seen endoscopically in 24% of their patients with ulcerative colitis. They concluded that double contrast examination and proctosigmoidoscopy are complementary, and both should be used in evaluating patients with inflammatory disease of the colon.

The histologic diagnosis of ulcerative proctitis/proctosigmoiditis can be difficult to differentiate from other types of proctitis.[21,22] In a biopsy study,[22] the following histologic features were found to be typical of the ulcerative colitis form of proctitis: distorted crypt architecture, villous surface abnormalities, surface erosions, crypt atrophy, lamina propria inflammation, and neutrophils in the surface epithelium. However, relatively few of these histologic features differentiated specifically ulcerative colitis from Crohn's disease, and the granuloma in Crohn's disease was, as one would expect, the most important differentiating feature. Thus, although the crypt abscess has been considered a major histologic feature of ulcerative colitis, this study[22] reemphasizes its nonspecificity and the difficulty in making a "specific" histologic diagnosis of proctitis.

CLINICAL COURSE

The clinical course of patients with ulcerative proctitis/proctosigmoiditis is characterized by remission and exacerbations.[1, 4, 12] Prediction of which patient might develop a relapse or recurrence (as well as prevention of them) has been one of the most difficult clinical problems encountered by physicians who treat such patients. It has been difficult to obtain "objective" evidence, for example, which relates to disease activity and correlation with symptoms. Powell-Tuck et al.[28] used the most obvious "objective" clinical feature, the appearance of the rectal mucosa visually, and cross-tabulated 225 observations of each of ten symptoms and signs with the sigmoidoscopic appearances in patients with ulcerative colitis. The visual appearance of the mucosa was graded as: nonhemorrhagic (grade 0), no bleeding spontaneously or on light touch; hemorrhagic (grade 1), bleeding on light touch, but no spontaneous bleeding seen ahead of the instrument; hemorrhagic (grade 2), spontaneous bleeding seen ahead of the instrument at initial inspection with bleeding on light touch. They concluded that "the subdivision of hemorrhagic mucosae into those which bleed spontaneously and those which bleed only on light touching or scraping is meaningful clinically."[28] Sigmoidoscopic appearances correlated better with clinical disease activity than histologic assessment, and no clinical variable predicted the extent of disease. The degree of mucosal inflammation correlated with the patient's sense of "well-being" judged by limitation of activities, bowel frequency, stool consistency, and these three symptoms combined with the sigmoidoscopic description gave a "good but simple measure" of disease severity for clinical assessment.[28] This has likewise been our clinical experience.[3, 12]

Following the initial diagnosis and treatment of the patient, the follow-up period is essential for determining extent, severity, and activity of disease, as well as dealing with relapses. Relapses are characterized by a recurrence of symptoms of proctitis with a return of rectal bleeding; this pattern may persist for many years.[1, 4] Thus, the determination of whether or not the disease has "resolved" becomes a function of the follow-up and duration of the period of observation of the patients. In our study,[12] we found that 70% of patients had complete resolution of symptoms after an 11-year follow-up.

Although extension of disease occurs in approximately 10% of patients,[1, 4, 12, 24, 29] severe complications, including toxic megacolon, are rare. Proctitis/proctosigmoiditis occurring in older patients may or may not have a more severe clinical course than other patients with distal colon ulcerative colitis. Among patients reported by Carr and Schofield,[14] there were no significant complications among those with proctitis and none required operation. In the study by Zimmerman and co-workers,[15] patients with proctosigmoiditis with onset beyond the age of 51 years had episodes which were "more protracted and the ensuing remission of shorter duration" than in patients with onset at a younger age. As both of these studies emphasize, it is the general health and other diseases present that correlate with the overall clinical problems encountered, a finding confirmed by our study.[12]

ULCERATIVE PROCTITIS IN CHILDREN

We recently reviewed our experience with ulcerative proctosigmoiditis with onset of symptoms before the age of 21 years.[13] There were 85 patients with a mean onset of symptoms at age 16 years. The clinical features that the time of diagnosis were similar to those in our experience generally.[12] Complications among this group of patients were significantly greater than observed in our previous studies in adults. Two groups of patients could be identified: in 62% of the patients the disease remained stable or did not extend during the follow-up period (mean of 14.6 years); 38% of patients had continuously active disease with subsequent extension despite initial localization to the distal colon. While rectal bleeding was present in all patients in both categories, diarrhea, anemia, joint symptoms, and skin lesions were more common in the continuously active disease group of patients. In addition, complications were much more common in the continuously active group of patients with acute intestinal bleeding in 9%, fulminant colitis in 8%, toxic megacolon in 6%, and operation necessary for 16%. While there were nine patients whose disease extended within 1 year following initial diagnosis (and who could have conceivably had extensive but undetectable disease initially), there was an extension rate of 28%, usually occurring within 5 years from the onset of symptoms. One patient developed rectal carcinoma; the disease had become extensive within 2 years from the onset of proctosigmoiditis, and total colitis was present at the time of colectomy.

In view of the different clinical course among children with proctosigmoiditis, one might speculate that etiologic factors other than those found in adults might be present. If so, allergic proctitis would likely be the most significant theoretical etiologic possibility, and this subject has been addressed recently with a review of 15 children with allergic proctitis.[30] However, the onset was at age 6 months or less and all were under the age of 2 years when they presented with rectal bleeding alone or in combination with diarrhea.[30] Rectal mucosal biopsy revealed a diffuse increase in eosinophils in the lamina propria associated with a focal infiltration of the epithelium by eosinophils. Thus, this report gives indirect support to our observation that proctosigmoiditis in children is a similar entity as that found in adults except with a more severe clinical course.[13]

The publication of our paper resulted in an editorial by Gryboski who reiterated the increased possibility of more severe disease and proximal extension, and noted that the disease will remain stable in only about a third of cases, and that if disease extension occurs it will do so within 5 years after initial diagnosis.[31] The editorial concluded that "the message (of our paper) is a clear one. The diagnosis of proctosigmoiditis is not secure, and children who have continued or increasing symptoms must be considered as having more proximal extension of their disease."[31]

TREATMENT

Treatment of ulcerative proctitis/proctosigmoiditis has been difficult for a number of reasons: (1) diagnostic uncertainty, particularly in comparison with self-limited forms of proctitis; (2) the empiric nature of the therapy, particularly so during the 30 years in which hydrocortisone enemas have been used[32]; (3) the spontaneous resolution of the bleeding at times with difficulty to correlate the clinical response and therapy; (4) the uncertainty as to the duration of therapy and the ability to suppress inflammation and prevent relapses; and (5) the considerable difficulty of controlled clinical trials with "objective" assessment comparison of one therapeutic modality versus another, or comparison of therapy versus placebo. Because of this, most therapeutic trials have been observational in nature, with various forms of therapy used and results subsequently ascertained. In addition to hydrocortisone enemas, the two most commonly used forms of therapy have been oral sulfasalazine and steroid suppositories; various forms of sulfa enemas and systemic steroids have also been used.

Following the advocacy of the use of hydrocortisone enemas by Truelove,[32] we began using this therapeutic approach for patients with proctitis.[3] In 1979, we reported the results of treatment of 62 patients with a mean follow-up of 7.7 years.[12] Complete resolution of symptoms and findings had occurred for 74% of the patients during the time they were receiving the hydrocortisone enemas. There was incomplete resolution of symptoms for 23% of patients with extension of disease in only 3%. These clinical results encouraged us to continue use of hydrocortisone enemas for treatment of ulcerative proctitis/proctosigmoiditis.

In addition to difficulty of assessment of clinical response and duration of therapy, concern continued that rectal installation of hydrocortisone enemas might be similar to oral use, with significant systemic absorption which would negate to a certain extent the "topical" effect of the steroids. Because of this, we performed steroid absorption studies with determination of pituitary-adrenal responsiveness for patients treated with 100 mg of hydrocortisone as nightly retention enemas over a 3-week period.[33] These studies indicated not only that such therapy was effective, but that approximately one third of the steroid was absorbed systemically, which led to minimal effect on the pituitary-adrenal axis if the therapy was continued for no longer than 3 weeks at one time. Thus, our concept of intermittent use of hydrocortisone enemas as therapy for ulcerative proctitis/proctosigmoiditis developed from these studies.

Because patients sometimes have difficulty administering hydrocortisone enemas, there has been an attempt to find another form of topical steroid beneficial in a similar manner, leading to the use of rectal hydrocortisone foam. A comparative study of hydrocortisone enemas and rectal hydrocortisone foam was carried out by Ruddell and colleagues.[34] Both agents were found to be effective and were similar in objective improvement, but subjective improvement was greater with the foam preparation. Assessment of the therapeutic efficacy of the foam preparations has been even more difficult than that of the hydrocortisone enema preparation; the foam preparation, like the steroid suppository, remains an alternative form of therapy for patients with ulcerative proctitis/proctosigmoiditis.

Oral sulfasalazine has been used in ulcerative colitis for many years, and, for patients with proctitis, sulfasalazine is "clearly efficacious and will lead to remission or significant improvement in up to 80 percent of patients."[35] Although oral sulfasalazine therapy has been the mainstay of treatment for patients with diffuse forms of ulcerative colitis, it has also been used for many years in patients with proctitis/proctosigmoiditis.[4] Only recently has the pharmacology of sulfasalazine been better understood. It is a conjugate of sulfapyridine and 5-aminosalicylic acid linked by a diazo bond, and it appears that the adverse side effects are associated with sulfapyridine moiety.[35] The relative lack of absorption of 5-aminosalicylate has led to new approaches to use of sulfasalazine derivatives. Campieri and his colleagues gave 5-aminosalicylic acid (5-ASA) orally in a slow release form or in enema form for patients who had previous allergic responses to oral sulfasalazine.[36] They studied plasma and urinary concentration of 5-ASA after rectal administration and found that 5-ASA concentration was dose and volume dependent, and no accumulation of 5-ASA was found in plasma after repeated daily administration. They concluded that the beneficial effect of 5-ASA enemas on the rectal mucosa may be "local" thus making the same assumption as we did regarding hydrocortisone.[33] There continues to be interest in the use of various forms of topical steroid agents, as well as nonglucocorticosteroid agents such as Tixocortil pivalate,[35] and a number of prospective studies are ongoing. Operation is seldom indicated for patients with ulcerative proctitis/proctosigmoiditis,[1, 4, 12] unless there is proximal extension[24] or severe rectal bleeding. If necessary, excision of the distal large bowel with sigmoid colostomy may be feasible.

PROGNOSIS

Although virtually all of the studies and reviews that include large numbers of patients have concluded that the clinical course of patients with ulcerative proctitis/proctosigmoiditis is benign, recurrences are common and extension occurs in 10% or more of patients.[1, 3, 4, 11, 12, 24, 38] The problem of prognosis for the individual patient was assessed by Ritchie and co-workers,[11] who observed 269 patients with ulcerative colitis. Their study underscored four pertinent questions frequently asked by patients: (1) "Is my condition dangerous?"; (2) "Will the inflammation spread?"; (3) "Will I need an operation?"; and (4) "Will I develop cancer?" While the physician can reassure the patient generally regarding these four questions, the 10% or so of patients who do develop more extensive disease can be difficult to predict at the outset or at the time of diagnosis. However, our experience[3, 12] indicates that when extension does occur, it usually does so before 2 years and almost invariably before 5 years of disease. This has been reaffirmed by our recent study[13] in children and supported by the accompanying editorial.[31] Further, increasing use of colonoscopy and assessment of the mucosa proximal to the inflamed area[25, 26] have further improved the ability to predict a favorable outcome.

Greenstein and co-workers[39] reported that patients with proctitis/proctosigmoiditis have no greater risk of developing colonic carcinoma than the general population; those with left-sided colitis have a higher risk than the general population, and the risk was still greater for patients with extensive ulcerative colitis. The relative lack of association of colonic cancer with longstanding proctitis has been emphasized by several large series.[1, 4, 11, 12, 38] As our previous experience[3, 12] and recent review of 82 cases of cancer in ulcerative colitis[40] indicate, colon cancer among patients with ulcerative proctitis/proctosigmoiditis is not significantly greater than that of the general population. Thus, although theoretically existing, the cancer risk in proctitis is not statistically nor numerically significant.

PROCTITIS: TRACTABLE AND INTRACTABLE

There remains a group of patients, variably estimated at about 15% to 30% of those with ulcerative proctitis/proctosigmoiditis, who have a course characterized by multiple recurrences but without significant extension of disease.[12] The reasons for this are poorly understood, and there is relatively little written about such patients, despite the difficulty created for the patient by the symptoms and the therapeutic dilemma posed to the physician attempting to deal with this problem. As noted previously, most of the therapeutic studies have been of patients with either new onset of disease or with a specific recurrence rather than attempting to evaluate therapy that deals with multiple recurrences. It is in this latter group of patients that "new drugs" are frequently used, that anecdotal results are given, and that clinical trials are especially difficult to perform. Nevertheless, from the perspective of long-term prognosis, these patients can be reassured, at least generally, provided the disease has been present for longer than 2 years (which it almost inevitably has in patients of this type) or, even more so, for patients whose disease has been present for greater than 5 years.[12] Likewise, these patients can be reassured concerning the lack of association of the development of cancer.[11, 39, 40]

From a personal perspective, having served as a consultant for patients with proctitis since the publication of our first paper on this subject in 1966,[3] there is a recurrent theme to such consultations. Although the patient referral is frequently made by a physician, encouragement to do so often comes from the patient or family. Seldom have I found that the diagnosis is incorrect or that some complication has occurred without the knowledge of the patient or the physician. By far the most frequent problem encountered has been the suboptimal response despite multiple therapeutic regimens. While the primary symptom for patients referred under these circumstances is almost always rectal bleeding, there frequently is associated tenesmus and occasionally mild diarrhea. However, other symptoms are usually absent and the response of the physician is frequently that the patient is exaggerating the severity of the symptoms. The response of the patient under these circumstances often is to request a "new drug" or to pay inordinate attention to such items as diet, allergic factors, or stress factors. Thus, the physician may become involved in tangential or even irrelevant clinical issues as well as inadequate therapeutic evaluation. Further, the patient's expectation that a consultant will produce either a dramatic or a "simple" solution often compounds the problem. Thus, the consultant physician may be in an adversarial relationship with the patient at the time of the initial visit! There are two important solutions to this dilemma from the perspective of the physician. The first is for the physician to determine the "role" he or she is playing with the patient—a specialist-consultant-expert, a counselor, or a continuing care physician. Second, the judicious use of statistical data, particularly that relating to long-term prognosis, can be particularly useful in reassuring the patient. What is to be avoided, of course, is the trivialization of the symptoms or an excessive (even obsessive) discussion of them. Certainly, this clearly requires the "art" as well as the "science" of medicine.

A physician dealing with a patient suspected of having ulcerative proctitis/proctosigmoiditis does have several dilemmas: the correctness of the diagnosis, the appropriateness of therapy, assessment of the therapeutic response, concern over recurrences, and consideration of the long-term prognosis. Because of these factors, there frequently will be a disproportionate physician–patient interaction, with multiple patient visits for an essentially benign condition. Thus, explanation to the patient of the nature and prognosis of the condition, understanding and rapport with the patient, and judicious use of therapy by the physician are extremely important, both to benefit the patient and to achieve a favorable clinical response.

References

1. Lennard-Jones JE, Cooper GW, Newell AC, et al: Observations on idiopathic proctitis. *Gut* 1962; 3:201–206.
2. Thaysen TEH: Simple hemorrhagic proctitis and proctosigmoiditis. *Acta Med Scand* 1934; 84:1–24.
3. Farmer RG, Brown CH: Ulcerative proctitis: Course and prognosis. *Gastroenterology* 1966; 51:219–223.
4. Nugent FW, Veidenheimer MC, Zuberi S, et al: Clinical course of ulcerative proctosigmoiditis. *Am J Dig Dis* 1970; 15:321–326.
5. Farmer RG, Brown CH: Emerging concepts of proctosigmoiditis. *Dis Colon Rectum* 1972; 15:142–146.
6. Calkins BM, Lilienfeld AM, Garland CF, et al: Trends in incidence rates of ulcerative colitis and Crohn's disease. *Dig Dis Sci* 1984; 29:913–920.
7. Gilat T: Incidence of inflammatory bowel disease: Going up or down? *Gastroenterology* 1983; 85:196–203.
8. Nordenvall B, Brostrom O, Berglund M, et al: Incidence of ulcerative colitis in Stockholm County 1955–1979. *Scand J Gastroenterol* 1985; 7:783–790.
9. Both H, Torp-Pedersen K, Kreiner S, et al: Clinical appearance at diagnosis of ulcerative colitis and Crohn's disease in a regional patient group. *Scand J Gastroenterol* 1983; 18:987–991.
10. Wright JP, Marks IN, Jameson C, et al: Inflammatory bowel disease in Cape Town, 1975–1980. Part 1. Ulcerative colitis. *S Afr Med J* 1983; 63:223–226.
11. Ritchie JK, Powell-Tuck J, Lennard-Jones JE: Clinical outcome of the first ten years of ulcerative colitis and proctitis. *Lancet* 1978; 1:1140–1143.
12. Farmer RG: Long-term prognosis for patients with ulcerative proctitis. *J Clin Gastroenterol* 1979; 1:47–50.
13. Mir-Madjlessi SH, Michener WM, Farmer RG: Course and prognosis of idiopathic ulcerative proctosigmoiditis in young patients. *J Pediatr Gastroenterol Nutr* 1986; 5:570–575.
14. Carr N, Schofield PF: Inflammatory bowel disease in the older patient. *Br J Surg* 1982; 69:223–225.
15. Zimmerman J, Gavish D, Rachmilewitz D: Early and late onset ulcerative colitis: Distinct clinical features. *J Clin Gastroenterol* 1985; 7:492–498.
16. Marshall JB, Butt JH: Proctitis: Approach to diagnosis, causes and treatment. *J Clin Gastroenterol* 1982; 4:431–444.
17. Quinn TC, Corey L, Chaffee RG, et al: The etiology of anorectal infections in homosexual men. *Am J Med* 1981; 71:395–406.
18. Quinn TC: Gay bowel syndrome. The broadened spectrum of nongenital infection. *Postgrad Med* 1984; 76:197–210.
19. Ritchie JK, Lennard-Jones JE: Crohn's disease of the distal large bowel. *Scand J Gastroenterol* 1976; 11:433–436.
20. Glotzer DJ, Glick ME, Goldman H: Proctitis and colitis following diversion of the fecal stream. *Gastroenterology* 1981; 80:438–441.
21. Rickert RR: The important "imposters" in the differential diagnosis of inflammatory bowel disease. *J Clin Gastroenterol* 1984; 6:153–163.
22. Surawicz CM, Belic L: Rectal biopsy helps to distinguish acute self-limited colitis from idiopathic inflammatory bowel disease. *Gastroenterology* 1984; 86:104–113.
23. Surawicz CM, Goodell SE, Quinn TC, et al:

Spectrum of rectal biopsy abnormalities in homosexual men with intestinal symptoms. *Gastroenterology* 1986; 91(3):651–659.
24. Powell-Tuck J, Ritchie JK, Lennard-Jones JE: Prognosis of idiopathic proctitis. *Scand J Gastroenterol* 1977; 12:727–732.
25. Das KM, Morecki R, Nair P, et al: Idiopathic proctitis: The morphology of proximal colonic mucosa and its clinical significance. *Am J Dig Dis* 1977; 22:524–528.
26. Farmer RG, Whelan G, Sivak MV Jr: Colonoscopy in distal colon ulcerative colitis. *Clin Gastroenterol* 1980; 9:297–306.
27. Williams HJ Jr, Stephens DH, Carlson HC: Double-contrast radiography: Colonic inflammatory disease. *Am J Roent* 1981; 137:315–322.
28. Powell-Tuck J, Day DW, Buckell NA, et al: Correlations between defined sigmoidoscopic appearances and other measures of disease activity in ulcerative colitis. *Dig Dis Sci* 1977; 27:533–537.
29. Sparberg M, Fennessy J, Kirsner JB: Ulcerative proctitis and mild ulcerative colitis: A study of 220 patients. *Medicine* 1966; 45:391–412.
30. Goldman H, Proujanski R: Allergic proctitis and gastroenteritis in children. Clinical and mucosal biopsy features in 53 cases. *Am J Surg Pathol* 1986; 10(2):75–86.
31. Gryboski JD: Extension of proctosigmoiditis in children. *J Pediatr Gastroenterol Nutr* 1986; 5(6):842–843.
32. Truelove SC: Treatment of ulcerative colitis with local hydrocortisone. *Br Med J* 1956; 2:1267–1272.
33. Farmer RG, Schumacher OP: Treatment of ulcerative colitis with hydrocortisone enemas; Relationship of hydrocortisone absorption, adrenal suppression, and clinical response. *Dis Colon Rectum* 1970; 13:355–361.
34. Ruddell WS, Dickinson RJ, Dixon MF, et al: Treatment of distal ulcerative colitis (proctosigmoiditis) in relapse: Comparison of hydrocortisone enemas and rectal hydrocortisone foam. *Gut* 1980; 21:885–889.
35. Peppercorn MA: Current status of drug therapy for inflammatory bowel disease. *Compr Ther* 1985; 11:14–19.
36. Campieri M, Lanfranchi GA, Boschi S, et al: Topical administration of 5-aminosalicylic acid enemas in patients with ulcerative colitis. Studies on rectal absorption and excretion. *Gut* 1985; 26:400–405.
37. Nakano G, Ritchie JK, Thomson JPS: Ulcerative colitis treated by excision of the distal large bowel alone. *Postgrad Med J* 1984; 60:278–279.
38. Edwards FC, Truelove SC: The course and prognosis of ulcerative colitis. *Gut* 1963; 4:299–315.
39. Greenstein AJ, Sachar DB, Smith H, et al: Cancer in universal and left-sided ulcerative colitis: Factors determining risk. *Gastroenterology* 1979; 77:290–294.
40. Mir-Madjlessi SH, Farmer RG, Easley KA, et al: Cancer in ulcerative colitis. *Cancer* 1986; 58:1569–1574.

Colonic Crohn's Disease:
What is a workable approach to management?

BURTON I. KORELITZ, M.D.

The classic description of ileitis reported in 1932 concerned 14 patients with granulomatous inflammatory process involving the terminal segment of the small intestine. It was established soon after, however, that this entity could cross the ileocecal valve, involve the colon in conjunction with the ileum (subsequently referred to as ileocolitis), or involve the colon without associated ileitis, now called Crohn's disease of the colon.

DEFINITION

The diagnosis of Crohn's disease of the colon implies an inflammatory process with gross and histologic features characteristic of Crohn's disease, involving any amount of the colon from a short segment to the entire organ. The process may be continuous or characterized by skip areas of involvement. Because Crohn's disease is characteristically an asymmetric process, one wall of the colon may be clearly involved while the opposite wall appears normal. Involved areas may be the sites of transverse fissures, fistulas, and pseudodiverticula. Grossly uninvolved areas may be the site of microscopic inflammation. Most commonly, the rectal segment appears normal or at least relatively uninvolved when compared with the more proximal colon. Crohn's disease of the colon most often affects some combination of areas including the right colon. This may be cecum to ascending, transverse, descending, or sigmoid colon. It may be transverse alone or extending to some point more distal. It may involve the left colon alone, with or without extension to the rectum. When the cecum is involved there is usually at least microscopic involvement of the terminal ileum as well; despite this, lack of gross involvement of the terminal ileum serves to retain colonic involvement under the classification of Crohn's colitis. There are cases of Crohn's disease limited to the rectal segment; these are prevalent in patients with onset at age 60 or older. Technically, these must be considered cases of Crohn's disease of the colon even though they are exceptional and should probably maintain their own identity.

Crohn's disease of the colon is the third most common form of Crohn's disease, accounting for approximately 25% of cases, following ileocolitis (40%) and ileitis (30%). Cases of Crohn's disease manifested by perirectal abscesses and fistulas, which remain unassociated with bowel involvement, and cases of Crohn's disease of the stomach, duodenum, or more proximal tissues, unassociated with more distal bowel disease, are uncommon. Although Crohn's disease limited to the colon has the same peak age of onset as other distributions (in the latter half of the second decade), in patients with onset after the age of 50, Crohn's colitis is more common than ileocolitis. This is accounted for mostly by cases of Crohn's disease of the left colon and the occasional cases of Crohn's proctitis previously mentioned. Crohn's disease is slightly more common in females than in males, and this is true of Crohn's disease of the colon as well as other distributions.

DIFFERENTIAL DIAGNOSIS

The differential diagnosis of Crohn's disease from ulcerative and other kinds of colitis is particularly difficult when the inflammatory process is limited to the left colon. An acute infectious colitis can usually be identified by history, culture, and the self-limited course. A postantibiotic or pseudomembranous colitis can be recognized by historic and endoscopic features aided by a positive *Clostridium difficile* titer. A parasitic colitis can be determined by historic features and stool examinations. Ulcerative colitis can easily be ruled out if the rectal segment is spared and the mucosa appears normal at sigmoidoscopy. If the rectal segment is involved, however, differential gross and microscopic features are helpful but not always absolute.[1] The most difficult problems in differential diagnosis occur in older patients with inflammatory processes involving the left colon. One is diverticular disease, which commonly involves the left colon and is often blamed for the passage of blood rectally even though it might not be the cause. The occasional appearance of longitudinal fistulas from diverticulum to diverticulum in the presence of other features of a colitis will help to clarify the diagnosis of Crohn's disease of the left colon. The other process is ischemic colitis, in which the diagnosis is supported by a sudden onset, associated degenerative diseases, and progressive deterioration or a self-limited course.

HISTOLOGIC FEATURES

Biopsies of rectal and colonic mucosa are important in the diagnosis of Crohn's disease. Even in those cases of Crohn's disease of the colon in which the rectal mucosa appears normal, rectal biopsies show nonspecific acute and chronic inflammation in about 60%.[2] They also reveal, however, indicators of inflammation more specific for Crohn's disease in about 40%. These include crypt abscesses, some with eosinophils or macrophages, preservation of the mucosal goblet cells, disproportionate inflammation in the submucosa, lymphoid nodules, and lymphangiectasia. In 20% to 35% of patients, characteristic granulomas and less well-developed microgranulomas are found.[3] When multiple biopsy specimens are taken and serial sections are studied, the yield of these diagnostic lesions increases.[4] They are more likely to be found when the mucosa appears grossly normal than when the biopsy specimen is taken from a site of obvious inflammation. On colonoscopy, biopsy specimens have also shown the inflammation in areas more proximal where the mucosa appears normal, increasing the extent of involvement beyond that seen on x-ray films. Because there is evidence that Crohn's disease involves the entire gastrointestinal tract, a definition of extent should include the diagnostic modality used to determine it (roentgenography versus endoscopy). Granulomas and microgranulomas seem to be found much less frequently in colonoscopic biopsies than rectal biopsies, whether the mucosa appears normal or inflamed.

CARCINOMA OF THE COLON

Carcinoma of the intestine occurs less commonly in bowel involved with Crohn's disease than with ulcerative colitis. Nevertheless, the incidence of carcinoma of the colon complicating Crohn's disease is approximately six times as great as in the average population, and the risk increases with duration of disease and extent of involvement just as it does in ulcerative colitis.[5] Crohn's disease of the colon does not lend itself to a surveillance program as readily as ulcerative colitis because of stricturing, shortening, nodularity, polyposis, and extensive deformity. Nevertheless, dysplasia is prevalent and signifies a premalignant state. Therefore, if the colonoscope can be passed through the colon, it should be done on a regular surveillance basis after 10 years of disease with biopsies performed throughout. Multiple synchronous neoplasms have been disclosed in resected specimens of Crohn's disease of the colon.

PREGNANCY AND FERTILITY

The fertility rate for women with Crohn's disease is not statistically different from that of the general population. In women with active Crohn's disease, however, the ability to conceive is reduced. One report concluded that fertility was even more compromised in patients with Crohn's disease of the colon than with other distributions of the disease.[6] Current evidence supports a program of drug therapy in anticipation of pregnancy to improve the likelihood of conception.

Once pregnancy occurs, there is an increased rate of premature delivery and spontaneous abortion attributable to active Crohn's disease. Again, disease activity should be suppressed with drug therapy throughout pregnancy to reduce this risk. Treatment with corticosteroids and sulfasalazine has been shown to be safe in regard to fetal outcome and nursing. The most favorable outlook for pregnancy depends on keeping Crohn's disease activity suppressed.[7]

Pregnancy does not serve to worsen the course of the Crohn's disease in the female patient. Should the need for surgical intervention arise, however, survival of the fetus is severely threatened and the risk to the mother is increased. Vigorous drug therapy is warranted for control of the disease for the sake of both the mother and the child.

MEDICAL MANAGEMENT

No one drug has been shown to be indefinitely effective in controlling Crohn's disease. Many drugs, however, have demonstrated their effectiveness in some distribution or some phase of activity. These include corticosteroids and adrenocorticotropic hormone (ACTH), sulfasalazine, 6-mercaptopurine, metronidazole, and broad-spectrum antibiotics. In general, all of these drugs have been more effective in Crohn's disease of the colon than in other distributions of Crohn's disease.

Adrenal Corticosteroids

Corticosteroids or ACTH almost always works well in Crohn's disease of the colon. When the patient is overtly or acutely ill, these drugs are almost always required to effect a remission. This creates a role for the chronic phase drugs, which otherwise might not have had the opportunity to be effective on confronting an overwhelming inflammatory process. Steroids serve to reduce inflammation rapidly; they eliminate fever, diarrhea, and pain and increase appetite and well-being. In some instances, the remission that follows will be long, but eventually there will be a recurrence if a chronic phase drug is not added to the program. In still more cases the symptoms of Crohn's disease of the colon will recur soon after stopping the steroids or even while the dosage is being reduced. When steroids are used on an ambulatory basis, the initial dose should be higher than that calculated to be effective. If prednisone is chosen, at least 60 mg daily should be prescribed, preferably in four divided doses. Once the favorable response, which occurs within 2 to 10 days, is evident, a formula is established for the rate of reduction as guided by the original severity of symptoms or physical findings and the rate of response. On the average, it should take about a month to eliminate the prednisone. This time should be used to plan chronic phase therapy and introduce the new drug or method of administration. Often it is necessary to reintroduce or raise the dose of steroids soon after their initial elimination or before the reduction schedule can be completed. Under these circumstances, the dose should once more be brought to a level calculated to suppress the disease.

Raising the dose by small increments involves the risk of not effecting a remission and permitting the disease to become more entrenched and more difficult to eliminate. The inflammation should be suppressed as early as possible to reduce the risk of chronicity and the temptation to administer steroids at some dosage level indefinitely. *Steroids should not be considered maintenance drugs.* When used for prolonged periods, these drugs cause many complications of their own, which then substitute for or add to the manifestations and infirmities of the primary bowel disease.

When Crohn's disease is severe enough to warrant hospitalization, intravenous ACTH should be favored over oral steroids. Crystalline ACTH may be administered continuously at a rate of 120 U given over 24 hours or as a bolus of 40 U given every 8 hours. Both forms seem to be equally effective. The volume of intravenous fluids in which the ACTH is given may be varied with the degree of dehydration. If hydration is not clinically necessary, the ACTH may be given in 500 ml of fluids, preferably water rather than saline to minimize salt retention. Otherwise, a volume of 1,000 to 3,000 ml may be used. Once a remission is secured, the dose of intravenous ACTH can be reduced and intramuscular ACTH or oral steroids or both can be substituted. Oral steroids can then be reduced according to the formula previously mentioned and eventually can be eliminated. Meanwhile, chronic phase therapy is introduced. *The specific goals of ACTH or steroid therapy should be determined for each case.*

Sulfasalazine

Sulfasalazine has been the chronic phase drug with the longest history of use in the treatment of Crohn's disease. Although its effectiveness against active Crohn's disease in general has been questioned, its favorable role in treating Crohn's disease of the colon has been confirmed.[8] This may best be explained by the need for colonic bacteria to split the diazo bond releasing the effective moiety, 5-aminosalicylic acid (5-ASA). Its effectiveness as a prophylactic agent in maintaining remissions of Crohn's disease of the colon, similar to its major role in ulcerative colitis, has not been clearly demonstrated but is most likely valid. Once remission is accomplished, whether attributable to sulfasalazine or not, this drug, again similar to the situation in ulcerative colitis, should be continued indefinitely unless it has been demonstrated in the individual case to be of no value. The maintenance dose of sulfasalazine is 4 gm per day to be administered in divided doses with meals and at bedtime. The full dose should be achieved slowly, however, to avoid nausea, headaches, and less common side effects. Starting with one tablet (0.5 gm) daily and adding one tablet daily until the full dose is reached or a side effect occurs has proved to be an effective method. Clinical experience must be used to achieve patient tolerance for this drug and to provide every opportunity for it to work. Even allergic skin eruptions caused by sulfasalazine should not serve to eliminate its use. Desensitization by starting with tiny doses (⅛ to ¼ tablet daily or drops of the suspension) and slowly increasing (every 3 to 7 days) has been successful in 80% of the cases, and the drug can be effective therapeutically for extended periods thereafter. Perhaps oral preparations of 5-ASA will have an effective role under the circumstances as well.

Immunosuppressives

It has been proven that 6-mercaptopurine effects remission in 65% to 70% of patients with active Crohn's disease,[9] and it should be used in selected patients as a chronic phase drug. This drug has been the most effective in Crohn's disease of the colon. The mean time after its introduction until it takes effect is 3.1 months. Therefore, it is often necessary to use ACTH or corticosteroids to effect a remission and allow time for the 6-mercaptopurine to work. The drug has served to permit elimination or at least reduction of the steroid dose, to close or improve all varieties of fistulas,[10] and to eliminate or reduce the primary bowel manifestations of the disease. Its favorable effect occurs independent of steroid therapy. Although 6-mercaptopurine is considered an immunosuppressive drug, the manner in which it achieves its success is not yet known. Leukopenia is a known side effect of the drug and should be expected at some time in each case. The initial dose is 50 mg daily, and complete blood count and platelets are monitored once weekly for the first 3 weeks. When it is shown that the patient tolerates the drug well, the frequency of monitoring can be reduced. If the blood count permits, the dose can then be increased to 50 mg on one day alternating with 50 mg twice daily, or to 50 mg twice a day.

Many patients and managing physicians fear the use of 6-mercaptopurine, mostly because of the high incidence of lymphomas and other malignancies when other immunosuppressive drugs have been used as part of a program for renal transplantations or chemotherapy. In those instances, however, multiple immunosuppressive agents have been used simultaneously, and doses have been larger than ever used in the treatment of Crohn's disease. Serious complications have been demonstrated infrequently coincident with the small doses of 6-mercaptopurine used in treating Crohn's disease.[11] Pancreatitis has occurred in about 5% of patients, but in all instances it was reversible.[12] Bone marrow depression has not occurred since experience has been acquired in management. The rate of important complications of all drugs used in the treatment of Crohn's disease, especially corticosteroids, has been higher. *When all information known and unknown about 6-mercaptopurine has been shared, and when the course of uncontrolled Crohn's disease of the colon has been described, most intelligent patients want an opportunity to try 6-mercaptopurine, and when compliance has been complete, they do so without mishap.* The drug is continued for an arbitrary period of 2 years once its effectiveness and its ease of management are demonstrated. Thereafter, some patients prefer to continue and others prefer to stop. Relapse is anticipated, the mean period being 6 months after stopping the 6-mercaptopurine, but the recurrence can be mild and amenable to other drugs, or it may not take place at all until much later. Normal childbirth has been experienced by women who became pregnant while taking 6-mercaptopurine. Nevertheless, women have been advised to avoid pregnancy and men have been advised not to impregnate their wives until 3 months after the drug has been stopped.

Metronidazole

Metronidazole has been demonstrated to be effective in reducing perirectal and perineal abscesses and fistulas.[13] Unfortunately, a dose of 1.5 to 2.0 gm daily is required to accomplish this, a level at which drug toxicity in the form of peripheral neuropathy often occurs. Even after the drug is stopped, the neuritis may persist for many months. Coincidentally, recurrence of the abscesses and fistulas occurs as the drug is stopped or reduced. Metronidazole has also been shown to have an effect approximately equivalent to sulfasalazine against the primary bowel symptoms at the lesser dosage of 250 mg three times a day.[14]

Broad-Spectrum Antibiotics

In addition to their supplemental role in treating the secondary infection accompanying perirectal and intra-abdominal abscesses, broad-spectrum antibiotics occasionally will be effective in the treatment of Crohn's disease of the colon when all other drugs have failed. In my experience the one most responsible for long remission is ampicillin, which I have continued to administer for more than a year in some patients. I have used cephalexin (Keflex) and tetracycline also, initially as supplemental drugs and then as primary therapy. Chronic antibiotic therapy is specifically warranted for ileo-vesical fistulas when the only clinical manifestation is pyuria.

Other Considerations in Medical Management

Drugs given for pain should be used cautiously and sparingly. Drug abuse and dependence are common in young people with Crohn's disease, and the situation is compounded during postoperative periods.[15]

Nonspecific antidiarrheal agents may be used to supplement a treatment program, but care should be taken to minimize the risk of dependence, addiction, and contribution to the development of colonic dilatation and megacolon.

A small bowel tube is sometimes used to treat colonic obstruction contributed to by a stricture, an abscess, or a mass.

Parenteral nutrition may accelerate the healing of the primary bowel inflammation, obstruction due more to inflammation than fibrosis, and even fistulas. If ACTH or a steroid is used at the same time, the value of stopping oral feedings is questionable. Parenteral nutrition does not lead to permanent reversal of the inflammatory process, and therefore *the temporary period of improvement should be used to initiate a new mode of chronic phase drug therapy.*

Emotional factors do not seem to be causative in Crohn's disease but clearly serve to aggravate its course. Although no generalization should be made, many patients will profit by consultation with a therapist, whether a psychiatrist or psychologist, a family therapist, or a psychiatric social worker. In this regard, the self-help groups offered by chapters of the National Foundation for Ileitis and Colitis have been extremely helpful.[16]

SURGERY

In the natural course of Crohn's disease, the extent of involvement originally demonstrated by roentgenography remains more or less stable independent of the severity of the local involvement. With clinical worsening, the disease might extend distally but not proximally. Once the bowel is transected for purposes of resection or diversion, however, Crohn's disease spreads proximally. The extension occurs earlier when the operation is performed for ileitis or ileocolitis, later for colitis involving the right colon, and still later for colitis grossly limited to the left colon. Regardless of the original extent, given enough time the proximal spread can be anticipated in all cases. By the time clinical symptoms of recurrent Crohn's disease occur, characteristic features are already present on x-ray films and have probably been visible there for varying periods of time. Should colonoscopy or ileoscopy be performed prior to recurrent symptoms, evidence of inflammation is frequently encountered in the new terminal ileum. If gross inflammation has not yet appeared, biopsy specimens are likely to show histologic features of inflammation, sometimes including granulomas.

Despite the provocation by resection or transection, surgical intervention has been indicated in approximately 70% of patients with Crohn's disease during their lifetimes. When Crohn's disease is grossly confined to the colon, many surgeons have managed the disease like ulcerative colitis with ileostomy and total proctocolectomy. One study showed that the rate of recurrent ileitis in the patients with ileostomy was no greater than in the patients with ulcerative colitis, even though ileostomy revisions might be required more often.[17] Other investigations, including my own,[18] have demonstrated that the ileostomy is no barrier to extension of the Crohn's disease proximally after transection. The issue is academic to the extent that if surgery, which includes ileostomy, must be done, then it must be done, but it should not be performed with the expectation that Crohn's disease of the colon can be cured in this manner.

The Kock, or continent ileostomy and the ileopouch-anal anastomosis are contraindicated for Crohn's disease because of the likelihood of recurrence in the pouch. Only with due regard for this high risk might these procedures be considered and then only in very special circumstances.

There are two alternatives to total proctocolectomy. When the rectal segment is grossly spared, resection with ileorectal anastomosis might be feasible. In some instances in which the distal extent of Crohn's disease of the colon is more proximal, and ileotransverse or ileodescending colostomy or an ileosigmoidoscopy might be considered. Surgeons are unwilling to perform an ileorectal anastomosis in the presence of grossly active disease in the rectal segment. Microscopic inflammation need not necessarily contraindicate an ileorectal anastomosis. Retention of the anal sphincter contributes to a better quality of life, even if the average number of stools per day increases with an anastomosis. If the Crohn's disease eventually extends to the previously normal or almost normal appearing rectal segment, the few additional years gained without need for an ileostomy warrant considering this option. Sometimes the clinical situation necessitating the colectomy is such that performing an anastomosis is contraindicated. The rectum under these circumstances is left in situ, and an ileostomy is performed with the intention of either leaving the rectum as is or doing the reanastomosis at a later date. The rectum, however, is subject to the same diversion proctitis that occurs when a temporary colostomy is performed for obstructing cancer of the colon or diverticular disease.[19] It has been shown that inflammatory changes that develop in the rectum can be reversed with reanastomosis. Whether the proctitis which occurs in the rectal segment is purely diversion or Crohn's disease accentuated by the diversion, a primary reanastomosis should be favored. If this is not feasible, then the reanastomosis should be performed as early as possible.

Prognosis and Indications for Surgery

Crohn's disease of the colon will most often require total proctocolectomy with ileostomy if surgical resection is warranted. This situation contrasts with a limited ileitis, for which minimal resection can be performed with reanastomosis and preservation of bowel continuity and sphincter control. In addition to having to cope with an ileostomy, the patient cannot be given the satisfaction of cure of the disease, as would be the case with ulcerative colitis. Therefore, every effort should be made to bring the disease into remission once again with nonoperative methods and to maintain that remission.

Fortunately, almost all current programs of drug therapy have been more effective for Crohn's disease of the colon than for any other type of Crohn's disease. Once ACTH or corticosteroids have reduced or eliminated the inflammatory process, sulfasalazine has been effective in completing and/or maintaining the remission for long periods in many cases. Once it is clear that sulfasalazine has failed, 6-mercaptopurine also has been more effective in Crohn's disease involving the colon than in ileal disease.[9] *Patients should be made aware of the opportunity to be treated with 6-mercaptopurine for Crohn's disease of the colon*, particularly as an alternative to surgical resection that would include an ileostomy as well as the risk of recurrent ileitis in the stoma.

There are few remaining absolute indications for surgical intervention in Crohn's disease. These include

1. Massive hemorrhage that cannot be reversed by large doses of intravenous ACTH or corticosteroids
2. Perforation of the colon
3. Toxic megacolon that cannot be reversed. In my experience dilatation of the colon in Crohn's disease responds even better than the same complication of ulcerative colitis to a nonoperative program of intravenous ACTH, broad-spectrum antibiotic coverage, small bowel tube and rectal tube decompression, and rolling the patient to both sides and into the prone position.[20]
4. Carcinoma of the rectum or colon. This diagnosis is rarely made preoperatively, but it has been done by both sigmoidoscopic and colonoscopic examinations and by biopsies.

Other indications for surgery in the course of Crohn's disease of the colon are *relative*.

1. The primary bowel symptoms usu-

ally respond to drug therapy, particularly when all drugs of proven value are used alone or in combination.
2. Colonic-vesical fistulas respond to 6-mercaptopurine in most instances.
3. Colonic-gastric, duodenal, jejunal, and ileal fistulas respond to 6-mercaptopurine in most instances.
4. Colonic and rectovaginal fistulas respond to 6-mercaptopurine in most instances. Surgical repair of a rectovaginal fistula without colectomy can be considered only in special cases, and even then it should be accomplished by a diverting ileostomy.
5. Colonic-abdominal wall abscess-fistula that does not respond to drainage, antibiotics, and a new program of drug therapy might require colonic resection.
6. Perirectal, perineal, vulval, and scrotal fistulas often improve with simple drainage, usually in conjunction with a drug program that emphasizes 6-mercaptopurine or metronidazole. When this approach is not satisfactory, a modified Park's procedure, with dissection of fistulas to their common source and eradication of the underlying intersphincteric abscess, has been effective in preventing recurrences in 75% of patients without the need to resort to bowel resection.[21] Extensive and destructive abscesses and fistulas eroding the perineum and buttocks have been successfully handled in this way, even as a primary procedure, thereby giving a new program on drug therapy the opportunity to concentrate on the primary bowel disease. *Diversion of the fecal stream* by either colostomy or ileostomy *is not effective therapy for this problem* and causes the additional risks of recurrent Crohn's disease proximal to the transection and development or accentuation of an inflammatory process in the rectal mucosa.
7. Rectal strictures, unless markedly advanced, can be dilated with the 11-mm rigid scope, the finger, or both. With an improved drug program and frequent dilatations, colectomy can be avoided. Suppository preparations of corticosteroids often aid this process.
8. Colonic strictures can sometimes be dilated via the colonoscope but infrequently cause obstruction. Only when there is a strong suspicion that the colonic stricture masks a carcinoma, and the region cannot be satisfactorily biopsied, should colectomy be considered for this indication. Colonic obstruction due to nodularity, erosions, or strictures has served as one of the most absolute indications for 6-mercaptopurine.
9. Pyoderma gangrenosum not responding to steroids or 6-mercaptopurine might require colectomy.
10. Poor quality of life sometimes warrants no further pursuit of an effective drug program and mandates surgical resection despite the risk of extension of disease.

In the past 8 years, I can recall only six patients with Crohn's disease of the colon who required surgical resection. One had a carcinoma of the rectum disclosed by rectal biopsy, and colectomy revealed multiple neoplasms. The second had a segmental resection of the descending colon for a long stricture associated with a mass causing pain, weight loss, and poor quality of life. A diverting ileostomy was performed and then closed 3 months later. The third had a fistula from the splenic flexure to the abdominal wall which was eliminated by a successful segmental resection. Two had segmental resections of rectal-sigmoidal strictures with diverting ileostomy and subsequent reanastomosis, despite the presence of Crohn's disease more proximal in the colon. The sixth had total proctocolectomy performed for ulcerative colitis, and pathologic examination of the resected specimen revealed histologic evidence favoring Crohn's disease of the colon. *The success rate for Crohn's disease of the colon treated with 6-mercaptopurine is so high that no patient with this distribution of Crohn's without a carcinoma should come to surgery without an opportunity for a trial on this drug.*

References

1. Korelitz BI, Sommers SC: Differential diagnosis of ulcerative colitis and granulomatous colitis by sigmoidoscopy, rectal biopsy and cell counts of rectal mucosa. *Am J Gastroenterol* 1974; 61:460–469.
2. Korelitz BI, Sommers SC: Rectal biopsy in patients with Crohn's disease. *JAMA* 1977; 237:2742–2744.
3. Rotterdam HZ, Korelitz BI, Sommers SC: Microgranulomas in grossly normal rectal mucosa in Crohn's disease. *Am J Clin Pathol* 1977; 67:550–554.
4. Surawicz CM, Meisel JC, Ylvisaker T, et al: Rectal biopsy in the diagnosis of Crohn's disease. Value of multiple biopsies and serial sectioning. *Gastroenterology* 1981; 80:66–71.
5. Korelitz BI: Carcinoma of the intestinal tract in Crohn's disease: Results of a survey conducted by the National Foundation for Ileitis and Colitis. *Am J Gastroenterol* 1983; 78(1):44–46.
6. de Dombal FT, Burtin IL, Goligher JC: Crohn's disease and pregnancy. *Br Med J* 1972; 3:550–553.
7. Baiocco PJ, Korelitz BI: The influence of inflammatory bowel disease and its treatment on pregnancy and fetal outcome. *J Clin Gastroenterol* 1984; 6:211–216.
8. Summers RW, Switz DM, Sessions JT Jr, et al: National Cooperative Crohn's disease study: Results of drug treatment. *Gastroenterology* 1979; 77:847–869.
9. Present DH, Korelitz BI, Wisch N, et al: Treatment of Crohn's disease with 6-mercaptopurine. *N Engl J Med* 1980; 302:981–987.
10. Korelitz BI, Present DH: Favorable effect of 6-mercaptopurine on fistulae of Crohn's disease. *Dig Dis Sci* 1985; 30(1):58–64.
11. Present DH, Meltzer SJ, Wolke A, et al: Short and long term toxicity to 6-mercaptopurine in the management of inflammatory bowel disease (abstract). *Gastroenterology* 1985; 88(5):1545.
12. Haber CJ, Meltzer SJ, Present DH, et al: Nature and course of pancreatitis caused by 6-mercaptopurine in the treatment of inflammatory bowel disease. *Gastroenterology* 1986; 91:982–986.
13. Bernstein LH, Frank MS, Brandt LJ, et al: Healing of perineal Crohn's disease with metronidazole. *Gastroenterology* 1980; 79:357–365.
14. Ursing B, Alm T, Barany F, et al: A comparative study of metronidazole and sulfasalazine for active Crohn's disease: The comparative Crohn's disease study in Sweden. II Result. *Gastroenterology* 1982; 83:550–562.
15. Kaplan MA, Korelitz BI: Narcotic dependence in inflammatory bowel disease. *J Clin Gastroenterol* 1988; 10(3):275–278.
16. Banks PA, Present DH, Steiner P: *The Crohn's Disease and Ulcerative Colitis Fact Book.* New York; Charles Scribner's Sons, 1983.
17. Nugent FW, Veidenheimer MC, Meissner WA, et al: Prognosis after colonic resection for Crohn's disease of the colon. *Gastroenterology* 1973; 65:398–401.
18. Korelitz BI, Present DH, Albert LI, et al: Recurrent regional ileitis after ileostomy and colectomy for granulomatous colitis. *New Engl J Med* 1972; 287:110–115.
19. Korelitz BI, Cheskin LJ, Sohn N, et al: Proctitis after fecal diversion in Crohn's disease and its elimination with reanastomosis: Implications for surgical management: Report of 4 cases. *Gastroenterology* 1984; 87:710–713.
20. Present DH: Management of toxic megacolon, in Korelitz BI, Sohn N (eds): *Inflammatory Bowel Disease: Experience and Controversy.* San Diego, Grune & Stratton, 1985, pp 217–222.
21. Sohn N, Korelitz BI, Weinstein MA: Anorectal Crohn's disease: Definitive surgery for fistulas and recurrent abscesses. *Am J Surg* 1980; 139:394–397.

34

Intractable Perineal Fistulae in Crohn's Disease:
Can life be made worth living?

LESLIE H. BERNSTEIN, M.D.

One of the most debilitating manifestations of Crohn's disease is involvement of the perineum by intractable and progressive fistulae. Although very rarely responsible for hospitalization, this indolent manifestation often leads to progressive isolation, celibacy, and the inability of its victims to engage in productive employment and social and physical intercourse. In its severest form, it remains a primary reason for proctocolectomy in Crohn's disease.[1] Even after such major surgery, it may continue to torture the patient in the form of cavernous unhealed wounds which may not only fail to heal, but may spread as an enlarging ulcer to involve the anterior perineum and external genitalia. Testimony to the frustrating nature of these unhealed proctectomy wounds is provided by the spate of operations that have been proposed in an attempt to close the defects and produce a healed wound; these range from simple skin grafting, to the implantation of musculocutaneous flaps, to coccygeal amputation. Many postoperative perineal wounds in patients with Crohn's disease remain unhealed years after the primary surgery.[2]

Even when the bowel disease has been controlled and the perineal disease is relatively quiescent, the patient may be left incontinent of gas, feces, or both due to progressive destruction of the anal sphincter, either by disease, or more often by repeated surgery performed by well-meaning physicians attempting to cure chronic fistulous disease.[3]

Experience, accumulated during the course of clinical studies on the effect of metronidazole in this problem, has led me and my associates to adopt certain principles in its treatment.[4]

SPECTRUM OF THE PERINEAL MANIFESTATIONS OF CROHN'S DISEASE

The perineal manifestations of Crohn's disease are rarely encountered in patients in whom the disease is confined to the small intestine. Perineal disease in such patients should cause the physician to consider the probability that the disease has spread to involve the colon. Rarely the perineal manifestations may be the first manifestation of Crohn's disease or the disease may be confined to only a short segment at the anorectal junction. In these situations, knowledge of the spectrum of perineal complications will raise the suspicion that Crohn's disease is the underlying problem.

The perineal manifestations of Crohn's disease include
1. Anal fissure
2. Perianal abscess
3. Anal fistulae—simple or complex and involving the urethra, scrotum, penis, etc.

4. Granulomatous hypertrophic tissue ("elephant ears")
5. Pseudo-Bartholin's gland abscess
6. Rectovaginal fistula
7. Unhealed proctectomy wound
8. Metastatic Crohn's disease involving the vulva[5]
9. Esthiomene—vulval elephantiasis

Several points should be stressed to alert the physician or surgeon that a local perianal condition might represent perineal Crohn's disease:

1. Crohn's perineal disease is usually quite painless unless collections of undrained pus (abscess) exist. Such a collection may exist in the ischiorectal fossae, as a pseudo-Bartholin's gland abscess, in the rectovaginal septum, or as a perianal or perirectal abscess.[6]

   Relief of pain is accomplished by simple incision and drainage, but the patient must understand that a fistula is likely to result; closure of an abscess or fistula following surgical drainage is unlikely. Further, in the patient with known Crohn's disease it is wise to caution the patient that new areas of drainage are to be expected, so that the appearance of other fistulous orifices is not thought to be the result of improper therapy.

2. Frequently a violaceous discoloration of the perineal skin is noted in patients with Crohn's disease—even at some distance from the apparent local involvement. I suspect this represents "congestion" from underlying edema and lymphatic involvement by the burgeoning subcutaneous process.

3. Painless "external hemorrhoids" in a patient with known Crohn's disease must be reevaluated. The perianal hypertrophic tissue in such patients is frequently misidentified as hemorrhoidal in origin with catastrophic results often following hemorrhoidectomy, including nonhealing of the hemorrhoidectomy wound, spreading ulceration and anal stricture, when and if healing takes place. Too often the pathologist is the first physician to make the diagnosis after review of the submitted specimen.

4. The Bartholin's gland abscess in a patient with colonic involvement by Crohn's disease is almost always a manifestation of perineal fistulous disease and not a primary infection of the gland. Although relief of pain is to be expected following surgical drainage, occasional or persistent discharge from the incision site is common.

5. Rectovaginal fistulae unassociated with obstectric trauma, surgery, or radiotherapy is Crohn's disease until proven otherwise. A corollary of this is that swelling within the rectovaginal septum in a patient with Crohn's disease represents a relative "therapeutic emergency," and metronidazole should be started immediately in an attempt to prevent breakdown of the septum and formation of a rectovaginal fistula. Fluctuant collections within the septum should not be drained vaginally, but back into the rectum under general anesthesia if at all possible.

   In patients who have undergone hysterectomy, one occasionally sees fistulae to the vaginal vault from colonic or ileal Crohn's disease. These are treated as other intra-abdominal fistulae with good results following resection of the segment of bowel from which the fistula originates.

6. Rectal bleeding or mucous discharge accompanying the passage of stool in a patient with quiescent colonic disease frequently represents drainage of a perirectal collection through an undetected rectoanal tract. The material is usually serosanguineous or sanguinopurulent, and the site can frequently be determined by careful anoscopy.

7. Perineal fistulae, whether they occur in a patient with underlying Crohn's disease or not, all begin in the same way, with an abscess or infection of the anal crypts; the extent and resistance to therapy are the hallmarks of

the perineal fistulae accompanying Crohn's disease.

Development of fistulae usually halts when suitable cutaneous drainage is established; the fistulous tract may then epithelialize, in part, and become chronic. Stool is virtually never passed through perineal fistulae after they epithelialize and become chronic.

In contrast to the usual course, the establishment of a cutaneous drainage site frequently fails to arrest the progress of the tract in Crohn's perineal disease. Burrowing continues and multiple openings develop along the branching tracts of the fistula, reaching the groin, genitalia, buttocks, thighs, and even the popliteal fossa.

Multiple weeping orifices along the course of the fistula result in the "watering can" perineum, which is the archetypical form of the disease. Involvement of the vulvar lymphatics leads to elephantiasis or esthiomene, formerly considered to be a manifestation only of the LGV strains of *Chlamydia*.

Throughout the natural progression of this disease, it is remarkable how little pain is experienced by the patient. Occasional episodes of pain or discomfort associated with impaired drainage are noted but are usually few and far between. However, problems with odor, stained underclothes, and reluctance to engage in sex on the part of the patient or partner are everyday concerns.

A PLEA FOR CONSERVATIVE THERAPY

In 1976, John Alexander-Williams reviewed the course of 109 patients with perineal involvement in Crohn's disease and made a plea for conservative surgical therapy.[7] He reviewed this same population subsequently with a longer follow-up of over 10 years and again renewed his plea.[8] Sixteen of his patients were incontinent; of these five were totally incontinent of feces and flatus. All such cases occurred following surgery for complicated fistulous tracts. He opined that "fecal incontinence in Crohn's disease is the result of aggressive surgeons and not of progressive disease."

Because a minor degree of incontinence becomes a major problem in a patient in whom diarrhea is a part of daily life, it cannot be stressed too strongly that in a patient with Crohn's disease, recurrent attempts to open fistulae in the usual manner, whereby a "few" sphincteric fibers are sacrificed, should be avoided. The addition of new drugs to the gastroenterologist's armamentarium and improved conservative approaches by the experienced proctologic surgeon allows this conservative course to be more easily followed. It should be remembered that the overwhelming majority of patients with Crohn's disease will have surprisingly little debility and virtually no pain from their fistulous disease, *if* anal stenosis and incontinence are avoided by conservative care.

MEDICAL THERAPY FOR PERINEAL CROHN'S DISEASE

Metronidazole

In 1975, Ursing and Kamme reported the use of metronidazole in patients with Crohn's disease.[9] At that time, metronidazole was employed in the United States as an antiprotozoal medication, but in Europe its potent antianerobic bactericidal properties were already being exploited. Because Ursing's initial five patients responded dramatically, numerous other investigators employed metronidazole with equivalent or somewhat lesser results. In many of these series, patients with perineal problems showed improvement independent of the course of the underlying bowel disease.

In view of the response of the perineal disease to metronidazole therapy noted in these series, a study of consecutive patients with progressive perineal fistulous problems associated with Crohn's disease was begun.[4] In a series of 21 patients, the average duration of the Crohn's disease was over 11 years, and the perineal disease had been present for an average of 5 years.

Gratifying results were obtained in most patients, including those with complex fistulae and ulceration, metastatic Crohn's ulcer, and unhealed proctectomy wounds. Advanced or complete healing was observed in 15 of 18 patients who maintained therapy for more than 2 months. The bowel disease also improved in many of these patients, as has been observed by others,[10, 11] including active disease with enteroenteric fistulae.

The eventual development of significant paresthesia[12, 13] in patients on long-term metronidazole has been the major problem in terms of its use as maintenance therapy. Paresthesia occurs in 50% to 100% of patients, depending on the series, and develops about 6 months after initiation of therapy. It appears to be dose related, and in some cases lowering dosage by as little as 20% can cause paresthesia to regress. Frequently, the drug must be withdrawn because of this troubling side effect, and in most of patients in whom this is done perineal disease will recur or worsen.

It is our policy at present to treat perineal disease with metronidazole until complete healing has occurred or the disease has improved and stabilized and at that point, to submit the patient to conservative "sphincter-saving" surgery if needed (see below). This policy has been particularly gratifying in episodes of threatened rectovaginal fistulization in which swelling and tenderness in the rectovaginal septum have responded to metronidazole with complete healing and no surgical intervention.

6-Mercaptopurine

Response of perineal fistulous disease to 6-mercaptopurine (6-MP) has been noted by Korelitz and Present[14] in their controlled study on the efficacy of this analogue of adenine. Their series included rectovaginal and perirectal fistulae with a response rate in the latter of at least 30% to 40%. As with metronidazole, the mechanism of action is unknown, but there is a marked similarity in the manner in which patients respond when the two drugs are compared. 6-mercaptopurine is usually well tolerated and safe if idiosyncratic pancreatitis (1% to 4%), drug allergy, and severe pancytopenia do not occur. Relapse is to be expected if the drug is withdrawn, but reinstitution of the drug has been consistently effective in gaining control of the fistulous disease. Clearly 6-MP can be carefully used in the patient with severe and progressive perineal fistulous disease, before more aggressive therapy is used.

SURGICAL APPROACHES

As I have indicated earlier, patients with Crohn's perineal disease are subject to recurrent episodes of perineal fistulous disease. Surgical therapy performed in the usual manner, which consists of laying open the fistulous tract to its origin, frequently has to be repeated, resulting in partial or total incontinence in a patient with chronic diarrheal disease. Therefore, surgical therapy, when undertaken, must be designed to spare as much of the sphincteric mechanism as possible.

Sohn and co-workers[15] have championed the partial internal sphincterotomy, introduced by Parks,[16] as the procedure of choice for patients with Crohn's perianal fistulae. In this approach, a small area of skin and mucosa overlying the internal opening of the fistula is removed followed by a portion of the underlying internal sphincteric muscle, thus draining the intersphincteric abscess. The procedure is performed under general anesthesia, and the external portion of the fistula can be curetted to promote healing of the tract. Incontinence has not been a problem according to the authors, or in my experience, in patients in whom this procedure has been employed.

Occasionally, patients with uncomplicated anterior fistulae have been successfully treated by the use of a seton passed through the fistulous tract. The seton consists of a nonabsorbable suture, which, when tied tightly on the perineal skin gradually cuts its way to the surface while the path behind it becomes fibrotic, preventing retraction of muscular (sphincteric) fibers. Unfortunately, the complicated nature of the tracts in patients with Crohn's disease makes this simple procedure rarely applicable.

The results of fecal diversion procedures performed to promote perineal healing have been unimpressive and of little benefit. Surgical attempts to close rectovaginal fistulae without bowel resection are similarly disappointing and occasionally disastrous. A newer procedure using rectal mucosal "advancement" has been advocated,[17] but I have no personal experience with this procedure.

CONCLUSION

Most cases of perianal fistulae associated with Crohn's ileocolitis or colitis will be slowly progresive or will stabilize after several years. They are rarely associated with severe pain or hospitalization.

Intractable, progressive disease associated with ulceration, increase in the number of fistulae, threat of rectovaginal fistualization, or an unhealed proctectomy wound should be treated initially with metronidazole or alternatively with 6-MP. Conservative surgery designed to protect the sphincteric mechanism should be undertaken if healing fails to occur or the process stabilizes. Failure to recognize the initial manifestations as part of the Crohn's disease symptom complex and to use sphincter-sparing surgical techniques is a major cause of morbidity in patients afflicted with this problem. The majority of patients will respond initially to metronidazole therapy, but maintenance is difficult because of the development of paresthesia. 6-MP represents an alternative for progressive perineal disease, although the response rate appears to be somewhat lower than with metronidazole.

References

1. Hellers G, Bergstrand O, Ewerth S, et al: Occurrence and outcome after primary treatment of anal fistulae in Crohn's disease. *Gut* 1980; 21:525–527.
2. Anderson R, Turnbull RB Jr: Grafting the unhealed perineal wound after coloproctectomy for Crohn disease. *Arch Surg* 1976; 111:335–338.
3. Alexander-Williams J, Buchmann P: Perianal Crohn's disease. *World J Surg* 1980; 4:203–207.
4. Bernstein LH, Frank MS, Brandt LJ, et al: Healing of perineal Crohn's disease with metronidazole. *Gastroenterology* 1980; 79:357–365.
5. Reyman L, Milano A, Demopoulos R, et al: Metastatic vulvar ulceration in Crohn's disease. *Am J Gastroenterol* 1986; 81:46–49.
6. Sohn N, Korelitz BI, Weinstein MA, et al: Anorectal Crohn's disease: Diagnosis and management. *Am J Surg* 1980; 139:394–397.
7. Alexander-Williams J: Fistula-in-ano: Management of Crohn's fistula. *Dis Colon Rectum* 1976; 19:518–519.
8. Buchmann P, Keighley MRB, Allan RN, et al: Natural history of perianal Crohn's disease. Ten year follow-up: A plea for conservatism. *Am J Surgy* 1980; 140:642–644.
9. Ursing B, Kamme C: Metronidazole in Crohn's disease. *Lancet* 1975; 1:775.
10. Jakobovits J, Schuster MM: Metronidazole therapy for Crohn's disease and associated fistulae. *Am J Gastroenterol* 1984; 79:533–540.
11. Eisenberg HW: Combined metronidazole and surgery in the management of complicated Crohn's disease. *Contemp Surg* 1982; 21:95–102.
12. Duffy LF, Daum F, Fisher SE, et al: Peripheral neuropathy in Crohn's disease patients treated with metronidazole. *Gastroenterology* 1985; 88:681–684.
13. Brandt LJ, Bernstein LH, Boley SJ, et al: Metronidazole therapy for perineal Crohn's disease: A follow-up study. *Gastroenterology* 1982; 83:383–387.
14. Korelitz BI, Present DH: Favorable effect of 6-mercaptopurine on fistulae of Crohn's disease. *Dig Dis Sci* 1985; 30:58–64.
15. Sohn N, Korelitz BI, Weinstein MA: Anorectal Crohn's disease: Definitive surgery for fistulas and recurrent abscesses. *Am J Surg* 1980; 139:394–397.
16. Parks AG: Pathogenesis and treatment of fistula in ano. *Br Med J* 1961; 1:463–469.
17. Farkas AM, Gingold BS: Repair of rectovaginal fistula in Crohn's disease by rectal mucosal advancement flap. *Mt Sinai J Med* (NY) 1983; 50(5):420–423.

# 35

Toxic Megacolon:
Is there a superior approach to management?

DANIEL H. PRESENT, M.D.

Toxic megacolon is one of the most difficult and dangerous medical problems that arise in the course of inflammatory bowel disease. Fortunately, most internists and gastroenterologists will see only a few cases during their careers, but when faced with this complication, the potential for a poor outcome is so great that it requires clear understanding of the medical and surgical options. It has been said that toxic megacolon should only be managed at specialist centers by physicians with extensive experience with this complication.[1] I would have to agree that the changing mortality data would bear out this recommendation.[2]

CLINICAL FEATURES

For toxic megacolon to be correctly diagnosed, the patient with colitis must show clinical signs of "toxicity" as well as the radiologic features of megacolon. Dilatation alone, in a patient with colitis who is not clinically ill, does not constitute this entity. For example, dilatation might occur with narcotic agents producing a motility disorder or with distal organic colonic obstruction. Likewise, patients may become "toxic" without developing colonic dilatation. By definition, both components should be evident before making this specific diagnosis.

The patient with toxic megacolon will manifest the following: increased bowel movements, usually over six daily, with gross blood present in the stools, elevated temperature above 100 F, and tachycardia with a pulse rate of 90 or greater.[3] It must be understood that many of the above features may be modified by medications (e.g., fever may be suppressed if the patient is on high doses of corticosteroids). Bowel movements may also be lessened with antidiarrheals. The erythrocyte sedimentation rate is 30 mm/hour or greater and in most studies there are other laboratory abnormalities described, such as leukocytosis, anemia, hypoalbuminemia, and elevated serum orosomucoid. Megacolon patients have also been shown to have elevated arterial pH and base excess as well as frequent low serum potassium and calcium.[4]

If the clinical condition worsens, the deteriorating patient may also show signs of dehydration, mental confusion, and hypotension. Findings on abdominal examination may vary greatly. The abdomen may not appear distended, may be nontender to palpation, and may be only slightly tympanitic to percussion. The findings can be significantly altered if the patient is taking intravenous or oral steroids. I have seen patients who have perforated their colons during an episode of toxic megacolon with absolutely no abnormal abdominal findings on examination. More commonly, however, with toxic megacolon the findings will include mild abdominal distention, usually in the upper abdomen, mild to moderate tenderness occurring most commonly in the left lower abdomen but which can occur over any area of the colon. Localized rebound tenderness is seen in severe cases. Tympany is often evident in the left upper quadrant and may also be present along the upper abdomen (over the area of transverse colon). In a patient with active colitis, tympany may be the earliest warning sign of an impending megacolon. The abdomen must be percussed for hepatic dullness at every physical examination. Loss of hepatic dullness may be the *only* clinical sign of a perforated toxic megacolon, especially if the patient is taking steroids.

RADIOGRAPHIC FEATURES

The clinical entity and radiographic features were first described by Marshak in 1950.[5] Dilatation is most evident in the transverse colon but can be seen throughout the colon depending on the positioning of the patient. The transverse colon is the most anterior portion of the colon, and during severe colitis activity, patients usually lie in bed in a supine position with the upper body elevated. This allows more air to accumulate in this segment. If the patient is rolled to a prone position, colonic air will redistribute to the ascending and descending colon, thus changing the radiographic picture.[6] Most authors state that there must be dilatation of the transverse colon beyond 6 cm to label the condition toxic megacolon. Other authors state that the 6-cm measure is not crucial if the rest of the clinical condition is present. I disagree with the latter concept and label this condition "toxic colitis." It is true that if untreated these severely ill toxic colitis patients often develop a megacolon, however I feel that by definition the 6-cm level must be reached to appropriately apply this label to the patient's condition. The average degree of colonic dilatation is close to 9 cm and may extend as high as 15 cm.[7] Equally important as the dilatation are the radiographic features of loss of normal haustral pattern, irregular contour of the bowel wall, and polypoid projections seen along the margins. Nodularity may be seen projecting through the colonic column of air which represents edematous mucosal islands surrounded by denuded and ulcerated mucosa. These "polypoid" changes can be seen in all areas of the colon depending on the extent of the colitis and the presence of air in that segment of bowel. Linear lucencies along the bowel wall have been described, which suggest imminent perforation, and, of course, free air under the diaphragm may be seen, indicating that the medical treatment has not succeeded and that emergency surgery must be performed. Recently, a new radiographic finding has been demonstrated, namely that of increased amounts of small bowel gas in about 50% of cases of severely active colitis.[8] In this group, about 25% went on to toxic megacolon, suggesting that increased small bowel gas is commonly seen in toxic megacolon. My personal experience agrees with this finding and must be taken into account in terms of the suggested medical management (Fig 35–1).

DIFFERENTIAL DIAGNOSIS

Toxic megacolon is not limited to patients with ulcerative colitis and Crohn's disease. The complication has been seen with other infectious colitides, such as amoebiasis, salmonellosis, shigellosis, and campylobacter. On presentation, all patients with active colitis must be immediately cultured for pathogens, and stools must be searched for parasites. History should be obtained as to the recent taking of antibiotics. In any event, stools should be sent to the laboratory and tested for *Clostridium difficile*. If a patient with well-documented ulcerative colitis or Crohn's disease has been quiescent for a protracted period and now exacerbates with the development of toxic megacolon, stools should again be carefully examined for a superimposed secondary infection. Toxic megacolon has also been reported with other conditions such as ischemic

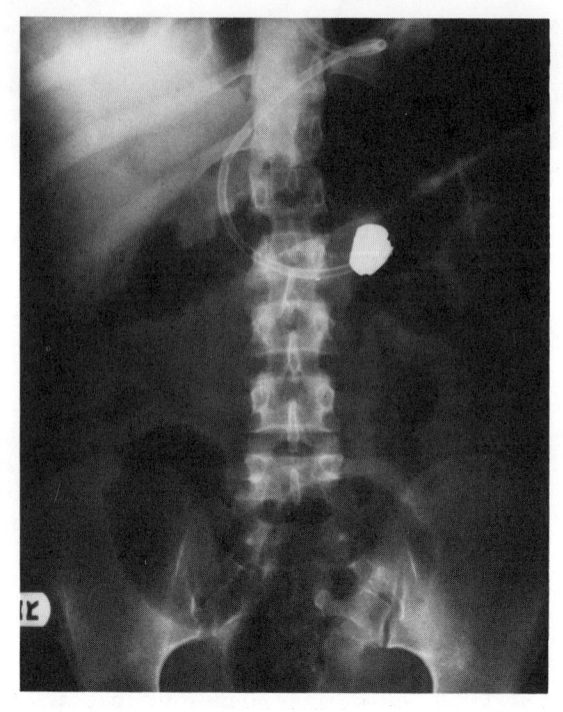

FIG 35–1.
Patient with toxic megacolon demonstrating increased small intestinal gas. The passing of a small intestinal tube will alleviate much of this gas and aid in decompression.

colitis, colitis secondary to gold therapy, and cytomegalic virus.

If the toxic megacolon patient has had colitis but has never been seen by the admitting physician, a careful history and review of prior endoscopies and barium enemas are mandatory. The differential diagnosis between ulcerative colitis and Crohn's disease can become extremely difficult during the acute inflammatory phase, and the medical management, surgical management, and prognosis differ in these two entities. Therefore, the questions of rectal involvement, presence or absence of chronic bleeding, and continuous type picture seen on endoscopy should all be answered, because they signify ulcerative colitis. Likewise, a history of small bowel involvement, clubbing, and oral aphthous ulcerations would tend to favor Crohn's disease.

PREDISPOSING FACTORS

Toxic megacolon may develop in the first attack of colitis, may be a complication in a patient with continuous low-grade activity, or may occur after many years of quiescent colitis. Therefore, duration of disease is not a predisposing factor to developing toxic megacolon. In the majority of reported series, toxic megacolon appears in the first attack of colitis in about 40% of cases.[9]

It has been noted that antidiarrheal drugs, including narcotics (codeine, deodorized tincture of opium), anticholinergics, and antidepressants may induce megacolon. I do not believe this is true, but rather, these drugs can trigger a megacolon only in the presence of *active* colitis.

The same speculation is centered on barium enemas precipitating toxic megacolon.[10] I and many other authors have observed the onset of megacolon soon after a barium enema. Once again, I believe it is the combination of significant disease activity plus the procedure that produces the megacolon. Parenthetically, the administration of strong laxatives as preparation for a barium enema and the use of double contrast techniques are to be avoided in patients with either Crohn's disease or ulcerative colitis who are manifesting severe clinical activity. Colonoscopy and flexible sigmoidoscopy also should not be performed when the bowel is showing increasing inflammatory signs. The preparation and introduction of air may be triggering factors. The value of the information to be derived is not equal to the risk of precipitating a toxic megacolon. A rigid sigmoidoscopy to 5 to 6 inches will provide the most vital information, that is, the degree of activity in ulcerative colitis, or rectal sparing indicating Crohn's disease. Other factors, such as electrolyte abnormalities triggering a megacolon, have been less well documented.

PATHOGENESIS AND PATHOLOGY

The extension of the inflammatory process from the mucosa through all layers of the bowel wall has been seen in surgical specimens. This transmural extension, perhaps with destruction of the myenteric plexus may be a pathogenetic mechanism. Extensive smooth muscle damage with subsequent loss of motility or an antecedent sealed off local perforation might also be pathogenetic factors, producing decreased motility and subsequent dilatation. The gross pathologic features are a repetition of the prior mentioned x-ray findings and show transmural inflammation and severe ulcerations with intervening edematous islands of mucosa. The bowel wall is often markedly thinned with some muscle wall destruction, and occasionally there are sites of sealed off perforations of the bowel.

MANAGEMENT

General

Admission to the hospital on an emergency basis is required if the patient develops a megacolon or is showing any of the prior listed criteria for toxicity. Baseline blood studies, including CBC, ESR, 12-channel chemistry and electrolytes, should be performed daily. Some centers have now added indium[III]-labeled leukocyte testing to evaluate extent and severity of activity. Repeat indium[III] testing may be helpful in gauging degree of improvement. Stools should be cultured, tested for ova and parasites and *Clostridium difficile*. Obstructive series must be performed daily until toxicity has abated. The films must include the diaphragms and be carefully scrutinized for signs of impending perforation (air in the bowel wall), or the presence of free air within the abdomen. Newer techniques of monitoring include a 24-hour measurement of fecal weight, which has been noted to be increased with severity. Fecal bicarbonate and fecal potassium/sodium ratios are lowest in severely ill patients.[11] Alkalosis worsens with severity and can be monitored with arterial pH samples. Monitoring of the patient also includes measurement of fluid intake and output. Stool charting for numbers of movements, amount of blood, and consistency can also be done either by patient or nurse. Vital signs have to be monitored at least four times daily.

It is essential that an experienced bowel surgeon be called to see the patient daily until the megacolon and toxicity have abated. All patients with toxic megacolon should be seen at least three times daily, usually by attending physician, surgeon, and house staff. In fact, most are seen twice daily by each of the above. Decisions as to management are made around the clock. Most symptomatic medications, including anticholinergics (for cramping), antidiarrheals (to slow the action of the bowel), and narcotic analgesics (for pain relief), should not be used during the acute phase of toxic megacolon. These agents will likely worsen the megacolon, promote distention, and cloud the clinical signs. Abdominal pain usually is not severe unless there is perforation and/or peritonitis. The usual low-grade type of pain will improve with decompression of the colon. Narcotics should be used sparingly because addiction may develop in some patients if the hospital course is prolonged. After there has been decompression of the colon and toxicity has subsided and the patient is eating, cautious administration of antidiarrheal agents can and should be used to control bowel movements.

Specific

Intravenous Fluids

Intravenous fluids are used to correct dehydration. Care should be taken, especially as regards excessive potassium wasting caused by the diarrhea and the concomitant use of steroids. Blood should be replaced as needed, and the hematocrit should be kept at a level of 30 or higher. In this era of alimentation, many centers will treat ulcerative colitis patients with total parenteral nutrition (TPN). TPN, in controlled trials, has shown no benefit in the outcome of an episode of fulminant colitis or toxic megacolon.[12, 13] Duration in the hospital and percentage of patients coming to surgery is the same with or without TPN in patients with chronic ulcerative colitis. This is in contrast to Crohn's colitis in which there has been some evidence of promotion of healing. Therefore, TPN should only be started to maintain nutrition in an ulcerative colitis patient who was depleted before the acute event or possibly prior to surgery to promote postoperative healing.

"Bowel rest" (i.e., nothing by mouth with IV or TPN replacement) has never been shown to be effective in ulcerative colitis. Early studies using ileostomy to rest the bowel showed no improvement in the inflammatory process. This is once again in contrast to patients with Crohn's disease in whom diversion has clearly been shown to quiet inflammation. I therefore treat all patients with nothing by mouth during the acute phase, but when toxicity has abated and distention has disappeared, I start oral feedings in both ulcerative colitis and Crohn's disease patients.

Steroids

Because no "controlled trial" has ever demonstrated the efficacy of steroids in toxic megacolon, and because steroids mask the clinical signs and symptoms, there has been debate whether steroids should be administered to toxic megacolon patients who have not been taking these agents prior to the acute episode.[14] Steroids, however, have been shown to be effective when orally administered in mild to moderate ulcerative colitis in a controlled trial.[15] For ethical reasons it is doubtful that a placebo-controlled trial will ever be performed in the treatment of fulminant colitis and toxic megacolon. I personally believe that it is a foolhardy approach not to administer steroids and that they are the drug of choice for moderate and severe active ulcerative colitis and Crohn's disease, and there is no rationale to deny their use in toxic megacolon. Oral administration is not advised because the bowel is often dilated and there is a question of malabsorption. Therefore, IV administration of corticosteroids is used to ensure effective blood concentration. A controlled double-blind trial demonstrated that 120 units of IV ACTH is more effective than 300 mg of IV Solucortef, if the patient has not been previously treated with steroids.[16] However, hydrocortisone was more effective if the patient had been receiving prior corticosteroids. I closely adhere to these principles of steroid administration.

There has been little discussion in the literature regarding whether intravenous steroids should be given by continuous drip or by a single intravenous pulse. Some clinicians advise the pulse technique to diminish steroid side effects, but this reason seems inappropriate in the acute situation. My clinical impression and those of my colleagues at the Mt. Sinai Hospital in New York is that continuous infusion is more effective. It is also the habit of many specialists to administer rectal as well as IV steroids in ulcerative colitis. There is no strong documentation of efficacy of this added modality in the controlled literature, and patients may also have difficulty retaining these enemas. I therefore delay routine administration of rectal steroids until the megacolon has been decompressed. If this has been accomplished, I administer 100 mg of Solucortef nightly in the form of a 60-ml enema.

Antibiotics

There is major controversy surrounding the role of antibiotic therapy in toxic megacolon. There is no controlled evidence demonstrating efficacy, and in fact, IV metronidazole[17] and oral vancomycin[18] have failed to show any benefit over placebo during an acute severe attack of ulcerative colitis. This, plus the failure to demonstrate any bacterial agents playing a major role in ulcerative colitis exacerbation, has led investigators to use antibiotics only prior to laparotomy and colectomy.[19] The opposing argument could cite the frequent operative finding of sealed off perforations in toxic megacolon complicating ulcerative colitis and would therefore suggest broad coverage to prevent and treat secondary infection. Also metronidazole has been shown to be an effective therapeutic agent in Crohn's disease, affecting the colon. As noted, in new cases of colitis, it is also difficult to quickly exclude amoebiasis. Therefore, despite the lack of controlled data I prefer to administer metronidazole (for possible amoebic infection and Crohn's coverage) plus an aminoglycoside and ampicillin directed at enterococci. The newer cephalosporins ultimately may prove to give adequate broad-spectrum coverage. I recheck patient stools for *Clostridium difficile* after 5 to 7 days of hospitalization to make sure this secondary complication has not occurred.

5-ASA Compounds

There is not good justification for starting sulfasalazine or one of the newer oral 5-ASA compounds in this acute situation. The patient is not taking oral foods, and the drug usually requires longer than 1 week to show efficacy. However, if the patient is taking these agents and the megacolon is decompressed, I reintroduce them as soon as food is tolerated.

DECOMPRESSION OF THE COLON

With significant distention of the colon, the greatest fear is that of perforation. It is stated that the colon is very inaccessible to decompression. In fact, surgical procedures were designed to decompress the colon with multiple stomas (blow hole technique).[20] My own experience and that of a few investigators is that a long tube is helpful in the management.[21] This would agree with the recent reports finding that increased small intestinal gas preceded megacolon in many cases.[8] I therefore have a long tube introduced at the time of hospital admission and have it positioned immediately in the duodenum or distal antrum. This is done fluoroscopically in the x-ray department. I believe the long tube helps in preventing entrance of some small bowel gas into the colon. As was noted earlier, because gas accumulates preferentially in the transverse colon, I have the patient roll into the prone position for 10 to 15 minutes every 2 to 3 hours.[22] This allows redistribution of colonic air, and I then encourage the patient to evacuate gas while lying prone. I have found that this simple technique results in significant decompression of the colon with lessening of abdominal distention and relief of patient discomfort. I believe that the combination of a long tube *plus* the rolling technique prevents further accumulation of colonic air and will almost always result in decreased colonic distention. Because the treating physician will observe this radiographic improvement, there will be less pressure for surgical intervention. This decompression technique will also allow more time for the steroids to be effective in diminishing the "toxic inflammatory" process. New, creative techniques to decompress megacolon, such as using endoscopic placement of colonic tubes, await further testing.[23]

DURATION OF TREATMENT AND OUTCOME

The Oxford group has suggested that a maximum of 5 days of therapy be allowed to show improvement in severe exacerbation of ulcerative colitis before colectomy is performed.[24] In fact, surgery is often advised earlier if the megacolon develops. Most experienced surgeons feel that the maximum therapeutic medical trial is 24 to 72 hours.[2] This is at variance with my personal experience and that of other gastroenterologists.[25] In a consecutive series of 19 toxic megacolons, I have decompressed all patients with the mean time of decompression of approximately 5 days. The rolling technique has allowed this extra time for improvement. Many major centers will allow 7 to 10 days of medical therapy for fulminant colitis, having found this time period to be safe.[19, 26] I would venture that the rolling technique will allow them to expand this time period to toxic megacolon. It must be stated emphatically that there are no hard and fast rules for individual patients. The suggested longer period of medical treatment does not apply to patients showing *no* signs of improvement or who in fact are worsening. Surgery should not be delayed in these situations. These decisions are made at the bedside using all available laboratory and clinical data. Because these are difficult decisions, toxic megacolon should be managed by an experienced team.

The literature is very variable as regards the long-term outcome. It will depend on whether the reporting investigator is a gastroenterologist or a surgeon and whether he or she has treated many or few patients. Strong teachers have imposed their views about early surgery on succeeding generations at some major institutions, despite improved medical and surgical techniques. Overall mortality rates using medical and surgical management vary greatly, and a review of over 600 cases reveals a medical mortality of 27% and a surgical mortality of 19.5%.[27] In the latter group the surgical mortality was 8.8% without perforation, but was 41.2% if the bowel was perforated. The more recent medical and surgical literature shows mortality rates as low as 0% and 1.2%, respectively.[25, 28]

The long-term fate of patients after an episode of megacolon has also changed over the years, with improvement in medical therapy. Although it was thought that colectomy was inevitable after megacolon, three large series showed that about 50% of patients will not lose their colons.[2, 22, 25] Salvaging the colon may be more likely to occur in patients who have megacolon during the first episode and Crohn's colitis patients who develop megacolon. Therefore, the long-term plan after decompression must be individualized. If the patient is young, has had the disease a short time, is not at risk for carcinoma, or has Crohn's disease, a long-term medical treatment plan should be strongly considered. If the patient has had extensive colitis for many years, has required frequent courses of intermittent or continued steroids, and then develops megacolon, he or she should undergo elective colectomy soon after the colon has been decompressed.

SURGERY

Surgical options have increased in the last 10 years. Initially the choices were those of total colectomy and ileostomy, or ileostomy and subtotal colectomy with a mucous fistula. As was noted, the blow hole technique with multiple stomas was also popular at a few centers. Ileostomies without colectomies were tried and abandoned because they were not effective in ulcerative colitis. If surgery is required either for persistent megacolon or perforation, the procedure of choice is subtotal colectomy and ileostomy, retaining the rectum as a Hartmann pouch. This allows the surgeon to perform an ileoanal anastomosis with proximal pouch after the patient has recovered from the acute attack. Rarely is the ileoanal anastomosis with proximal pouch performed during an acute situation. If pan proctocolectomy is required, such as with severe bleeding from the rectal segment, a continent pouch can be considered electively after the patient has made a full recovery. In Crohn's disease preservation of the rectum is essential for future anastomosis. This can be done during the acute phase at the surgeon's discretion with or without protective ileostomy, however in most patients it is usually performed in two stages.

In summary, toxic megacolon is a potentially fatal complication of ulcerative colitis and Crohn's disease. However, with an experienced medical and surgical team, with careful monitoring, and with a comprehensive medical treatment plan for decompression, mortality can be lowered below 10% and the colon can be saved with restoration of good health in over 50% of cases.

References

1. Bucknell NA, Lennard-Jones JE: How district hospitals see acute colitis. *Lancet* 1979; i:1226–1229.
2. Grant CS, Dozois RR: Toxic megacolon: Ultimate fate of patients after successful medical management. *Am J Surg* 1984; 147:106–110.
3. Truelove SC, Witts LJ: Cortisone in ulcerative colitis. Final report on a therapeutic trial. *Br Med J* 1955; 2:1041–1048.
4. Caprilli R, Vernia P, Colaneri O, et al: Risk factors in toxic megacolon. *Dig Dis Sci* 1980; 25:817–822.
5. Marshak RH, Lester LJ, Friedman AI: Case reports: Megacolon, a complication of ulcerative colitis. *Gastroenterology* 1950; 16:768–772.
6. Kramer P, Wittenberg J: Colonic gas distribution in toxic megacolon. *Gastroenterology* 1981; 80:433–437.
7. Norland CC, Kirsner JB: Toxic dilatation of the colon (toxic megacolon): Etiology, treatment and prognosis in 42 patients. *Medicine* 1969; 48:229–250.
8. Caprilli R, Vernia P, Latella G: Early recognition of toxic megacolon. *J Clin Gastroenterol* 1987; 9:160–164.
9. Jalan KN, Sircus W, Card WI, et al: An experience in ulcerative colitis. I. Toxic dilatation in 55 cases. *Gastroenterology* 1969; 57:68–82.
10. Goldberg HI: The barium enema and toxic megacolon: Cause–effect relationship? *Gastroenterology* 1975; 68:617–618.
11. Caprilli R, Frieri G, Latela G, et al: Fecal excretion of bicarbonate in ulcerative colitis. *Digestion* 1986; 35:136–142.
12. Dickinson RJ, Ashton MG, Axton ATR, et al: Controlled trial of intravenous hyperalimentation and total bowel rest as an adjunct to the routine therapy of acute colitis. *Gastroenterology* 1980; 79:1199–2004.
13. McIntyre PB, Powell-Tuck J, Wood SR, et al: Controlled trial of bowel rest in the treatment of severe acute colitis. *Gut* 1986; 27:481–485.
14. Meyers S, Janowitz HD: Systemic corticosteroid therapy of ulcerative colitis. *Gastroenterology* 1985; 89:1189–1191.
15. Lennard-Jones JE, Longmore AJ, Newel AC, et al: An assessment of prednisone, salazopyrine and topical hydrocortisone hemisuccinate used as outpatient treatment for ulcerative colitis. *Gut* 1960; 1:17–222.
16. Meyers S, Sachar DB, Goldberg JD, et al: Corticotropin versus hydrocortisone in the intravenous treatment of ulcerative colitis. A prospective, randomized, double-blind clinical trial. *Gastroenterology* 1983; 85:351–357.
17. Chapman RW, Selby WS, Jewell DP: Controlled trial of intravenous metronidazole as an adjunct to corticosteroids in severe ulcerative colitis. *Gut* 1986; 27:1210–1212.
18. Dickinson RJ, O'Connor HJ, Pinder I, et al: Double-blind controlled trial of oral vancomycin as adjunctive treatment in acute exacerbations of ulcerative colitis. *Gut* 1985; 26:1380–1384.
19. Jarnerot G, Rolny P, Sandberg-Gertzen H: Intensive intravenous treatment of ulcerative colitis. *Gastroenterology* 1985; 89:1005–1013.
20. Turnbull RB Jr, Hawk WA, Weakly FL: Surgical treatment of toxic megacolon. Ileostomy and colostomy to prepare patients for colectomy. *Am J Surg* 1971; 122:325–331.
21. Neschis M, Siegelman SS, Parker JG: Diagnosis and management of megacolon of ulcerative colitis. *Gastroenterology* 1968; 55:251–259.
22. Present DH, Wolfson D, Gelernt IM, et al: The medical management of toxic megacolon: Technique of decompression with favorable long term followup. *Gastroenterology* 1981; 80:1255.
23. Banez AV, Yamanishi F, Crans CA: Endoscopic decompression of toxic megacolon, placement of colonic tube, and steroid colonclysis. *Am J Gastroenterol* 1987; 82:692–694.
24. Truelove SC, Jewell DP: Intensive intravenous regimen for severe attacks of ulcerative colitis. *Lancet* 1974; i:1067–1070.
25. Katzka I, Katz S, Morris E: Management of toxic megacolon: The significance of early recognition in medical management. *J Clin Gastroenterol* 1979; 1:307–311.
26. Meyers S, Lerer K, Feuer J, et al: Predicting the outcome of corticoid therapy for acute ulcerative colitis. Results of a prospective, randomized double-blind clinical trial. *J Clin Gastroenterol* 1987; 9:50–54.
27. Strauss RJ, Flint GW, Platt N, et al: Surgical management of toxic dilatation of the colon. A report of 28 cases and review of the literature. *Ann Surg* 1976; 184:682–688.
28. Flatmark A, Fretheim B, Gjone E: Early colectomy in severe ulcerative colitis. *Scand J Gastroenterol* 1975; 10:427–431.

36

Intestinal Surgery:
How can we choose between pouches and stomas?

KEITH A. KELLY, M.D.
BRUCE G. WOLFF, M.D.

A Brooke ileostomy, while simple and safe to construct, is completely incontinent of both gas and stool. An appliance must be worn day and night to collect the output from the stoma. The appliances are unsightly, uncomfortable, and odoriferous. Embarrassing noises may issue from the stoma during times of fecal discharge. There is also the ever-present danger of leakage at the site of attachment of the appliance to the skin. In addition, the appliances are expensive. Some patients estimate the cost of maintaining the appliance and servicing the ileostomy to be in the neighborhood of $500 per year. Thus, an alternative to the incontinent Brooke ileostomy would be well received.

Until recently, few alternatives were available. Today, however, a number of continence-preserving operations have emerged,[1] the most attractive of which are the ileal pouch–anal anastomosis[2–6] and the continent ileostomy (Kock pouch).[7–9] These newer operations are performed mainly for ulcerative colitis and familial polyposis coli. The operations are not advised for Crohn's disease, because of the risk of recurrence of Crohn's disease in the small bowel remaining after operation. They are done for the intestinal or extraintestinal complications of the colitis and the polyposis coli, and to treat or prevent the development of cancer of the large intestine.

ILEAL POUCH–ANAL ANASTOMOSIS

The current preferred operative approach to ulcerative colitis and familial polyposis coli is colectomy, mucosal rectectomy, and ileal pouch–anal anastomosis. The rationale behind the operation is that it removes the disease via the colectomy and mucosal rectectomy, and yet it preserves anal sphincter function, voluntary transanal defecation, and anal continence. No permanent ileostomy is required. The ileal pouch provides sufficient reservoir to prevent excessive stooling. Moreover, because the mucosal rectectomy is done from the luminal side of the rectum, operative injury of the perirectal nerves to the bladder and genitalia is minimized. Thus, there is little likelihood of postoperative urinary or sexual dysfunction. In addition, the anus and rectum are not excised, so that no perineal wound is present after the procedure, a wound that is sometimes difficult to heal.

Patient Selection

This operation can be done in children, young adults, or middle-aged adults. Patients older than 65 years are less likely to be candidates because their anal sphincters may be less competent than those of younger patients. Patients should have good anal sphincteric function and good continence prior to operation. Anorectal manometry may be useful in determining rectal compliance and sphincter competence and may have some predictive value in the results after ileal pouch–anal anastomosis. Frequently, in patients with a diseased rectum with submucosal scarring, compliance will be low and elasticity will be lost. Fecal urgency and even incontinence can result. This may lead patients to believe they are not candidates for the operation, when in fact they are. In many of these patients, the noncompliant, diseased rectum can be satisfactorily replaced with a nondiseased, compliant ileal pouch.

The patient should not be obese, because the added fat in the ileal mesentery may restrict mobility and prevent a pouch from reaching the anus. In addition, stomas in such patients are difficult to construct and manage. Also, the operation is more likely to be successful if there is no perianal disease, such as an abscess or an anal fistula, and if there has been no previous anal surgery. However, severe illness, inanition, and the taking of corticosteroids do not prevent use of the procedure. The procedure has been safely performed in cases of fulminant colitis but should not be done in patients with toxic megacolon. In these patients, a colectomy, ileostomy, and Hartmann rectal pouch should be performed. At a later time, the ileal pouch–anal anastomosis can be accomplished. The procedure should also not be performed in patients having cancers of the mid or lower rectum, although it can be done in patients with cancers of the proximal rectum or colon, providing these cancers can be completely removed. The 17 such patients in our series have had an acceptable mortality and morbidity and comparable functional results to those of patients without cancer.

Operative Management

The patients are placed on a clear liquid diet the day before operation and given laxatives, enemas, and an antibiotic preparation of neomycin sulfate, 250 mg four times a day, and erythromycin estolate, 250 mg four times a day. Alternatively, a lavage preparation, using 4 to 5 L of Golytely or a similar solution, can be used on the day before operation. The lavage is administered from 11:00 A.M. to 5:00 P.M., and then 2 g of neomycin sulfate and 2 g of metronidazole are given by mouth at 7:00 P.M.. This dose is repeated at 11:00 P.M. The lavage preparation may be tolerated better than the laxative-enema preparation in patients with severe colonic disease or with perianal disease. Also, results from the lavage preparation, in terms of postoperative infection rate, are comparable to the enema preparation. Cephalothin sodium, 0.5 g, is administered intravenously just before the operation, during the operation, and in the immediate postoperative period. This is common practice, although concrete benefit of adding intravenous antibiotics to a mechanical and oral antibiotic preparation has not been clearly shown.

The patient is anesthetized and placed in a modified lithotomy position to provide access to both the abdomen and the perineum.[10] A vertical, midline abdominal incision is made, the abdominal contents are inspected, and the presence of ulcerative colitis or polyposis coli is verified. In many cases, the diagnosis of ulcerative colitis or familial adenomatous polyposis will have been verified preoperatively. In 10% of cases, Crohn's colitis may be mistaken for ulcerative colitis and vice versa. The small bowel should be carefully examined for evidence of Crohn's disease upon initial exploration. In cases where the pathologist is not able to discriminate Crohn's disease from ulcerative colitis (i.e., in cases of indeterminant colitis), the the ileal pouch–anal procedure can still be performed. In our series, these patients have done as well as those with clear-cut ulcerative colitis.

The large intestine is mobilized from the cecum to the levator ani and its blood supply is divided. The mid rectum is stapled closed and transected at a point about 7 cm proximal to the levator ani. The cecum, colon, and proximal rectum are removed. The operator then positions himself at the perineum and injects a solution of Marcaine, hyaluronidase, and epinephrine submucosally into the lower rectum to facilitate removal of the diseased rectal mucosa.[11] The rectal mucosa is stripped from the underlying tunica muscularis and internal anal sphincter using the cautery or scissors. The dissection begins at the dentate line and extends to a point 5 cm orad to the line or to a point at the top of the puborectalis sling and levator ani. At this level, the rectal wall is transected and the rectum proximal to the transection is removed.

The operator returns to the abdominal side where an ileal pouch is constructed from the terminal 30 cm of ileum. The 30 cm are fashioned into the shape of a J, and the anterior and posterior layers of the J is anastomosed using two layers of continuous 2-0 chromic catgut or stainless steel staples (Fig 36–1). With construction of the pouch complete, the most dependant portion of the pouch is brought down endorectally to the anal canal and sewn to the canal at the dentate liner. A proximal diverting loop ileostomy in the right lower quadrant completes the initial operative procedure.

Alternatively, an S-shaped or a W-shaped pouch can be made instead of J-shaped pouch. S-shaped or W-shaped pouches may increase reservoir size and reduce frequency of bowel movements compared to the J pouch, but no clear-cut data are present. The S and W pouches must be hand-sewn, and they often require the use of more small bowel than the J pouch. Care must be taken not to construct an efferent limb longer than 3 cm when using an S pouch; a longer efferent limb may obstruct pouch outflow and so require the patient to intubate in order to empty the pouch.

In centers where the procedure is frequently performed, the proximal diverting ileostomy is sometimes avoided in carefully selected patients.[12, 13] Our criteria are that the patient has minimal rectal disease, has not been on a steroid medication, has an anastomosis completely without tension, and has had a smooth operation. Polyposis patients are more likely to have this option than colitis patients. When no ileostomy is used, a silastic number 28F tube may be inserted transanally into the pouch to decompress the pouch for several days postoperatively.

When an ileostomy is used, the patient is allowed 2 to 3 months to recover from the initial procedure, at which time roentgenographic studies of the ileal pouch and the anastomosis and sometimes anorectal manometry are performed to ascertain the degree of healing and the integrity of anorectal function. A well-healed anastomosis, absence of intrapelvic sepsis or fistulas, and a good anal sphincter indicate that the diverting ileostomy can be closed at a second operation.

After closure of the ileostomy, the patients are placed on loperamide hydrochloride and a psyllium preparation until thickening of the enteric content is obtained and satisfactory stooling frequency is present. These medications usually can be gradually decreased over a 3-month to 4-month period.

The main complications of the operations are perianastomotic sepsis and intestinal obstruction. Perianastomotic sepsis can be minimized by using the bowel preparation outlined above and by constructing the diverting loop ileostomy. Obtaining excellent hemostasis prior to

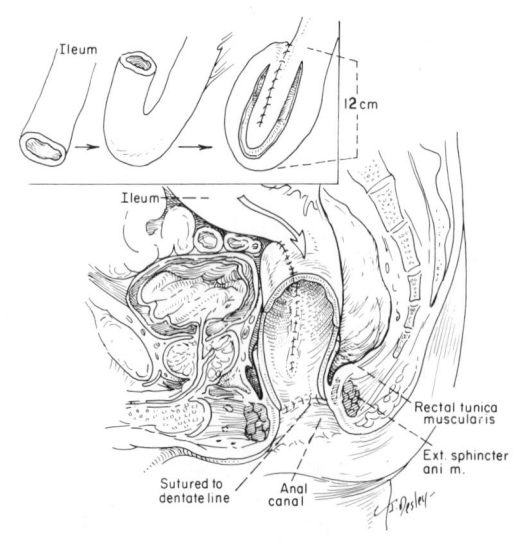

FIG 36–1.
Construction of J-shaped ileal pouch with ileal pouch–anal anastomosis.

closure and the use of the pelvic drain will remove serum and blood in the area of operation and so minimize abscess formation. The drain should be placed well away from the ileal pouch–anal anastomosis so as to not hinder healing of the anastomosis.

Intestinal obstruction is combatted again by careful hemostasis prior to closure; intra-abdominal irrigation to remove necrotic material, debris and blood; and construction of the ileostomy in the right lower quadrant using the loop method. The proximal ileum is positioned intra-abdominally to the left of the stoma, and the distal ileum is placed to the right of the stoma and laterally. This positioning of the bowel helps to prevent herniation of the proximal bowel into the space lateral to the ileostomy. An intestinal tube is also placed into the proximal bowel via the stoma at the operation. The tube prevents kinking and volvulus of the proximal bowel in the early postoperative period, after which the tube is removed.

Outcome

The operation is generally safe. Over 750 patients have been operated on at Mayo in the last 7 years with but one postoperative death—a patient who died of a pulmonary embolism at home 3 weeks after operation. The long-term success of the procedure has also been good, with only 5% of patients having to have a permanent ileostomy reestablished.

In regard to the physiologic outcome, four principal factors regulate fecal continence after the operation: the reservoir capacity of the pouch, the internal and external anal sphincters, the ileal pouch–anal angulation, and the volume and consistency of the stool.[14] The importance of a pouch reservoir was clearly shown several years ago in a study comparing ileoanal anastomosis without a pouch to a similar anastomosis with a pouch.[15] The pouch patients had better continence and fewer stools.

In discussing the anal sphincters, it is important to remember that the anal canal can be divided into either an "anatomical anal canal" or a "surgical anal canal." The anatomical anal canal describes the area from the anal verge to the dentate line, whereas the surgical anal canal also includes the area between the dentate line and the puborectalis sling. The surgical anal canal has a length of 3 to 4 cm. The internal anal sphincter is a thin circular layer of muscle that surrounds the surgical anal canal. It provides a substantial part of the resting tone of the anal canal, perhaps two-thirds. The internal sphincter is carefully preserved during the ileal pouch–anal anastomosis operation, and so resting anal tone is normal, or nearly so.[16] The voluntarily controlled, external anal sphincter, consisting of the puborectalis, the superficial external sphincter, and subcutaneous external sphincter, provides another major mechanism of continence. The external sphincter allows the subject to squeeze the anal canal tightly closed on demand, and so prevent sudden leaks of fecal content. The external anal sphincter is also well preserved by the ileal pouch–anal anastomosis operation.[15, 16]

The anorectal angle, or the angle formed between the anal canal and the rectum, is created by the puborectalis muscle pulling the anorectal junction anteriorly toward the pubis. An angle of 90 degrees or less is formed. The angle acts as a barrier to anal soiling, especially during sudden increases in intra-abdominal pressure. Loss of the angle means a straight channel between rectum and anus, and loss of the barrier to anal soiling. Fortunately, the ileal pouch–anal anastomosis preserves the angle.

The operation, however, does not preserve the fourth factor, the volume and consistency of stool. The volume of the stool is increased fourfold after operation, and the consistency of the stool is decreased. The fecal output of the patients averages about 650 ml per day, and the stool is semisolid or mushy. Both volume and consistency can be controlled to some extent with the addition of the stool bulking agents (psyllium) and drugs that decrease small bowel motility and increase absorption (Imodium). The control, however, is incomplete. The continuing changes in the volume and consistency of stool account to a large extent for the increase in frequency of bowel movements after the operation.

In regard to bowel habit, the patients are nearly always completely continent during the day, when they pass four to eight bowel movements. The patients can usually discriminate gas from feces prior to and during the passage of enteric content. At night during sleep, there may be some minor fecal leakage because of the more fluid nature of the enteric content and the propulsive force of the distal ileal contractions. About one-half of the patients have at least one bowel movement during the night. Bowel habits can also change suddenly should inflammation develop in the pouch, so-called pouchitis. Diarrhea, fever, malaise, and weakness are the main symptoms. About one in seven patients develops this condition, thought to be related to the overgrowth of bacteria in the pouch.[2, 17] The condition can almost always be treated satisfactorily with an antibacterial agent, such as metronidazole, 250 mg given four times per day, after which the symptoms of the pouchitis subside. Recurrent bouts, however, can occur.

In contrast to alterations in bowel habit, sexual function is well preserved and often improved by the operation. The incidence of postoperative impotence among males after the operation is only about 1%. Female patients also enjoy normal sexual and reproductive function. A number have become pregnant and have delivered vaginally without incidence.[18]

In summary, the procedure does achieve its objective of maintaining fecal control without the need for permanent ileostomy and with voluntary transanal passage of fecal content. The main disadvantages of the procedure are frequent bowel movements, occasional leakage of stool at night, and an associated perineal or perianal irritation when leakage does occur. Outcome is based on many factors, including the surgeon's familiarity and experience with the procedure, the hospital support system, including enterostomal therapy, and the patient's own desire to achieve an acceptable result.

THE CONTINENT ILEOSTOMY (KOCK POUCH)

The continent ileostomy or Kock pouch consists of three parts: a pouch made of distal ileum, a valve made of terminal ileum interposed between the pouch and the exterior, and an efferent ileal limb leading from the valve to the stoma.[7] For patients who require an ileostomy, the Kock pouch provides fecal continence and eliminates the need for an ileostomy appliance. The rationale behind the procedure is that the pouch collects and holds fecal content until it is emptied by passing a catheter through the stoma and valve into the pouch. The content then drains through the catheter directly into the toilet bowl, after which the catheter is removed. The catheter is rinsed after its use and placed in a purse to be carried in the patient's pocket during the day. A small dressing is placed over the stoma to prevent mucus secreted by the surface epithelium of the ileum from soiling the clothes. Between intubations, no gas or stool leaks, and so no ileal appliance need be worn. The patient has complete control over fecal discharge.

Patient Selection

This operation is suitable for young or middle-aged adults who already have an incontinent Brooke ileostomy after proctocolectomy for colitis or polyposis coli or who require proctocolectomy and do not wish to have the increased frequency of stooling present with the ileal pouch–anal anastomosis. An example of such a patient is a dental student, recently referred to us for colectomy and restorative surgery, who found it easier to perform his work with the Kock pouch intubation schedule of three times per day, rather than the six movements which might be expected with the ileal pouch–anal anastomosis procedure. Patients must have sufficient understanding, intelligence, and physical dexterity to deal with catheterization and care of the pouch. Thus, children or patients over 70 years of age are often not candidates. Also, construction of a Kock pouch is difficult in obese patients.[8,9]

Operative Management

The operation is done in one stage and is performed with the patient in the modified lithotomy position. The proctocolectomy is accomplished, after which the pouch is fashioned from the terminal 45 cm of ileum. The anterior and posterior walls of the pouch are constructed with two layers of continuous 2-0 chromic catgut. The terminal ileum is intussuscepted into the newly formed pouch for a distance of 5 cm to form the valve (Fig 36–2). The intussuscepted ileum is anchored in place with four cartridges of stainless steel staples, while additional sutures of 4-0 Dacron are taken at the exit of the efferent limb from the pouch to further anchor the valve in place. The efferent ileal limb leading to the stoma is made as short as possible, and the stoma is placed just above the hairline in the right lower quadrant. The pouch is sewn to the anterior abdominal wall just beneath the stoma, again with interrupted 4-0 Dacron sutures. The ileostomy is made flush with the skin. The space lateral to the pouch is closed by approximating the ileal mesentery to the parietal peritoneum of the right lower quadrant of the abdomen. This obviates volvulus of the pouch and peripouch herniation of the more proximal small intestine.

The pouch is intubated for a period of 1 month postoperatively to ensure that the pouch and valve remain in the appropriate position while the fibrous tissue of healing fixes the structures in place. The tube is then removed, and the patient begins intermittent intubation of the pouch. At first, the intubations are done every 2 hours during the day, while the catheter

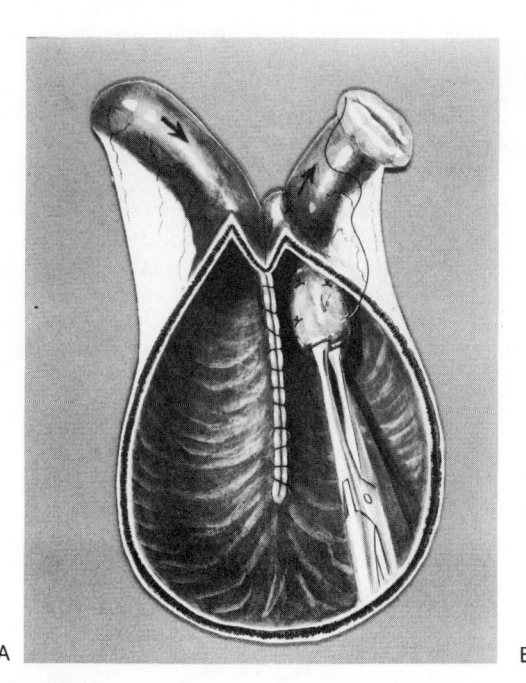

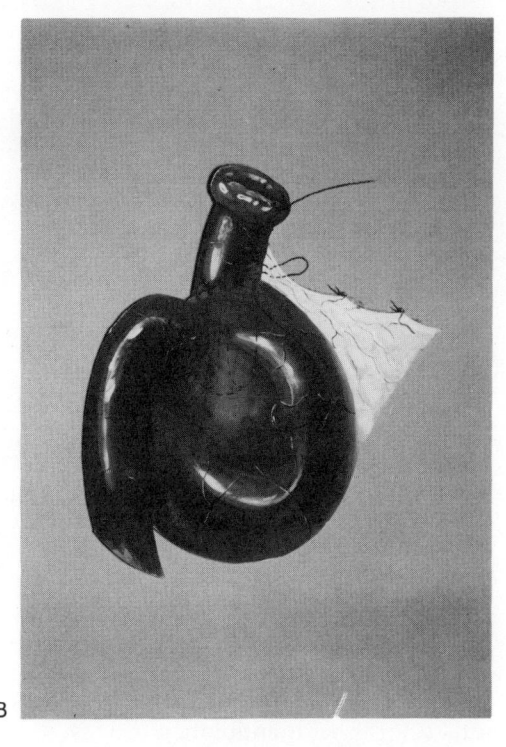

FIG 36–2.
Construction of ileal pouch and valve (Kock pouch) placed in a prestomal location. **A,** a valve is created by intussuscepting the terminal ileum into the newly forming pouch and anchoring the valve in place with sutures or staples (staples not shown). **B,** after closure of the anterior wall of the pouch, additional sutures are taken to fix the efferent limb of the pouch to the adjacent pouch wall.

is left in place continuously overnight. The interval between intubations is increased gradually, until after a second month the patient is intubating the pouch four times a day, but not at night. The patients require no medication and can eat a general diet, providing that they masticate thoroughly. Poorly masticated, indigestible materials, such as mushrooms, kernels of corn, string beans, and cabbage, plug the catheter during intubations and delay emptying.

Outcome

The procedure does achieve its objective of providing complete control over fecal discharge. The patients, however, do have an ileostomy, and they must intubate the ileal pouch to empty it. In addition, two complications of the Kock pouch have appeared: malfunction of the valve and diarrhea.

Malfunction of the valve occurs because the intussusceptum of terminal ileum which forms the valve sometimes reduces partially, resulting in a tortuous tract leading from the pouch to the exterior. The patient then has two problems: difficulty intubating the pouch and leakage of content from the pouch. Reoperation is usually required, at which time the valve must be replaced within the pouch and reanchored with stainless steel staples and sutures. Reoperation is necessary today in about 15% to 20% of patients and is usually successful. However, reoperation does not guarantee that the valve will function perfectly henceforth. A second reoperation may be required in an additional 15% to 20% of patients.

Diarrhea, which occurs in about 5% of patients, likely results from "pouchitis" and bacterial overgrowth in the pouch, just as with the ileal pouch–anal anastomosis operations. The diarrhea, when symptomatic, can usually be managed satisfactorily with antibiotics.

Satisfactory continence in a long-term follow-up of a large group of patients with the Kock pouch has been achieved in 95% of the patients, even though many have had reoperation with nipple valve revision. The procedure remains an alternative, but has given way in our practice to the ileal pouch–anal procedure which is preferred by most patients.

ILEORECTOSTOMY

Ileorectostomy has been used infrequently at Mayo. The operation does not excise the diseased rectal mucosa, which continues to ulcerate, bleed, and cause pain and diarrhea in ulcerative colitis.[19, 20] In addition, the risk of carcinoma developing in the rectal mucosa remains in patients with colitis or familial polyposis coli.

Patient Selection

Nonetheless, there are some patients who have such minimal involvement of the rectum that an ileorectostomy is a reasonbale choice, especially if these patients are young and anxious to avoid any type of ileostomy or the disabilities and minimal risk to sexual or urinary function occasioned by an ileoanal anstomosis.

Operative Management

The operation is done in the supine position through a midline abdominal incision. After excision of the cecum and colon, the ileum is anastomosed end-to-end to the rectum using continuous 3-0 chromic catgut on the mucosal layer and interrupted 4-0 Dacron sutures on the seromuscular layer. Alternative sutures are 3-0 and 4-0 polyglycolic acid sutures. The 25-mm circular stapler can also be used.

Outcome

Less than one-half of patients undergoing this operation will have a satisfactory result over a 5- to 15-year follow-up. Those with a good result experience less than eight bowel movements a day, are continent, require no systemic steroids, and maintain a satisfactory life-style. They require yearly proctoscopic examinations to ascertain the presence or absence of

TABLE 36–1.
Outcome of Operations for Ulcerative Colitis and Polyposis Coli

Procedure	Fecal Continence Preserved	Stoma Present	Intubations Required	Disadvantages
Brooke ileostomy	No	Yes	No	Ileostomy bag required
Ileal pouch–anal anastomosis	Yes	No	No	Frequent stooling, occasional fecal leakage
Kock pouch	Yes	Yes	Yes	Valve malfunction, diarrhea
Ileorectostomy	Yes	No	No	Rectal mucosa may cause symptoms, develop cancer

continuing inflammation in their rectal mucosa and also to check for dysplasia, polyps, or other signs of malignancy in this mucosa. The other one-half of the patients have more disabling symptoms that require treatment, threaten life, and may eventually mandate excision of the remaining rectal mucosa.

SUMMARY

The pros and cons of the various operations for ulcerative colitis and familial polyposis coli are outlined in Table 36–1. On the balance, we advise and most patients elect ileal pouch–anal anastomosis. Its major advantages, which include total excision of the disease, avoidance of the ileostomy, maintenance of voluntary transanal defecation, and reasonable continence, recommend it over the other options.

References

1. Dozois RR: *Alternatives to Conventional Ileostomy,* Chicago, Year Book Medical Publishers, Inc. 1985.
2. Utsunomiya J, Iwama J, Imaho H, et al: Total colectomy, mucosal proctectomy and ileoanal anastomosis. *Dis Colon Rectum* 1900; 23:459–466.
3. Parks AG, Nicholls RJ, Belliveau P: Restorative proctocolectomy with ileal reservoir and ileoanal anastomosis. *Br J Surg* 1980; 67:533–538.
4. Metcalf AM, Dozois RR, Kelly KA, et al: Ileal "J" pouch–anal anastomosis: Clinical outcome. *Ann Surg* 1985; 202:735–739.
5. Nicholls RJ, Lubowski DZ: Restorative proctocolectomy: The four loop (W) reservoir. *Br J Surg* 1987; 74:564–566.
6. Pemberton JH, Kelly KA, Beart RW Jr, et al: Ileal pouch–anal anastomosis for chronic ulcerative colitis: Long-term results. *Ann Surg,* 206:504–513, 1987.
7. Kock N, Darle H, Hulten L, et al: Ileostomy. *Curr Probl Surg* 1977; 14:1–52.
8. Dozois RR, Kelly KA, Beart RW Jr, et al: Improved results with continent ileostomy. *Ann Surg* 1980; 192:319–324.
9. Dozois RR, Kelly KA, Ilstrup D, et al: Factors affecting revision rate after continent ileostomy. *Arch Surg* 1981; 116:610–613.
10. Ballantyne GH, Pemberton JH, Beart RW Jr, et al: Ileal J pouch–anal anastomosis: Current technique. *Dis Colon Rectum* 1985; 28:197–202.
11. O'Connell PR, Pemberton JH, Weiland LH, et al: Does rectal mucosa regenerate after ileoanal anastomosis: *Dis Colon Rectum* 1987; 30:1–5.
12. Metcalf AM, Dozois RR, Kelly KA, et al: Ileal pouch–anal anstomosis without temporary, diverting ileostomy. *Dis Colon Rectum* 1986; 29:33–35.
13. Metcalf AM, Dozois RR, Beart RW Jr, et al: Temporary ileostomy for ileal pouch–anal anastomosis: Function and complications. *Dis Colon Rectum 1986;* 29:300–303.
14. Beart RW Jr, Dozois RR, Wolff BG, et al: Mechanisms of rectal continence: Lessons from the ileoanal procedure. *Am J Surg* 1985; 149:3134.
15. Taylor BM, Cranley B, Kelly KA, et al: A clinicophysiological comparison of ileal pouch–anal and straight ileoanal anastomoses. *Ann Surg* 1983; 198:462–468.
16. O'Connell PR, Pemberton JH, Brown ML, et al: Determinants of stool frequency after ileal pouch–anal anastomosis. *Am J Surg* 1987; 153:157–164.
17. O'Connell PR, Rankin DR, Weiland LH, et al: Enteric bacteriology, absorption, morphology and emptying after ileal pouch–anal anastomosis. *Br J Surg* 1986; 73:909–914.
18. Metcalf AM, Dozois RR, Beart RW Jr, et al: Pregnancy following ileal pouch–anal anastomosis. *Dis Colon Rectum* 1985; 28:859–861.
19. Farnell MB, Van Heerden JA, Beart RW Jr, et al: Rectal preservation in nonspecific inflammatory disease of the colon. *Ann Surg* 1980; 192:249–253.
20. Wolff BG, Beahrs OH: Preservation of the anorectum. *Adv Surg* 1984; 18:1–35.

Colon Cancer:
Which therapeutic measures prolong life?

NICHOLAS J. PETRELLI, M.D., F.A.C.S.
LEMUEL HERRERA, M.D., F.A.C.S.

This year colorectal carcinoma will be the second leading cause of cancer deaths in males and the third leading cause in females. Approximately 60,000 persons will die from the disease in the ensuing 12 months. The American Cancer Society statistics states that the survival rates for colorectal carcinoma following surgical resection have not changed significantly during the past four decades.[1] However, these statistics are misleading and do not take into consideration the individual stages of the disease. The title of this chapter asks the question "Which therapeutic measures prolong life?". The answer to this question is a simple one: Surgery will prolong life in patients with primary colorectal carcinoma and in a subgroup of patients with distant metastases spcifically liver, lung, and local perineal pelvic recurrence.

Another question this chapter will attempt to answer is: "Which therapeutic measures can improve the quality of life of a patient with colon carcinoma?". A review of the present status of chemotherapy in metastatic colon carcinoma will also be discussed.

Adenomatous polyps will be reviewed because these lesions establish an environment in which their removal may decrease the subsequent development of colon carcinoma. This has already been shown in a nonrandomized study by Gilbertsen[2] in which the prophylactic excision of adenomatous polyps of the rectosigmoid led to a reduction in the incidence of carcinoma. With the era of fiberoptic endoscopy, polypectomy has become a common procedure.

THE SIGNS AND SYMPTOMS OF COLON CANCER: ARE THEY SPECIFIC FOR THIS DISEASE?

There is no question that the public lacks confidence that colorectal cancer can be detected early. People correctly recognize that colorectal cancer cannot be prevented. As a result, the public distinguishes between colon cancers and cancers of the lung and skin which can be prevented by specific behavioral measures such as avoiding cigarette smoking or overexposure to sunlight. It is not uncommon for even physicians to believe that once a colon cancer is diagnosed, its growth is fairly well advanced and survival chances remain poor. However, survival rates with early detection are perceived to be more pessimistic than the facts would support. Public attitudes can be corrected with educational programs on colon cancer and with the help of community physicians.

National programs sponsored through the American Cancer Society can make the public aware of the signs and symptoms of colorectal carcinoma. Table 37–1 lists the signs and symptoms of colorectal cancer. However, physicians and the public assume that these signs and symptoms are due to benign conditions such as diverticulosis, hemorrhoids, or irritable bowel syndrome. If one looks at the signs and symptoms of right-sided colon cancer one would have to admit that these are nonspecific except for a palpable mass in the right lower quadrant which would lead to the suspicion of a carcinoma. The vague dull uncharacteristic pain and anemia are nonspecific and certainly can be related to other disease processes. In reviewing the signs and symptoms of left-sided colon cancer, the most specific signs are bright red blood coating the surface of the stool and a decrease in stool caliber. Acute large bowel obstruction can certainly be due to carcinoma but also diverticulitis. The signs and symptoms of rectal carcinoma are nonspecific. The most outstanding sign is that of blood on the stool. Our belief at Roswell Park Memorial Institute is that although the majority of these signs and symptoms are nonspecific, patients in their fourth, fifth, sixth, and early seventh decade should have a full evaluation of their large bowel to rule out carcinoma.

The stool blood test is a relatively simple and inexpensive procedure to detect hidden blood (discussed in Chap 38). The present problem with the stool blood test is that it cannot distinguish between human and animal blood. However, present research to solve this dilemma is ongoing at Roswell Park Memorial Institute in collaboration with Smith Kline Diagnostics, Inc.

Despite the nonspecificity of the majority of signs and symptoms in colon cancer, the clinical picture in right and left colon carcinoma correlates with the pathophysiologic features. For example, right colonic tumors are usually polypoid and exophytic in nature and have a tendency for chronic bleeding subsequently leading to anemia. Left colonic lesions are usually ulcerative and annular in character, and because the lumen of the sigmoid colon is narrower than that of the cecum, patients with sigmoid lesions often present with large bowel obstruction.

Physicians in their daily practice may have noted a change in the signs and symptoms of colon cancer due to a shift in tumor sites. In addition to the increase in the incidence of colorectal carcinoma in the United States, statistics from Tumor Registries of the National Cancer Institute and other agencies have shown a shift from left- to right-sided lesions.[3] Between 1940 and the early 1970s the incidence of colonic cancer rose higher than that of rectal carcinoma. In the past 30 years, the incidence of right colonic involvement has increased. Several explanations have been offered for this left-to-right shift: the formation of a new environmental agent, the late expression of carcinogens affecting the right colon, a shift in the age distribution of the at-risk population, or an absolute decrease in the incidence of left colon cancers. The reason for this shift appears to be academic at the present

TABLE 37–1.
Signs and Symptoms of Colorectal Cancer

Right Colon	Left Colon	Rectal
Pain—Vague/dull	Pain—Cramping	Pain is a late feature
Stool—Mixed with dark or mahogany-colored blood	Stool—Surface coated with bright red blood; decrease caliber	Stool—Surface coated with bright red blood
Anemia	Change in bowel habits; increased use of laxatives	Tenesmus
Mass—Right lower quadrant	Large bowel obstruction, abdominal distention, pain, vomiting, constipation	

time, and early detection and close follow-up of patients at high risk for the development of colon cancer must be a priority in the medical community.

Our recommendations for asymptomatic individuals in terms of large bowel evaluation are similar to those of the American Cancer Society (Table 37–2).

ADENOMATOUS POLYPS: AN OPPORTUNITY TO PREVENT THE DEVELOPMENT OF COLORECTAL CARCINOMA

It is currently accepted that the vast majority of colonic cancers arise in preexistent adenomatous polyps. However, polyp (Greek—*Polypous:* a morbid excrescence) is a clinical term that refers to any protruding growth from the mucous lining of the colon. The origin of colonic cancer in adenomatous polyps may be divided into direct and indirect evidence. Direct evidence is the observation of minute cancers within adenomas or of adenomatous changes in larger carcinomas. The main reason the changes are not seen is because as the carcinoma grows, it destroys the premalignant adenoma. Also, numerous block sections made from large carcinomas will show evidence of residual adenoma. Indirect evidence is provided by epidemiologic studies. They have demonstrated a correlation between the incidence of adenoma and carcinomas in low and high incidence areas of the world. If adenomas precede carcinomas one would expect them to occur at an earlier age. Indeed, the incidence of adenomas is at a maximum 7 to 8 years earlier than the carcinoma.

TABLE 37–2.
Recommendations for Large Bowel Evaluation in Asymptomatic Individuals

1. Men and women over the age of 40 years should have a rectal examination every year.
2. Men and women over the age of 50 should have a stool blood test every year.
3. Men and women over the age of 50 should have a sigmoidoscopic (preferably 65-cm flexible endoscopy) examination every 3 to 5 years after two initial negative examinations 1 year apart.

Retrospective studies have confirmed that the adenoma, regardless of size, histologic type (tubular, villous, or tubulovillous) or its degree of dysplasia (mild, moderate, or severe) is a marker for increased cancer risk. This is not surprising in view of our experience with familial adenomatous polyposis where the risk of cancer with time reaches 100%. If the adenomas contribute significantly to the development of carcinomas one would expect that their systemic removal would result in a reduction in the expected number of carcinomas. Indeed, Gilbertsen has reported his experience with proctosigmoidoscopy which over the last decade has accumulated 100,000 patient years. In his experience only 13 cancers of the rectal ampulla have been found, and 8 were confined to the mucosa and could be termed "in situ." Four cancers invaded the submucosa, and only one invaded the muscular layer. These 13 cancers are significantly less than one would expect statistically. Not one person who has entered the program of annual physical examinations with proctosigmoidoscopy has died of rectal cancer in 30 years, and no rectal cancer has surfaced for an additional 8 years after patients have left the program.[2]

Although de novo carcinomas can occur, they are more likely to occur in experimental models and are rare at the clinical level. The mechanism of direct dysplasia is only operative in exceptional circumstances. However, this may pertain to those unusual families who present with a predisposition for a high incidence of colorectal cancer associated with an autosomal dominant inheritance, absence of synchronous adenomatous polyps, prevalence of right-sided colon lesions, and young age. This is the so-called cancer family syndrome.

We and others have previously indicated that patients in whom colorectal cancers and synchronous adenomatous polyps are demonstrated are at an increased risk for developing metachronous polyps and cancer. Close postoperative surveillance of the colon is imperative because there is a risk of new polyp formation with malignant degeneration. The rationale behind this surveillance is that detection and removal of metachronous neoplasias may produce results similar to those of Gilbertsen. Changes toward a smaller size and to a more differentiated histology of lesions removed during follow-up endoscopy indicate that prevention of metachronous cancer is possible. Colon cancer is a potentially multicentric disease. Therefore, one should expect a certain number of patients to develop a second metachronous tumor. The problem is to identify those groups of patients at high risk for developing a subsequent cancer. One has to consider this risk against the potential morbidity or mortality of an abdominal colectomy versus a segmental colectomy, periodic colonoscopy, and follow-up compliance. The size and distribution of polyps, and the presence of atypical changes or carcinomas in situ are factors that also must be carefully weighed. A subtotal colectomy leaving 15 to 20 cm of rectosigmoid will remove the diseased organ leaving the patient with a tolerable number of stools and no impairment of bladder or sexual function, and will result in a large bowel easy to follow with proctosigmoidoscopy, a more cost-effective method than colonoscopy.

Biopsy followed by endoscopic polypectomy has become the procedure of choice in the initial management of colonic adenomatous polyps. A problem may arise if the final pathologic examination demonstrates a carcinoma. If the carcinoma is in situ, then no further treatment is necessary. Malignant cells deep to the muscularis mucosa and into the submucosa denote an invasive carcinoma. This lesion has been labeled as "early" invasive cancer because only 10% to 15% have been found to have metastases to lymph nodes. Based on these figures, some physicians consider endoscopic resection a curative treatment especially when there is a margin free of cancer, a well-differentiated cancer, and no vascular invasion. We believe that many of these lesions have been previously understaged due to the lack of recognition of metastases to small lymph nodes, and, therefore, we recommend a standard colon resection to ensure the removal of any involved regional lymph nodes in physically fit patients.

In summary, there is a well-established body of evidence that indicates that the sequence of adenoma to carcinoma occurs in the large bowel. This is relevant not only in the pathogenesis of colorectal cancer, but it has implications in the postoperative management of patients who have undergone surgery with a curative intent for a previous cancer and for patients in whom an adenomatous polyp discloses a biologic predisposition for neoplastic development of the large bowel.

IS ADJUVANT TREATMENT NECESSARY FOLLOWING SURGERY?

Tumor recurrence in patients with colorectal cancer represented by either local or distant metastases must be attributed to our current failure to detect foci of micrometastases already present at the time of the initial surgery. For the physician who has experienced this event, there is a compelling urge to do something in addition to the surgery in an effort to increase treatment effectiveness.

The patterns of recurrence found at second look surgery indicate that from transverse colon 38% are locoregional, 13% are peritoneal seedings, and 25% are disseminated metastases. From primary carcinomas of the cecum, 49% are locoregional, 16% are peritoneal seedings, and 30% are widely disseminated metastases. From the ascending and descending colon, recurrences are 50% locoregional, 28% peritoneal seedings, and 30% disseminated metastases. Thus, it is clear that the pattern of recurrence may be affected by the administration of an effective systemic cytotoxic drug following surgery of the primary colon cancer.

The basic concept of adjuvant chemotherapy after the eradication of all gross tumor is appealing because of its simplicity. If recurrences are caused by undetected foci of tumor cells and if they can be reached by a cytotoxic drug, then they could be destroyed. Experimentally, a small focus of tumor is much more easily destroyed as compared to large bulky tumors. The introduction of fluorinated pyrimidines in 1958 signaled a breakthrough in the management of gastrointestinal cancer. Since then 5-fluorouracil (5-FU) has become the standard drug for advanced colorectal cancer. Most physicians accept a response rate of only 20% to 25% and often short-lived (9 months). Other chemotherapeutic agents such as methyl CCNU and mitomycin C have also shown evidence of activity, however, their close therapeutic toxicity ratio associated with a low response rate precludes clinical use on a large scale either singly or in combination. Studies in which 5-FU has been used for advanced colon carcinoma in addition to either mitomycin C or methyl CCNU have demonstrated that there is no additive effect whereas the toxicity has been found synergistic and not well tolerated.

The Gastrointestinal Tumor Study Group (GITSG) reported a four-arm adjuvant colon study carried out from 1975 to 1979. It included 621 patients with a modified Dukes' stage: B_2—tumor through the bowel wall; C_1—one to four lymph nodes positive; and C_2—five or more lymph nodes with metastases regardless of bowel wall penetration by tumor. Patients were randomized following surgery to receive (1) 5-fluourouracil (5-FU) and semustine (methyl-CCNU), (2) methanol extraction residue (MER) bacille Calmette Guérin (BCG), (3) 5-FU, methyl-CCNU and MER, or (4) surgery alone. The treatment groups continued for 70 weeks. The results at 5 years revealed that the recurrence rate and survival were not significantly different in all groups. This prospective study also demonstrated a 5-year survival of the Dukes' B_2 control group of 77% rather than the historical control survival of 45%. Had a historical population been chosen as a "control" group for the treated patients, a conclusion of the effectiveness of treatment against colon cancer could have been reached. Also, this study led to the conclusion that only patients with surgically resected colon cancer and positive lymph nodes should be included in adjuvant chemotherapy trials because these individuals are the highest risk for recurrence. Other adjuvant studies such as the Southwest Oncology Group (SWOG) included 626 patients who were randomized to surgery alone, surgery plus 5-FU and methyl-CCNU with or without BCG. Again, no overall difference in survival was seen at the 7-year median follow-up. A study conducted by the National Surgical Adjuvant Breast and Bowel Project (NSABP) randomized 6,166 patients to surgery alone versus surgery plus BCG or MOF (methyl-CCNU, vincristine (oncovin), and 5-FU). At the 5-year median follow-up there is a suggested disease-free survival advantage in the adjuvant chemotherapy arm. At present, we feel strongly that the use of adjuvant chemotherapy following surgery for colon cancer should only be offered to patients entered into a prospectively randomized trial after appropriate histologic stratification.

Before embarking on a study of adjuvant therapy one has to clearly define its objectives taking into consideration all prognostic variables. The importance of optimal stratification of patients by disease stage and the knowledge of the therapeutic limitations cannot be underscored enough. Patient stratification is affected by (1) the biologic characteristics of the malignancy, (2) the histologic stage of the tumor, and (3) the performance of a skillful surgical procedure that accomplishes the complete removal of the primary cancer and its lymphovascular anatomy. One must fully realize that the vast majority of patients with Dukes' A and B carcinomas can be cured by surgery alone, therefore it is not justified to include them in an adjuvant treatment protocol.

It is also important to underline that the goal of adjuvant therapy is to significantly prolong survival while maintaining an acceptable quality of life. Therefore, all adjuvant protocols must clearly set timely evaluations to judge the effect of therapy on overall survival, the disease-free interval, and the patient's quality of life.

In summary, the current status of adjuvant chemotherapy for colon cancer must be regarded as investigational. The main reason for its primitive stage of development is the lack of a drug with a predictable high response rate and tolerable toxicity.

CHEMOTHERAPY FOR METASTATIC COLON CARCINOMA: IS IT WORTH GIVING?

None of the chemotherapeutic trials applied to metastatic colon cancer in the literature has shown an improvement in survival. Whether this changes with the era of biochemical modulation, which will be discussed further in this section, can only be answered with maturation of presently ongoing controlled trials.

Pending these controlled trials in biochemical modulation, we at Roswell Park Memorial Institute still consider 5-fluorouracil (5-FU) the standard chemotherapeutic agent for the treatment of advanced colon carcinoma. The fact that this agent is suboptimal makes the problem even more frustrating. Other single chemotherapeutic agents have been tried inclusive of drug combinations with 5-fluorouracil, resulting in no success. Contradictory experiences have been reported within all these therapeutic programs, and none of them has shown an advantage over 5-fluorouracil alone.

5-Fluorouracil has been given as an intravenous bolus, orally, as a continuous infusion, and even intralumenally for colon cancer with a wide range of responses. However, in controlled trials, the objective response rates have ranged between 15% and 20% demonstrating its suboptimal activity.[4-11] In the past the most common used schedule has been 450 mg/m^2 intravenous bolus for 5 days repeated every 5 weeks.

Every conceivable drug has been tried to increase the response rates in patients with metastatic colon carcinoma. However, essentially all have been failures. Among these agents mitomycin C, the nitrosoureas, and methotrexate have been the most common. Since its introduction, mitomycin C has exhibited an objective response rate at least equal to 5-fluorouracil.[12] However, the most serious drawback to the use of mitomycin C has been its ability to produce prolonged hematologic suppression and occasional renal injury. Although a number of schedules have been tried in an attempt to reduce this toxicity, the most common is 10 to 20 mg/m^2 intravenous once every 6 weeks. Toxicity may be seen as early as after the second course of treatment. The nitrosoureas, consisting of CCNU, methyl-CCNU, BCNU, and streptozotocin, have had even more extensive use in clinical trials. The Mayo Clinic has been the most active in evaluating these agents in metastatic colon carcinoma.[13] However, in previously untreated patients a response rate of only 10% to 15% has been noted. The dose-limiting toxicity for the nitrosoureas has been myelosuppression with renal toxicity, nausea and vomiting having limited the more extensive use of streptozotocin. Recently, another potential serious toxicity associated with methyl-CCNU reported in an adjuvant trial has been acute myelogenous leukemia.[14]

No combination of agents has been superior to 5-fluorouracil alone for metastatic colon carcinoma.[15-20] The most widely used chemotherapeutic combinations have been 5-fluorouracil, vincristine, and methyl-CCNU (MOF); methotrexate, Oncovin, 5-fluorouracil, and streptozotocin (MOF-STREP); and 5-fluorouracil and cisplatin.[21-23]

After three unsuccessful decades of trying to find an agent or combination of agents that would improve the survival of patients with metastatic colon carcinoma, the era of biochemical modulation has arrived. The therapeutic activity of 5-fluorouracil in colon carcinoma may be enhanced by increasing the tumor cell reduced folate pools in vivo.[24-27] One of the mechanisms of action of 5-FU is its conversion into fluorodeoxyuridylate (FdUMP), which inhibits thymidylate synthetase (TS). FdUMP binds tightly to TS in the presence of the cofactor L-5, 10-methylene tetrahydrofolate (CH_2FH_4). High levels of inhibition of TS and a slow recovery of this enzyme activity can occur only in the presence of sufficient intracellular concentrations of reduced folates.

The initial work with biochemical modulation in patients with metastatic colorectal carcinoma was reported by Machover et al.[27] In view of this study, our group at Roswell Park Memorial Institute completed a phase I–II trial of 5-fluorouracil and leucovorin (folinic acid) in which partial responses were seen in 9 of 23 patients (38%).[26] The recommended dose of 5-FU for a phase III study was 600 mg/m^2 and leucovorin 500 mg/m^2 weekly for 6 weeks followed by a 2-week rest period. The leucovorin was given as an intravenous 2-hour infusion, and 1 hour after this infusion was begun the 5-fluorouracil was given as an intravenous bolus. A completed phase III study with 74 previously untreated patients with metastatic colorectal carcinoma has been published.[28] Table 37-3 illustrates the three regimens of randomization. The combined complete and partial response rates in the three regimens were 11%, 5%, and 48%, respectively ($p = 0.0009$). The median duration of response in the 5-fluorouracil and leucovorin regimen was 10 months. However, there was no statistically significant difference between the treatment regimens with respect to survival ($p = 0.6$). Also, the toxicity in the 5-fluorouracil and leucovorin regimen was predominantly diarrhea as opposed to myelosuppression in the 5-fluorouracil alone regimen and the 5-fluorouracil and methotrexate regimen. Perhaps the reason that no improvement in survival time was noted was the fact that one would not expect survival to be effected by a treatment program that does not produce significant numbers of complete responses.

Other investigators have reported various regimens in which 5-fluorouracil and reduced folates (leucovorin) were administered to colorectal patients with varying responses.[24, 29-32] However, the majority of these reports reveal response rates double that of 5-fluorouracil alone.

Despite these encouraging response rates with the modulation of 5-fluorouracil and leucovorin we at Roswell Park Memorial Institute still feel that this drug program is investigational. The question of whether 5-fluorouracil and leucovorin will replace 5-fluorouracil alone as the standard treatment for metastatic colorectal carcinoma can hopefully be answered by a present ongoing prospective multicenter phase III trial organized by the Gastrointestinal Tumor Study Group. Originally this trial consisted of the four regimens illustrated in Table 37-4. Regimen number two of this phase III trial has been stopped, and patient accrual was closed June 1, 1987.

REGIONAL LIVER INFUSION: IS IT STANDARD TREATMENT?

The development of hepatic metastases will occur in 20% of the 60,000 patients who will die from advanced colorectal carcinoma in a year. A small percentage of patients will be able to undergo surgical resection for liver metastases, however, the majority of patients at the time of diagnosis of liver metastases will have surgically unresectable disease. In approaching unresectable liver metastases there are basically three treatment modes: (1) systemic chemotherapy which has been described previously in this chapter, (2) hepatic artery infusion with a portable

TABLE 37-3.
Phase III Study of 74 Previously Untreated Patients With Metastatic Colorectal Carcinoma

1. 5-Fluorouracil 450 mg/m^2 as an intravenous bolus daily for 5 days or toxicity, then 200 mg/m^2 intravenous bolus every other day for six doses every 4 weeks
2. Methotrexate 50 mg/m^2 as an intravenous infusion over 4 hr followed by an intravenous bolus of 5-fluorouracil 600 mg/m^2 administered weekly for 4 weeks then every 2 weeks
3. Leucovorin 500 mg/m^2 in a 2-hr intravenous infusion with 5-fluorouracil 600 mg/m^2 as an intravenous bolus 1 hr after the leucovorin every week for six weeks

TABLE 37-4.
Gastrointestinal Tumor Study Group Phase III Trial

1. 5-Fluorouracil alone 500 mg/m^2 intravenous bolus days 1-5 with escalation every 4 weeks
2. 5-Fluorouracil 1000 mg/m^2 intravenous bolus beginning 1 hr after leucovorin 25 mg/m^2 given as a 10-min infusion every 3 weeks. This regimen had escalating doses of leucovorin to 250 mg/m^2 and subsequently 500 mg/m^2
3. 5-Fluorouracil 600 mg/m^2 intravenous bolus beginning 1 hr after leucovorin 500 mg/m^2 in a 2-hr infusion weekly for six weeks
4. 5-Fluorouracil 600 mg/m^2 intravenous bolus beginning 1 hr after leucovorin 25 mg/m^2 as a 10-min infusion weekly for 6 weeks

pump, implantable pump, or percutaneously, and (3) hepatic artery ligation alone or with dearterialization or hyperthermia or concomitant chemotherapy infusion.

The question of how best to deal with unresectable liver metastases from adenocarcinomas of the colon and rectum is very often faced by the practicing physician, and, despite the extremely widespread nature of this problem, this question for the most part does not have a definitive answer. No prospective randomized trials of the above three approaches have been reported, and no large series exist for some of these forms of treatment. Where trials have been done, patient populations and criteria of response have varied widely.

It is clear, despite the presence of other organ involvement, that hepatic metastases exert a substantial adverse influence on the course of the underlying disease in the above patients. Hepatic metastases are present in 40% to 80% of patients at autopsy, and, in a significant number of these patients, this regional metastases causes morbidity and eventual death. Thus, the thinking is that successful treatment of liver metastases may provide palliation for many patients despite the presence of other sites of metastases and may increase the possibility of cure for the few patients having unresectable tumor confined to the liver.

There have been numerous series in the literature concerning intra-arterial chemotherapy using an implantable pump.[33-37] Phase II studies for colorectal liver metastases with a totally implantable pump reveal response rates in the range of 29% to 88% with a median duration of response from 6 to 13 months. One of the most important reasons for the variability in response rates is that total liver perfusion has not been adequately documented in many of the series. Also, modifications in the regimens because of toxicity can be expected to alter the response rates.

Despite these problems, the chemotherapeutic intra-arterial approach for liver metastases from colorectal carcinoma is attractive because of the ability to deliver a high dose of drug to a particular target organ (liver) without subsequent development of systemic side effects (e.g., myelosuppression). However, local regional toxicity, such as biliary sclerosis and gastroduodenal ulcers, has been noted.[35, 37, 38] These studies also have illustrated that there are certain patient prognostic factors which must be taken into account when comparing different treatment modalities. These are liver function tests, specifically alkaline phosphatase and total bilirubin; the performance status of the patient; the presence of extrahepatic intra-abdominal metastases as opposed to liver metastases alone; and the degree of liver replacement by metastases at the time of laparotomy.

More importantly, in the series of trials using the implantable pump for intra-arterial chemotherapy, the relapse sites of metastases revealed a large number of patients failing in sites other than the liver. For example, in the series by Niederhuber and co-workers,[37] 78% of patients failed in the lung and porta hepatis. The report by Balch and co-workers[33] revealed the majority of patients relapsed in the lung. Of the patients who showed evidence of tumor progression, only 23% of them progressed in liver alone.

Recently the Northern California Oncology Group randomized trial compared intravenous Floxuridine (FUDR) and intra-arterial FUDR in 143 patients with liver metastases alone from colorectal carcinoma.[39] The intravenous group consisted of 76 patients receiving FUDR 0.75 mg/kg/day for 14 days, and the intra-arterial FUDR group consisted of 67 patients receiving FUDR 0.2 mg/kg/day for 14 days through an implantable pump. Of these 143 patients, 110 were evaluated for response, toxicity, and time to progression. Six of 59 patients in the intravenous regimen were responders (10%), whereas 19 of 51 patients were responders in the intra-arterial regimen (37%) ($p < 0.002$). The median time to liver progression was 7 months in the intravenous group and 22 months in the intra-arterial group ($p < 0.0003$). It is too early to report survival data.

The bottom line is that a new systemic drug or combination is needed for the treatment of advanced colorectal carcinoma. Whether the biochemical modulation of 5-fluorouracil with leucovorin will be the answer to this problem can only be solved with time. At present, one must still consider the intra-arterial administration of chemotherapy to the liver via an implantable pump as investigational.

Since better control of liver tumor has been achieved, distant disease in other organ systems has clearly become a greater factor in determining survival. This again emphasizes the systemic nature of colorectal carcinoma and the need for multimodality treatment. The reason for the propensity of metastases to the liver remains speculative but among the various factors are (1) routes of blood flow, (2) selective portal venous filtration before pulmonary filtration, (3) a selectivity for the particular organ by various cellular features as yet unknown that allows cells to "home" in on specific target organs, (4) angioneogenesis, (5) trauma both mechanical and chemical, and (6) host immunologic factors.

SUMMARY

It is obvious from this overview of therapeutic measures that may prolong life in colon cancer that the primary modality that may prolong life is surgery, especially in primary disease. The development of national screening programs to detect this disease at an early stage and a premalignant stage will contribute to improved survival. The contribution of the biochemical modulation of 5-fluorouracil (5-FU) and leucovorin in advanced colon carcinoma to increased survival will soon be determined with completed trials. Regional liver infusion for metastases cannot be considered standard treatment, and patients should be treated in a controlled trial environment.

References

1. Silverberg E, Lubera J: Cancer statistics. *CA* 1987; 37:2–19.
2. Gilbertsen VA: Proctosigmoidoscopy and polypectomy in reducing the incidence of rectal cancer. *Cancer* 1974; 34:936–939.
3. Greene FL: Distribution of colorectal neoplasms: A left to right shift of polyps and cancer. *Am Surg* 1983; 49:62–65.
4. Douglass HO Jr, Lavin PT, Woll J, et al: Chemotherapy of advanced measurable colon and rectal carcinoma with oral 5-fluorouracil, alone or in combination with cyclophosphamide or 6-thioguanine, with intravenous 5-fluorouracil or beta-2'-deoxythioguanosine or with oral 1(2-chlorethyl)-1-nitrosourea. A phase II–III study of the Eastern Cooperative Oncology Group (EST 4273). *Cancer* 1978; 42:2538–2545.
5. Hahn RG, Moertel CG, Schutt AJ: A double-blind comparison of intensive course 5-fluorouracil by oral vs. intravenous route in the treatment of colorectal carcinoma. *Cancer* 1975; 35:1031–1035.
6. Bateman JR, Pugh RP, Cassidy FR: 5-Fluorouracil given once weekly: Comparison of intravenous and oral administration. *Cancer* 1971; 28:907–913.
7. Engstrom P, MacIntrye J, Mittelman A, et al: Chemotherapy of advanced colorectal carcinoma with 5-fluorouracil alone vs 2 drug combination using 5-FU, hydroxyurea, semustine, decarbazine, razoxane, mitomycin. A phase III trial by the Eastern Cooperative Oncology Group (EST 1278). *Am J Clin Oncol* 1984; 7:313–318.
8. Moertel CG, Schutt AJ, Reitemeier RJ, et al: Comparison of 5-fluorouracil administered by slow injection and rapid injection. *Cancer Res* 1972; 32:2717–2719.
9. Seifert P, Baker LH, Reed ML, et al: Comparison of continuously infused 5-fluorouracil with bolus injection in treatment of patients with colorectal adenocarcinoma. *Cancer* 1975; 36:123–125.
10. Ansfield F, Klotz J, Nealon T, et al: A phase III study comparing the clinical utility of four regimens of 5-fluorouracil. A preliminary report. *Cancer* 1977; 39:34–40.
11. Lahiri SR, Boileau G, Hall TC: Treatment of metastatic carcinoma with 5-fluorouracil by mouth. *Cancer* 1971; 29:902–906.
12. Crooke ST, Bradner WT: Mitomycin C: A review. *Cancer Treat Rep* 1976; 3:121–139.
13. Moertel CG: Clinical management of advanced gastrointestinal cancer. *Cancer* 1975; 36:675–682.
14. Gastrointestinal Tumor Study Group: Adjuvant therapy of colon cancer—Results of a prospectively randomized trial. *N Engl J Med* 1984; 310:737–743.
15. Kemeny N, Yagoda A, Braun D Jr: A randomized study of two different schedules of methyl-CCNU, 5-FU and vincristine for metastatic colorectal carcinoma. *Cancer* 1979; 43:78–82.
16. Lokich JJ, Skarin AT, Mayer RJ, et al: Lack of effectiveness of combined 5-fluorouracil and methyl-CCNU therapy in advanced colorectal cancer. *Cancer* 1977; 40:2792–2796.
17. Kisner D, Schein P, Smith L: 5-Fluorouracil, methyl-CCNU and vincristine (FMV) for colorectal carcinoma. Confirmation of increased response rate using weekly 5-FU. *Proc Am Soc Clin Oncol* 1976; 17:264.
18. Moertel CG, Schutt AJ, Hahn RG, et al: Therapy of advanced colorectal cancer with a combination of 5-fluorouracil methyl-1-3 3 cis (2 chlor-

ethyl), 1-nitro-sourea and vincristine. *J Natl Cancer Inst* 1975; 54:69.
19. Falkson G, Falkson HC: Fluorouracil, methyl-CCNU and vincristine in cancer of the colon. *Cancer* 1976; 38:1468–1470.
20. Baker LH, Talley RW, Matter R: Phase III comparison of treatment of advanced gastrointestinal cancer with bolus weekly 5-FU vs methyl-CCNU plus bolus weekly 5-FU. *Cancer* 1976; 38:1–7.
21. Einhorn LH, Williams D, Loehrer P: Combination chemotherapy with platinum (p) plus 5-FU in metastatic colorectal carcinoma. *Proc Am Soc Clin Oncol* 1984; 3:133.
22. Shepard K, Bitran J, Sweet D, et al: Treatment of metastatic colorectal carcinoma with cisplatin and 5-fluorouracil. *Proc Am Soc Clin Oncol* 1984; 3:147.
23. Petrelli N, Madejewicz S, Rustum Y, et al: Combination chemotherapy of cisplatinum and 5-fluorouracil for advanced colorectal adenocarcinoma. *Cancer Chemother Pharmacol* (in press).
24. Machover D, Goldschmidt E, Chollet P, et al: Treatment of advanced colorectal and gastric adenocarcinoma with 5-fluorouracil and high dose folinic avid. *J Clin Oncol* 1986; 5:685–696.
25. Houghton JA, Maroda SJ, Phillips JO, et al: Biochemical determinants of responsiveness to 5-fluorouracil and its derivatives in xenografts of human colon adenocarcinomas in mice. *Cancer Res* 1981; 41:144–149.
26. Madajewicz S, Petrelli N, Rustum YM, et al: Phase I–II trial of high dose calcium leucovorin and 5-fluorouracil in advanced colorectal cancer. *Cancer* 1984; 44:4667–4669.
27. Machover D, Schwarzenberg L, Goldsmith E, et al: Treatment of advanced colorectal and gastric adenocarcinoma with 5-FU combined with high dose folinic acid: A pilot study. *Cancer Treat Rep* 1982; 66:1803–1807.
28. Petrelli N, Herrera L, Rustum Y, et al: A prospective randomized trial of 5-fluorouracil versus 5-fluorouracil and leucovorin versus 5-fluorouracil and methotrexate in previously untreated patients with advanced colorectal carcinoma, *J Clin Oncol* 1987; 10:1559–1565.
29. Cunningham J, Bukowski R, Budd T, et al: 5-Fluorouracil and folinic acid: A phase I–II trial in gastrointestinal malignancy. *Invest New Drugs* 1984; 2:391–395.
30. Bruckner HW, Roboz J, Spigelman M, et al: An efficient leucovorin and 5-fluorouracil sequence: Dosage escalation and pharmacological monitoring. *Proc Am Assoc Cancer Res* 1983; 24:138.
31. Byrne P, Smith F, Treat J, et al: 5-Fluorouracil and higher dose folinic acid treatment of colorectal carcinoma patients. *Proc Am Soc Clin Oncol* 1983; 2:121.
32. Rosso R, Nobile MT, Sertoli MR, et al: Therapy of metastatic colorectal carcinoma with high dose N^5 methyl-tetrahydro-folate (MTHF) and 5-fluorouracil (FU). *Proceedings Second Euro Conf Clin Oncol* 1983; Vol. 1, 199.
33. Balch CM, Urist MM, Soong SJ, et al: A prospective phase II clinical trial of continuous FUDR regional chemotherapy for colorectal metastases to the liver using a totally implantable drug infusion pump. *Ann Surg* 1983; 198:567–573.
34. Shepard KV, Levin B, Karl RC, et al: Therapy of metastatic colorectal cancer with hepatic artery infusion of chemotherapy using a subcutaneous implanted pump. *J Clin Oncol* 1985; 3:161–169.
35. Kemeny N, Daly J, Oderman P, et al: Hepatic artery pump infusion: Toxicity and results in patients with metastatic colorectal carcinoma. *J Clin Oncol* 1984; 2:595–600.
36. Weiss GR, Garnick MC, Osteen RT, et al: Long-term hepatic arterial infusion of 5-fluorodeoxyuridine for liver metastases using an implantable infusion pump. *J Clin Oncol* 1983; 1:337–344.
37. Niederhuber JE, Ensminger W, Gyves J, et al: Regional chemotherapy of colorectal cancer metastatic to the liver. *Cancer* 1984; 53:1336–1343.
38. Hohn D, Melnick J, Stagg R, et al: Biliary sclerosis in patients receiving hepatic arterial infusions of floxuridine. *J Clin Oncol* 1985; 3:98–102.
39. Hohn D, Stagg R, Friedman M, et al: NCOG randomized trial of intravenous (IV) vs hepatic arterial (IA) FUDR for colorectal cancer metastatic to the liver. *Proc Am Clin Oncol* 1987; 6:333.

38

Heme-Positive Stool:
What is the appropriate evaluation?

JOHN H. BOND, M.D.

Occult bleeding from the gastrointestinal tract is defined as bleeding into the esophageal, gastric, or intestinal lumen that is insufficient to cause noticeable changes in the color or consistency of stool. Occult bleeding is usually detected using one of several available chemical slide tests for fecal occult blood.[1] Other abdominal or systemic symptoms may or may not be present. Likewise, the patient may or may not have microcytic anemia. A patient found to have occult gastrointestinal bleeding often represents a diagnostic challenge for the physician for three reasons. First, a large number of conditions throughout the alimentary tract may result in loss of small volumes of blood. Second, the cause of bleeding of this magnitude may be trivial and of no consequence to the patient's health or it may represent an early manifestation of a potentially life-threatening disease. Last, the clinician must always remember that even with an elaborate and expensive work-up, no certain cause of occult bleeding may be identified. Therefore, considerable clinical judgment and a systematic approach is required to effectively rule out important pathology, while at the same time not performing unnecessary tests or examinations.[2]

This chapter first discusses some of the precautions and limitations of the most commonly employed qualitative slide tests for fecal occult blood. The most common and clinically important causes of occult gastrointestinal bleeding are then reviewed. Lastly, a rational, systematic approach to the patient with this important clinical sign is presented.

FECAL OCCULT BLOOD TESTS

The slide tests most frequently used to detect occult blood in the stool employ a colorless indicator, guaiac, which in the presence of hemoglobin undergoes oxidation to form a blue color. Because hemoglobin acts as a pseudoperoxidase, the reaction is catalyzed by the addition of hydrogen peroxide (Fig 38–1). Previously, a liquid guaiac solution was used to perform the tests, but this method was unreliable and excessively sensitive, causing a high frequency of false-positive tests.[3] Most commercially available fecal occult blood tests (e.g., Hemoccult) now use guaiac-impregnated filter paper which is more standardized and reliable and which has a sensitivity roughly one-fourth to one-fifth that of the older liquid tests.[3] Using these slide tests, a patient may prepare his or her own test at home in an easy and aesthetically acceptable manner by simpling smearing the slide window with a wooden spatula which has been touched to a freshly passed stool. The slide specimen may then be brought in or mailed to a medical facility for developing.

Table 38–1 lists causes of a false-positive or false-negative guaiac slide test for fecal occult blood. False-positive reactions

$$2H_2O_2 \xrightarrow{\text{Hemoglobin}} 2H_2O$$

$$\text{Colorless guaiac} \xrightarrow{O_2} \text{Blue, oxidized guaiac}$$

FIG 38–1.
The guaiac reaction.

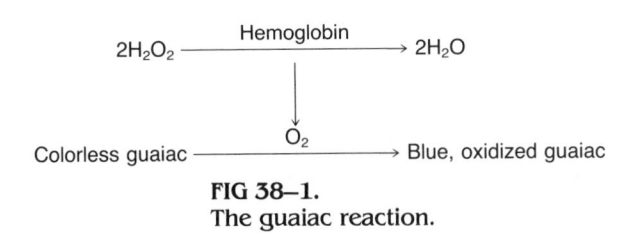

are a serious problem when the test is used for screening, because it results in the performance of many costly and unnecessary diagnostic examinations. Dietary sources of peroxidase present in red meat and certain fruits and vegetables (Table 38–2) may render the test positive, especially when the rehydration technique is required.[4] In this situation, patients should avoid eating red meat and large portions of the foods listed for 24 to 48 hours before testing. Iron supplements can cause false-positive guaiac reactions and should be avoided for several days prior to testing.[5] Presumably, this is the result of a direct effect of iron compounds on the guaiac reaction.

There are several reasons why the guaiac test might be negative even though a clinically important gastrointestinal lesion or condition is present. The lesion may not bleed or it may bleed intermittently. Even if active bleeding is present, the blood may not be evenly distributed throughout the stool so that the samples taken for testing might not contain blood. Because of these sampling problems, testing is usually done by taking two samples from each of three consecutive stools. Another reason for a false-negative test is that bleeding from the proximal gastrointestinal tract, or even in some instances from the right colon, may not be detected because hemoglobin loses its peroxidase activity if it passes too slowly through the intestinal tract. Supplemental vitamin C suppresses the hemoglobin–guaiac reaction and therefore should not be taken for several days prior to testing.[6] Lastly, slides that contain blood may test negative after storage for more than 3 days.[7] Adding water to the slide before developing will prevent this change. However, this "rehydration" of slides also increases the sensitivity of the test and therefore the incidence of false-positive reactions. It should be employed only if storage for more than 3 days is necessary and the patient has observed strict dietary precautions.

Barium, laxatives, and commercial products added to toilet water during flushing do not appear to alter the guaiac slide test results. Patients are generally asked to increase their fiber intake during testing. Although the value of this has not been shown in controlled studies, a lesion in the colon may be more likely to bleed during testing if it is in contact with more solid, higher bulk stool.

Incorrect processing or interpretation of the guaiac slides may be a cause of either a false-positive or a false-negative test. Training and experience using standards of known reaction are important for individuals charged with processing of this laboratory determination.

TABLE 38–1.
Causes of False-Positive and False-Negative Guaiac Slide Tests for Fecal Occult Blood

False-Positive	False-Negative
Dietary peroxidase	Lesion not bleeding
Iron supplements	Lesion bleeding intermittently
Processing error	Sampling error
	Proximal bleeding
	Vitamin C supplements
	Storage over 3 days
	Processing error

TABLE 38–2.
Dietary Sources of Peroxidase

Red meat	Cantaloupe	Grapefruit
Turnip	Cucumber	Cabbage
Cauliflower	Artichoke	Pumpkin
Radish		

CAUSES OF OCCULT GASTROINTESTINAL BLEEDING

Table 38–3 lists the numerous conditions that must be considered when investigating the cause of occult gastrointestinal hemorrhage. Preliminary results from the University of Minnesota Colon Cancer Screening Program,[8] as well as data from smaller studies involving both asymptomatic and symptomatic individuals,[9,10] indicate that most clinically important causes of occult gastrointestinal bleeding are located in the large bowel or perianal area. Of greatest importance are colorectal cancers and potentially premalignant neoplastic polyps. Other causes of a positive fecal occult blood test found in the lower intestinal tract include benign perianal disease (e.g., hemorrhoids, anal fissures), acute and chronic colitis, vascular ectasia, radiation mucosal injury, and diverticulosis. Upper gastrointestinal pathology is implicated less frequently as a cause of occult blood loss, especially in asymptomatic patients. Conditions that should be included in a differential diagnosis include esophagitis, gastritis, duodenitis, peptic ulcer disease, vascular ectasia, and benign or malignant tumors. Lesions of the remainder of the small bowel which occasionally need to be considered include Crohn's disease, vascular ectasia, and, rarely, benign or malignant tumors.

DIAGNOSTIC APPROACH

The diagnostic approach to a patient with occult gastrointestinal bleeding will be modified by the patient's age, health, and the known presence of acute or chronic conditions likely to cause bleeding. Because occult bleeding is such a common early manifestation of curable colorectal cancer, most patients over the age of 40 should first undergo a thorough examination of the entire large bowel. Even if a likely cause for bleeding is found in the perianal area or rectum, the entire colon should be examined for synchronous colonic neoplasms. If these studies fail to reveal the cause, or if other signs or symptoms suggest upper gastrointestinal tract pathology, examination of the upper tract may then be indicated. Small bowel studies are needed only in the rare patient with an otherwise negative evaluation who has persistent bleeding or bleeding sufficient to cause microcytic anemia.

Evaluation of the Colon and Rectum

A digital rectal examination with a thorough inspection of the anal area is a quick, safe, and inexpensive way to diagnose a significant fraction of benign or malignant perianal or low-rectal disease. Approximately 5% to 10% of colorectal cancers are detectable by digital examination.

In performing the evaluation of the rest of the large bowel, a physician will have to choose between a barium x-ray study, endoscopic examination of the colon, or some combination of x-ray and endoscopic procedures. This choice should be based on the following considerations of the comparable accuracy, safety, comfort

TABLE 38–3.
Differential Diagnosis of Occult Gastrointestinal Bleeding

Upper GI Tract	Small Bowel	Lower Intestinal Tract
Esophagitis	Crohn's disease	Colorectal cancer
Gastritis	Vascular ectasia	Colorectal polyps
Duodenitis	Tumors	Perianal disease
Peptic ulcer		Inflammatory bowel disease
Vascular ectasia		Radiation colitis
Tumors		Vascular ectasia
		Diverticulosis

or convenience, and the cost of the alternative strategies.

Barium enema. The standard single-column barium enema examination is a low-resolution, relatively inaccurate method for detecting curable colonic cancers and polyps in most patients. Because the colon has a wide diameter, appreciable redundancy, and frequent areas of stasis or spasm, this technique often fails to provide a detailed outline of much of the mucosa, and small cancers and polyps may be missed. In the large cancer screening trial at the University of Minnesota, single-column barium enemas diagnosed only 60% of cancers and 40% of neoplastic polyps that were above the reach of the rigid proctoscope.[11]

The double-contrast (air contrast) barium enema, which uses higher density barium followed by air insufflation, usually provides clearer, more detailed pictures of the mucosal outline and is currently considered the radiologic procedure of choice for demonstrating large bowel neoplasms.[12] A recent study from the Netherlands compared the accuracy of single-column and double-contrast barium enema examination in 425 consecutive patients for the detection of colonic polyps and stricturing carcinomas.[13] Each patient was examined with both techniques during the same session. Although there was no difference between the two methods in the detection rate of carcinomas, the double-contrast technique was far superior to single-contrast for the detection of polyps.

Several other studies have shown that small lesions (cancers and polyps) are frequently missed by barium enema even when double-contrast techniques are employed, espcially in the left colon in the presence of diverticulosis.[14-16] The lower rectum is often poorly visualized by x-ray studies; therefore, proctosigmoidoscopy should always accompany the barium enema examination.

Aside from accuracy considerations, the main limitation of barium enema as a means of evaluating the entire colon is that it, of course, does not allow for biopsy of suspicious lesions or resection of polyps. Therefore a positive study usually necessitates the subsequent performance of colonoscopy.

Flexible Sigmoidoscopy. One of the main values of flexible sigmoidoscopy appears to be in screening asymptomatic individuals for colonic neoplasms.[17] Comparative studies indicate that flexible sigmoidoscopy detects an average of three times as many polyps and cancers and is a more acceptable procedure to patients than rigid sigmoidoscopy.[18] Obviously, if a decision is made to perform total colonoscopy, there is no need to perform flexible sigmoidoscopy. The combination of a double-contrast barium enema and flexible sigmoidoscopy has been promoted as a reasonable compromise to complete colonoscopic examination of the colon. Flexible sigmoidoscopy provides an accurate examination of the rectosigmoid colon, which, especially in patients with diverticulosis, is a difficult area for the radiologist to examine accurately. Double-contrast barium enema appears to be more accurate in the proximal colon in most patients. Although flexible sigmoidoscopy allows biopsy of left colonic lesions, it should not be used for polypectomy unless the entire colon is adequately prepared to eliminate the risk of electrocautery-induced explosion.

Colonoscopy. Colonoscopy is the most accurate means of diagnosing neoplasms of the large bowel and provides a means of biopsying suspicious lesions and resecting most colonic polyps. In a carefully controlled comparison study of air contrast barium enema vs colonoscopy in the diagnosis of colonic polyps, Hogan and co-workers reported an accuracy of 94% for colonoscopy vs 67% for air contrast barium enema.[19]

Although previously a common practice, performance of barium enema is no longer considered a prerequisite to the safe and accurate performance of colonoscopy. Furthermore, the complication rate for colonoscopy and colonoscopic polypectomy performed by experienced endoscopists is very low.

Despite its obvious advantages, colonoscopy has some limitations. Certain areas proximal to major curves or flexures and the ileocecal valve may be difficult to visualize. Furthermore, in 5% to 10% of patients, usually those with diverticular disease or previous pelvic surgery or radiation, the endoscopist may not be able to comfortably or safely pass the instrument to the cecum. Therefore, barium enema and colonoscopy will continue to be complementary, rather than competitive, procedures in the evaluation of the colon.

Cost Considerations. The cost comparisons in Table 38–4 were derived from a Midwestern university hospital endoscopy unit; thus, in a direct comparison, the strategy of performing air contrast barium enema plus flexible sigmoidoscopy appears to be less expensive than performing primary colonoscopy in the evaluation of the patient with possible colorectal neoplasia. However, cost comparisons should also consider the need to perform a subsequent colonoscopy in most patients with a positive barium enema or flexible sigmoidoscopy. For example, in the initial screening of asymptomatic individuals for fecal occult blood in the Minnesota study, patients with a positive test had an incidence of colorectal cancer and polyps of 7.8% and 32%, respectively.[20] Therefore, if we add the cost of performing an additional colonoscopy in nearly 40% of patients, the average cost of the barium enema plus flexible sigmoidoscopy strategy exceeds the average cost of primary colonoscopy ($633 vs $620).

Based on the above considerations, primary colonoscopy without a prior barium x-ray study is recommended for most patients undergoing evaluation for occult gastrointestinal bleeding. The procedure is very accurate in the diagnosis of large bowel neoplasia, has a satisfactorily low complication rate when performed by skilled and experienced examiners, and allows for both immediate biopsy and polypectomy when these are indicated. The entire preparation and evaluation can be completed in a day, minimizing patient inconvenience and loss of work time. While the alternative strategy of performing flexible sigmoidoscopy and a barium x-ray study is initially less costly, the need to do subsequent colonoscopy in the 30% to 40% with a positive work-up makes this approach, on the average, more expensive.

Evaluation of the Upper Gastrointestinal Tract

Health-threatening disease of the upper gastrointestinal tract is much less common than colonic disease as a cause of occult gastrointestinal bleeding, especially in asymptomatic individuals. When a thorough examination of the colon fails to reveal a source of bleeding, a decision must be made as to whether it is necessary to rule out upper tract pathology. If mucosal inflammation of the esophagus, stomach, or duodenum is suspected because of the use of nonsteroidal anti-inflammatory drugs (NSAID), alcohol abuse, or viral infection, a trial of therapy may be successful and obviate the need for further, expensive tests. However, if positive tests for fecal occult blood persist, or if the patient develops iron deficiency anemia, a thorough evaluation of the upper tract is indicated. Obviously, any suspicion of obstruction or malignant disease warrants immediate investigation, although esophageal and gastric cancer appear to be exceedingly rare causes of occult bleeding in asymptomatic individuals.

TABLE 38–4.
Cost Comparisons between Colonoscopy and Barium Enema plus Flexible Sigmoidoscopy

	Colonoscopy	Barium Enema	Flexible Sigmoidoscopy
Hospital charges	$190	$160	$65
Professional fee	$430	$ 70	$90
Total	$620		$385

Upper Gastrointestinal Barium X-Ray Studies vs Endoscopy. If evaluation of the upper tract is indicated, a choice is usually made between an initial barium x-ray study and endoscopy. For upper tract lesions presenting with occult bleeding, direct endoscopic examination of the esophagus, stomach, and proximal duodenum is much more likely to reveal the source than indirect x-ray methods. For example, in one study, barium x-ray studies failed to detect 65% of cases of superficial mucosal inflammation diagnosed by endoscopy.[21]

A radiologic diagnosis of a peptic ulcer requires the demonstration of barium within an ulcer crater. Secondary signs of duodenal ulcers include deformity of the duodenum due to spasm, edema, or scarring. In the presence of this deformity, ulcer craters may be difficult to detect.[22] False-positive readings may result from accumulations of barium between folds. In studies comparing endoscopy and radiology in the diagnosis of gastric and duodenal ulcers, radiology has an error rate ranging from 7% to 33%, including a false-positive rate of 2% to 11% and a false-negative rate of 5% to 27%.[23] The lowest error rate for x-ray was reported by experienced radiologists using air contrast techniques.

The accuracy of endoscopy is high; however, even in skilled hands lesions are missed in 2% to 4% of cases.[24] Endoscopy allows diagnosis of vascular ectasia and direct biopsy of abnormal mucosal areas or suspicious mass lesions. Endoscopy is extremely safe and well tolerated. Its major limitation is its cost which is approximately double that of barium x-ray studies.

Radionuclide Scanning. The use of radionuclide scanning to detect gastrointestinal hemorrhage is relatively inexpensive, noninvasive, and safe. The tests are capable of detecting active bleeding into the alimentary tract at rates as low as 0.1 ml/minute. Unfortunately, occult gastrointestinal bleeding often is too slow or too intermittent to be detected using available methods.

Two methods using two different technetium-99m-labeled substances, sulfur colloid and erythrocytes, are currently used. Intravenously injected ^{99m}Tc–sulfur colloid is cleared rapidly by the reticuloendothelial system, and therefore background activity decreases rapidly after administration, facilitating imaging of even small amounts of extravasated radioactivity at a bleeding site.[25] The test requires only 20 to 30 minutes to complete and is most useful for the evaluation of active, acute gastrointestinal hemorrhage of unknown cause and location. False-negative scans may result from intense liver and spleen uptake which obscures part of the upper abdominal area.

The second method employs ^{99m}Tc-labeled erythrocytes and may be more useful in the evaluation of intermittent gastrointestinal bleeding.[26] An aliquot of the patient's blood is mixed with the isotope and reinfused intravenously. Attached to circulating erythrocytes, the radioactivity remains in the circulation for over 24 hours. Therefore, the test is potentially able to detect intermittent bleeding that occurs during that period. Serial scans are obtained after a single injection until a collection of radioactivity is detected in the bowel lumen.

These radionuclide tests are positive only in the presence of active bleeding and therefore are not employed routinely in the evaluation of occult stool blood. An exception would be the rare case in which the disease course is interrupted by possible episodes of more active hemorrhage.

Arteriography. As is the case with radionuclide scans, arteriography detects only the site and not the cause of active bleeding. Bleeding into the upper and lower gastrointestinal tract of greater than 0.5 ml/minute is readily identified.[27] Selective infusion of vasoconstricting drugs and embolic therapy have been effective in the management of acute, active upper or lower tract hemorrhage. However, arteriography is rarely helpful in the average patient with occult stool blood. Arteriography may occasionally be useful in the diagnosis of chronic intermittent bleeding severe enough to cause iron deficiency anemia. Because extravasation of blood into the intestinal lumen is rarely seen in these patients, the value of arteriography is the demonstration or exclusion of otherwise undetected vascular dysplasia, vascular tumors, or chronic inflammatory bowel disease.

Chronically Positive Fecal Occult Blood Tests

The patient with persistently positive tests for occult stool blood poses a difficult problem for the clinician because of concern about the possibility of a missed colorectal cancer. Causes of chronically positive fecal occult blood tests include hemorrhoids, especially with chronic constipation; chronic inflammatory bowel disease; radiation colitis; heavy use of NSAID or alcohol; and postgastrectomy inflammation of the gastric remnant. It is obviously not wise to repeat a complete gastrointestinal evaluation every time a positive fecal occult blood test is found in these patients. For those in the colon cancer age range, an initial thorough examination of the colon should always be done, and if no pathology is found, repeat colonic studies might be performed at about 5-year intervals.

References

1. Winawer SJ: Fecal occult blood testing. *Dig Dis Sci* 1976; 21:885–888.
2. Bond JH, Peterson WL: Evaluation of occult bleeding from the gastrointestinal tract. *Pract Gastroenterol* 1983; 7:15–21.
3. Ostrow JD, Mulvaney CA, Hansell JR, et al: Sensitivity and reproducibility of chemical tests for fecal occult blood with an emphasis on false-positive reactions. *Dig Dis Sci* 1973; 18:930–940.
4. Stroehlein JR, Fairbanks VF, Go VLW, et al: Hemoccult stool tests: False-negative results due to storage of specimens. *Mayo Clin Proc* 1976; 51:548–552.
5. Macrae FA, St. John DJ, Caligiore P, et al: Optimal dietary conditions for hemoccult testing. *Gastroenterology* 1982; 82:899–903.
6. Jaffe RM, et al: False negative stool occult blood tests caused by ingestion of ascorbic acid (vitamin C). *Ann Intern Med* 1975; 83:824–826.
7. Wells HJ, Pagano JF: Hemoccult test: Reversal of false negative results due to storage. *Gastroenterology* 1977; 72:A125/1148.
8. Gilbertsen VA, McHugh R, Schuman L, et al: The early detection of colorectal cancers. *Cancer* 1980; 45:2899.
9. Glober GA, Peskoe SM: Outpatient screening for gastrointestinal lesions using guaiac-impregnated slides. *Am J Dig Dis* 1974; 19:399.
10. Winawer SJ, Andrews M, Flehinger B, et al: Progress report on controlled trial of fecal occult blood testing for the detection of colorectal neoplasia. *Cancer* 1980; 45:2959.
11. Gilbertsen VA, Williams SE, Schuman L, et al: Colonoscopy in the detection of carcinoma of the intestine. *Surg Gynecol Obstet* 1979; 149:877.
12. Miller RE: Detection of colon carcinoma and the barium enema. *JAMA* 1974; 230:1195.
13. DeRoos A, Hermans J, Shaw P, et al: Colon polyps and carcinomas: Prospective comparison of the single- and double-contrast examination in the same patients. *Radiology* 1985; 154:11–13.
14. Beggs I, Thomas BM: Diagnosis of carcinoma of the colon by barium enema. *Clin Radiol* 1983; 34:423–425.
15. Kelvin FM, Gardiner R, Vas W, et al: Colorectal carcinoma missed on double contrast barium enema study: A problem in perception. *AJR* 1981; 137:307–313.
16. Schnyder P, Moss AA, Thoeni RF, et al: A double-blind study of radiologic accuracy in diverticulitis, diverticulosis, and carcinoma of the sigmoid colon. *J Clin Gastroenterol* 1979; 1:55–56.
17. Winawer SF, Leidner SD, Byle C, et al: Comparison of flexible sigmoidoscopy with other diagnostic techniques in the diagnosis of rectocolon neoplasia. *Dig Dis Sci* 1979; 24:277.
18. Winnan G, Berci G, Panish J, et al: Superiority of the flexible to the rigid sigmoidoscope in routine proctosigmoidoscopy. *N Engl J Med* 1980; 302:1011.
19. Hogan WJ, Stewart ET, Geenen JE, et al: A prospective comparison of the accuracy of colonoscopy vs air-barium contrast exam for detection of colonic polypoid lesions. *Gastrointest Endosc* 1977; 23:230.
20. Bond JH, Gilbertsen VA: Early detection of colonic carcinoma by mass screening for occult stool blood: Preliminary report. *Gastroenterology* 1977; 72:1031.
21. Martin TR, et al: A comparison of upper gastrointestinal endoscopy and radiography. *J Clin Gastroenterol* 1980; 2:21.
22. Goldberg HI: Radiographic evaluation of peptic ulcer disease. *J Clin Gastroenterol* 1981; 3:57.
23. Laufer I: Assessment of the accuracy of double contrast gastroduodenal radiology. *Gastroenterology* 1976; 71:874.
24. Tedesco FJ, et al: "Skinny" upper gastrointestinal endoscopy: The initial diagnostic tool. A comparison of upper gastrointestinal endoscopy and radiology. *J Clin Gastroenterol* 1980; 2:27–30.
25. Alavi A, Ring EJ: Localization of gastrointestinal bleeding: Superiority of the ^{99m}Tc–sulfur colloid compared with angiography. *Am J Roentgenol* 1981; 137:741–748.
26. McKusick KA, et al: ^{99m}Tc red blood cells for detection of gastrointestinal bleeding. *Am J Roentgenol* 1981; 137:1113–1118.
27. Ring E: Current status of angiographic techniques in the management of gastrointestinal bleeding. *J Clin Gastroenterol* 1980; 2:99–103.

39

Massive Rectal Bleeding:
What is a rational approach?

NAURANG M. AGRAWAL, M.D.
ATILLA ERTAN, M.D.

Management of lower gastrointestinal (GI) bleeding requires a coordinated effort by multiple disciplines of medicine in order to make an accurate diagnosis. Treatment of lower GI bleeding differs according to severity of bleeding. Thus, it becomes a challenging problem for the attending physician to make an accurate diagnosis and initiate treatment immediately. Lower GI bleeding is defined when the source of bleeding is below the ligament of Treitz. It has few specific features: patients, who are relatively older, present with hematochezia, rarely melena. Technologic advances in diagnostic approach have led to important changes in therapy and appear to have reduced morbidity and mortality. While the majority of patients with lower GI bleeding spontaneously stop bleeding, massive bleeding poses both diagnostic and therapeutic problems. In recent years many new diagnostic and therapeutic modalities have become available for patients with massive rectal bleeding, namely radionuclide scanning; angiography; transcatheter embolization; colonoscopy; and endoscopic therapeutic thermal modalities, such as laser photocoagulation, heater probe, and bicap electrocoagulation. This chapter will discuss rational use of the various modalities available to a practicing physician for making an early diagnosis in a patient with massive lower GI bleeding in order of least discomfort and risk to the patient.

Massive lower GI bleeding is a medical emergency and requires prompt diagnosis and management. Lower GI bleeding is usually painless. Because of frightening nature of presentation, patients seek medical attention early. Weakness or syncope following lower GI bleeding suggests losses greater than 20% of the total blood volume. Resuscitative measures should begin immediately with fluid and electrolyte replacement with a large size catheter. Frequent monitoring of vital signs by a central venous catheter will give an indication of amount and rapidity with which blood loss is taking place, and a Foley catheter should be inserted to monitor urine output. Transfusion requirements should be met on an emergency basis. If there is any indication of bleeding diathesis, this should be evaluated and corrected accordingly.

DIAGNOSTIC APPROACH

The cause of lower GI bleeding will be found during a good history and physical examination in the majority of cases. Painless bleeding in a middle-aged or elderly patient usually signifies bleeding from diverticular disease, vascular malformations, or neoplasms; in a child or a young patient it may suggest bleeding from colonic polyps, specific or nonspecific colitis, or Meckel's diverticulum. History of previous arterial graft surgery in abdominal vessels may lead to bleeding from graft-enteric fistula. On rare occasions symptoms of dyspepsia in either age group may be associated with massive rectal bleeding which may be related to peptic ulcer disease. Obviously, recent history of colonoscopic excision of polyp will make one consider diagnosis of postpolypectomy bleeding. Abdominal pain and diarrhea will suggest inflammatory bowel disease.

A rectal examination can lead toward certain diagnoses, particularly bleeding from anal fissure and hemorrhoids. This should be followed by flexible sigmoidoscopic examination. While some may prefer rigid proctoscopic examination, we prefer flexible sigmoidoscopic examination because of its ability to visualize rectum, sigmoid, and descending colon as well as its ability to be retroflexed in the rectal ampulla to look for any bleeding lesions of the anal canal. If a bleeding lesion is found during flexible sigmoidoscopy, it then also offers opportunity for therapeutic intervention at the same setting depending on the nature of bleeding lesion.

If flexible sigmoidoscopy determines a source of bleeding beyond its reaches, as a routine we like to exclude bleeding from the upper GI tract. Passage of a nasogastric tube in the gastric lumen and lavage prevent major pitfalls in further management of a few patients who are massively bleeding from the upper GI tract. In some patients with duodenal ulcer or graft-enteric fistula, hematemesis may not be the presenting symptom; rapid transit through small bowel from an arterial bleeding lesion may present as lower GI bleeding. Even these patients may present with hematochezia without a positive nasogastric aspirate. Therefore, when bowel sounds are active and BUN is elevated, upper GI endoscopy should be performed.

Barium enema has no place in the management of massive lower GI bleeding. Not only may the bleeding lesion be missed, but results may be very misleading if only diverticula are seen. Furthermore, a colon full of barium makes subsequent colonoscopy and/or angiography impossible.

Radiologic evaluation of massive GI bleeding can be performed either with radionuclide scan or angiography. Both of these tests can be effective depending on the patient's clinical condition and availability of personnel. Radionuclide scan is excellent as a screening test. Under experimental conditions this method has been reported to detect bleeding as small as 0.05 to 0.1 ml per minute. Thus, this method has very high sensitivity in detecting bleeding sites but has very low specificity in identifying the lesion and exact location of active bleeding from lower GI tract.

Currently there are two radionuclide techniques in use: (1) technetium-99m sulfur colloid and (2) technetium-99m or indium-111 labeled erythrocytes. Following IV injection, the technetium-99m sulfur colloid is picked up by the reticuloendothelial system and cleared from the blood within 12 to 15 minutes in patients with normal liver function. In diffuse liver disease, clearance of the tracer may be prolonged. If there is active bleeding, sulfur colloid will extravasate and collect at the bleeding site. The chance of detecting the bleeding site with this method is better than with angiography because the intraarterial time of the radionuclide is between 12 and 15 minutes versus only 8 to 10 seconds for angiographic contrast medium. Localization of the extravasated tracer may change with intestinal peristalsis, permitting it to be distinguished from background activity. However, this shift may also be responsible for a number of incorrect interpretations. The second method requires in vitro labeling of erythrocytes with either technetium-99m or indium-111.

Intravenous injection of a radioactive substance with detection of intestinal extravasation by an isotope counter is, theoretically, an attractive, noninvasive way to localize the site of active bleeding, although the precise lesion and location cannot be determined. There is one exception—Meckel's diverticulum. In this special situation, technetium-99 pertechnate may extravasate from an actively bleeding lesion and may also be taken up by ectopic gastric mucosa in patients with ceased bleeding. However, it should be remembered that this technique can produce false-positive and false-negative results. Focal accumulation of activity is interpreted as a bleeding site. The most common cause of inaccuracy of localization of technetium-labeled erythrocytes is the propulsion of extravasated radionuclide by bowel peristalsis. This finding is more likely to be complicated in patients who have received or who are receiving vasopressin.

Enthusiasm for radionuclide scanning should be viewed in the context of practical consideration. The time required to prepare the tracer and image the patient is longer than that required by angiography. However, if emergency angiography is not available, then radionuclide scanning becomes the test of choice. The advantage of radionuclide evaluation lies in its ability to detect minimal bleeding. It is also clear that a negative radionuclide examination obviates the necessity for emergency angiography.

Angiography is a safe and effective method to localize the site of acute massive GI bleeding and offers an opportunity to treat acute massive bleeding by infusion of vasopressin or transcatheter embolization of bleeding vessels. Clinical experience suggests that in most instances a rate of bleeding greater than 0.5 ml per minute is necessary for angiography to show the site of bleeding. Reports of overall accuracy of angiography for detection of GI bleeding vary between 58% and 86%, influenced by experience of the vascular radiologist as well as patient selection (Table 39–1). Angiography may define lesions with abnormal vasculature even if extravasation is not seen, such as vascular malformations, colonic cancers, colonic leiomyomas, or leiomyosarcomas. Angiography also offers therapeutic modality of infusion of vasopressin (0.1 to 0.5 units/minute, into the artery supplying the bleeding site) when a bleeding site is identified. Intra-arterial infusion of vasopressin has been successful in cessation of bleeding in 70% to 91% of patients in various studies. However, this form of treatment is also associated with high incidence of rebleeding episodes which varies from 22% to 71% during the same admission. Side effects of vasopressin, such as intestinal ischemia, hypertension, myocardial infarction, angina pectoris, hyponatremia, and fluid retention, should be considered. Transcatheter embolization with Gelfoam or other agents may stop the bleeding in selected patients who are unresponsive to vasopressin therapy.

Thus, radionuclide scanning and angiography can be complementary in identifying the site of bleeding as well as the type of abnormality from which the bleeding is occurring. When both radionuclide scanning and angiography are available, the patient's clinical condition may direct one toward selection of one of these two diagnostic tests. In our experience, a patient with massive lower GI bleeding may be a candidate for angiography rather than radionuclide scanning, because if a bleeding site is demonstrated on angiography the patient can also undergo immediate therapy.

Contrary to widespread belief, emergency colonoscopy can be performed in the majority of patients with massive lower GI bleeding after a fluid purge. While intensive resuscitative measures and transfusions are continuing, patients are given saline purge per nasogastric tube, to avoid nausea and vomiting. Jensen and Machicado (1979) were able to perform complete colonoscopy up to the cecum in 15 of 16 patients by this method. In addition to localization of the site of bleeding, colonoscopy offers multiple therapeutic thermal modalities such as laser photocoagulation, heater probe or bicap electrocoagulation for various bleed-

TABLE 39–1.
Detection of Massive Lower GI Bleeding Site by Angiography

Author	Number of Patients	Positive Angiography (%)
Browder et al, 1986	50	36 (72)
Britt et al, 1983	40	23 (58)
Nath et al, 1981	14	12 (86)
Boley et al, 1979	43	28 (65)
Wright et al, 1979	14	12 (86)

ing lesions and also offers choice of polypectomy in patients who are bleeding from polyps.

Thus, by using the above mentioned approach, diagnosis of massive lower GI bleeding can be made in the majority of patients (Figure 39–1). The most common causes of acute massive lower GI bleeding (Table 39–2) are colonic diverticula and colonic vascular malformations.

Rectal bleeding may be evident in 15% to 30% of patients with diverticular disease; acute massive lower GI bleeding from colonic diverticula, reported to occur in 3% to 5% of those with diverticulosis, is considered probably to be the most common cause of life-threatening lower GI bleeding in the elderly. Massive painless lower GI bleeding from uninflamed diverticula occurs predominantly in right colon, even though 70% to 90% of diverticula are located in the sigmoid and descending colon. The increased frequency of lower GI bleeding from right-sided diverticula is puzzling because of the anatomical relationship of the vasa recta. The diverticula are similar throughout the colon, although the right-sided diverticula have wider necks and domes. Histologic sections of the vasa recta associated with bleeding diverticula consistently show a vascular lesion characterized by eccentric intimal thickening, altered internal elastic lamina, and focal attenuation of the media. Usually massive lower GI bleeding occurs in an uninflamed diverticulum, in contrast to the mild and often intermittent bleeding secondary to colonic diverticulitis. Natural history of bleeding from colonic diverticula suggests that 20% of patients will continue bleeding, 20% will stop and rebleed during the same hospitalization, and the remaining 60% will cease and probably never have another bleeding episode. For those with massive bleeding, selective mesenteric angiography locates the site and, if vasopressin is infused, the bleeding ceases at least temporarily in the majority of patients. Many of these patients do not require further therapy during the follow-up. Surgery is indicated for those patients who fail a trial of intra-arterial vasopressin infusion, who rebleed during the same hospitalization, or who have had previously proven diverticular bleeding episodes.

Colonic vascular malformations (angiodysplasias or vascular ectasias) occur mostly in patients over age 60 and are not associated with vascular malformations of the skin or other viscera. The etiology of the angiodysplasias remains unknown. The fact that the disorder is usually found in elderly patients has led to the suggestion that it is a vascular degenerative process related to aging. Approximately 50% of patients with angiodysplasias have a history or clinical diagnosis of cardiac disease, and 15% to 25% have aortic stenosis. Angiodysplastic lesions vary in size

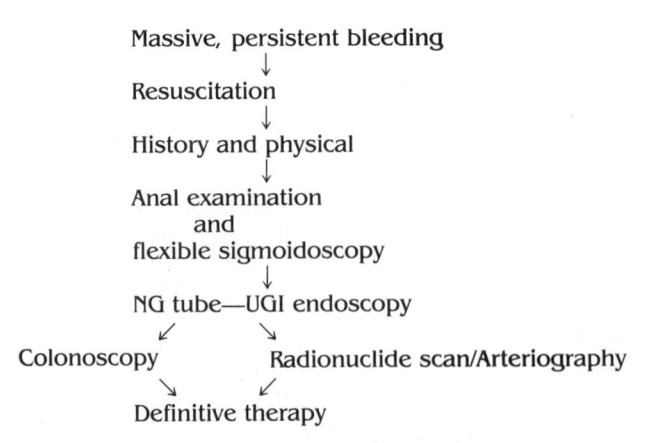

Massive, persistent bleeding
↓
Resuscitation
↓
History and physical
↓
Anal examination
and
flexible sigmoidoscopy
↓
NG tube—UGI endoscopy
↙ ↘
Colonoscopy   Radionuclide scan/Arteriography
↘ ↙
Definitive therapy

FIG 39-1.
Management of massive lower gastrointestinal bleeding.

TABLE 39–2.
Causes of Lower Gastrointestinal Bleeding

Diseases	Massive Acute	Recurrent, Chronic
Perianal diseases	−	+
Colonic diverticula	+	−
Vascular malformations	±	+
Colon cancer	±	+
Colon polyp	±	+
Solitary colonic ulcer	−	+
Colonic varices	+	−
Postpolypectomy	+	−
Ischemic colitis	±	−
Inflammatory bowel disease	±	+
Radiation colitis	−	+
Meckel's diverticulum	+	−
Graft-enteric fistula	+	−
Peptic ulcer disease	+	−

+ = usually; ± = occasionally; − = usually not.

but rarely exceed a few millimeters in diameter, and the lesions do not protrude appreciably into the lumen of the bowel. Microscopically, they consist of dilated, distorted, thin-walled vessels, mostly lined only by endothelium; structurally, they appear to be ectatic veins, venules, and capillaries. Lesions begin submucosally, and, as they become more extensive, they show increasing numbers of dilated and deformed vessels traversing the muscularis mucosa and involving the mucosa until, in most severe lesions, the mucosa is replaced by a maze of distorted, dilated vascular channels. Clinically, the bleeding is usually chronic, recurrent, and self-limited. In some cases, there is an evidence of massive lower GI bleeding. The angiodysplasias have been most often in the cecum and ascending colon. However, they also occur in the sigmoid colon and other parts of GI tract. These lesions are very common, producing bleeding only in those individuals with more striking mucosal involvement. When visualized endoscopically, they are single or multiple and usually flat, bright red, and fern-like. Intraoperative colonoscopy may be helpful in defining lesions on the mucosal surface because angiodysplasias are not generally visible on serosal surface. Selective mesenteric angiography with enhancement magnification has been of great value in establishing the diagnosis. Positive findings include the demonstration of a vascular tuft of dilated irregular small vessels, which fill rapidly during the arterial phase. This is followed by a localized "blush" during the parenchymal phase, and an unusually early or delayed draining vein may be seen. Only occasionally will bleeding be brisk enough for extravasation of contrast material to be noted. The structure of the lesions with massive bleeding makes it unlikely that permanent, good results will be achieved by selective infusion of vasopressin. Endoscopic therapeutic thermal modalities may be alternatives to surgery in the management of bleeding angiodysplasias. Right hemicolectomy is considered the procedure of choice when the source of massive bleeding is thought to be either diverticula or vascular malformations of the right colon. Subtotal colectomy is recommended for good-risk patients with pancolonic diverticulosis or with right-sided vascular malformations plus left-sided diverticula in whom the bleeding site is not identified with available methods.

Bibliography

1. Athanasoulis CA: Angiography in the management of patients with gastrointestinal bleeding (review). *Adv Surg* 1983; 16:1–23.

2. Barrett JF, Jamieson MH: Massive lower gastrointestinal bleeding. A review (review). *S Afr J Surg* 1985; 23:110–113.
3. Baum S: Angiography and the gastrointestinal bleeder. *Radiology* 1982; 143:569–572.
4. Boley S, DiBiase A, Brandt L, et al: Lower intestinal bleeding in the elderly. *Am J Surg* 1979; 137:57–64.
5. Britt L, Warren L, Moore O: Selective management of lower gastrointestinal bleeding. *Am Surg* 1983; 49:121–125.
6. Browder W, Cerise EJ, Litwin MS: Impact of emergency angiography in massive lower gastrointestinal bleeding. *Ann Surg* 1986; 204:530–536.
7. Cello JP, Grendeil JH: Endoscopic laser treatment for gastrointestinal vascular ectasias. *Ann Intern Med* 1986; 104:352–354.
8. Colacchio TA, Forde KA, Patsos TJ, et al: Impact of modern diagnostic methods on the management of active rectal bleeding. Ten year experience. *Am J Surg* 1982; 143:607–610.
9. Ertan A, Hollander A: Vascular malformations of the gastrointestinal tract (review). *Surv Dig Dis* 1985; 3:42–48.
10. Forde KA: Colonoscopy in the diagnosis and management of colonic bleeding (review). *Bull NY Acad Med* 1983; 59:301–305.
11. Hagihara PF, Sachatello CR, Matting SS, et al: Massive rectal bleeding of colonic origin: Localization of the bleeding site. *Surgery* 1982; 92:589–597.
12. Hillemelier C, Gryboski JD: Gastrointestinal bleeding in the pediatric patient (review). *Yale J Biol Med* 1984; 57:135–147.
13. Jensen D, Machicado G: Emergent colonoscopy in patients with severe lower gastrointestinal bleeding (abstract). *Gastroenterology* 1979; 80:1184.
14. Kadir S, Ernst CB: Current concepts in angiographic management of gastrointestinal bleeding. *Curr Probl Surg* 1983; 20:281–343.
15. Lawler G, Bircher M, Spencer J, et al: Embolisation in colonic bleeding. *Br J Radiol* 1985; 58:83–84.
16. Leuchter RS, Petrilli ES, Dwyer RM, et al: YAG laser therapy of rectosigmoid bleeding due to radiation injury. *Obstet Gynecol* 1982; 59:65S–67S.
17. Markisz JA, Front D, Royal HD, et al: An evaluation of 99mTc-labeled red blood cell scintigraphy for the detection and localization of gastrointestinal bleeding sites. *Gastroenterology* 1982; 83:394–398.
18. Nath R, Sequeira J, Weitzman F, et al: Lower gastrointestinal bleeding: Diagnostic approach and management conclusions. *Am J Surg* 1981; 141:478–481.
19. Orecchia PM, Hensiey EK, McDonald PT, et al: Localization of lower gastrointestinal hemorrhage. Experience with red blood cells labeled in vitro with technetium Tc. 99m. *Arch Surg* 1985; 120:621–624.
20. Rosenkrantz H, Bookstein JJ, Rosen RJ, et al: Postembolic colonic infarction. *Radiology* 1982; 142:47–51.
21. Scott HJ, Lane IF, Glynn MJ, et al: Colonic haemorrhage: A technique for rapid intra-operative bowel preparation and colonoscopy. *Br J Surg* 1986; 73:390–391.
22. Spiller RC, Parkins RA: Recurrent gastrointestinal bleeding of obscure origin: Report of 17 cases and a guide to logical management. *Br J Surg* 1983; 70:489–493.
23. Wright H, Pellicia O, Higgins E, et al: Controlled semi-elective segmental resection for massive colonic hemorrhage. *Am J Surg* 1980; 139:535–538.

40

The Chronic Abdomen

W. GRANT THOMPSON, M.D., FRCPC

Few medical practices do not include patients with chronic, undiagnosed abdominal pain. Such patients pose difficult and frustrating problems in diagnosis and management. Imprecise diagnosis is disappointing to both patient and physician. Terms like "abdominal pain N.Y.D.," "functional" or "psychogenic abdominal pain" may sustain the doctor's mystical sense of omniscience but do little to clarify the cause or indicate useful treatment. Such patients risk two harmful extremes of management. First, the doctor, unable to understand the nature of the complaint may minimize its importance, forcing the patient to seek advice elsewhere. There are charlatans who prey on such patients.[1] At the other extreme, repeated complaints of abdominal pain may generate costly consultations, hazardous investigations and treatments (even surgery) that serve to exaggerate the importance of the pain and the patient's concern.

This is not a discussion of the acute abdomen, which is usually handled by the surgeon. Nor will I discuss in any detail chronic recurrent abdominal conditions, such as peptic ulcer or biliary colic, except to differentiate them from the chronic abdomen. This chapter will discuss the prevalence of chronic abdominal pain, the various chronic pain syndromes, etiology, pathogenesis, diagnosis, and management.

PREVALENCE

The chronic abdomen might be defined as abdominal pain of more than 6 months' duration for which no pathophysiologic explanation is found. There is evidence that chronic abdominal pain is very common. Apley and Nash reported that 11% of one thousand school children had recurrent abdominal pain at least three times in 3 months, sufficiently severe to interfere with their activities.[2] Twenty percent of 301 apparently healthy adults had nonmenstrual abdominal pain at least six times in the 12 months prior to interview[3] (Table 40–1). This prevalence has been confirmed by other authors.[4-6] Some of these pains may be due to organic causes, but the majority occur in the absence of any demonstrable pathology.

Series of consecutive patients with abdominal pain seen in hospital[7] or clinic[8, 9] indicate that 85% have no organic cause for their pain. Many of these patients could not be considered chronic, but the figures demonstrate the frequency with which abdominal pain occurs without organic cause. Even one emergency room series indicates no organic cause in 41%[10] (Table 40–1).

It should also be mentioned that although many suffer from abdominal pain, most do not report it to a doctor.[3, 4] Therefore, the reason that the patient has sought medical advice is important. Often it is not the severity of the pain that troubles the patient but rather fear, depression, or guilt, which may be important clues to management.

TABLE 40–1.
Functional Abdominal Pain: Prevalence in Population and in Patient Groups Complaining of Pain

	Author	Number	Pain	Functional
In the population	Thompson[3]	301	21%	Most or all
	Drossman[4]	789	24%	Most or all
	Bommelaer[6]	1200	14%	Most or all
Patient groups				
In the clinic	Gomez[8]	96	84%	All
	Woodhouse[9]	20	85%	All
In the hospital	Sarfeh[7]	64	85%	All
In the emergency room	Brewer[10]	1000	41%	All

CHRONIC PAIN SYNDROMES AND PSEUDOSYNDROMES

Syndromes

Irritable Bowel Syndrome (IBS)

The irritable bowel is the most common complaint seen by gastroenterologists.[11, 12] It may be defined as abdominal pain, altered bowel habit, and bloating for which no pathophysiology can be proven.[13] In many patients alterations in bowel habit are prominent, and the diagnosis presents no problem. When the abdominal pain is the patient's main complaint, the other features may not be obvious. Careful attention to historic details that connect the pain with bowel habit, such as "pain-related defecation,"[14, 15] should permit a diagnosis of IBS.

Gas

Sufferers of gas seldom call their discomfort a pain. Bloating, fullness, postprandial abdominal discomfort usually accompanied by belching, borborygmi, or gas per rectum lead the sufferer to feel he is full of gas. As we shall see, intestinal gas is not increased in such situations.[16] The discomfort is a component of IBS.

Nonulcer Dyspepsia (NUD)

Dyspepsia defies definition. It may cover abdominal complaints as widely or as narrowly as one wishes. Even the term "ovarian dyspepsia" has been used.[17] For the purpose of this discussion, dyspepsia is defined as chronic recurrent epigastric pain with features, such as relationship to meals, relief of pain with food or antacids, nocturnal occurrence, burning quality, or spring and fall periodicity, that lead the physician to suspect a peptic ulcer. When no ulcer is found, the patient is said to have NUD.

Biliary Dyskinesia

Some patients with an acalculus gallbladder, normal biliary tree, and recurrent attacks of right upper-quadrant pain consistent with biliary colic have "manometric abnormalities" of the common bile duct and sphincter of Oddi.[18–20]

Pelvic Pain

Chronic pelvic pain in women without evidence of organic disease is frequently encountered by the gynecologist and is the most common indication for laparoscopy.[21] In some cases the pain is associated with menstruation, ovulation, or intercourse, and the phenomenon has been linked, without controlled study, to vascular congestion of the pelvic organs[22] or pelvic varicosities.[23] Heaton[24] has suggested that many such patients are suffering from IBS and has emphasized the importance of historic factors that link the pain to bowel dysfunction. Both disorders have been attributed to anxiety and depression,[21, 22] but pelvic pain has not been studied in any systematic controlled manner.

The Abdominal Woman (or Man)

There remains in everyone's experience a group of patients with chronic abdominal pain, often described in colorful phrases, unassociated with any bodily function, alleviated by nothing and clearly dominating the patient's life. Sixty years ago Hutcheson[25] described the doctor's dilemma with such a patient, which he called "the abdominal woman":

> Incessant demand for sympathy and understanding makes the abdominal woman a veritable vampire, sucking the vitality out of all who come near her. Half an hour with her reduces her doctor to the consistency of chewed string and is more exhausting to him than all the rest of his daily visits put together, for she is always discovering fresh symptoms, will not admit to any improvement in her condition, and has an objection to everything that is proposed.

Such chauvinism would not survive today. There are "abdominal men." Male or female, such pain-prone patients challenge the physician's management skill and test one's resolve to avoid further tests, drugs, or even surgery.

Münchausen's Syndrome

Some patients have such bizarre medical and personal histories that Asher named the syndrome after Baron Münchausen. This eponym is taken from a legendary 18th-century German army officer, Baron Münchausen, noted for his tall tales of the Russian campaign.[26] The Münchausen patient's fantastic histories often center on abdominal pain, which may lead to costly and hazardous investigations and fruitless laparotomy.[26, 27]

Pseudosyndromes

The descriptions of a number of chronic pain syndromes seem to infer causation. Because they mislead or encourage inappropriate management, reference to these pseudosyndromes should be avoided (Table 40–2).

TABLE 40–2.
Chronic Functional Abdominal Pain

Somatic Syndromes	Somatic Pseudosyndromes
Irritable bowel	Splenic flexure
Gas	Celiac artery
Nonulcer dyspepsia	Adhesions
Biliary dyskinesia	Postcholecystectomy
Abdominal woman/man (pain-prone)	Chronic appendicitis
Münchausen's syndrome	Diverticular pain

Splenic Flexure Syndrome

Gas trapped in the splenic flexure is said to generate pain[28, 29] in the left upper abdomen or even chest. Frequently such a mechanism is proposed for anginalike chest pain or postcholecystectomy pain. This phenomenon must be rare, if it occurs at all. One should at least demonstrate a greatly dilated splenic flexure during the pain, and that is seldom the case. Dworken showed that distention of the splenic flexure may reproduce the pain.[30] Later work by Lasser and co-workers[16, 31] and Swarbrick and co-workers[32] suggests that this is a manifestation of a hypersensitive gut. It is best regarded as a variant of IBS.

Celiac Artery Syndrome

Intermittent epigastric pain has been attributed to compression of the celiac artery and treated with division of the median arcuate ligament.[33] The syndrome is accompanied by a long, loud epigastric bruit. However, editorials[34, 35] point out that bruits occur in 30% of normal people.[36] The follow-up is short-term, and no physiologic abnormality has been demonstrated that is corrected by surgery. There are no controls to show that compression does not occur in asymptomatic individuals, or that sham operation might be as effective as the division of the ligament. This proposed syndrome should be distinguished from the apparent duodenal obstruction by the superior mesenteric artery. The latter phenomenon is likely due to chronic intestinal pseudo-obstruction and will not be discussed further.

Adhesions

"Adhesions!" the exhausted cry of the diagnostically destitute, are often blamed for the chronic abdomen. No doubt adhesions are a cause of bowel strangulation, a surgical emergency, but their importance in chronic recurrent abdominal pain is doubtful. It is well known that patients with IBS are prone to surgery[37, 38] at which no pathology is found. Symptoms following such surgery may continue to be those of IBS. In a retrospective review of a hundred laparoscopies for chronic pelvic pain and 88 for infertility, no difference in the prevalence of adhesions was demonstrated.[39] The distinguished British surgeon, Alexander-Williams, states, "I believe it to be a poorly substantiated myth that adhesions can cause abdominal or pelvic pain."[40] Any who claim miraculous cures after lysis of adhesions, "should be aware of the powerful placebo affect of the procedure."[40]

Chronic Appendicitis

Sometimes patients suffer continuous or recurrent right lower-quadrant abdominal pain that convinces them that they have chronic appendicitis. However, appendixes removed for this diagnosis are as likely to be normal as those removed incidentally at non-GI operations.[41] Sixty to ninety percent of appendixes removed from young females with right lower iliac fossa pain are normal histologically.[42-44] In 1940 Alvarez[45] stated that of 255 patients who had previously undergone appendectomy without any attack of acute appendicitis only 2 were cured of the pain. Sixty-seven percent of 130 who had true acute appendicitis were cured. Thus, the chronic appendix is a pseudosyndrome.

Postcholecystectomy Syndrome

Distinct from the biliary colic/dyskinesia syndrome is dyspepsia associated with gallstones. This epigastric distress is less distinct than biliary colic and more constantly present. It is often described as bloating, burning, or indigestion. However, fatty food intolerance and dyspeptic symptoms are no more common in those with or without gallstones.[46, 47] Price showed 25 years ago that among patients referred for cholecystogram, dyspepsia was equally prevalent whether stones were present or not.[48] A patient with such symptoms can, therefore, expect no relief with cholecystectomy. Thus, the postcholecystectomy syndrome implies that the operation was done for incorrect reasons in the first place.

Painful Diverticulosis (Diverticular Pain)

A perforated diverticulum leads to painful complications. However, abdominal pain occurs in some but not all patients with uncomplicated colonic diverticula.[49] Two studies of patients undergoing barium enema demonstrate no difference in the prevalence of abdominal pain between those with normal x-rays and those with uncomplicated diverticular disease.[50, 51] Other IBS symptoms were also equally present in the two groups. Thus, when pain occurs in uncomplicated diverticular disease it is likely due to a coexistent IBS. Such coincidence should not surprise. Abdominal pain occurs in 14% to 24% of adults,[3-5] and colonic diverticula occurs in 50% of the elderly.

ETIOLOGY AND PATHOGENESIS

The cause of the chronic abdomen is unknown. Many claim to understand the mechanism of some of the syndromes, but no view has achieved any substantial support. Putative physiologic or psychologic markers have not been validated. The following discussion will deal with these theories and markers under physiology, psychology, and factitious pain. Because more research has centered around IBS, and this is likely the most common type of chronic abdomen, it will receive special emphasis.

Physiology

Gut Motility

The study of gut motility has many hazards. Although it is now possible to access most of the gut, the technology employed to measure gastrointestinal movements is not standardized. Some studies are done with empty intestines, others not. Diet and other environmental conditions are not controlled. The exact symptomatology of the patients studied is unclear. Finally abdominal pain, even IBS itself, does not seem likely to have a single mechanism.

Early attempts to relate gut symptoms to physiology include those of Connell and others in the 1960s.[52] He made the apparently paradoxical observation that the sigmoid motility index (amplitude times frequency) was greater in patients with constipation and abdominal pain and less in those with diarrhea. One might, therefore, attribute abdominal pain and constipation to "spasm" of the sigmoid. Unfortunately, many patients do not fit this pattern. Furthermore, gut function cannot be measured representatively in the last 25 cm of the colon. Wingate, using a radiotelemetry device, recorded small-bowel activity in IBS patients and controls who were submitted to severe environmental stress which included driving in London traffic.[53] He observed small-bowel motor abnormalities under these circumstances in 19 out of 20 IBS patients and only 1 out of 15 controls. This is cited as evidence that small gut function is disturbed in the irritable bowel.

Myoelectric Activity

Snape and co-workers[54] and Hyland and co-workers[55] reported 10 years ago that the normally dominant six-cycle-per-minute colonic myoelectric activity was replaced by a three-cycle-per-minute dominant pattern in IBS patients. Subsequently, Latimer[56] found this pattern in psychoneurotic patients without irritable bowel symptoms. Although work continues in this area, there is much to be established before we accept the three-cycle-per-minute pattern as an IBS marker. European workers using a different recording technology found two types of action potentials: long- and short-spike bursts associated with longitudinal and circular muscle fibers.[57] The short-spike bursts appeared to correlate with abdominal pain. As stated by Latimer, however, "There is no convincing physiologic model to explore how the finding of an abnormal electrical control activity can account for the clinical features of the IBS."[56]

Gas

Many patients relate their abdominal discomfort or pain to "gas." Typically the complaint is of bloating, distention, and relief with belching or passing gas from below. Using an argon washout technique, Levitt demonstrated that patients complaining of gas have no more gas in their gut than controls, but retrograde movement of gas is more common in those complaining of gas.[16] Aerophagia may play a role. Recent work suggests that emotional arousal increases spontaneous swallowing.[58] Bloating, "flatulence," and "distention" are important features of the irritable bowel.[3, 14, 15] By itself, however, gas, either ingested or produced by colon bacteria, is an unlikely explanation of the chronic abdomen.

Gastroduodenal Function

The cause of the epigastric discomfort of nonulcer dyspepsia is unknown. Pyloroduodenal dysmotility is frequently blamed.[17, 59] Infusion of duodenal contents into the stomach of postoperative patients reproduces their symptoms,[60] but extrapolation of this information to nonulcer dyspepsia is not justified. Perhaps dyspeptic symptoms are due to dysmotility of the upper gut, in a manner analogous to lower gut dysmotility thought to cause IBS. Antral tachygastria has been reported to cause postprandial upper abdominal distress, usually with vomiting.[61, 62] These motility abnormalities cannot be demonstrated in most dyspeptics.

Bile Ducts

Balloon distention of the common bile duct produces pain in the epigastrium, right hypochondrium, and sometimes the back—a distribution similar to that of biliary colic.[19] The characteristic abnormalities of biliary dyskinesia are said to include an elevated sphincter of Oddi (SO) pressure and even retrograde peristalsis.[18, 20] Although this seems to be an entity, great caution is needed in interpretation of the pain or manometry. Most patients with such pain do not have SO abnormalities. Indeed, 21 of 22 patients with acalculus gallbladders and much investigated recurrent upper abdominal pain had the symptom reproduced exactly by small bowel distention.[63] In such cases focus on the biliary tree is misplaced.

Other

It seems likely that nerves and hormones are important in chronic abdominal pain. However, attempts to show specific abnormalities in gut hormone levels in IBS and other functional disturbances have been futile.[64] IBS subjects have increased sigmoid motility in response to parasympatheticomimetic drugs,[65] but the significance of this is unknown. The abnormality, if there is one, may be in the afferent or efferent nervous system.

Ritchie[66] inflated a balloon in the rectum of IBS patients and nonpatients and sometimes reproduced abdominal pain, urgency, and gaseousness. Discomfort occurred with less balloon distention in the IBS patients. The advent of colonoscopy permitted one to distend the colon at all levels. Of 48 patients with painful irritable bowel, 29 had their pain reproduced by distention of certain segments in the colon.[32] Although the pain tended to overlay the region with the distended colon, it could be referred anywhere in the abdomen and indeed to the chest, back, sacroiliac, thigh, and perineum. Further studies employing gut distention indicate that patients with chronic abdominal pain may have "trigger points" in the small bowel as well.[63, 67]

This fascinating work reinforces the notion that the gut is a seat of much chronic abdominal pain, but does not settle the afferent or efferent issue. Is chronic abdominal pain a normal perception of abdominal gut physiology or an abnormal perception of normal gut physiology?[68]

Psychology

Thus, abdominal pain does not infer the presence of structural disease. Many observers are convinced that it may occur as a result of psychologic trauma, which may be entirely central or might act via the enteric nervous system to alter physiology or one's perception of physiology.

It is a common experience that acute emotion alters gut function. Examinations, interviews, or tragedies may be accompanied by a variety of symptoms ranging from butterflies to abdominal pain. Forty years ago, Almy demonstrated that emotional or physical distress produces spasm, engorgement, and excessive mucous secretion in the sigmoid colon.[69–71] Others have confirmed that psychologic stress can be accompanied by disturbed intestinal motility[65, 72, 73] or myoelectric activity[74] and that such disturbance may be more pronounced in patients with an irritable bowel. It is not known, however, whether motility changes are mechanisms of pain or epiphenomena.

Many studies claim that IBS patients have more depression, anxiety, or neuroticism than controls or patients with other conditions.[13, 75–77] However most IBS sufferers do not see a doctor for their symptoms, and newer work seems to demonstrate that IBS noncomplainers, unlike IBS patients, have a psychologic makeup similar to asymptomatic people.[78–80] It may be that the IBS sufferer is motivated to see his physician by psychologic or personality factors rather than symptom severity.

Environmental stresses or threatening life events have been observed to be more likely prior to onset of the IBS,[75, 81, 82] or inorganic abdominal pain[83, 84] than those without pain or those with pain due to organic gastrointestinal disease. Clinic visits by IBS patients may be precipitated by death in the family (cancer), a marriage break-up, or loss of job. Talley was unable to show such a connection in patients with nonulcer dyspepsia.[85] Ingram et al.[44] pointed out that among women with right iliac fossa pain who had an appendectomy, those with a normal appendix were more likely to have emotional problems and a less satisfying outcome 1 year later than those with an inflamed appendix. In a more recent report, Creed[86] again showed that removal of an uninflamed appendix for abdominal pain was more likely to be preceded by a serious life event, to occur in females, to be accompanied by psychologic symptoms or depression and to be followed by persistent gut complaints.

Psychiatrists and psychologists describe learned illness or learned pain behavior.[87] Perhaps at a young age some patients were rewarded for being ill by sympathy or avoidance of unpleasant activities. Those with nonorganic abdominal pain were more likely to have parents with abdominal pain.[83] Whitehead,[5] in a random telephone survey, found that subjects with painful irritable bowel were more likely than peptic ulcer sufferers or those with no pain to have multiple somatic complaints, to view their colds as more serious than those of other people, and to consult a physician for minor illnesses. They also tended to have received gifts and special food when ill as children. Germane to this is the tendency of recurrent abdominal pain in childhood to persist into adult life.[88, 89]

Engel[90] in his classic paper "Psychogenic Pain and the Pain-Prone Patient" states that guilt is an invariable factor in the choice of pain as a symptom. Personality features include masochism, abuse as a child, onset when things were going well, and life-long continued pain and suffering. "The relish with which the pain-prone patient recounts his tale of suffering alerts the physician that such is an unconscious source of gratification."[90]

No doubt such a process is at work in the introspective, hypochondriacal, self-important, sympathy-craving, "abdominal" women described by Hutcheson.[25] Although no physiologic research has been done in this area, it seems unlikely that such patients have a primary motility disorder as the basis of their pain. Some may be hypochondriacal—convinced they have a disease, fearing the disease, and preoccupied with their bodies.[91] Some are hysterical.[92] Many others are simply depressed.[76, 92]

Factitious Pain

Some complainers of abdominal pain are malingering. Often there is an obvious secondary gain dependant upon the outcome of a disability ruling or a damage suit. Here the physician is in a bind because the pain will not resolve until the legal issue is settled, and the patient's continued complaints delay the settlement.

More obscure is the Münchausen syndrome.[26] Some patients have bizarre medical and personal histories that are somehow plausible in the context of a bustling emergency department attended by a physician who naturally gives the patient the benefit of the doubt.[26, 93] Such patients submit themselves to an awesome array of costly and dangerous procedures including laparotomy.[29, 94] Once their "game is up," Münchausen patients usually sign themselves out of the hospital and move on to another center, leaving their physician perplexed. No coherent physiologic or psychologic mechanism has been forthcoming, and there is no satisfactory treatment.

DIAGNOSIS

Say ye, oppress'd by some fantastic woes,
Some jarring nerve that baffles your repose;
. . . Who with sad prayers the weary doctor tease,
To name the nameless ever new disease.
                                    Crabbe[95]

It goes without saying that one should be alert to the possibility of chronic recurrent abdominal pain due to organic illness. Cholelithiasis, cholecystitis, peptic ulcer, nephrolithiasis, pylonephritis, Crohn's disease, diverticulitis, and subacute obstruction due to tumor may produce episodes of pain over many months or years. Attention to the details of history and physical examination and notation of fever, weight loss, melena, anemia, or an elevation of the erythrocyte sedimentation rate (ESR) should alert one to a treatable medical or surgical disorder. Often patients with the chronic abdomen will have features resembling one or two of these illnesses and will require their exclusion.

Nonulcer Dyspepsia

The greatest difficulty in the diagnosis of the chronic abdomen is uncertainty, which engenders insecurity in the physician. Without the conviction of a positive diagnosis, the physician carries little credibility with the patient, who usually seeks a ready answer. To begin with, one should attempt to relate pain temporally and anatomically with body function. Epigastric pain that is associated with eating, occurs at night, and is relieved by antacids suggests peptic ulcer.[96, 97] Abdominal tenderness is no guide because it is equally prevalent in ulcer and nonulcer dyspepsia.[98] Endoscopy will best settle the issue, and those with no ulcer may be said to have nonulcer dyspepsia.[17] It has been argued that dyspeptic patients should be given a trial of therapy for 6 to 8 weeks and only endoscoped if there is no improvement.[99] This may be a rational policy if endoscopy costs are high or the patient cannot afford it. I submit, however, that such an approach is false economy. Nonulcer dyspepsia is a chronic, recurrent condition with a high placebo response to any drug. Therefore, improvement on medication does not prove the existence of a peptic ulcer.[17] Rather it may hook the patient for life to an inappropriate drug, creating an expense that overtakes that of an initial definitive diagnosis.

Biliary Type Pain

Biliary tract pain is rarely colicky.[100, 101] Recurrent, often nocturnal,[101] attacks of steady epigastric or right upper-quadrant abdominal pain lasting 15 minutes or 1 to 2 days points to the biliary tree. An ultrasound examination is necessary to rule out cholelithiasis. If no stones are found and the pain is unrelated to meals or bowel habit, it may not be possible to make a diagnosis. Some may have "biliary dyskinesia," and sphincter of Oddi dysfunction may be suspected if there is a transient rise of liver enzymes or bilirubin during an attack.[20] Note again, however, that in many, such pain may be reproduced by intraluminal balloon distention of the upper gut.[63]

The Irritable Bowel

The irritable bowel syndrome may be defined as abdominal pain and altered bowel habit often accompanied by gaseousness for which no pathophysiology may be proven.[13] There are now data that establish that a positive diagnosis can be made with a high degree of accuracy[14, 15] (Table 40–3). A diagnosis of irritable bowel made by an experienced physician needs no change over time provided new symptoms do not intervene.[102–104] To enhance one's credibility, one should do a sigmoidoscopy as part of the irritable bowel work-up.[105] Because carcinoma of the colon and the irritable bowel syndrome are both common, they may occur coincidentally in the elderly patient. Thus, the prudent physician will do a barium enema in most individuals over age 40 complaining of bowel dysfunction.

Other Chronic Pain Syndromes

In those whose pain is unrelated to bodily function, a precise functional diagnosis is impossible. Frequently, the pain is continuous and may radiate beyond the abdomen. Sometimes it is vague and moves from place to place. In others, it is described with "relish"[90] in colorful detail. One should look for a secondary gain, re-

TABLE 40–3.
Symptoms Found to be More Common in the Irritable Bowel Than in Organic Disease*

Abdominal pain eased after bowel movement
Looser stools after onset of pain
More frequent stools after onset of pain
Abdominal distention
Mucus per rectum
Feeling of incomplete emptying
Abdominal pain plus flatulence plus irregularity
Symptoms more than 2 years
Diarrhea *and* constipation
Pellety stools or mucus

*Data from Manning AP, Thompson WG, Heaton KW, et al: Towards positive diagnosis of the irritable bowel. *Br Med J* 1978; 2:653–654 and Krvis W, Thieme CH, Weinzierl M, et al: A diagnostic score for the irritable bowel syndrome: Its value in the exclusion of organic disease. *Gastroenterology* 1984; 87:1–7.

---

cent stressful events, and, most importantly, signs of depression. The only physical signs are the facial expression of depression and multiple abdominal scars resulting from fruitless surgery to which such patients are prone.[25, 106, 107] Persistent pain, hysteria, pain-proneness as described by Engel, and the use of narcotics are more likely in those who have had multiple surgery.

> We see too many scarred abdomens with persistence of symptoms, too many "re-operation" and operations undertaken for pain.
> JA Ryle[37] 1928

Patients with the chronic abdomen may have a psychologic or personality disorder. In the case of the IBS, gas, or NUD; anxiety or depression may bring the patient to the doctor. In those bizarre or persistent pains that make little physiologic sense, the psychiatric condition may be an integral part or cause of the pain. There is still a stigma attached to mental symptoms, and many consider them an indication of personal failure. It is unacceptable for some to regard themselves as emotionally ill. Thus, their psychiatric illness may assume a physical guise.[92] The physician must, therefore, be alert to the presence of depression or depressive equivalent, hypochondriasis (needs the illness to cover for failure), hysteria (symbolic disability), pain proneness (masochism to atone for guilt),[90] and paranoid schizophrenia.[92] In the latter case, a psychiatrist is necessary. Most other patients must usually be managed by the physician.

MANAGEMENT

Those caring for the chronic abdomen must be mindful of Osler's dictum to do no harm. As defined here the chronic abdomen is benign in a physical sense, but invasive tests and even surgery can cause real morbidity and undermine confidence in the diagnosis.

Therefore, one should develop a strategy of management based on a diagnosis that confidently excludes organic disease, sympathetic exploration of psychosocial factors, explanation and reassurance, minimal use of drugs and tests, and a follow-up plan designed to support the patient without further investigation or harmful therapy[105] (Table 40–4). Most physicians suspect the chronic abdomen without organic disease on the first or second visit. One may either identify one of the symptom patterns such as IBS or be impressed by bizarre features that do not follow any pathologic pattern. It is impor-

TABLE 40–4.
A Strategy for Managment of the Chronic Abdomen*

First clinical visit
  A positive diagnosis
  Reason for visit (psychosocial factors)
  Explanation
  Avoid drugs, minimize tests
  Bulk or appropriate alternative at least for placebo effect
Follow-up visit
  Ensure compliance and comprehension
  New strategy for unimproved patient
  Consider alternate diagnosis, but avoid unnecessary tests
  Selected drugs for specific symptoms
The unsatisfied patient
  Provide emotional support and continued care
  Referral options

*Adapted from Thompson WG: A strategy for management of the irritable bowel. *Am J Gastroenterol* 1986; 81:95–100.

tant to do the necessary diagnostic tests in the first instance, both to reassure the patient and to avoid the necessity of having them done later in a way that weakens the patient's confidence in the diagnosis.

Time spent discussing the patient's problem with him or her and attempting to explain how symptoms can occur without any structural disease should pay dividends later. In some patients with the chronic abdomen, it is the insistence that there *must* be something wrong that makes them so difficult to handle.

The individual with the irritable bowel, particularly if constipated, may notice some improvement in bowel function with the use of bran. This helps build up confidence even though it may not help pain. Studies of bran and other bulking agents in the irritable bowel show little benefit compared with placebo (aside from constipation). However, the placebo response is up to 71%, and, because bran is harmless, this is a desirable result.[108] Similarly, in nonulcer dyspepsia, many patients benefit from a placebo response through the use of antacids even though there is no rationale of their use. Certainly, this is preferable to systemic drugs.

One small, blinded 4-year study provides evidence that sphincterotomy improved the pain in patients with SO motor abnormalities.[18] This is still experimental. More experience is necessary before this hazardous procedure can be recommended for regular use. It is likely that most biliary-type pain in acalculus patients is not biliary dyskinesia.

In patients with functional abdominal pain, especially if no associated gut symptoms exist, one should look for psychiatric or personality disorders. Pfeiffer[92] emphasizes five disorders: depression, hypochondriasis, hysteria, pain-proneness, and paranoid schizophrenia, and offers some suggestions for management (Table 40–5).

The depressed patient may benefit from a tricyclic antidepressant.[76] Even if the depression is not obvious, the drug may have a salutary effect. If not successful after several weeks or if there is a threat of suicide, consider psychiatric referral.

TABLE 40–5.
The Chronic Abdomen*

Psychiatric Entity	Management
Depression, or depressive equivalent	Tricyclic antidepressants
Hypochondriasis	Regular brief visits (placebo)
Conversion/hysteria	Follow-up visits Family therapy
Pain-prone (masochism)	Minimize tests, drugs Management of guilt feelings
Somatic delusions (paranoid schizophrenia)	Psychiatric referral

*Adapted from Pfeiffer E: Treating the patient with confirmed functional pain. *Hosp Phys* 1971; 6:68–72.

Hypochondriacs have a sense of personal failure or inadequacy. Unable to admit this to themselves, they unconsciously present as physically rather than psychologically impaired. Telling such patients that they obviously are not sick is of no avail. Such a patient needs to be in someone's care and is often satisfied by regular brief appointments several weeks apart. Inert placebos with no side effects help demonstrate this care until the patient trusts the doctor enough to discuss his or her problems of living.

Hysterical patients have abdominal pain or other disability for complex reasons. In spite of "la belle indifference," the pain likely carries great symbolic meaning, which may take psychiatric methods to unravel. The best that the physician can do is to try to help these patients deal with the conflicts they encounter in their lives. Family involvement seems important.

Hutcheson[25] described assumption of the pain-prone patient's care as a "bleak prospect." He suggests the need for ". . . something which will dislocate the patient's mind from its perpetual revolution of her umbilicus and set it open to wider horizons." Engel observed that such patients are worse when things are going well for them; their histories are a litany of painful illnesses and injuries with redundant tests and therapies including surgery. It is as if some personal disaster serves to assuage their guilt.[90] A psychiatric consultation may be helpful, but it is usually the physician or the general practitioner who must provide ongoing care. In the individual with learned illness behavior one needs to stop the reward for being sick. This usually involves the complicity of friends or relatives.[87]

Pain-prone patients are often highly critical of previous physicians. Some suffer so vividly and cry out for relief of pain so plaintively that they "stir rescue fantasies in the most case-hardened doctor."[92] As succinctly put by Tryer,[87] "To attempt to change the habits of a lifetime—particularly if these remain advantageous to the patient and his family—may prove an unreasonable contract; the therapist is entitled to retire to the wings if no progress is possible." Notwithstanding, the physician, however limited the realistic goals might be, must continue to support the patient and at least defend him or her from iatrogenic illness.

In the case of IBS, one controlled study demonstrated that psychotherapy was effective. One hundred and one patients were allocated to two treatment groups, both of which received the same medical therapy.[109] One group received 10 hour-long psychotherapy sessions over 3 months, following which there was a significant improvement in somatic symptoms including abdominal pain. The improvement was even more pronounced a year later. Supportive psychotherapy and stress management are important components of management of patients with nonorganic abdominal pain.

Other treatment options include hypnotherapy,[110] biofeedback,[111] and psychiatric consultation. The former two require special expertise and validation, while the latter will be of little assistance to those who refuse to accept the mental component of their symptoms. In most cases cure is an unrealistic goal. One should try to help the patients cope with stress and offer continued concern and care.

To cure sometimes, to relieve often, to comfort always.

Anonymous

SUMMARY

Chronic abdominal pain is common. Recurrent attacks of organic disease such as peptic ulcer or biliary colic can be identified by a careful history. Most of the remaining cases will have no pathology. One should attempt to identify and treat syndromes such as the irritable bowel or functional dyspepsia. The remaining patients who have pain with no connection to gastrointestinal function or even those with the irritable bowel who fail to improve with the usual measures may be suffering from depression, hypochondriasis, hysteria, pain-proneness, or schizophrenia. The latter requires psychiatric consultation. The others must be managed by the physician, who may find the exercise frustrating. A positive diagnosis of functional abdominal pain is essential in order to avoid unnecessary tests and drugs. Some patients respond to reassurance that no serious disease exists, but most require continuing care with repeated visits which aim to reassure, help to cope with stressful situations, and attempt to modify the illness behavior.

References

1. Smart HL, Mayberry JF, Atkinson M: Alternative medicine consultations and remedies in patients with the irritable bowel syndrome. *Gut* 1986; 27:826–828.
2. Apley J, Nash N: Recurrent abdominal pain: A field survey of 1000 school children. *Arch Dis Child* 1958; 33:165–170.
3. Thompson WG, Heaton KW: Functional bowel disorders in apparently healthy people. *Gastroenterology* 1980; 79:283–288.
4. Drossman DA, Sandler RS, McKee DC, et al: Bowel dysfunction among subjects not seeking health care. *Gastroenterology* 1982; 83:529–534.
5. Whitehead WE, Winget C, Fedaravicius AS, et al: Learned illness behaviour in patients with irritable bowel syndrome and peptic ulcer. *Dig Dis Sci* 1982; 27:202–208.
6. Bommelaer G, Rouch M, Dapoigny M, et al: Epidemiologie des troubles fonctionnels dan une population apparement saine. *Gastroenterol Clin Biol* 198; 10:7–12.
7. Sarfeh JI: Abdominal pain of unknown etiology. *Am J Surg* 1976; 132:22–25.
8. Gomez J, Dally P: Psychologically mediated abdominal pain in surgical and medical outpatient clinics. *Br Med J* 1977; 1:1451–1453.

9. Woodhouse CRG, Bockner S: Chronic abdominal pain: A surgical or psychiatric symptom? *Br J Surg* 1979; 66:348–349.
10. Brewer RJ, Golden GT, Gitch DC, et al: Abdominal pain: An analysis of 1,000 consecutive cases in a university hospital emergency room. *Am J Surg* 1976; 131:219–223.
11. Switz DM: What the gastroenterologist does all day. *Gastroenterology* 1976; 70:1048–1050.
12. Harvey RF, Salih SY, Read AE: Organic and functional disorders in 2,000 gastroenterology outpatients. *Lancet* 1983; 1:632–634.
13. Thompson WG: The irritable bowel. *Gut* 1984; 25:305–320.
14. Manning AP, Thompson WG, Heaton KW, et al: Towards positive diagnosis of the irritable bowel. *Br Med J* 1978; 2:653–654.
15. Kruis W, Thieme CH, Weinzierl M, et al: A diagnostic score for the irritable bowel syndrome: Its value in the exclusion of organic disease. *Gastroenterology* 1984; 87:1–7.
16. Lasser RB, Bond JH, Levitt MD: The role of intestinal gas in functional abdominal pain. *N Engl J Med* 1975; 293:524–526.
17. Thompson WG: Non ulcer dyspepsia. *Can Med Assoc J* 1984; 130:565–569.
18. Geenen JE, Hogan WJ, Dodds WJ, et al: Long term results of endoscopic sphincterotomy for treating patients with sphincter of Oddi dysfunction: A prospective study (abstract). *Gastroenterology* 1987; 92:1401.
19. Doran FSA: The sites to which pain is referred from the common bile-duct in man and its implication for the theory of referred pain. *Br J Surg* 1967; 54:599–606.
20. Meshkinpour H, Mollot M, Eckerling GB, et al: Bile duct dyskinesia: Clinical and manometric study. *Gastroenterology* 1984; 87:759–762.
21. Beard RW, Reginald PW, Pearce S: Pelvic pain in women. *Br Med J* 1986; 293:1160–1163.
22. Mills WG: The enigma of pelvic pain. *J Roy Soc Med* 1977; 71:257–259.
23. Beard RW, Highman JH, Pearce S, et al: Diagnosis of pelvic varicosities in women with chronic abdominal pain. *Lancet* 1984; 2:946–949.
24. Heaton KW: Pelvic pain in women. *Br Med J* 1986; 293:1504.
25. Hutcheson R: The chronic abdomen. *Br Med J* 1923; 1:667–669.
26. Asher R: Munchausen syndrome. *Lancet* 1951; 1:339–341.
27. Bardsley JE, Gibson JE: The Munchausen syndrome. *Mod Med Can* 1975; 30:984–988.
28. Roth JL: The symptom patterns of gaseousness. *Ann NY Acad Sci* 1968; 150:109–125.
29. Grosberg SJ: The diagnostic significance of intestinal gas. *Am Geriatr A* 1969; 17:400–403.
30. Dworken HJ, Biel FJ, Machella TE: Supradiaphragmatic reference of pain from the colon. *Gastroenterology* 1952; 22:222–231.
31. Lasser RB, Levitt MD, Bond JH: Studies of intestinal gas after ingestion of a standard meal. *Gastroenterology* 1976; 70:906.
32. Swarbrick ET, Hegarty JE, Bat L, et al: Site of pain from the irritable bowel. *Lancet* 1980; 2:443–446.
33. Watson WC, Sadikali F: Celiac axis compression; Experience with 20 patients and a critical appraisal of the syndrome. *Ann Intern Med* 1977; 86:278–284.
34. Sleisenger MH: The celiac artery syndrome—again. *Ann Intern Med* 1977; 86:355–356.
35. Editorial: Celiac axis compression—a treatable cause of persistent abdominal pain? *Lancet* 1977; 1:1240–1241.
36. Watson WC, Williams PB, Duffy G: Epigastric bruits in patients with and without celiac axis compression: A phonoarteriographic study. *Ann Intern Med* 1973; 79:211–215.
37. Ryle JA: Chronic spasmodic affections of the colon. *Lancet* 1928; 2:1115–1119.
38. Fielding JF: Surgery and the irritable bowel syndrome: The singer as well as the song. *Ir Med J* 1983; 76:33–34.
39. Rapkin AJ: Adhesions and pelvic pain: A retrospective study. *Obstet Gynecol* 1986; 68:13–15.
40. Alexander-Williams J: Do adhesions cause pain? *Br Med J* 1987; 294:659–660.
41. Thackrey AC: Chronic appendicitis—some pathological observations. *Br J Radiol* 1959; 32:180–182.
42. Rang EH, Fairbourn AS, Acheson ED: An inquiry into the incidence and prognosis of undiagnosed abdominal pain treated in hospital. *Br J Prev Soc M* 1970; 24:47–51.
43. Harding HE: A notable source of error in the diagnosis of appendicitis. *Br Med J* 1962; 2:1028–1029.
44. Ingram PW, Evans G, Oppenheim AN: Right iliac fossa pain in young women. *Br Med J* 1965; 2:149–151.
45. Alvarez WC: When should one operate for chronic appendicitis: *JAMA* 1940; 114:1301–1306.
46. Bainton D, Davies GT, Evans KT, et al: Gallbladder disease: Prevalence in a South Wales industrial town. *Lancet* 1981; 1:1147–1149.
47. Koch JP, Donaldson RM: A survey of food intolerance in hospitalized patients. *N Engl J Med* 1964; 271:657—660.
48. Price WH: Gall bladder dyspepsia. *Br Med J* 1963; 2:138–141.
49. Thompson WG, Patel DG: Clinical picture of diverticular disease of the colon. *Clin Gastroenterol* 1986; 15:903–916.
50. Thompson WG, Patel DG, Tao H, et al: Does uncomplicated diverticular disease produce symptoms? *Dig Dis Sci* 1982; 27:605–608.
51. Sim GPG, Scobie BA: Large bowel diseases in New Zealand based on 1118 air contrast enemas. *N Zealand Med J* 1982; 95:611–613.
52. Connell AM, Jones FA, Rowlands EN: Motility of the pelvic colon. IV abdominal pain associated with colonic hypermotility after meals. *Gut* 1965; 6:105–112.
53. Kumar D, Wingate DL: The irritable bowel syndrome: A paroxysmal motor disorder. *Lancet* 1985; 2:973–977.
54. Snape WJ, Carlson GM, Matarazzo SA, et al: Evidence that abnormal myoelectrical activity produces abnormal colonic motor dysfunction

in the irritable bowel syndrome. *Gastroenterology* 1977; 72:383–387.
55. Hyland JMP, Darby CF, Hammond P, et al: Myoelectric activity of the sigmoid colon in patients with diverticular disease and the irritable colon syndrome suffering from diarrhea. *Digestion* 1980; 20:293–299.
56. Latimer P, Sarna S, Campbell D, et al: Colonic motor and myoelectric activity: A comparative study of normal subjects, psychoneurotic patients, and patients with IBS. *Gastroenterology* 1981; 81:893–901.
57. Bueno L, Fioramonti J, Ruckebush Y, et al: Evaluation of colonic myoelectric activity in health and functional disorders. *Gut* 1980; 21:480–485.
58. Fonagy P, Calloway SP: The effect of emotional arousal on spontaneous swallows. *J Psychosom Res* 1986; 30:183–188.
59. Johnson AG: Pyloric function and gallstone dyspepsia. *Br J Surg* 1972; 59:449–454.
60. Meshkinpoor H, Marks JW, Schoenfield LJ, et al: Reflux gastritis syndrome: Mechanism of symptoms. *Gastroenterology* 1980; 79:1283–1287.
61. Reynolds RPE, Bardakjian BL, Diamant NE: A case of antral tachygastria: Symptomatic and myoelectric improvement with gastroenterostomy and domperidone therapy. *Can Med Assoc J* 1983; 128:826–829.
62. You CH, Chey WY, Lee KY, et al: Gastric and small intestinal myoelectric dysrhythmia associated with chronic intractable nausea and vomiting. *Ann Intern Med* 1981; 95:449–451.
63. Kingham JGC, Dawson AM: Origin of chronic right upper quadrant pain. *Gut* 1985; 26:783–788.
64. Besterman HS, Sarson DL, Rambaud JC, et al: Gut hormone responses in the irritable bowel syndrome. *Digestion* 1981; 21:219–224.
65. Chaudhary NA, Truelove SC: Human colonic motility: A comparative study of normal subjects, patients with ulcerative colitis and patients with the IBS. *Gastroenterology* 1961; 40:18–26.
66. Ritchie J: Pain from distension of the pelvic colon by inflating a balloon in the irritable bowel syndrome. *Gut* 1973; 14:125–132.
67. Moriarty KJ, Dawson AM: Functional abdominal pain: Further evidence that whole gut is effected. *Br Med J* 1982; 1:1670–1672.
68. Ford MJ: The irritable bowel syndrome. *J Psychosom Res* 1986; 30:399–410.
69. Almy TP, Kern F, Tulin M: Alteration in colonic function in man under stress. ii: experimental production of sigmoid spasm in healthy persons. *Gastroenterology* 1949; 12:425–436.
70. Almy TP, Hinkle LE, Berle B, et al: Alterations in colonic function in man under stress. iii: experimental production of sigmoid spasm in patients with spastic const. *Gastroenterology* 1949; 12:4371–4379.
71. Almy TP, Abbot FK, Himkle LE: Alterations in colonic function under stress. *Gastroenterology* 1950; 15:95–103.
72. Cann PA, Read NW, Cammack L, et al: Psychological stress and the passage of a standard meal through the stomach and small bowel in man. *Gut* 1983; 24:236–240.
73. Welgan P, Meshkinpoor H, Hoehler F: The effect of stress on colon motor and electrical activity in irritable bowel syndrome. *Psychosomat Med* 1985; 47:139–149.
74. Narducci F, Snape WJ, Battle WM, et al: Increased colonic motility during exposure to a stressful situation. *Dig Dis Sci* 1985; 30:40–44.
75. Chaudhary NA, Truelove SC: The irritable colon syndrome. *Q J Med* 1962; 31:307–323.
76. Hislop IG: Psychological significance of the irritable colon syndrome. *Gut* 1971; 12:162–166.
77. Young SJ, Alpers DH, Norland CC, et al: Psychiatric illness and the irritable bowel syndrome. *Gastroenterology* 1976; 70:162–166.
78. Welch GW, Stace NH, Pomare EW: Specificity of psychological profiles or irritable bowel syndrome patients. *Aust N Z J Med* 1984; 14:101–104.
79. Drossman DA, McKee DC, Sandler RS, et al: Psychosocial factors in the irritable bowel syndrome: A multivariate study of patients and nonpatients with IBS. *Gastroenterology* In press.
80. Whitehead WE, Bosmajian L, Zonderman A, et al: Role of psychological symptoms in irritable bowel syndrome: Comparison of community and clinic samples (abstract). *Gastroenterology* 1987; 92:1693.
81. Mendeloff AI, Monk IM, Seigel CI, et al: Illness experience and life stresses in patients with irritable colon and with ulcerative colitis. *N Engl J Med* 1970; 282:14–17.
82. Ford MJ, Miller P McC, Eastwood J, et al: Life events, psychiatric illness and the irritable bowel syndrome. *Gut* 1987; 28:160–166.
83. Hill OW, Blendis L: Physical and psychological evaluation of non-organic abdominal pain. *Gut* 1967; 8:221–229.
84. Craig TKJ, Brown GW: Goal frustration and life events in the etiology of painful gastrointestinal disorder. *J Psychosom Res* 1984; 28:411–421.
85. Talley NL, Piper DW: Major life event, stress and dyspepsia of unknown cause. *Gut* 1986; 27:127–134.
86. Creed F: Life events and appendectomy. *Lancet* 1981; 1:1381–1385.
87. Tyrer SP: Learned pain behaviour. *Br Med J* 1986; 292:1–3.
88. Christensen MF, Mortensen O: Long-term prognosis in children with recurrent abdominal pain. *Arch Dis Child* 1975; 50:110–114.
89. Apley J, Hale B: Children with recurrent abdominal pain: How do they group up? *Br Med J* 1973; 2:7–9.
90. Engel GL: Psychogenic pain and the pain-prone patient. *Am J Med* 1959; 26:899–918.
91. Appleby L: Hypochondriasis: An acceptable diagnosis (editorial). *Br Med J* 1987; 294:857.
92. Pfeiffer E: Treating the patient with confirmed functional pain. *Hosp Phys* 1971; 6:68–72.
93. Thompson WG, Schuster J, Williams RL, et al: Munchausen syndrome: A cause of pyrexia of unknown origin. *Can Med Assoc J* 1964; 91:1021–1023.

94. Chapman JS: Perigrinating problem patients—Munchausen's syndrome. *JAMA* 1957; 195:927–933.
95. Crabbe G: *The Village*. New York, Penguin. 1973, p 26.
96. Crean GP, Card WI, Beattie AD, et al: Ulcerlike dyspepsia. *Scand J Gastroenterol* 1982; 79:9–15.
97. Lawson MJ, Grant AK, Paull A, et al: Significance of nocturnal abdominal pain: A prospective study. *Br Med J* 1980; 1:1302.
98. Priebe WM, DaCosta LR, Beck IT: Is epigastric tenderness a sign of peptic ulcer disease? *Gastroenterology* 1982; 82:16–19.
99. American College of Physicians. Endoscopy in the evaluation of dyspepsia. *Ann Intern Med* 1985; 102:266–269.
100. French EB, Robb WAT: Biliary and renal colic. *Br Med J* 1963; 2:13–18.
101. Torosis J, McDougall CJ, Spiro HM, et al: Circadian periodicity of biliary pain (abstract). *Gastroenterology* 1987; 92:1972.
102. Holmes IM, Salter RH: Irritable bowel syndrome—a safe diagnosis. *Br Med J* 1982; 285:1533–1534.
103. Svendsen JH, Munck LK, Andersen JR: Irritable bowel syndrome—prognosis and diagnostic safety. *Scand J Gastroenterol* 1985; 20:415–418.
104. Harvey RF, Mauad AC, Brown AM: Prognosis in the irritable bowel syndrome: A 5-year prospective study. *Lancet* 1987; 1:963–965.
105. Thompson WG: A strategy for management of the irritable bowel. *Am J Gastroenterol* 1986; 81:95–100.
106. Ryle JA: Chronic spasmodic affections of the colon. *Lancet* 1928; 2:1115–1119.
107. Fielding JF: Surgery and the irritable bowel syndrome: The singer as well as the song. *Ir Med J* 1983; 76:33–34.
108. Lucey MR, Clark ML, Lowndes JO, et al: Is bran efficacious in irritable bowel syndrome? A double blind placebo controlled study. *Gut* 1987; 28:221–225.
109. Svedlund J, Sjoden I, Ottosson JO, et al: Controlled study of psychotherapy in irritable bowel syndrome. *Lancet* 1983; 2:589–591.
110. Whorwell PG, Prior A, Faragher EB: Controlled trial of hypnotherapy in the treatment of severe, refractory irritable bowel syndrome. *Lancet* 1984; 2:1232–1234.
111. Marzuk PM: Biofeedback for gastrointestinal disorders: A review of the literature. *Ann Intern Med* 1985; 103:240–244.

41

Infectious Colitis:
What is an effective approach?

VALERIE JAGIELLA, M.D.
BERNARD M. SCHUMAN, M.D.
FRANCIS J. TEDESCO, M.D.

Infectious colitis is caused by a variety of infectious agents including viruses, bacteria, and parasites. In order to select appropriate therapy, it is important to distinguish infectious colitis from other colitides. Sometimes diagnosis is difficult because colonic infections can clinically, endoscopically, and radiographically mimic inflammatory bowel disease, ischemic colitis, and colitis that is associated with systemic disease.

EPIDEMIOLOGY

Types of Transmission and Sources

Transmission of the organism can occur by means of the fecal–oral route or by direct person-to-person contact, as in *Shigella* and *Campylobacter* infections. Other agents are transmitted via contaminated food or water. For example, *Salmonella* infections have developed after the ingestion of unpasteurized milk and contaminated meat. *Campylobacter jejuni*, *Shigella*, and *Yersinia enterocolitica* have been transmitted by means of untreated water.[1] Moreover, animals, including pets, can also be reservoirs of enteric pathogens, as has been reported with *Campylobacter jejuni*.[2]

Seasonal Variations

Viral infectious agents are most common in winter months, whereas bacterial infections predominate in the summer and fall. An exception is *Yersinia enterocolitica*, which is more frequently isolated during the winter months. Parasitic colitis is more common in the warmer or rainy seasons in tropical climates.

Patient Population

Although infectious colitis affects all age groups, there are age-associated disease patterns as well as variations related to patient population. Enteropathogenic *Escherichia coli* has often been reported as the causative agent in nursery outbreaks.[1,3] In babies, toddlers, and older children, *Shigella*, *Yersinia*, and *Campylobacter* are common enteropathogens. In the elderly, *Salmonella* and *E. coli*, specifically serotype 0157:H7, may behave more virulently.[4-6]

Homosexual men with and without gastrointestinal symptoms have been shown to have a high prevalence of intestinal infections such as *Entamoeba histolytica*, *Chlamydia trachomatis*, herpes simplex virus, and *Neisseria gonorrhoeae*. Up to a quarter of the symptomatic homosexual male patients have been found to have multiple pathogens. Hence, the presence of nonpathogens indicates a search for another enteric "treatable" pathogen.[7, 8]

The patient with acquired immune deficiency syndrome (AIDS) presents unique challenges for the diagnosis of enteric infections. AIDS may be associated with multiple opportunistic colonic infections such as *Salmonella typhimurium*, *Cryptosporidium*, and *Cytomegalovirus*.[8, 9]

ETIOLOGY AND PATHOGENESIS

A wide variety of viral, bacterial, and parasitic agents have been shown to cause enterocolitic infections. The virulence traits of these pathogens can be categorized into three basic types (Fig 41–1). The majority of the infections are of the noninflammatory or secretory type. Typical examples include *Vibrio cholerae*, enterotoxigenic *E. coli* (observed in the tropics), *Clostridium perfringens*, *Staphylococcus aureus*, rotavirus, Norwalk-like viruses, and possibly *Giardia lamblia*.

Inflammatory diarrhea, on the other hand, is caused by direct invasion of the colonic mucosa by the organism and cytotoxic effect which induce an inflammatory response occasionally leading to bloody diarrhea. In these infections, fecal polymorphonuclear leukocytes are found on microscopic examination of the stool. Causative agents include *Salmonella* and *Shigella* species, *Campylobacter jejuni*, invasive *E. coli* as well as cytotoxigenic *Clostridium difficile*.

Organisms that fit into the third category of virulence are those that act by "penetration" of the mucosa, usually of the Peyer's patches in the ileum, where they multiply intracellularly and cause systemic disease. This enteric fever syndrome is exemplified by typhoid fever, but sometimes *Yersinia* or *Campylobacter fetus* infections behave in this fashion. Stool examination occasionally reveals mononuclear leukocytes. The diagnosis is frequently made from blood, bone marrow, or lymph node biopsy culture.[1, 6, 10, 11]

DIAGNOSTIC APPROACH

Distinguishing between the various causes of colitis, proctocolitis, and proctitis is well suited to the primary care physician because specialized radiologic procedures such as barium enema studies and colonoscopy are rarely indicated. Infectious colitis is usually self-limited, and, by the time a causative agent is identified, specific treatment is rarely needed. Thus diagnostic studies are usually reserved for patients with persistent disease, dysentery, debilitating diarrhea, or significant systemic complaints requiring hospitalization. In those patients with chronic diarrhea or in outbreaks that require public health investigation, the diagnostic clues are derived from the history, physical examination, sigmoidoscopy, rectal biopsy, stool examination and cultures, and serology. The patient can then be classified as either high risk, requiring hospitalization and treatment, or someone who can

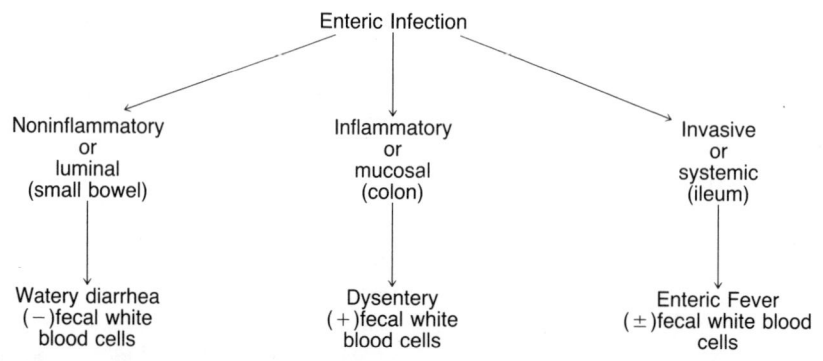

FIG 41–1.
Virulence traits of enterocolitic pathogens.

be evaluated and treated as an outpatient.

Obtaining a comprehensive medical history is important, and inquiries should be made about childhood health, previous surgery, and a family history of gastrointestinal disease. Particular attention should be paid to a history of contact with individuals with similar symptoms or with animals or household pets, of ingestion of particular foods or use of drugs, and of foreign travel. The character of the diarrhea or rectal discharge, and the presence of abdominal pain, nausea, vomiting, fever, and weight loss should be assessed.

Physical examination will ascertain if there is fever, anemia, skin rash, or jaundice. Careful attention should be given to the degree of hydration and nutrition. On examining the abdomen, a search for masses should be carried out, and tenderness, distention, and bowel sounds should be evaluated. Perianal inspection may reveal fissures, fistulas, or an abcess. Rectal examination and sigmoidoscopy should be done unless the patient has such severe perianal disease that he or she cannot tolerate the procedure.[11, 12]

Laboratory tests include a complete blood count, evaluation of serum electrolytes, urinalysis, and stool examination. Stool specimens should be collected in a container and examined within 30 minutes of passage.[13] If no bowel prep has been done, the stool sample can be obtained during sigmoidoscopy by attaching a "trap" specimen container to the suction tubing. The collected stool can then be divided into several samples for different studies. Visual inspection may confirm the presence of blood, mucus, or pus. The stool should be tested for occult blood, which is frequently present in inflammatory infections. Microscopically, pus cells, ova, cysts, and parasites may be seen.

If parasites are a consideration, two to three specimens, one of which is a purged specimen, should be collected. Each sample should be placed in a different preservative, one in polyvinyl alcohol (PVA) alone, the other in PVA with 5% or 10% formalin. Culture of bacteria is not possible from a specimen in parasitic preservative. For motile organisms, such as amoeba, the best results are obtained with direct examination of fresh stool.[13, 14]

Microscopic examination of stool for leukocytes with methylene blue stain may be diagnostic. Positive smears have 50 or more polymorphonuclear cells per high power field (PMN/HPF) and are found in infections with *Shigella*, enteroinvasive *E. coli*, *E. coli* 0157:H7, and *Campylobacter*. However, the absence of leukocytes does not preclude bacterial infections (Table 41–1). If leukocytes are present, stool cultures should be done.

For stool cultures, transport depends on the climate and organisms suspected. High ambient temperature makes isolation of pathogens difficult due to the competition between pathogenic and nonpathogenic bacteria. Low temperatures, as with refrigeration, injure some *Shigella* and, to a lesser extent, *Salmonella* species. Bacterial cultures may cost from $15 to $35[10] or more per culture and routinely recover only *Shigella*, *Salmonella*, and, depending on the laboratory, *Campylobacter*, which is one of the most common causes of diarrhea. The laboratory culture of *Campylobacter* is complex and not done everywhere. When available, selective media are necessary to isolate the organism, and its identification may take a few days to several weeks. However, Gram staining the stool may demonstrate a curved Gram-negative bacteria consistent with *Campylobacter*. Unless specifically requested, organisms such as enteropathogenic *E. coli*, *Clostridium difficile*, *Yersinia*, and *Vibrio cholerae* will not be cultured.[10, 13, 15] Moreover, enteropathogenic *E. coli* testing is expensive, is only done in reference laboratories, and is rarely clinically applicable. If *E. coli* is suspected in cases of epidemiologic interest, stool specimens should be frozen for eventual serotyping.[4, 16] Viral cultures are also expensive, and rarely are they clinically useful in adults. Moreover, cytomegalovirus infection is not diagnosed by culture but by demonstrating cytomegalic inclusion in tissues or by serial serum antibody titers.[9, 11, 13]

Clostridium difficile-induced colitis almost exclusively occurs in the presence of antibiotics[17-19] or chemotherapy.[9] There is an increasing frequency with advancing age, and the organism is often identified in hospital-acquired enteric infections[20]

TABLE 41–1.
Fecal Leukocytes in Enteric Infections

	Viral	Bacterial	Parasitic
Positive		Shigella, Campylobacter, Escherichia coli: enteroinvasive and enterohemorrhagic (0157:H7)	
Variably positive		Salmonella, Yersinia, Vibrio cholerae-non 01 Clostridium difficile, Vibrio parahaemolyticus	Entamoeba histolytica
Negative	Rotavirus Norwalk agent Adenovirus Cytomegalovirus Herpes simplex virus	Escherichia coli: enteropathogenic, enterotoxigenic; Vibrio cholerae; Clostridium perfringens, Bacillus cereus, Staphylococcus aureus	Giardia lamblia Strongyloides Cryptosporidium

and among residents of chronic-care facilities.[21] In such cases the stool sample should be refrigerated until processed. Delays of more than 24 hours are not acceptable for these anaerobic cultures.[13] The isolation of Clostridium difficile is not necessarily diagnostic of pseudomembranous colitis, but, when present, the strain should be tested for cytotoxic production in vitro and the patient should be considered for treatment.

When sexually transmitted infections are suspected, the rectum should be swabbed for both Gram stain and Neisseria gonorrhoeae culture. Rapid detection of Chlamydia trachomatis with Chlamydiazyme® can be performed directly on swab specimens collected from urethral, rectal, and cervical sites.[22] Direct immunofluorescent staining of scrapings from the base of active herpes simplex viral lesions offers specific and relatively rapid diagnosis (yield is 85% to 88%[22]). Serum antibody titers may be helpful as in cases of Y. enterocolitica, invasive amebiasis (by indirect hemagglutination), and lymphogranuloma venereum (LGV) serotypes of Chlamydia trachomatis.[10, 13]

Sigmoidoscopy with or without rectal biopsy may be diagnostic particularly in cases of pseudomembranous colitis and should be performed without bowel preparation, because enemas may distort or cause edema of the mucosa and remove pus, blood, and exudates. Rectal biopsy may delay a barium enema study for 1 week; nevertheless, if the rectal or colonic mucosa is abnormal or a lesion is noted, a biopsy is vital. If amebiasis is suspected, the mucosal ulcer should also be scraped and examined on a wet mount. Endoscopic biopsy can be of great value in diagnosing more unusual cases (e.g., schistosomal and tuberculous colitis). Although acid-fast bacilli are rarely identified, granulomas are usually found on biopsy of tuberculous lesions.[23]

Endoscopically, acute infectious colitis commonly mimics chronic ulcerative colitis and less frequently Crohn's disease.[24–27] The histologic appearance of acute self-limiting colitis can be diagnostic[28–31] especially if the biopsies are taken during the first 4 days after the onset of bloody diarrhea (Table 41–2) because the histology evolves rapidly. By days 6 through 9 there may only be scattered residual crypt lesions with regeneration (focal cryptitis) by biopsy, and within 2 weeks complete healing can occur. Resolution, however, can take more than 30 days as in some cases of Campylobacter colitis.[29]

In most cases of infectious colitis, the primary causes of morbidity and mortality are dehydration and electrolyte abnormalities. Rehydration and replacement of essential salts are the primary goals of therapy. In most cases oral rehydration can be accomplished.[10, 11, 32, 33] The use of antimotility drugs such as opium, diphenoxy-

TABLE 41–2.
Histologic Features Differentiating Acute Self-Limiting Colitis (ASLC) from Chronic Ulcerative Colitis (CUC).*

ASLC	Active CUC
Diffuse mucosal edema	Edema of lamina propria often obscured by hypercellularity
Cryptitis, crypt ulcers, or abscesses	Cryptitis, crypt ulcers or abscesses, crypt atrophy
Depletion of the mucous content of the crypts and surface epithelium (±) Regenerative features	Depletion of mucous content of crypt and surface epithelium (+) Regenerative changes
Superficial ulcers or erosions with little or no underlying granulation tissue	Possible ulcers with underlying granulation tissue
Hypercellular lamina propria (+) neutrophils (±) lymphocytes, eosinophils	Hypercellular lamina propria (+) plasma cells, lymphocytes eosinophils (±) neutrophils
No plasmacytosis	Diffuse plasmacytosis extending to the base of the mucosa
No mucosal distortion	Mucosal distortion

*Distinction between these two entities should be made at the time of presentation because histologic changes rapidly evolve in ASLC.

late, and loperamide hydrochloride, is controversial. They are contraindicated in shigellosis, salmonellosis,[6, 32] and *E. coli* infections particularly the 0157:H7 strain[34] in which the use of such agents may prolong excretion of the organism and toxin.

In certain infections, antimicrobial therapy can reduce the severity and duration of the diarrhea (Table 41–3). However, antibiotics in infections such as nontyphoidal species of *Salmonella* may prolong the intestinal carrier state without changing the clinical course.[6, 10, 34] The physician should also be cognizant of the emergence of many antibiotic-resistant bacteria, especially *Shigella* and *Salmonella* species, possibly requiring the use of newer, investigational drugs.[10, 34, 37, 39]

SPECIAL PROBLEMS

Certain groups of patients are at high risk for infectious diarrhea and may pose difficult problems in diagnosis and management. International travelers, the homosexual male population, and the elderly are of particular interest to the primary care physician.

Travelers' Diarrhea

High-risk areas for acquiring travelers' diarrhea include Africa, Asia, the Middle East, and South and Central America.[11, 40] In the Third World countries the most frequent agents of travelers' diarrhea are enterotoxigenic *E. coli*, less commonly *Salmonella*, *Shigella*, Norwalk agent, and rotavirus (Fig 41–2).[11, 41–43] In Asia, *Aeromonas, Plesiomonas, Vibrio parahaemolyticus,* and *Vibrio cholerae* (non 01) are the more common culprits causing diarrhea.[11] The onset of diarrhea is usually 2 to 6 days after the traveler has arrived in the country. The diarrhea is watery (four to five loose stools per day) sometimes accompanied by abdominal cramps, nausea, vomiting and fever. In most cases the symptoms last 3 days. The initial treatment carried out by the patient may be all that is required.[11, 43] The physician will generally become involved with the patient who has failed symptomatic therapy with antimotility agents or bismuth subsalicylate or had inadequate response to trimethoprim/sulfamethoxazole, trimethoprim alone,[44] doxycycline, or nalidixic acid. In such cases antibiotic-resistant bacteria and parasites[45] especially *Entamoeba histolytica*

TABLE 41-3.
Antimicrobial Therapy for Infectious Colitis

Organism	Primary	Alternative
Campylobacter sp.	Erythromycin 250 mg qid × 7 days	Tetracycline 250 mg qid × 7 days
Shigella sp.	Trimethoprim 160 mg/ sulfamethoxazole 800 mg bid × 7 days	Ampicillin 500 mg qid × 5 days Tetracycline 2.5 gm × one dose Norfloxacin 400 mg bid × 5 days*
Clostridium difficile	Vancomycin 125 mg po q6hr	Metronidazole 250 mg q6hr
Salmonella sp.† (nontyphoidal)	Chloramphenicol 500 mg IV q6hr‡	Ampicillin 1 gm IV q6hr Norfloxacin 400 mg bid to tid*
Yersinia enterocolitica†	Gentamicin or tobramycin 1.5 mg/kg IV q8hr, or amikacin 5 mg/kg IV q6hr	Third generation cephalosporin 1–2 gm IV q6hr
Yersinia pseudotuberculosis†	Ampicillin 1 gm IV q6hr	Tetracycline 500 mg q6hr
Neisseria gonorrhoeae§	Aqueous procaine penicillinG 4.8M units IM with probenecid 1 gm po	Spectinomycin 2 gm IM, Norfloxacin*
Chlamydia trachomatis	Tetracycline 500 mg qid × 7 days (× 3 weeks for LGV strains)	Erythromycin 500 mg qid × 7 days (× 3 weeks for LGV strains)
Entamoeba histolytica	Metronidazole 750 mg q8hr × 10 days (combine with iodoquinol 650 mg tid × 20 days in severe cases)	Emetine 1 mg/kg/day 5–10 days

* Investigational drug.[35, 36]
† Treat severe cases only.
‡ Resistance to this drug has emerged in the United States.[37]
§ Treat contacts; up to 35% of cases are penicillinase-producing *Neisseria gonorrhoeae*.[38]

should be suspected. Stool specimens should be obtained for examination and cultures. Sigmoidoscopy may reveal edema and ulcerations, which should be biopsied. Acute and convalescence serologies may be helpful. Therapy will include rehydration, nutritional support, and appropriate antibiotic therapy (Table 41–4). At present there are bacterial strains of *Shigella, Salmonella,* and *E. coli* that are resistant to the usual drugs of choice. Recent studies with new antimicrobial agents, such as Norfloxacin and Ciprofloxacin, have demonstrated promising results against such enteropathogens.[32, 35–37, 39]

Diarrhea in the Homosexual Male

The traditional list of venereal pathogens such as *Neisseria gonorrhoeae, Trepo-*

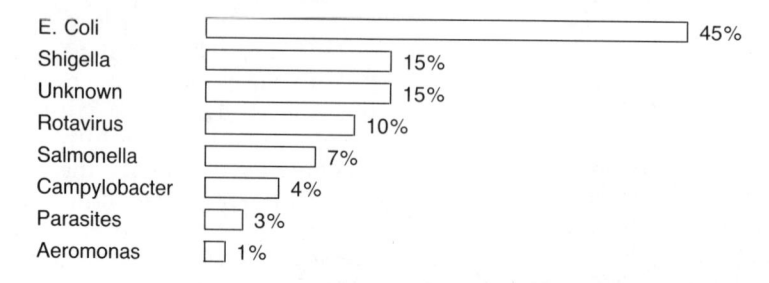

E. Coli — 45%
Shigella — 15%
Unknown — 15%
Rotavirus — 10%
Salmonella — 7%
Campylobacter — 4%
Parasites — 3%
Aeromonas — 1%

FIG 41–2.
Typical infectious agents responsible for travelers' diarrhea in Mexico.

nema pallidum, *Chlamydia trachomatis* (particularly LGV strains), and herpes simplex virus not only cause anorectal disease but also infectious colitis, the latter much less frequently. A rather difficult problem for the homosexual male is sexual transmission of enteric pathogens, including *Shigella, Salmonella, Campylobacter, Giardia,* and *Entamoeba histolytica*.[7,8] A careful history and physical examination are necessary. Serologic testing for syphilis, hepatitis B, and human immunodeficiency virus (HIV) antibody should be performed. In those patients with enteritis, stools should be examined for *G. lamblia*,[46] *Isospora, Cryptosporidium,* and cultures should be obtained for *Yersinia, V. parahaemolyticus,* and enterotoxigenic *E. coli*.[7,47]

Rectal material for examination and culture for *N. Gonorrhoeae* and *Chlamydia trachomatis* should be obtained with a swab. If an ulcer is observed anoscopically, dark field examination of scrapings of the ulcer base may reveal syphilis.[8] In the presence of edematous mucosa, a sterile cotton-wool-tipped applicator stick should be rolled over the rectal mucosa and then placed in transport medium for herpes virus culture. Sigmoidoscopy should then be done, and biopsies should be obtained if abnormal mucosa is found.

Histologically, some of the most marked pathologic alterations are in men with syphilis. The architecture remains intact, but plasma cells are markedly increased in the lamina propria. In more severe cases there may be neutrophils on the epithelial surface or in the lamina propria and crypt abscesses. On the other hand, biopsies of rectal gonorrhea are frequently normal.[48]

In cases of proctocolitis, examination and culture of stool specimens may reveal *Entamoeba histolytica, Chlamydia trachomatis* (LGV strain), *Shigella, Salmonella,* and *Campylobacter* sp. Serology may be useful in cases of *Chlamydia trachomatis*, and acute invasive amebic infections. The prevalence of *Entamoeba histolytica* is between 25% and 40% in homosexual men.[8] Greater than half of the infected individuals are asymptomatic carriers. Therefore treatment is indicated for symptomatic disease but disputable for the carriers.

Despite abnormal findings on sigmoidoscopy and biopsy, an infectious agent may not be identified, in which case repetitive sampling may be required to establish the diagnosis. In the absence of infectious etiology, trauma or irritation from chemicals contained in the lubricants used during anal intercourse may explain the abnormal findings.[8,48]

Patients with AIDS are more susceptible to intestinal infections by unusual pathogens (Table 41–5).[9,11] Cytomegalovirus, a herpes virus, usually causes asymptomatic infections, but in the immunosuppressed, clinical features vary from a mild nonspecific febrile illness to pneumonitis, hepatitis, and retinitis. Gastrointestinal involvement may be associated with these manifestations or may be the salient feature of the infection leading to intractable diarrhea. Proctocolitis may be present. Complications of perforation or massive hemorrhage have occurred in

TABLE 41–4.
Treatment of Travelers' Diarrhea

Mild Diarrhea	Severe Diarrhea
Bismuth subsalicylate (Pepto-Bismol 30 ml q1hr for eight doses or, 2 tablets q1hr as needed up to eight doses/day	Trimethoprim 160 mg/ sulfamethoxazole 800 mg bid for 3 days or,
	Doxycycline 100 mg bid for 3 days
	Norfloxacin,* Ciprofloxacin*

*Investigational drug.

TABLE 41–5.
Opportunistic Pathogens That
Cause Diarrhea

Cryptosporidium
Mycobacterium avium-intracellulare
Mycobacterium tuberculosis
Cytomegalovirus
Salmonella
Herpes simplex virus
Clostridium difficile
Candida sp.

a few cases with cecal ulcerations. In light of the high morbidity and mortality in the immunosuppressed patient with cytomegalovirus infection an effective therapeutic agent is needed. A promising new drug, Ganciclovir, is presently under investigation.[49, 50]

The parasite, *Cryptosporidium*, has been associated with diarrheal infections in both immunosuppressed and immunocompetent hosts. Cryptosporidia have been demonstrated by histopathologic examination of biopsies from various gastrointestinal sites. Although the illness is usually self-limited with profuse watery diarrhea, the severity and duration are a function of the immunologic status of the patient. In AIDS patients, the diarrhea may be severe, chronic, and unresponsive to therapy. Diagnosis can be by examination of fecal concentrations, direct and indirect fluorescent staining procedures, and direct wet preparations of fecal material. Tissue biopsies of the gastrointestinal tract may reveal nonspecific inflammation as well as cryptosporidia. These patients should be isolated to prevent spread of the disease. There is no known effective treatment for cryptosporidiosis although spiramycin is often tried.[9, 51–54]

Other infectious agents, such as *Salmonella* may lead to life-threatening diarrhea and bacteremia in AIDS patients. Despite appropriate antibiotic therapy, many patients have persistent or recurrent infection.[9, 55] *Mycobacterium avium-intracellulare* infection occurs late in the course of AIDS. Gastrointestinal symptoms may begin as esophagitis or diarrhea. Intestinal biopsy may mimic Whipple's disease, but the macrophages contain acid-fast bacilli. Sometimes the organisms are identified on fecal smears. This mycobacterium is highly resistant to the usual antitubercular agents. The infection in AIDS patients is extremely difficult if not impossible to eradicate with the available agents, ansamycin and clofazimine.[9]

The Elderly Patient

In the elderly, the most common type of colitis is infectious followed by ischemic colitis. *Salmonella* may act more virulently in these patients and is therefore more likely to lead to sepsis. Because there is increased morbidity and mortality in the older patients antibiotic therapy is more frequently indicated.[5] *Escherichia coli* 0157:H7 (verotoxin-producing) has recently been identified as a major cause of outbreaks of colitis in nursing homes.[4] The spectrum of illness can range from asymptomatic infection to nonbloody diarrhea to hemorrhagic colitis, hemolytic uremic syndrome, and death.[56–58] Diagnosis cannot be made unless stools for culture and *E. coli* serotyping are obtained early in the course of illness. The organism clears from the stool in 5 to 7 days; therefore, an early stool specimen should be frozen for eventual serotyping in case no other pathogen is found during the preliminary work-up. Arrangements must be made through state epidemiologists and laboratories to examine the stool for type-specific identification. Presently there is no proven effective antimicrobial therapy.[4] Moreover, antimotility agents, which have been shown to increase the severity of *Shigella* infections, may also increase the mortality and morbidity of *E. coli* 0157:H7 infections by allowing the organisms to multiply and produce the vero-cytotoxin (a Shiga-like toxin).[4, 34]

Pseudomembranous (antibiotic-associated) colitis caused by *Clostridium difficile* is a special type of infectious colitis most frequently found in the elderly patient, especially when confined for chronic care. Older patients are at increased risk for infection and, therefore, are more likely to

TABLE 41-6.
Criteria for the Diagnosis of *Clostridium difficile*-Associated Colitis*

1. Detection of *Clostridium difficile* in the stool
2. Detection of *Clostridium difficile* cytotoxin in the stool
3. Endoscopic (or biopsy) evidence of pseudomembranous colitis

*One or more of these tests should be positive.

receive antibiotic therapy.[21] Furthermore, epidemiologic studies strongly suggest hospital acquisition via person-to-person and common-source spread.[20] A recent study has demonstrated the association of previous infection and antibiotic therapy (particularly clindamycin) and therapy with multiple antibiotics and antacids.[20, 21, 59, 60] *Clostridium difficile* in adults usually causes symptomatic disease. The clinical picture is characterized by non-bloody mucoid diarrhea, low-grade fever, mild abdominal pain, and tenderness. Diagnosis is usually made at proctosigmoidoscopy which classically demonstrates slightly raised small yellow-white plaques that are sometimes confluent. The mucosa between the plaques is typically edematous but not ulcerated. In contrast, the rectal mucosa may be normal or may reveal only mild edema while the pseudomembranes are located in more proximal regions of the colon.[17-19] Therefore, in patients with less typical findings on sigmoidoscopy, determination of *Clostridium difficile* toxin and isolation of the organism from stool cultures using selective media are essential.

Although the best criteria for the diagnosis of *Clostridium difficile*-associated colitis are the presence of *Clostridium difficile* in the stool with detection of stool cytotoxin in patients with appropriate clinical findings, the diagnostic parameters are not always positive (Table 41-6). Several factors contribute to the variability of the results, including laboratory technique, quality of the stool specimen, the fastidious bacilli, and the difference in the toxigenic potential of the many strains of *Clostridium difficile*.[61, 62] Patients with *Clostridium difficile* isolated in stool that is cytotoxin-negative may demonstrate a toxin when the same stool is cultured.[59] Such patients should receive specific antimicrobial therapy, and the implicated antibiotic should be discontinued.[63, 64] Although oral vancomycin is almost uniformly successful, relapses after initial response to therapy have been documented. In such cases a course of metronidazole should be given. Should another relapse occur, a tapering dose of oral vancomycin for 21 days followed by a pulse dose of vancomycin for 21 days has been shown to be effective.[65]

In conclusion, numerous infectious agents can cause colitis, which can mimic other diseases such as chronic ulcerative colitis and Crohn's disease. Factors to be considered in the diagnosis include the patient population encountered, previous antimicrobial or antimetabolite therapy, and recent travel. Frequently, infectious colitis is of brief duration, and the patient will not seek medical attention. The physician generally becomes involved in the more difficult cases which require complete evaluation and, eventually, antibiotic therapy.

References

1. Guerrant RL, Lohr JA, Williams EK: Acute infectious diarrhea. I. Epidemiology, etiology, and pathogenesis. Pediatr Infect Dis 1986; 5(3):353–359.
2. Elliot DL, Tolle SW, Goldberg L, et al: Pet-associated illness. N Engl J Med 1985; 313(16):985–995.
3. Levine MM: *Escherichia coli* that cause diarrhea: Enterotoxigenic, enteropathogenic, enteroinvasive, enterohemorrhagic, and enteroadherent. J Infect Dis 1987; 155(3):377–389.
4. Ryan CA, Tauxe RV, Hosek GW, et al: *Escherichia coli* 0157:H7 diarrhea in a nursing home:

Clinical, epidemiological, and pathological findings. *J Infect Dis* 1986; 154(4):631–638.
5. Brandt LJ: Colitis in the elderly. *Hosp Pract* 1987; 22(6):99–122.
6. Rennels NB, Levine MM: Classical bacterial diarrhea: Perspectives and update—*Salmonella, Shigella, Escherichia coli, Aeromonas,* and *Plesiomonas. Pediatr Infect Dis* 1986; 5(1):S91–S100.
7. Weller IVD: The gay bowel. *Gut* 1985; 26:869–875.
8. Quinn TC: Clinical approach to intestinal infections in homosexual men. *Med Clin North Am* 1986; 70(3):611–634.
9. Bodey GP, Fainstein V, Guerrant R: Infections of the gastrointestinal tract in the immunocompromised patient. *Annu Rev Med* 1986; 37:271–281.
10. Williams EK, Lohr JA, Guerrant RL: Acute infectious diarrhea. II. Diagnosis, treatment and prevention. *Pediatr Infect Dis* 1986; 5(4):458–465.
11. Quinn TS, Bender BS, Bartlett JG: New developments in infectious diarrhea. *DM* 1986; 32(4):165–244.
12. Cooper BT: Diarrhoea as a symptom. *Clin Gastroenterol* 1985; 14(3):599–613.
13. Adler PM: Stool examination: Culture versus Gram stain. *Ann Emerg Med* 1986; 15(3):337–341.
14. Thomson RB Jr, Haas RA, Thompson JH Jr: Intestinal parasites: The necessity of examining multiple stool specimens. *Mayo Clin Proc* 1984; 59:641–642.
15. Simmonds SD, Noble MA, Freeman HJ: Gastrointestinal features of culture-positive *Yersinia enterocolitica* infection. *Gastroenterology* 1987; 92:112–117.
16. Ratnam S, March SB: Stool survey for *Escherichia coli* 0157:H7. *J Infect Dis* 1986; 153:1176–1177.
17. Tedesco FJ, Barton RW, Alpers DH: Clindamycin-associated colitis. A prospective study. *Ann Intern Med* 1974; 81:429–433.
18. Tedesco FJ: Antibiotic-associated pseudomembranous colitis: 1980. *Compr Ther* 1980; 5(13):15–17.
19. Tedesco FJ: Pseudomembranous colitis: Pathogenesis and therapy. *Med Clin North Am* 1982; 66(3):655–664.
20. Gerding DN, Olson MM, Peterson LR, et al: *Clostridium difficile*-associated diarrhea and colitis in adults. *Arch Intern Med* 1986; 146:95–100.
21. Bender BS, Laughon BE, Gaydos C, et al: Is *Clostridium difficile* endemic in chronic-care facilities? *Lancet* 1986; I:11–13.
22. Needham CA: Rapid detection methods in microbiology: Are they right for your office? *Med Clin North Am* 1987; 71(4):591–605.
23. Radhakrishnan S, A Nakib B, Shaikh H, et al: The value of colonoscopy in schistosomal, tuberculous and amebic colitis. Two-year experience. *Dis Colon Rectum* 1986; 29(12):891–895.
24. Tedesco FJ, Moore S: Infectious diseases mimicking inflammatory bowel disease. *Am Surg* 1982; 48(6):243–249.
25. Tedesco FJ, Hardin RD, Harper RN, et al: Infectious colitis endoscopically simulating inflammatory bowel disease: A prospective evaluation. *Gastrointest Endosc* 1983; 29(3):195–197.
26. Brown R, Tedesco FJ, Assad RT, et al: *Yersinia* colitis masquerading as pseudomembranous colitis. *Dig Dis Sci* 1986; 31(5):548–551.
27. Itzkowitz SH: Conditions that mimic inflammatory bowel disease. Diagnostic clues and potential pitfalls. *Postgrad Med* 1986; 80(6):219–231.
28. Surawicz CM, Belic L: Rectal biopsy helps to distinguish acute self-limited colitis from idiopathic inflammatory bowel disease. *Gastroenterology* 1984; 86:104–113.
29. Nostrant TT, Kumar NB, Appelman HD: Histopathology differentiates acute self-limited colitis from ulcerative colitis. *Gastroenterology* 1987; 92:318–328.
30. Van Speeuwel JP, Duursma GC, Meijer CJLM, et al: *Campylobacter* colitis: Histological, immunohistochemical and ultrastructural findings. *Gut* 1985; 26:945–951.
31. Boyd JF: Pathology of the alimentary tract in *Salmonella typhimurium* food poisoning. *Gut* 1985; 26:935–944.
32. Levine MM: Bacillary dysentery. Mechanisms and treatment. *Med Clin North Am* 1982; 66(3):623–637.
33. Black RE: The prophylaxis and therapy of secretory diarrhea. *Med Clin North Am* 1982; 66(3):611–621.
34. Marques LRM, Moore MA, Wells JG, et al: Production of Shiga-like toxin by *Escherichia coli*. *J Infect Dis* 1986; 154(2):338–341.
35. Lee C, Ronald AR: Norfloxacin: Its potential in clinical practice. *Am J Med* 1987; 82(Suppl 6B):27–34.
36. Dupont HL, Corrado ML, Sabbaj J: Use of Norfloxacin in the treatment of acute diarrheal disease. *Am J Med* 1987; 82(Suppl 6B):79–83.
37. Bryan JP, Rocha H, Scheld WM: Problems in salmonellosis: Rationale for clinical trials with newer β-lactame agents and quinolones. *Rev Infect Dis* 1986; 8(2):189–207.
38. Boslego JW, Tramont EC, Takajufi ET, et al: Effect of spectinomycin use on the prevalence of spectinomycin-resistant and of penicillinase-producing *Neisseria gonorrhoeae*. *N Engl J Med* 1987; 317(5):272–277.
39. Cherubin CE, Eng RHK, Smith SM, et al: Cephalosporin therapy for salmonellosis. Questions of efficacy and cross resistance with ampicillin. *Arch Intern Med* 1986; 146:2149–2152.
40. Steffen R, van der Linde F, Gyr K, et al: Epidemiology of diarrhea in travelers. *JAMA* 1983; 249(9):1176–1180.
41. DuPont HL, Ericsson CD, Johnson PC, et al: Antimicrobial agents in the prevention of travelers' diarrhea. *Rev Infect Dis* 1986; 8(S2):S167–S171.
42. Gorbach SL: Travelers' diarrhea. *N Engl J Med* 1982; 307(14):881–883.
43. Dupont H, Ericsson CD, Murray BE: Travelers' diarrhea: Can it be eluded? *JAMA* 1983; 249(9):1193–1194.
44. Dupont H, Reves RR, Galindo E, et al: Treatment of travelers' diarrhea with trimethoprim/sulfamethoxazole and with trimethoprim alone. *N Engl J Med* 1982; 307(14):841–844.
45. Poland GA, Navin TR, Sarosi GA: Outbreak of parasitic gastroenteritis among travelers return-

ing from Africa. *Arch Intern Med* 1985; 145:2220–2221.
46. Dupont HL, Sullivan PS: Giardiasis: The clinical spectrum, diagnosis and therapy. *Pediatr Infect Dis* 1986; 5(4):S131–S138.
47. Owen WF Jr: The clinical approach to the male homosexual patient. *Med Clin North Am* 1986; 70(3):499–535.
48. McMillan A, Lee FD: Sigmoidoscopic and microscopic appearance of the rectal mucosa in homosexual men. *Gut* 1981; 22:1035–1041.
49. Laskin OL, Cederberg DM, Mills J, et al: Ganciclovir for the treatment and suppression of serious infections caused by cytomegalovirus. *Am J Med* 1987; 83(2):201–207.
50. Chachoua A, Dieterich D, Krasinski K, et al: 9-(1,3-dihydroxy-2-propoxymethyl) guanine (Ganciclovir) in the treatment of cytomegalovirus gastrointestinal disease with the acquired immunodeficiency syndrome. *Ann Intern Med* 1987; 107:133–137.
51. Soave R, Armstrong D: *Cryptosporidium* and cryptosporidiosis. *Rev Infect Dis* 1986; 8(6):1012–1023.
52. Rolston KVI, Fainstein V: Cryptosporidiosis. *Eur J Clin Microbiol* 1986; 5(2):135–137.
53. Mata L: Cryptosporidium and other protozoa in diarrheal disease in less developed countries. *Pediatr Infect Dis* 1986; 5(4):S117–S130.
54. Sterling CR, Arrowood J: Detection of *Cryptosporidium* sp infections using a direct immunofluorescent assay. *Pediatr Infect Dis* 1986; 5(4):S139–S142.
55. Fischl MA, Dickinson GM, Sinave C, et al: *Salmonella* bacteremia as manifestation of acquired immunodeficiency syndrome. *Arch Intern Med* 1986; 146:113–115.
56. Ratnam S, March SB, Sprague WD: Are humans a source of *Escherichia coli* 0157:H7, the agent of hemorrhagic colitis? *N Engl J Med* 1986; 315(25):1612–1613.
57. Neill MA, Agosti J, Rosen H: Hemorrhagic colitis with *Escherichia coli* 0157:H7 preceding adult hemolytic uremic syndrome. *Arch Intern Med* 1985; 145:2215–2217.
58. Gransden WR, Damm MAS, Anderson JD, et al: Further evidence associating hemolytic uremic syndrome with infection by verotoxin-producing *Escherichia coli* 0157:H7. *J Infect Dis* 1986; 154(3):522–524.
59. Broitman SA: *Clostridium difficile* antibiotic-associated colitis. *Am J Gastroenterol* 1986; 81:1005–1006.
60. Bowman RA, Riley TV: *Clostridium difficile* in diarrheal disease. *J Infect Dis* 1986; 153:1177–1178.
61. Lashner BA, Todorczuk J, Sahm DF, et al: *Clostridium difficile* culture-positive toxin-negative diarrhea. *Am J Gastroenterol* 1986; 81:940–943.
62. Church JM, Fazio VW: The significance of quantitative results of *C. difficile* cultures and toxin assays in patients with diarrhea. *Dis Colon Rectum* 1985; 28(10):765–769.
63. Young GP, Ward PB, Bayley N, et al: Antibiotic-associated colitis due to *Clostridium difficile:* Double-blind comparison of vancomycin with bacitracin. *Gastroenterology* 1985; 89:1038–1045.
64. Tedesco F, Gorwith M, Markham R, et al: Oral vancomycin for antibiotic-associated pseudomembranous colitis. *Lancet* 1978; II:226–228.
65. Tedesco FJ, Gordon D, Fortson WC: Approach to patients with multiple relapses of antibiotic-associated pseudomembranous colitis. *Am J Gastroenterol* 1985; 80:867–868.

42

Obstipation:
What is the appropriate therapeutic approach?

GHISLAIN DEVROEDE, M.D.
JACQUES POISSON, M.D.
JEAN-CLAUDE SCHANG, M.D.

The purpose of this chapter is not to review extensively all aspects of constipation. This has been done elsewhere.[1] Rather, it will focus on the problems presented by the recognition, evaluation, and management of intractable constipation.

WHEN IS CONSTIPATION OBSTIPATION?

Constipation is a symptom. It is not a disease, nor a sign.

As a symptom, constipation may be indicative of many diseases, and a differential diagnosis[1] should be made as would be for abdominal pain. This chapter does not deal with these diseases, but with chronic idiopathic constipation: it implies, of course, that among this group of patients, some will be found, in the future, to suffer from specific etiologies, hitherto unrecognized.

A symptom is the experience of a sign by a patient; not only is the subjective appreciation highly variable from patient to patient, but previous unpleasant experiences of the same nature, both physical and emotional, interfere with the perception of the present experience. The difference between sign and symptom is that the scientific method, which relies on observations and measurements, is only applicable to the sign. Dismissing the symptom as unimportant as compared to the sign and dismissing the associated emotions as irrelevant are bound to lead to an oversimplified approach to constipation. It also explains the persistent symptomatology of some patients in whom little objective evidence of constipation has been found.

Constipation has different meanings for different patients. It may imply that their stools are too small, too hard, too difficult to expel, or that they have a feeling of incomplete evacuation after defecation. These symptoms are difficult to quantify.

Stool frequency is the easiest parameter of constipation to quantify. To avoid potential exaggeration of the problem,[2,3] a meticulous prospective count of stools should be made over a period of weeks. Recent studies show that less than five (and not three as previously thought) stools per week should be considered as a sign of constipation.[4,5] Whites defecate more often than blacks, and males more than females[5] (Fig 42–1). In Senegal on the contrary, people usually defecate in the morning and evening, and consider themselves constipated if they only have one stool per day.[6] In the Western world, one-third of "normal" subjects complain of symptoms suggestive of an irritable bowel syndrome, constipation being one

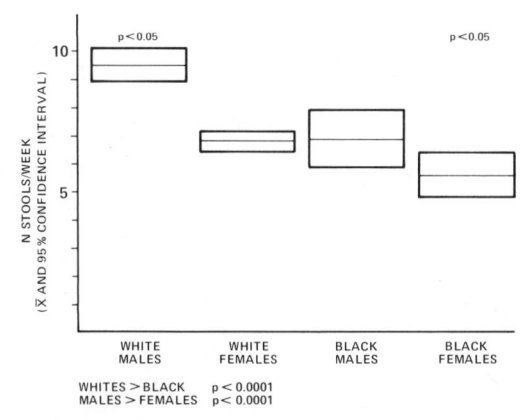

FIG 42–1.
Stool frequency of normal subjects. (Adapted from Sandler RS, Drossman DA: Bowel habits in apparently healthy young adults. *Dig Dis Sci*, in press.)

which may range from a completely flaccid, ineffective musculature in colonic inertia to a marked spasticity such as in Hirschsprung's disease and some patients with the irritable bowel syndrome.

The word obstipation should be reserved to characterize the following categories of patients:

Those who deny they defecate

Those who keep complaining of constipation despite little evidence for it in terms of stool frequency or large-bowel transit time, and who claim treatment does not modify the symptoms

Those who have persistent evidence of prolonged large-bowel transit time, irrespective of treatment; clinically, these patients will often complain of total absence of stools and flatus

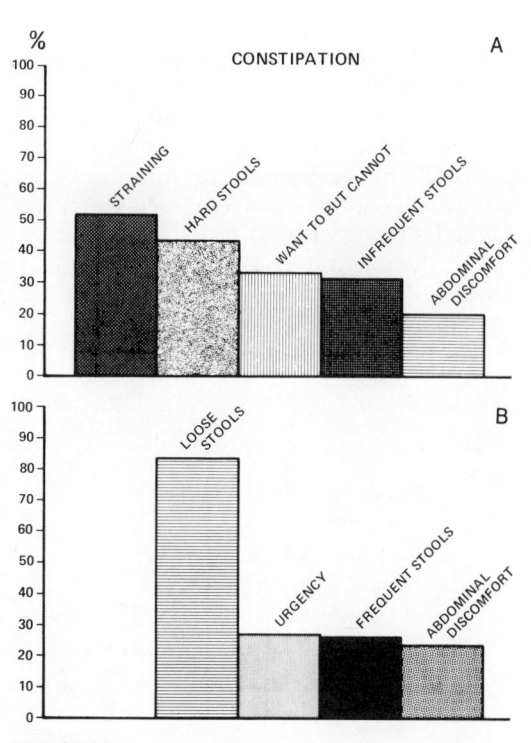

of its cardinal symptoms.[7] Finally, frequency per se is not of much concern to people who worry more about efforts to defecate, excessive stool consistency, and incapacity to defecate at will[5] (Fig 42–2). Normality does not change along secular trends and is not necessarily what most people do; thus, any complaint of constipation, even within "normal" range, should be listened to.

With this background in mind, how should the symptom "obstipation" be defined? The choice of words we use is never neutral,[8] and "obstipation" sounds very much like "obstinacy." This is even more evident in French, in which "obstinacy" translates into "obstination," and we know both these English and French terms derive from Latin. The linguistic analysis of "constipation" and "obstipation" reveals differences in the prefix only. *Stipare*, in Latin, means to cram, pack, to crowd. The prefix "con" comes from the latin *"cum,"* which means together, while the prefix "ob" means against. There is therefore only a difference in intensity, although more violence is implied in the term against. Interestingly, both words presume that constipation and obstipation result from a narrowing of the bowel, or from a compaction of feces, and do not reflect the spectrum of abnormal bowel function in constipation,

FIG 42–2.
People are more concerned by symptoms than by numbers.[5] For physicians, the reverse is true. This may be a cause of major misunderstandings and poor relationships. Medicine, if it is to be helpful, should be patient based, rather than physician based. **A** refers to constipation; **B** refer to diarrhea.

Overall, there are in "obstipation" many of the subjective components of "constipation," regardless of the objective, scientifically measurable components.

RISKS OF OBSTIPATION

Constipation is associated with many symptoms that are sources of discomfort.[9] This is even more so for obstipation. But constipation is not innocuous and also carries some risks.

Urinary tract infections, enuresis and vesicoureteral reflux may be associated with constipation and may disappear when the latter is treated.[10] It should be remembered, however, that association is not causation and that the pelvic floor is one neuromuscular unit traversed by the urinary, genital, and intestinal tract.[11] A disorder of the pelvic floor could induce both constipation and bladder dysfunction, without the former being the cause of the latter.

Potentially hazardous dilated loops of sigmoid are often associated with constipation.[12] Stercoraceous perforation is a potentially lethal consequence of prolonged storage of hard feces.[13]

As demonstrated by four controlled studies,[14–17] there is increased risk of cancer of the colon and rectum in patients with constipation, particularly for women. This is particularly so when patients defecate less than three times a week for a long period of time[16, 17] (Fig 42–3). However, the magnitude of risk for a given patient to develop cancer of the bowel is not known. In studies investigating geographic differences of cancer risk, a low prevalence of cancer of the large bowel was associated with greater stool weight but not with differences in rates of transit.[18, 19]

A socially inconvenient complication may result from chronic straining, which probably occurs quite often in patients with obstipation. Stretching of the pudendal nerve results in a weak and lax pelvic floor, where striated muscles are denervated, and this is conducive to fecal incontinence.[20]

The incidence of epithelial dysplasia in mammary secretions is in reverse correlation with stool frequency[21] (Fig 42–4). This suggests the possibility of an association between breast disease, benign and malignant, and bowel function.

Constipated patients are at high risk of unnecessary surgery, and this is probably even more true when constipation is obstipation. There is an excess of appendectomy in young women as compared to young men,[22] and this compares well to the predominance of women among constipated subjects. Few constipated patients present with an acute abdominal

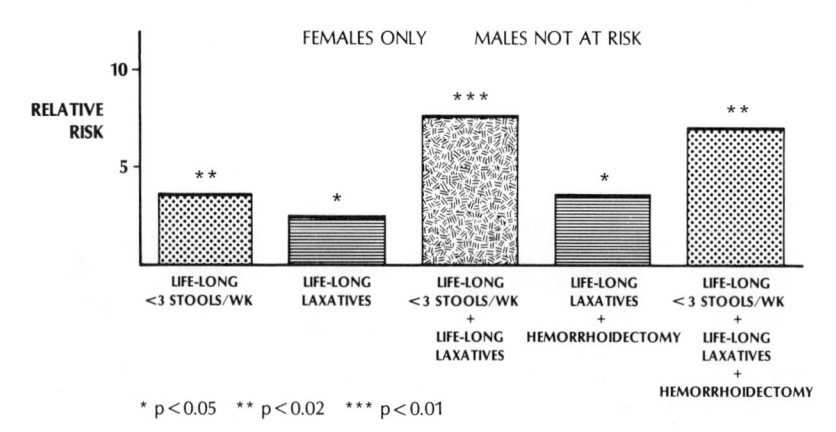

FIG 42–3.
Severe constipation is associated with a risk of large bowel cancer. (Adapted from Vobecky J, Caro J, and Devroede G: A case control study of risk factors for large bowel carcinoma. Cancer 1983; 51:1958–1963.)

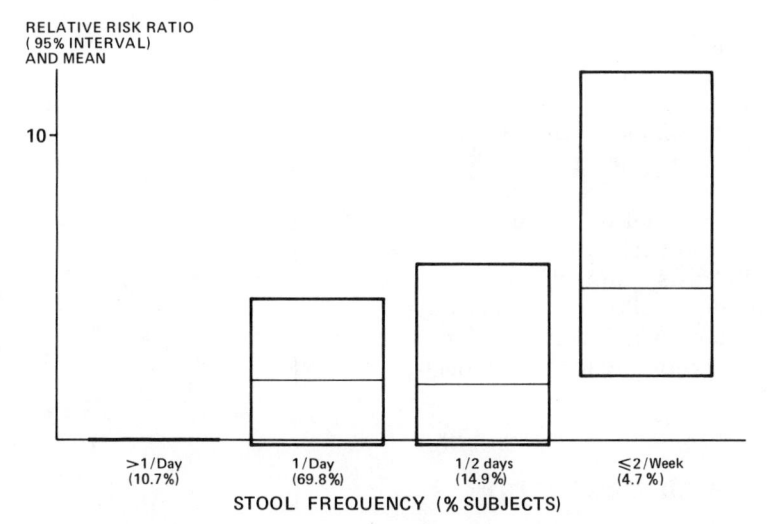

FIG 42–4.
There is an association between mammary dysplasia and a low stool frequency. (Adapted from Petrakis NL, King EB: Cytological abnormalities in nipple aspirates of breast fluid from women with severe constipation. *Lancet* 1985; Nov. 28:1203–1205.)

pain, but when they do, the physician should not rush to surgery. Unnecessary laparotomy is also performed much more often in patients with the irritable bowel syndrome than in controls.[23–26] Patients with slow-transit constipation are all women, and they undergo, ovarian cystectomy and hysterectomy more often as compared to controls[27] (Fig 42–5). Similarly, women with megarectum who were not constipated at birth also often undergo hysterectomy, and when studied microscopically, the specimen is normal.[3] It is easy to understand why unnecessary laparotomies are performed because of the frequent association of chronic lower

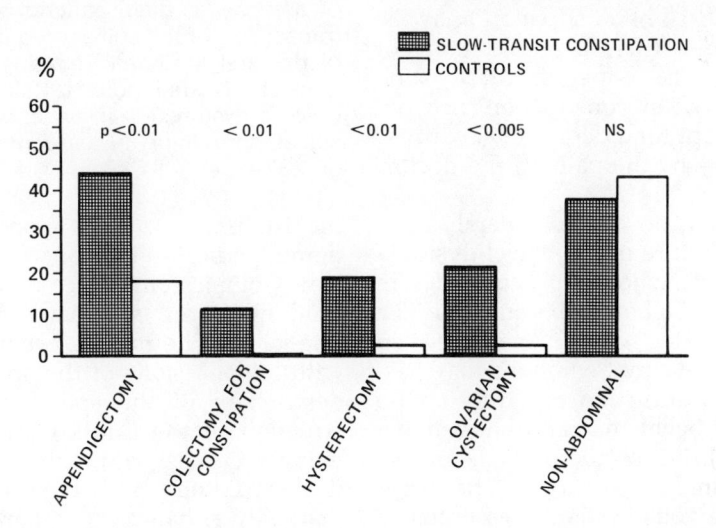

FIG 42–5.
A constipated woman runs an unnecessary risk of surgery. (Adapted from Preston DM, Lennard-Jones JE: Severe chronic constipation in young women: Idiopathic slow transit constipation. *Gut* 1986; 27:41–48.)

abdominal pain with constipation, but there is a danger of converting a functional problem into a real iatrogenic disease. Many physicians are unaware that psychiatric illness is often present in subjects with irritable bowel syndrome (IBS). This precludes optimal treatment. For example, hysteria seems not to be recognized by internists, and because it is a polysymptomatic illness, unnecessary surgery is often performed and more medications and more hospitalizations are prescribed.[28–30]

ETIOLOGY OF OBSTIPATION

Constipation and obstipation may be secondary to diseases that are inborn or acquired later in life. The vast majority of known etiologies will be recognized through a good differential diagnosis. The scope of this chapter does not allow review of all specific causes, which have been described thoroughly elsewhere.[1] We probably will learn a lot in the future about organic disorders of the intrinsic innervation of the bowel, but our present understanding is very poor.

It is within the group of patients suffering from chronic idiopathic constipation that a diagnosis of obstipation may be made. Of course there is ample room for subjectivity, because per se there is no difference between constipation and obstipation, except for a degree of severity—or frustration—by the patient, the doctor, or both.

An exception to these general statements is the nature of the bowel dysfunction in subjects who have a disorder in innervation of the bowel, because this is a source of agitated controversy between those who believe that emotions may trigger organic dysfunction and those who have another belief, namely that a material cause will be found to all disorders, whether organic or functional. The integrity of the nervous system is essential to maintain normal defecation. In patients with traumatic transection of the spinal cord above the level of the first lumbar vertebra there is no colonic response to

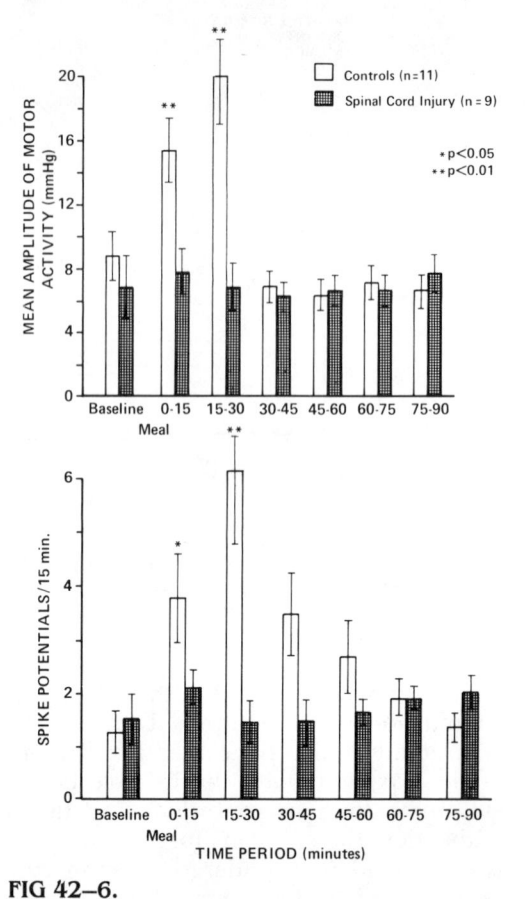

FIG 42–6.
The colon is not stimulated by the ingestion of a meal, in male patients with traumatic transection of the spinal cord above the level of the first lumbar vertebra. (Adapted from Glick ME, Meshkinpour H, Haldeman S, et al: Colonic dysfunction in patients with thoracic spinal cord injury. *Gastroenterology* 1984; 86:287–294.)

meal (Fig 42–6), while response to Prostigmin indicates the muscle itself is normal. Colonic compliance and tolerance to fluid filling are also markedly reduced[31] (Fig 42–7). The reverse occurs in patients with lower lesions of the spinal cord and destruction of the spinal cord and destruction of the cauda equina: pressure-volume curves within the colon are flat during filling, and the compliance is markedly enhanced.[32, 33] Parasympathetic innervation is also essential for normal bowel function.[34–36] Resection of the nervi erigentes leads to obstipation, loss of rectal sensation, and delayed transit through

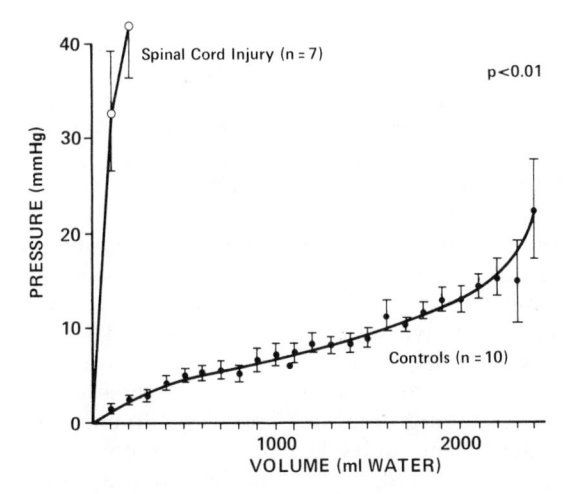

FIG 42–7.
The accommodation properties of the large bowel are markedly reduced in male patients who had traumatic transection of the spinal cord above the level of the first lumbar vertebra. (Adapted from Glick ME, Meshkinpour H, Haldeman S, et al: Colonic dysfunction in patients with thoracic spinal cord injury. *Gastroenterology* 1984; 86:287–294.)

the large bowel. Rectal sensation is lost, and rectal capacity to distention is increased after bilateral sacrifice of sacral nerves but not unilateral. Bypass of the hindgut restores transit, which suggests that sacral parasympathetic outflow exerts no influence on the ascending colon. Trauma to the cauda equina also results in constipation, even in the absence of paraplegia.[35] The anal canal becomes hypertonic. The rectoanal inhibitory reflex persists, but its amplitude is maximal for minimal levels of rectal distention, in contrast to health, where there is a linear relationship between level of rectal distention and degree of anal canal relaxation.[4] The rectoanal contractile reflex of the external anal sphincter also becomes much weaker than normal. An internal anal sphincter relaxing in presence of minimal rectal distention, associated to a poorly functioning external anal sphincter, of course, offers little protection against fecal incontinence if laxatives or enemas are used to overcome this type of constipation.

From this review of the importance of extrinsic innervation of the bowel in terms of function, we can conclude that diseases of innervation do induce constipation. We may also hypothesize that these same pathways may be followed in cases of functional disorders, and that they are not necessarily indicative of disease. For instance, it has been recently demonstrated that the electric activity of the human colon is markedly reduced during periods of sleep,[37] and thus it is not too surprising to learn that the irritable bowel syndrome is influenced by hypnotherapy.[38,39] Of course, the latter two experimental conditions demonstrate that diseases are not always present when there is a bowel disorder and that there is a mind–gut interaction.

OBSTIPATION AS A BODY CLUE: DISEASE OF THE PERSON

The relationship among emotions, the psyche, and bowel habits is poorly known. That such a relationship could be involved in constipation was proposed over 50 years ago by Groddeck.[40] Many will question the relationships between mind and body. The "tomato effect"[41] is the reverse of the "placebo effect." Many good treatments have been ignored or abandoned because they were not "supposed" to work. The field of psychosomatic relationships is going to produce a lot of "tomato" effects.

There is some support for the idea that a conflict between parent and child at the time of bowel training may modify bowel habits,[42] and voluntary repression of defecation is said to lead to chronic rectal distention and megarectum. This is a little simplistic, because some children with chronic idiopathic constipation may pass unfrequent stools even before they reach the age of toilet training.

There is a relationship between stool output and personality: Healthy individuals who display a greater degree of self-esteem and are more outgoing tend to produce more frequent and heavier stools.[43]

Megacolon is found in psychotic patients,[44] and this also suggests the possibility of a link between mind and body. Schizophrenics appear to be particularly at risk; this should be placed in perspective with the fact that, in patients with constipation by colonic inertia, transit time in the ascending colon correlates to the score of paranoia in the Minnesota Multiphasic Personality Inventory (MMPI).[45]

There is a very close relationship between the levels of anxiety and transit time in the ascending colon in constipated patients who have a delayed colonic transit, most of whom are obstipated.[45] This suggests the possibility that constipation may simply reflect anxiety, which is not expressed via the mind but through physical dysfunction. Cure from constipation by a psychologic approach is the ultimate necessary proof that the basic mechanism is not organic.[46,47]

Constipated patients with delayed transit through the ascending colon have a different personality than arthritic controls.[45] They score higher on several scales of the MMPI: hypochondria, hysteria, control, and low back pain. They score lower on the masculinity–femininity (MF) scale, which means they are more feminine. The two groups can be differentiated by discriminant analysis; use of the MMPI data alone yields 83% correct answers; addition of age raises this to 95%! This means the computer can recognize a constipated patient versus an arthritic one just with personality and age, regardless of medical investigation! Of course, this does not prove that constipation leads to personality disorder or the contrary, but it demonstrates there is a link between the two.

There are two dangers in medicine to avoid: medicalization and psychiatrization, and this is particularly true for constipation and obstipation. To medicalize is to reduce a suffering human being to a diseased organ or organs. Psychiatrization, conversely, is the attribution of all problems to emotional disorders. It would be a folly to treat a patient with autonomic neuropathy, or with hindgut dysgenesis[48] by psychotherapy. Conversely, it would be a major disservice to the patient who is hysterical and constipated to perform a colectomy for cure. Not unfrequently, the remaining bowel "takes over" the dysfunction; thus, in some patients who underwent colectomy for colonic inertia, no ileal content may exude from an ileostomy even if, preoperatively, small-bowel function was normal, as evidenced by the fact that swallowed radiopaque markers were in the caecum within 24 hours. This does not make sense if one only takes into account the measurable organic elements in the patient.

The Life of Martha

Our conduct for patients with severe obstipation is more and more to be careful and not to rush to surgery. We can exemplify by a brief case report. A patient consulted us at the age of 35 because of severe constipation; she claimed she had a bowel movement only every 2 months. She also told us during this first visit that she was going to commit suicide if we did not cure her. Finally, we learned that she had been raped by her father at the age of 16.

Her past medical history was quite extensive, in that she had been hospitalized at least once a year, from 1 to 30 days, for the past 10 previous years. She had undergone multiple abdominal operations, including a hysterectomy that proved to be for functional problems, because the specimen was normal. On two occasions, she had had evidence of self-inflicted injury, in the vagina and in the rectum. Diarrhea (7 to 25 liquid stools per day) had been present up to 1 year prior to the consultation. Constipation had began when a duodenal ulcer was diagnosed in her husband.

Recorded stool frequency, on a high-fiber diet, was indeed one per 1 to 2 months. A transit study of radiopaque markers[1] provided objective evidence of the constipation (Fig 42–8). Because transit was normal through the ascending colon, the mechanism of constipation seemed to be related to a hindgut dysfunction, rather than to colonic inertia.[1] Electromyography of the colon was performed (see further in the text for details of the technique).[1] It showed little propagating activity at rest (0.42 propagating potentials/hour) and no postprandial increase, as normally expected (0.50/hour).[49,50]

A diagnosis of Münchhausen's syndrome, with psychogenic constipation and depression, was made. Objective evidence of the depression was provided by an MMPI study. The highest score (normalized values should be under 70) was that of scale 2 (D, depres-

COLONIC MOTOR ACTIVITY IN A PATIENT WITH SEVERE CHRONIC IDIOPATHIC CONSTIPATION

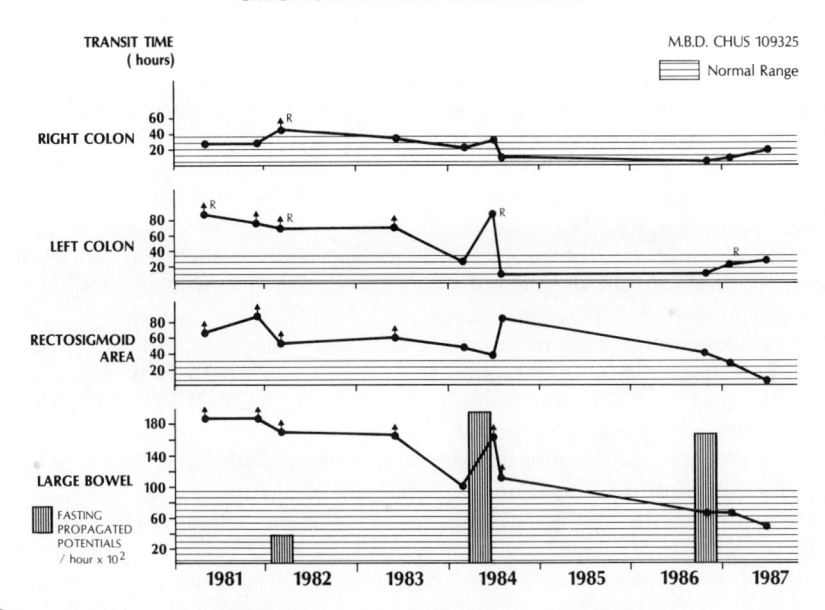

FIG 42–8.
The sign ↑ means the transit time exceeds the recorded value, because markers were still present in the examined site of bowel when radiographs were not taken any more for fear of excessive radiation (see text for details). The sign R means there is evidence of reflux of markers (and thus feces) from the distal regions of large bowel.

This figure shows data from a severely constipated patient whose abnormality was always mainly in the hindgut. The only delayed transit in the ascending colon (February 1982) was associated with reflux of markers from left to right colon. Until February 1984, the patient never excreted any marker within 1 week of ingestion, and this confirms the severity of constipation, as described in the text. Since 1986, total colorectal transit time is normal. The latest study shows segmental transit time is also normal in all bowel segments. Propagating electric activity in the distal large bowel is virtually absent in 1982. Latest studies are normal. There were no stationary potentials at first recording, either before or after meal. Subsequent studies showed some, with a postprandial increase.

sion): 98; followed by scale 8 (Sc, schizophrenia): 94; scale 1 (Hs, hypochondria): 87; scale 3 (Hy, hysteria): 84; scale 4 (Pd, psychopathic deviate): 83; scale 0 (Si, social introversion-extroversion): 83; scale 7 (Pt, psychasthenia): 79; and scale 9 (Ma, hypomania): 78.

Because of the history of self-inflicted injuries, and despite the exposure to radiation, transit studies of radiopaque markers were used as the sole means of follow-up evaluation. Figure 42–8 shows the sequence of data obtained over the years. This confirmed the fact that the function of the right colon was normal, because the single recorded delay in this site was associated to reflux of markers from left to right colon. Thus, her constipation was due to distal bowel spasticity rather than an inert colonic musculature in the ascending colon. This was confirmed by rectal accommodation studies, which showed the maximum tolerable volume was only 90 ml in 1981 (normal values: 170 to 440).

The constipation of this patient was managed symptomatically. She was given a lot of time and attention and was seen 50 times on an outpatient basis between March 28, 1981 and October 28, 1986, at which time she reported normal bowel habits. She was hospitalized in 1982 and in 1984, but only for specialized investigations, on an elective basis. During the follow-up, we learned that the rape by the father had been a sodomy. The change towards normal bowel habits occurred quite suddenly. Her father died in October 1986, and she was encouraged by telephone to ventilate her rage at him. She did so by writing a six-page letter which she placed in his suit, prior to burial; change in bowel habits was instantaneous. In December 1986, she recorded 26 stools over 34 days. She had between four and seven stools per week and never went more than 3 successive days without defecation. Figure 42–8 shows the improvement in transit times. The latest figures are still slightly longer than normal if stress-free controls are taken as a basis of comparison: mean right-colon transit time is now 22 hours (N < 18), left colon 32(N < 13), rectosigmoid 7(N < 20) and overall large-bowel transit time 55(N < 34). There was a concomitant improvement in propagating electric activity at rest (Fig 42–8). Rectal spasticity was decreased—in January 1987 maximum tolerable volume had increased to 140 ml. This value is normally reproducible within 10 ml. There was also an improvement in the MMPI. The latest score for depression is now 75. Scores for hypochrondria (78), hysteria (75), psychopathic deviate (64), schizophrenia (84), hypomania (70), and social introversion-extroversion (63) are all improved. Score of psychasthenia is still high at 79.

The patient has been seen 19 times since the turnabout, and she is now ventilating her anger at her husband because of his marital infidelity. Constipation is not discussed any more.

This sort of anecdote does not make science. However, it is one among many. One such story is enough to incite physicians to a lot of caution in patients with obstipation. Martha, indeed, needed more caring than colectomy.

MECHANISMS AND MANAGEMENT OF OBSTIPATION

Denial of Defecation

In 1968, Hinton and Lennard-Jones[51] described briefly three patients who denied having a bowel movement despite clear evidence to the contrary, as shown by the passage of radiopaque markers through the large bowel. The term "denied bowel movement syndrome" was applied to this situation. The label Munchausen's syndrome has been used for patients who consistently produce false stories and fabricate evidence, thus causing themselves needless medical investigations, operations, and treatment.[52] Meadow's syndrome, a Munchausen syndrome by proxy, occurs when parents fabricate false evidence and consult for their child.[53] Patients who deny they defecate belong to this class of patient, but they do not really fabricate false evidence of "disease"; the manipulation of the doctor is restricted to the symptomatology, and because this is purely mental, it is possibly more amenable to treatment through a good doctor–patient relationship. Confrontation, provocation, and, of course, rejection by the doctor are likely to produce a change in consultant. Allowing oneself to be manipulated for a while, during which time data-gathering is associated with verbal and nonverbal exchanges, permits the physician time to find the occasion of another subject of discussion.

The following case report is an example of a patient who denied defecation, even when transit time of markers was quite normal.

A 19-year-old girl was referred for evaluation of her constipation of 2 years' duration. Onset was subsequent to a crash diet with abundant laxative intake. Mean total gastrointestinal transit time of radiopaque markers was measured and found to be 39 hours, and on repeat examination 11 hours, both values considered well within normal limits.[3,54,55] Despite contrary evidence, the patient denied defecating, asked for surgery, and, upon refusal, left. She came back 3 years later with the same demand, underwent another evaluation with similar objective evidence, was refused surgery again, and left again. With the threat of suicide she managed to find herself a surgeon who transsected the ileum and anastomosed its proximal part to the sigmoid colon, leaving the bypassed large bowel in situ. Symptoms worsened, and she did a lot of doctor shopping, for variable lengths of time, before she finally had a psychiatric evaluation and was again referred to us.

At first encounter, her hands were cold and wet; there were tears in her eyes. She said she just had been abandoned by her lover. A probable important detail was that she said she always had had dyspareunia.[56] She cried about the death of her father several years before and about the fact she felt no emotional contact with her mother. The doctor–patient relationship was difficult, but it was facilitated because she had already had surgery. Frustrations were important both for her and the doctor, but she soon began to express a lot of grief which she had not done at the time of the death of her father when she was 13. She also remembered how, as a child, she used to constantly hold the hand of her teacher, who had told her—and she remembered—she did not get love at home. She spoke openly about her suicidal thoughts and her anguish when the many doctors she consulted told her they could not do anything for her. She refused to be followed by a psychologist or psychiatrist. Transference to the doctor was enhanced when he celebrated her birthday with due emphasis. Thereafter, a "contract" could be made with her, and the previous surgery was "undone." Postoperative course was not stormy (all objective parameters being normal) but laborious (the patient complaining bitterly of constipation). A first study with markers again revealed a transit of 48 hours. Recovery was slow, and visits became more spaced. The patient had used her prolonged stay as a way of reflecting about her condition, while being away from her mother (with whom she was still living); she mentioned also that constant praise by the doctor, despite the moments of confrontation, had rendered her more secure. Eventually she stopped consulting but sent the message through common acquaintances that she was now well and had a daily satisfying defecation. The entire process had lasted 5 years. However, when contacted 4 years later, she said she was still constipated. She again had been dismissed by a lover after a 2-year period of living together, because of her heavy alcohol intake, which she attributed to the constipation. Of note, during these 4 years she had stopped consulting physicians.

Patience and serenity are in order if such patients are to be helped. Asking for a consultation in psychiatry is often equivalent to dismissal; the patient denies any emotional or psychiatric problem, resents the hint there is one because a consultation in psychiatry was requested, feels rejected, and does not come back. One might say that reporting a story like that described above is not "scientific" and does not have its place in the present text. That's basically the problem; being just "scientific" misses the essential element of the doctor–patient relationship. A true science should be all-inclusive.

Constipation with Normal Transit

It is not known how many patients who consult for "constipation" (not otherwise defined) have objective evidence of delayed colonic transit. We have discussed above the limitations of what "normal" means. We also pointed out that what is normal for the doctor may not be for the patient. For all diseases and illnesses (the subjective experience of diseases), there is a long process of selection prior to consultation. Self-selection by the patient is an important part of this process, and there is a greater tendency in the population, today, for self-help. The referral pattern plays another role, important and variable according to the various communities.

It has been pointed out above that stool frequency per se is not the source of concern for people, and that they will complain more about the associated symptoms.[5] It has also been pointed out that among nonreporters with irritable bowel syndrome, there is a higher incidence of people with low stool frequency than among reporters; it is the addition of abdominal pain to constipation that leads people to consult.[57]

With this in mind, it is easy to understand why a sizable number of "constipated" people who consult have normal gastrointestinal transit times.[50, 58, 59] In contrast to the previous group; they do not deny defecation, but complain of being constipated. The percentage amounts to at least a third of individuals, but good epidemiologic data are still lacking.

There is evidence of psychosocial dysfunction in this group of patients.[58] Their prognosis also does not seem as good as for those patients who have a delayed transit in the left colon.[58]

As said above, people who are constipated consult when they also have abdominal pain. This is interesting because constipated patients who have abdominal pain have a faster transit time than those who are painless and thus are not more, but less sick![60] It is also known that, in constipated children, the presence of abdominal pain is a good prognostic omen.[61]

We tend to consider the constipation of these people, who may be very demanding, as an "admission ticket," a term coined by Thomas Almy when referring to the emotional problems associated in people with the irritable bowel syndrome. We try to integrate the "case" history into the "life" history. This can be done with a loosely structured interview,[47] or in a psychoanalytic way through associations made from either verbal or nonverbal messages. Basically, patients fall into two categories.[62] Psychofunctional personalities are those capable of expressing emotions and of having true relationships and who, with little help, will readily accept they have abdominal symptoms associated to specific stressful situations. This can then become the starting point of interviews focusing more on the stress than the constipation. We often point out that people accuse "the outside world" of being stressful for them, but that by doing this they focus on the "match," rather than the "dynamite" that is in them. The nature and source of the "dynamite" become the subject of subsequent encounters. In our experience, such patients eventually "forget" to speak about their bowels. In contrast to people with a psychofunctional personality, those with a psychosomatic structure tend to accuse their bowel dysfunction of being the cause of their mental ill-being—if they recognize it, which is not always the case. These patients are as difficult to treat as those who deny they defecate, and they tend to be alexithymic. We use medications to help them, even if most of those available are known to have a strong placebo effect, and follow them loosely. Occasionally, with trust, nonverbal behavior or slips of the tongue can be analyzed and become the source of insight. A quick way, in our experience, to sort out patients with psychofunctional from those with psychosomatic personality structures is to ask them if they remember their dreams; the latter don't.

Anismus

A recently described mechanism of constipation has been labeled anismus, spastic pelvic floor syndrome, or sphincteric disobedience syndrome. A broader term without implication of etiology (psychologic or organic) might be rectosphincteric dyssynergia, similar to the term vesicourethral dyssynergia used by urologists, who deal with similar problems in the bladder and urethra that lead to bladder retention and infections.[63] An even wider umbrella, because these patients also often have many sexual difficulties such as frigidity, dyspareunia, and anorgasmy,[56] would be the term abdominoperineal dyssynergia.

What is this abnormality?

Normally, during defecation the pelvic floor, which at rest is in a state of constant activity and contraction, relaxes completely.[64–66] Some patients, on the contrary, contract the external anal sphincter during straining, and this abnormality has been associated to constipation. Records of electromyographic activity show a transient increased activity at onset and end of straining, or a highly increased level of activity during the entire duration of the defecation act. A few subjects exhibit bursts of repetitive tetanic-like grouped action potentials succeeding each other in a fast (8/sec) rhythm and completely different from those recorded during voluntary contraction of the perianal musculature.[67] The clinical counterpart of this abnormality was initially labeled the puborectalis syndrome. Constipation, incomplete evacuation of the rectum, and anorectal pain were the presenting symptoms; the length of the anal canal was increased and spasm was present at the level of the puborectalis muscle; the posterior rectal pouch was unusually deep because of the angulation at the anorectal ring and any attempt to pull the puborectalis sling posteriorly triggered more spasm and pain.[68] More recently the term anismus has been used to describe patients in whom no inhibition of electric activity occurs in either the puborectalis or external anal sphincter muscles during straining, but rather an increased activity in one or both of these muscles, associated with a rise in anal canal pressure[69] (Fig 42–9). In a few subjects, this excess activity may persist up to 2 minutes after the straining effort has ceased. Thus, despite a rise in intrarectal pressure conducive to defecation, the anorectal pressure barrier persists, and patients are unable to defecate a balloon filled with 50 ml of water and placed in the rectum. The term anismus is quite appropriate because of its analogy to vaginismus, in which a spasm of the pelvic floor muscles also occurs, the difference of course being that vaginismus is resistance to penetration and anismus to expulsion. The findings have been confirmed in patients complaining of severe difficulty to pass formed stools and having no megarectum.[70]

Anismus was originally described in female patients with severe constipation,

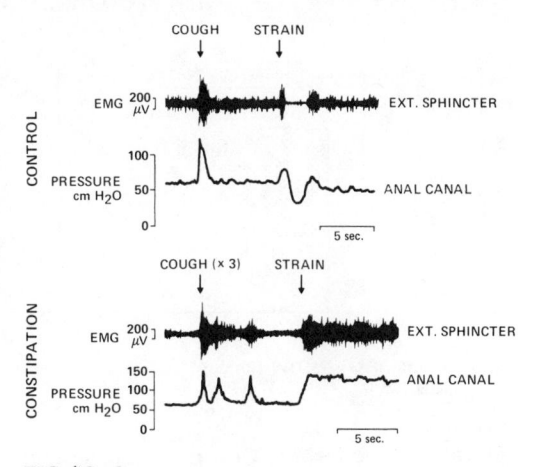

FIG 42–9.
Anismus. This patient, when asked to strain, squeezes the anal canal instead of relaxing it. (Adapted from Preston DM, Lennard-Jones JE: Anismus in chronic constipation. *Dig Dis Sci* 1985; 30:413–418.)

who all had delayed transit of radiopaque markers.[69] However, some patients with anismus have normal segmental and overall large-bowel transit times[71] (Fig 42–10). Moreover, anismus has been recently described in patients with idiopathic perineal pain and in patients with solitary rectal ulcer[66, 72] (Fig 42–11). Still, paradoxical puborectalis contraction is associated to a failure to defecate a small rectal balloon.[69, 72, 73] An association between constipation and abnormal external anal sphincter activity has also been reported in patients with megarectum.[74] A larger volume of rectal distention, enough to cause abdominal pain but no rectal sensation, was needed to produce total inhibition of the striated muscle activity of the pelvic floor, and occasionally an attempt to defecate caused an intense contraction of the floor. Defecation straining was also found to induce a grossly abnormal overactivity in the puborectalis muscle, usually with little change in the superficial external anal sphincter, in patients with the descending perineum syndrome.[66]

Is it possible to have a unifying concept of all this? Patients with the solitary rectal ulcer syndrome have an internal rectal prolapse and complain of obstructed defecation: they feel a complete blockage of the anal canal. Patients with the descending perineum syndrome have a weak pelvic floor, and when they strain it can be easily seen to bulge; they may at least in the early stages of dysfunction contract the pelvic floor at the same time they push it out. Patients with either condition thus must defecate through an unrelaxed puborectalis sling. It must be noted that the puborectalis muscle is innervated in part by a branch of the sacral nerve that lies above the pelvic floor; the pudendal nerve only supplies the ipsilateral external anal sphincter.[75] There may thus be distinct pathologies of the puborectalis muscle (and its associated iliococcygeal and pubococcygeal muscles) and of the external anal sphincter. Pudendal block, indeed, does not abolish the increase in resting pressure of the upper and lower anal canal that results from maximal voluntary contraction.[76] Why anismus would lead to internal rectal prolapse and perineal descent versus rectal enlargement is not known.

Chronic pelvic tensions have been said to result from psychologic conflicts during childhood and lead to urinary control

LARGE BOWEL TRANSIT TIME IN CONSTIPATED PATIENTS WITH RECTOSPHINCTERIC DYSSYNERGIA

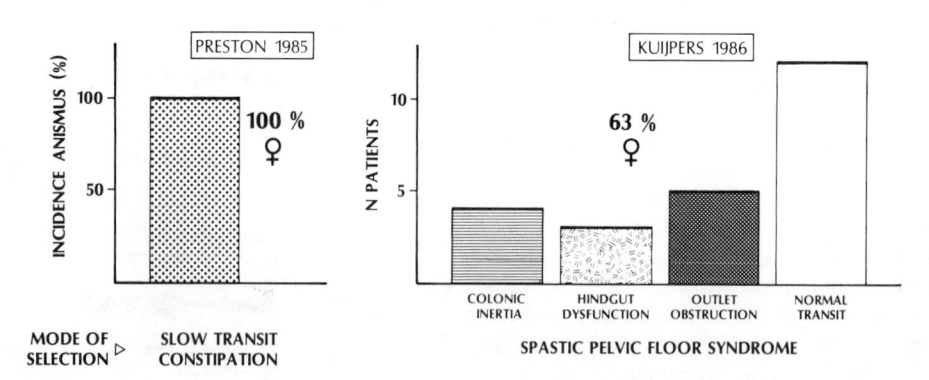

FIG 42–10.
Although patients with anismus were initially described as being all women and having all delayed transit of radiopaque markers in the large bowel,[69] this is not necessarily so. Patients with the spastic pelvic floor syndrome, a similar abnormality, may be males and may have normal transit. (Adapted from Kuijpers HC, Bleijenberg G, De Morree H: The spastic pelvic floor syndrome. Large bowel outlet obstruction caused by pelvic floor dysfunction: A radiological study. *Int J Colorectal Dis* 1986; 1:44–48.)

PARADOXICAL PUBORECTALIS CONTRACTION

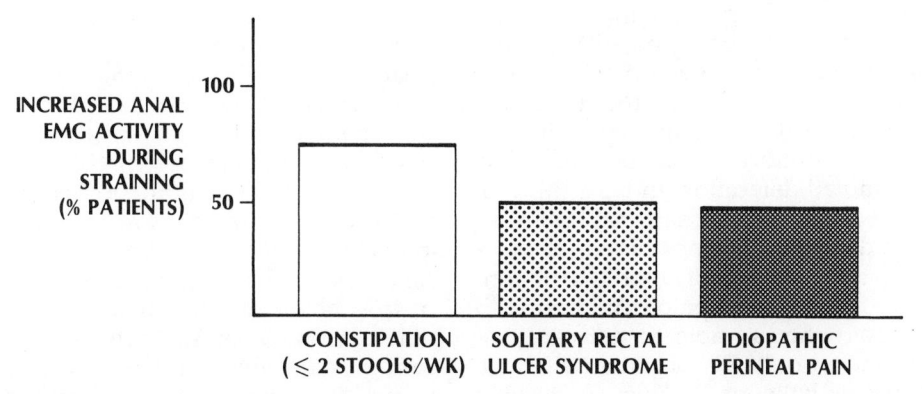

FIG 42–11.
A rectosphincteric dyssynergia is not only associated to constipation, but to internal rectal prolapse and to idiopathic perineal pain. (Adapted from Jones PN, Lubowski DZ, Swash M, et al: Is paradoxical contraction of puborectalis muscle of functional importance? *Dis Colon Rectum* 1987; 30:667–670.)

problems and diminished orgasmic response.[77, 78] In an interesting study of a large group of predominantly heterosexual college graduate women, the contractile strength of the pelvic floor muscles was demonstrated to be in relationship with both urinary control and orgasmic response.[11] The relationship of the posterior section of the pelvic floor to these concerns has not been investigated yet, but preliminary data suggest sexual difficulties in severely constipated women.[56] Therefore, the old suggestion of gynecologists that the pelvic floor should be treated as a neuromuscular unit, which takes into account the interrelationships between muscular motility and supportive, sphincteric, sensorimotor, and sexual functioning, may be pertinent for physicians dealing with patients complaining of constipation and found to have outlet obstruction by rectosphincteric dyssynergia.

The cause of anismus is not known. Organic malfunction of the anorectal structures is a remote possibility, because the only successful treatment found to date for this disorder has been biofeedback.[56, 79, 80] This suggests anismus is of the nature of an abnormal learning process rather than of a disease. In a large series of children with chronic idiopathic constipation, one-fourth were found to strain when asked to squeeze, one-fourth to squeeze when asked to strain (as in anismus), and 5% to do both and thus reverse the command; therefore the term "sphincteric disobedience syndrome" was coined to describe the findings. It is not known if the child does not want to do what is asked or does not understand what is asked.[81]

Anismus may be diagnosed in several different ways. The simplest way to detect it is to ask the patient to strain during a rectal examination: it is easy to feel the contraction of the external anal sphincter and/or the puborectalis muscle, while normally a relaxation would be expected. Defecography is a radiologic technique used to observe the dynamics of defecation, the morphology of the anorectal structures during this process, and the anorectal angle at rest, during squeeze, and during straining. In some constipated patients, the anorectal angle does not open and increase during straining but remains at 90 degrees. On rare occasions, the angle becomes even narrower. The barium paste in the rectum cannot be excreted. The term spastic pelvic floor syndrome has been proposed to describe this abnormality[82] and is akin to anismus. The clinical counterpart of the spastic pelvic clinical symptoms includes a sensation of perineal fullness and urge, straining for prolonged periods of time, and difficult and painful evacuation. Several patients insert a finger into the anal canal to initiate defecation. Electromyographic evidence of pelvic floor contraction may be found during attempted defecation and is a third diagnostic method. External anal sphincter activity decreases during the act of bearing down for defecation in 100% of controls, in 58% of constipated children with encopresis who are able to defecate balloons, and in only 7% of patients unable to defecate balloons.[83] This suggests a very strong association between increased external anal sphincter activity during defecation attempts, as recorded by electromyography, and failure to defecate a rectal balloon filled with 30 to 100 ml of water. A fourth way to search for anismus is to record the anal resting pressure during straining. Control subjects have an anal relaxation, but in anismus, there is an increase in pressure.[80, 84] This abnormality is often associated with other rectoanal disorders such as anal hypertonia, increased rectal compliance, and impaired rectal conscious sensitivity, but this is not overly surprising. The more tests are performed on constipated patients, the greater the likelihood to find a functional abnormality[59, 85] (Fig 42–12). A fifth and final method is to evaluate the configuration of the rectoanal inhibitory reflex during rectal distention; occasionally, it is possible to record an external anal sphincteric contraction in the midst of the reflex.[47] This contraction is also found in 45% of encopretic children (who exhibit external anal sphincter contraction during expulsion) and is thought, of course, to contribute to fecal retention.[86] No study has been done to compare these different diagnostic modalities of anismus.

Biofeedback techniques may be used when specific measurable functional abnormalities are found in patients with chronic idiopathic constipation, such as anismus. Biofeedback cured eight out of ten such patients with prolonged history of constipation, inability to defecate without enemas or laxatives, no defecation

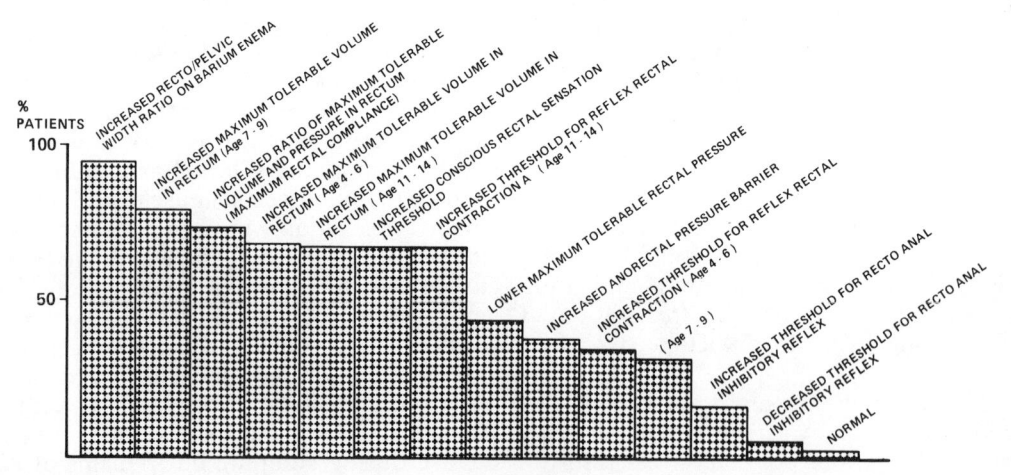

FIG 42–12.
Very few patients who are suffering from chronic idiopathic constipation have no functional abnormality. This is why more than one test is needed in these subjects. (Adapted from Meunier P, Louis D, Jaubert de Beaujeu M: Physiologic investigation of primary chronic constipation in children: Comparison with the barium enema study. *Gastroenterology* 1984; 87:1351–1357.)

urge, and difficult and painful defecation once every 4 to 14 days.[79] An anal-plug electrode is inserted to record the electromyographic activity of the external anal sphincter. Numeric and graphic feedback is produced to the patient asked to strain. This, in anismus or the spastic pelvic floor syndrome, increases muscular activity. To help the patient understand that straining must be carried out in a different manner, without pelvic floor contraction, a balloon is inserted into the rectum, distended with 60 cc of water, and slowly pulled out to have the patient recognize the feeling that the pelvic floor is relaxing and stool is coming. The next step, when the patient correctly relaxes the pelvic floor during straining, consists in learning to defecate artificial feces introduced into the rectum. Another biofeedback approach uses anorectal pressure recordings at rest and during rectal distention as a modality of feedback source.[46, 47, 56, 80, 87] There are predictors of outcome with regards to biofeedback techniques. For instance a depression score above 67 and a psychasthenia score above 57 on the MMPI are highly predictive of a failure of biofeedback-relaxation training outcome. Individuals who tend to like responsibility and are more executive and independent generally benefit more than doubtful, obedient, and depressed individuals.[88] This has not been studied specifically in subjects with anismus.

Surgery for this functional problem should be abandoned, and this is one of the reasons why we stress so much the need to recognize anismus, if present, in patients with obstipation. Puborectalis resection was advocated long ago to treat patients with the puborectalis syndrome.[68] Initial gratifying results were confirmed in subsequent uncontrolled observations.[89] In a group of women, however, who had surgery with the preoperative functional diagnosis of anismus, posterior division of the puborectalis muscles provided no benefit; incontinence for solid stool was not reported but there was some leakage of flatus, liquid stool, and mucus.[90] A more drastic approach, subtotal colectomy, also failed to cure patients with anismus.[71, 74]

Colonic Inertia and Colonic Pseudo-obstruction

Mechanisms of constipation can be studied in two different ways: following the progress of feces along the large bowel, or evaluating the bowel wall muscular activity and tone. The first method provides an estimate of the end-results induced by abnormalities demonstrated by the second method. On the basis of radiopaque marker studies, patients with constipation may be divided into different groups. There may be delay in the colon,[9, 27, 50, 51, 91] or feces may pass normally along the colon but may be stored too long in the rectum.[3, 50, 51] Relatively few patients have a delayed transit in the ascending colon. Thus, a study had to cover a 10-year period to yield 54 subjects.[91] In a recent study of 21 patients with less than two stools per week, 38% were found to have a prolonged transit in all three segments of large bowel.[58]

In patients with colonic inertia, markers stagnate along the entire large intestine.[91] However, delayed transit in the ascending colon may be merely secondary to a distal obstacle, which counteracts an effective colonic musculature in the ascending colon.[48] The term constipation by delayed colonic transit has been proposed when the delay is not due to bowel paralysis but distal obstruction. Hindgut (the embryologic distal bowel that goes from the left third of the transverse colon to the anorectal junction) dysfunction may exist as an isolated congenital abnormality[48] but probably also exists on a functional basis. Evidence for a delay in the ascending colon secondary to distal obstacle would be provided by retrograde movement of feces, demonstrated by radiopaque marker studies: The markers can be seen to travel back and forth from right to left colon, in the ascending colon, they disappear not in an exponential but a bumpy fashion. Electromyographic recordings have shown that in chronic idiopathic constipation by outlet obstruction, the propagation of the electric activity occurred not in the anal but in the oral direction.[55] This is the counterpart of retrograde movement of markers. In a recent study, two groups of patients with delayed transit in the ascending colon were identified. In the first, the abnormality was reproducible 1 year apart and there was no observable reflux of markers from descending to ascending colon; in the second, there was reflux, or the abnormality was not reproducible, suggesting the possibility of distal spasm.[45] One should thus probably reserve the term colonic inertia for the situation, in which transit time in the ascending colon is prolonged and no reflux or markers from the left colon are demonstrated.

Patients labeled as suffering from slow-transit constipation are similar: Transit time is prolonged in the large bowel, which is of normal size and configuration.[27] It is probably this kind of subject who, at the beginning of the century, underwent colectomy for protracted obstipation.[92]

Slow-transit constipation and colonic inertia are found quasi-exclusively in women, regardless of bowel size at barium enema. In contrast, megacolon is found in both sexes, suggesting that proportionally more constipated men have an easily distensible colon.[93, 94]

Very little is known about the mechanisms conducive to delayed passage of feces through the colon. In women with slow-transit constipation and those with colonic inertia, decreased bowel frequency is severe (one stool per week) and together with other symptoms begins around the age of puberty.[27, 91] In a few patients, symptoms begin suddenly after an abdominal operation or accident and are the consequence of a physical or emotional trauma. The latter possibility is rendered more plausible because these subjects have cold hands, clear signs of anxiety, and blackouts.[27]

Colonic motility, as measured with miniature balloons, does not differ in patients with slow-transit constipation and controls. However, the introduction of bisacodyl into the colonic lumen, which usually stimulates the appearance of powerful peristaltic waves in normal subjects, does not do so in slightly less than half of those with slow-transit constipation[95] (Fig

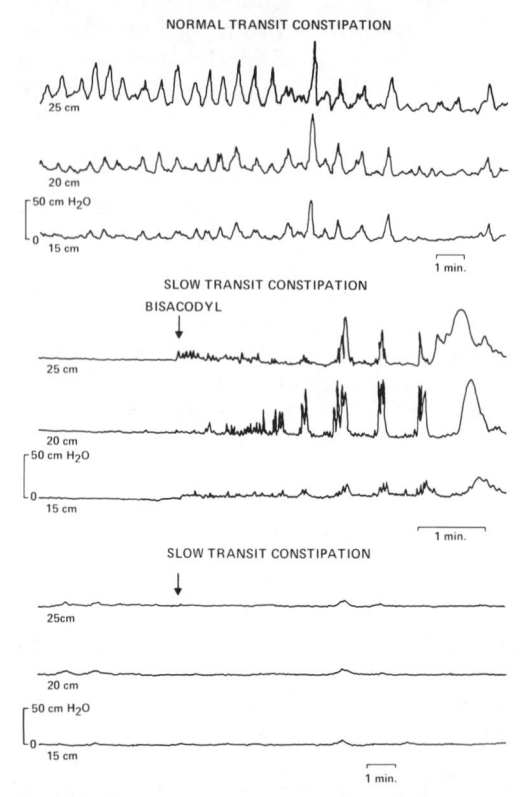

FIG 42–13.
Some patients with slow transit constipation have a colon that is not stimulated by bisacodyl. (Adapted from Preston JE, Lennard-Jones JE: Pelvic motility and response to intraluminal bisacodyl in slow-transit constipation. *Dig Dis Sci* 1985; 30:289–294.)

42–13). The response or absence of response of colonic motility to bisacodyl may perhaps in the future help physicians to recognize patients who have a very inert colonic musculature. In some constipated subjects, motor activity of the sigmoid colon increases to an abnormal degree after a meal, suggesting spasticity; in others, it is the reverse, and hypomotility is observed postprandially.[96] This again suggests two families of constipated subjects who have delayed transit in the colon: the hypomotor and the hypermotor subjects.

Myoelectric spiking activity of the descending and sigmoid colon has been measured in patients with constipation who have prolonged transit time in the right colon. The number of propagating electric potentials is significantly decreased in the fasting conditions, and no postprandial increase in their number is observed.[50] Unfortunately, this study did not distinguish patients with colonic inertia from those with constipation by delayed colonic transit. No abnormality was found in the number of rhythmic spike potentials, which are repetitive and stationary, nor in terms of the sporadic spike potentials, which are long spike bursts that do not propagate. Similarly, there is no postprandial increase of the propagating electric potentials in patients with the irritable bowel syndrome who have less than three stools per week[97] (Fig 42–14).

Dysphagia and gastroesophageal reflux, present in 40% of patients, are associated with both hypertonicity of the pharyngoesophageal sphincter and a weak gastroesophageal sphincter in patients with colonic inertia. There is also a high incidence of simultaneous contractions of the esophagus (tertiary contractions).[91] Nausea (53%) and vomiting (40%) are frequent. Pollakiuria (44%), frequent urinary tract infections (41%), urinary incontinence (31%), nycturia (31%), a feeling of incomplete bladder emptying (29%), a burning sensation at voiding (25%), and difficulties to initiate voiding (19%) all suggest urinary tract dysfunction. The evidence for this is provided by urodynamic studies that demonstrate a hypersensitivity of the bladder to urecholine.[91] Thus, there is abnormal function of the esophagus, large bowel, and bladder in these patients. There is a similar high incidence of nocturia and difficulty in starting to pass urine in patients labeled as having slow transit constipation.[27] Other common symptoms in patients with colonic inertia are migraine headaches (31%), constant rhinorrhea (18%), and orthostatic hypotension (28%). Finally, there is a high incidence of galactorrhea with normal prolactin levels in both women with colonic inertia and women with slow transit constipation.[27, 91] Reproductive hormones may be involved, because patients often complain of irregular, painful menstruation, have difficulties becoming pregnant, and undergo a lot of gynecologic surgery.[27] No fewer than 41% of women with colonic inertia are sterile, 27% had miscarriages, and 36% had hysterectomies. In some, raised serum prolactin levels, low urinary estrogens, and low plasma estradiol levels have been found.[98]

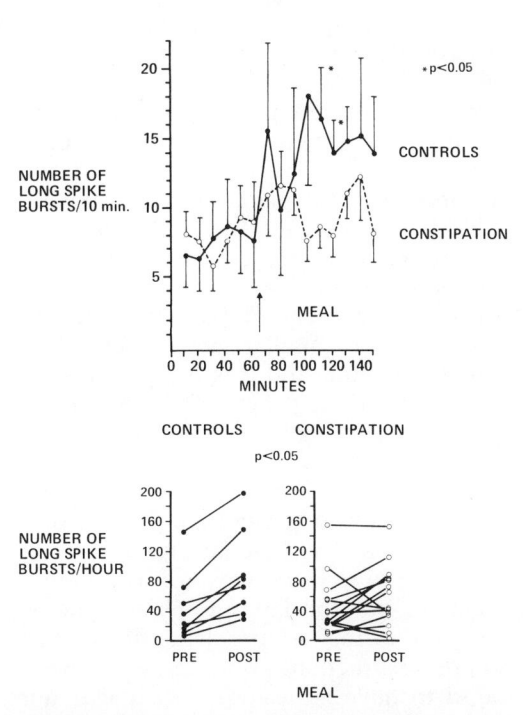

This all points out to a systemic disease or disorder. Some patients who undergo surgery for severe chronic idiopathic constipation have abnormalities of the neurologic structures in the bowel.[91, 99–101] However, most have a history of laxative intakes. It is, therefore, difficult in many

FIG 42–14.
The number of long spike bursts, which is an electric activity propagating along the distal large bowel, does not increase postprandially in severely constipated subjects, in contrast to controls.[97] Compare this abnormality, found in patients labeled as suffering from the irritable bowel syndrome, to that found in patients who had a traumatic transection of the spinal cord at the thoracic level, shown in Fig 42–6, and who clearly have an organic lesion.[31]

cases, to conclude whether the neurologic abnormalities are primary or secondary. Moreover, in similar patients evidence has also been produced of a correlation between transit time in the ascending colon and anxiety levels.[45] Together with markedly different personalities between constipated women with colonic inertia and controls,[45] this evidence may indicate the presence of a disorder of the person rather than a diseased body. Mechanisms, whether pharmacologic or neurogenic, remain to be clarified.

The management of patients with colonic inertia or similar syndromes is extremely difficult, and it is not possible today to provide a simple problem-solving approach. The high incidence of abdominal catastrophes in patients with colonic inertia is clear evidence of the severity of the problem. No fewer than 71% have a history of an abdominal operation. In 16%, the procedure was for bowel obstruction, but the laparotomy was negative, indicating a problem of colonic pseudo-obstruction. Another 20% were found to have adhesions, but it was not evident they were the cause of a mechanical obstruction. This is an area of medicine in which the personalities of the attending physicians and their own biases will play a major role in the choice of treatment. Those who believe only in organic diseases will probably resort to bowel resection. Those who believe in psychosomatic disorders will lean on psychotherapy with additional medication. Over the years, and because of many unhappy experiences with surgery, we have moved from the former to the latter attitude, but without mutual exclusion. We have also learned a lot from a single patient with severe colonic inertia, a poor childhood with much unhappiness and psychosocial problems,[102] and an abnormal MMPI.[45] Despite the recommendation to the contrary, she insisted on undergoing a palliative colectomy rather than psychotherapy. She had seen many consultants in the United States and Canada. She said she could not live the way she was any more and threatened to commit suicide. Reluctantly and with due warning about the possible outcomes of surgery: (normal function, severe diarrhea and incontinence, or pseudo-obstruction), we performed a subtotal colectomy with ileorectal anastomosis. Postoperatively, she had a psychotic episode that was both for her and us a mind-opener. The outcome of surgery was, as dreaded, chronic idiopathic pseudo-obstruction. She refused a Levin tube and was confused about her manipulative behavior. Insertion of the Levin tube triggered instant psychosis. She recovered both physically and mentally, and thereafter had three normal stools per day.

Megarectum

The association of megarectum with constipation has been recognized for some time.[103–105] In this condition, the rectal wall has little elasticity and can easily be distended to accommodate large amounts of fluid.[3] Although impaired rectal sensation has been reported in these patients,[106] the level of pressure at which sensation occurs is the same regardless of rectal volume, and this suggests that the nature of the problem is not impaired rectal sensation but inelasticity of the musculature: A greater stretch is needed before sufficient tension occurs and sensation begins.[3] The rectoanal inhibitory reflex is also impaired because it is triggered by rectal accommodation.[107] The reflex's amplitude is decreased, and the reflex can even be absent at low levels of distention. It is easy to understand that rectal deformation by a distended rectal balloon is minimal if the rectal wall is flaccid.

When the reflex is absent, it is absolutely necessary to rule out Hirschsprung's disease, in which it is also absent. Patients with constipation from birth who were found later to have a megarectum seem to differ from those who became constipated later in life: colonic transit is normal and storage occurs exclusively in the rectum, which accommodates huge volumes and is more flaccid than in any other situation. Rectal bypass offers some hope of cure, while it should be discouraged in patients with acquired megarectum. In latter groups, a greater recorded (as compared to recalled) stool frequency, clinical improvement by vastly different treatment modalities such as surgery or psychotherapy, delayed transit at the colonic as well as rectal level, and absence of correlation between colonic transit and rectal capacity all point to a functional problem akin to the irritable bowel syndrome, but without spasticity.[3]

EVALUATION OF OBSTIPATION

The restricted space of this chapter does not allow more than a superficial description of the evaluation of patients with obstipation and of those with constipation.[1] This evaluation not only serves a role in diagnosis, but conveys the nonverbal message that the problem being investigated is important. As a consequence, the foundations are laid for a trustful relationship between doctor and patient.

A first stage should be to rule out organic diseases. Organic disease is rarely the case in patients with obstipation: In most situations, no organic cause (or better-said, no known cause,) will be found. At history, a search should be made for the severity and chronicity of the problem. The association of urinary dysfunction and sexual problems may point to anismus and similar syndromes. Patients with megarectum may at times defecate huge stools that plug the toilet bowl. At colonic endoscopy, signs should be looked for to indicate a huge capacity of the rectum or colon. Anismus may be detected during the rectal examination. Rectal biopsies have little clinical practical value except in cases of Hirschsprung's disease, which is not the subject of this chapter. Barium enema would be expected to diagnose capacious large bowels, again will little practical implications.

The second stage consists in a functional evaluation.

Studies of Colonic Transit Times

To measure colonic transit times, subjects ingest radiopaque markers, remain on a high-residue diet, and refrain from laxatives, enemas, and all nonessential drugs. The markers are commercially available, but may be simply cut from a radiopaque nasogastric tube. Stools may be radiographed,[108, 109] or, to distinguish between the different types of constipation, the progression of markers along the colon may be followed by daily radiographs of the abdomen.[4, 9, 51, 53, 58, 110] Films are taken until total expulsion of markers, for a maximum of 7 days after ingestion. Markers are counted in the right colon, left colon, and rectosigmoid area by using the bony landmarks of the spine and pelvic contours. A simplified formula to calculate segmental transit time can be obtained if the patient swallows 20 markers and a film is obtained every 24 hours. Markers are counted in the segment of colon, each day, until distal total progression; these numbers are added and the sum multiplied by 1.2.[54] Normal values in adults have been obtained under strict dietary conditions.[54] To avoid radiation, it has recently been proposed to multiply marker ingestion and decrease the number of abdominal radiographs.[111, 112] This permits measurement of bowel transit time, but reflux of markers from left to right colon cannot be evaluated.

This test detects patients who lie or misrepresent their complaint. Markers disappear from the abdomen, even if patients deny they defecate. Transit studies may also be used to evaluate segmental colonic transit time in order to detect specific areas of the bowel that are not functioning properly. During follow-up, marker studies also serve the purpose of providing objective data reflecting the clinical course.

Electromyography of the Colon

Recording the electric activity of the bowel smooth muscle is of interest because spike bursts are the electric counterpart of smooth muscle contraction. An important advance has been to use an intraluminal tube, introduced by flexible colonoscopy and equipped with ring electrodes, which can pick up the signals by simple contact with the bowel wall.[49, 113, 114] Signals are filtered with short time constants, because there appears to be a better chance to obtain practical data when spiking activity only is recorded.[115] This consists basically of two types: (1) "Rhythmic and stationary bursts" ("short spike bursts"[115] and "discrete electrical response activity"[116]) are of short duration and occur in sequences lasting for several minutes; (2) "Sporadic bursts" ("long spike bursts"[115] and "continuous electrical response activity"[116]) are bursts with much more variable duration, ranging from 5 to 120 seconds. These sporadic spike bursts can be divided into two subgroups: Some show evidence of propagation from one recording site to another over long distances[49] or even the entire length of the colon;[115] the others do not seem to propagate and are seen at only one or two electrode sites. The sporadic bursts, particularly when propagating, are associated with both intraluminal pressure waves and significant propulsion or bowel content; the rhythmic bursts on the other hand do not seem to be involved in colonic propulsive activity.[117]

In colonic inertia, what appears to be practical and useful is the decrease in propagating electric activity and the lack of increase of this activity in response to meal.[50, 97]

Anorectal Pressure Studies

When the normal rectum is transiently distended, a sampling reflex occurs in the anal canal. It consists of the conjunction of a rectoanal inhibitory reflex (internal sphincter relaxation) and a rectoanal contractile reflex (external sphincter contraction).[4, 118] These reflexes do not have a normal configuration in patients with obstipation, but this is still a field for research.

Viscoelastic properties of the rectum differ in health and disease[3, 119–122] and should be studied to distinguish outlet obstruction induced by a hypo- or hypertonic rectum from simple anal achalasia. This type of study investigates the accommodation properties of the rectum to rapid (with air) or slow (with water) distention. Viscous properties reflect accommodation of the rectum to distention, and elastic properties reflect the residual tension after accommodation.

Anal Sphincter Electromyography

The search for anismus has provided some impetus to more routine performance of electromyography of the external anal sphincter and the puborectalis muscle. This can be performed with needle electrodes or with a less invasive method of plug electrodes. Reflexes between the perineal skin and the pelvic muscle floor can also be investigated to determine the integrity of the innervation to and from the cauda equina.

Dynamic Evaluation of Defecation

Balloon defecation is a new method for investigating the rectoanal dynamics during defecation. Impaired expulsion correlates to the mechanisms of constipation.[69, 83, 123]

The balloon proctogram permits evaluation of the anorectal angle and its relationship with the pubococcygeal level.[124] Balloon topography, in addition to this, yields opening pressures of the anal canal during distention and anal canal length.[125]

Defecography is another practical way to investigate anorectal morphology and dynamics during defecation. The most popular technique uses a barium paste which reproduces stool consistency.[126, 127]

The role of these techniques in the evaluation of obstipation is not known.

Who is the Patient?

During the organic and functional evaluation, one should never forget that the colon is within a person. The scientific approach to medicine does not take into account the fact that the unconscious representation of the body is largely imaginary.[128] Physicians must constantly keep in mind that constipation is not only the passage of hard and infrequent stools via different investigatable mechanisms, but also what this process or condition does subjectively to the patient. Not to be forgotten is the fact that physicians may obtain a selfish pleasure in the practice of medicine, through satisfying their curiosity for interesting "cases," through exercising their control over disease and patient, and through their thoroughness of investigation.[129] Often, the constipated patient is not a "good" obedient patient, and this may trigger unpleasant feelings, frustration, or even anger in the physician. It may lead to a break in doctor–patient relationship or unnecessary surgery. This, of course, is particularly true when dealing with obstipation.

Recording a life history as well as a case history is essential. An interview reviewing in depth all life experiences serves this purpose.[47, 130] It may trigger marked emotional responses, which contribute to the release of long repressed conflicts.[47] A cruder approach consists in using the MMPI and relating to the patient the findings and profile interpretation.[45] Some patients resent even the idea of having a psychologic problem, and caution must be exerted in this regard for fear of the patient "shopping" for another doctor.[57]

TREATING OBSTIPATION

Some indications of the best way to treat obstipated patients have already been given. We need an *effective* manner to treat them. What has been said about constipation[1] is even truer in obstipation. There is no gold standard of treatment. Thus biofeedback, behavioral therapy, dietary manipulations, any kind of psychotherapy, and even surgery have all been used. Colectomy with or without anastomosis has not been the subject of random trial, and patient selection is important to evaluate results. Staying in a spa temporarily accelerates transit time[131] (Fig 42–15). Moreover, even if patients remain clinically improved, the functional derangements may persist over a long period of time[87, 132] (Fig 42–16). These two observations should be kept in mind and

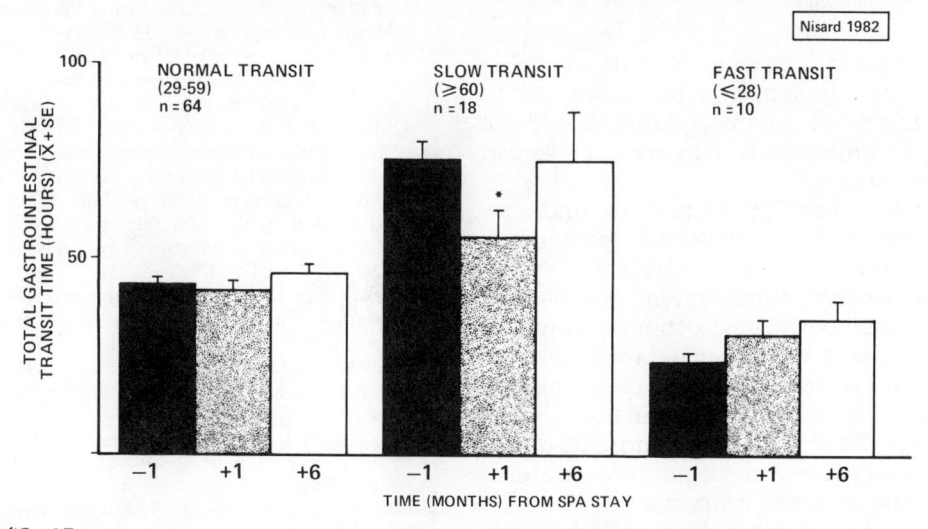

FIG 42–15.
Staying in a spa station accelerates transit time of constipated patients! The improvement is only temporary (* $p < 0.05$). (Adapted from Nisard A, Jian R, Chevalier J, et al: Effet d'une cure thermale à Châtel-Guyon sur le temps de transit intestinal total de patients atteints de colopathie fonctionnelle. *Rev Fr de Gastroentérologie* 1982; 175:5.)

LONG TERM PERSISTENCE (3 YEARS) OF ABNORMAL ANORECTAL MOTILITY IN CHILDREN WITH SEVERE CHRONIC CONSTIPATION AND ENCOPRESIS ($\bar{X}$ + SE)

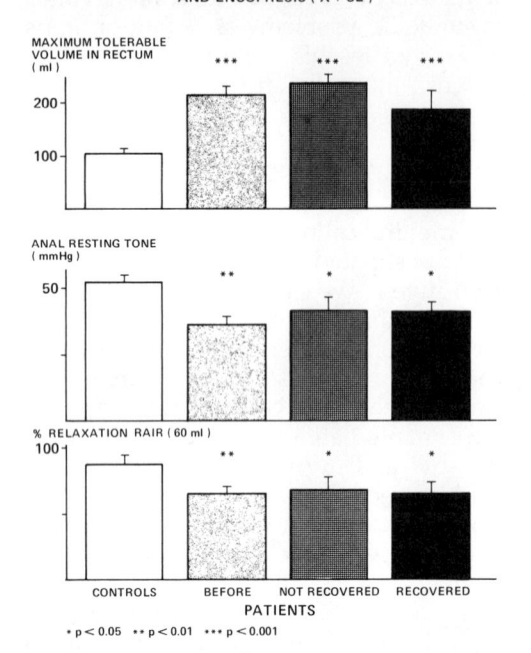

MAXIMUM TOLERABLE VOLUME IN RECTUM (ml)

ANAL RESTING TONE (mmHg)

% RELAXATION RAIR (60 ml)

CONTROLS   BEFORE   NOT RECOVERED   RECOVERED
PATIENTS

* $p < 0.05$ ** $p < 0.01$ *** $p < 0.001$

FIG 42–16.
Even when children recover from severe chronic idiopathic constipation with encopresis, functional abnormalities persist in their anorectal area. (Adapted from Loening-Baucke VA: Abnormal rectoanal function in children recovered from chronic constipation and encopresis. *Gastroenterology* 1984; 87:1299–1304.)

should encourage us to be cautious. Being rendered impotent by a frustrating condition is a source of anxiety; this should not lead to unnecessary surgery or rejection of the patient.

No less than 50% of patients undergoing colectomy and ileorectal anastomosis for severe constipation subsequently require further intervention because of acute small bowel obstruction; in contrast, the incidence rate of small bowel obstruction after resection for large bowel tumors is only 2% and for inflammatory bowel disease 9%.[133] Why such enormous differences after identical surgical procedures?

In the end, an important notion we must have in mind is that, while we should strive to find demonstrable objective abnormalities, we cannot dismiss patients who complain but have no demonstrable abnormality. Even when there is one, its interpretation must be very careful, particularly when a surgical procedure is contemplated.

References

1. Devroede G: Constipation, in *Gastrointestinal Diseases*, ed. 4 Sleisenger-Fordtran, Saunders, in press.
2. Manning AP, Wyman JB, Heaton KW: How trustworthy are bowel histories? Comparison of recalled and recorded information. *Br Med J* 1976; 2:213–214.
3. Verduron A, Devroede G, Bouchoucha M, et al: Megarectum. *Dig Dis Sci*, in press.
4. Martelli H, Duguay C, Devroede G, et al: Some parameters of large bowel function in normal man. *Gastroenterology* 1978; 75:612–618.
5. Sandler RS, Drossman DA: Bowel habits in apparently healthy young adults. *Dig Dis Sci*, in press.
6. Epelboin A: Selles et urines chez les Fulbe Bande du Sénégal Oriental. Un aspect particulier de l'ethnomédecine. Cah. Orstom, *Ser Sci Hum* 1981–1982; 18(4):515–530.
7. Thompson WG, Heaton KW: Functional bowel disorders in apparently healthy people. *Gastroenterology* 1980; 79:283–288.
8. Irigaray L: *Parler n'est jamais neutre*. Paris, Les éditions de minuit, 1985.
9. Martelli H, Devroede G, Arhan P, et al: Mechanisms of idiopathic constipation: Outlet obstruction. *Gastroenterology* 1978; 75:623–631.
10. O'Regan S, Yazbeck S, Schick E: Constipation, bladder instability, urinary tract infection syndrome. *Clin Nephrol* 1985; 23:152–154.
11. Meier E: *Pubococcygeal Strength: Relationship to Urinary Control Problems and to Female Orgasmic Response* (PhD thesis). California School of Professional Psychology, 1977. Published by University Microfilms International, Ann Arbor, Michigan, USA, London, England.
12. Riedl P: Radiological morphology of the sigmoid colon in the Ethiopian population with reference to the occurrence of volvulus. *East Afr Med J* 1978; 55:470–476.
13. Gekas P, Schuster MM: Stercoral perforation of the colon: Case report and review of the literature. *Gastroenterology* 1981; 80:1054–1058.
14. Bjelke E: Epidemiologic studies of cancer of the stomach, colon and rectum. *Scand J Gastroenterol* 1974; 9(Suppl 31):1–235.
15. Higginson J: Etiological factors in gastrointestinal cancer in man. *J Natl Cancer Inst* 1966; 37:527–545.
16. Wynder EL, Shigematsu T: Environmental factors of cancer of the colon and rectum. *Cancer* 1967; 20:1520–1561.
17. Vobecky J, Caro J, Devroede G: A case control study of risk factors for large bowel carcinoma. *Cancer* 1983; 51:1958–1963.
18. The International Agency for Research on Can-

cer Intestinal Microecology Group: Dietary fibre, transit time, faecal bacteria, steroids, and colon cancer in two Scandinavian populations. *Lancet* 1977; 2:207–211.
19. Glober GA, Nomura A, Kamiyama S, et al: Bowel transit-time and stool weight in populations with different colon-cancer risks. *Lancet* 1977; 2:110–111.
20. Kiff ES, Barnes PRH, Swash M: Evidence of pudendal neuropathy in patients with perineal descent and chronic straining at stool. *Gut* 1984; 25:1279–1282.
21. Petrakis NL, King EB: Cytological abnormalities in nipple aspirates of breast fluid from women with severe constipation. *Lancet* 1985; Nov. 28:1203–1205.
22. Creed F: Life events and appendicectomy. *Lancet* 1981; I:1381–1385.
23. Chaudhary NA, Truelove SC: The irritable colon syndrome. A study of clinical features, predisposing causes, and prognosis in 130 cases. *Q J Med* 1962; 31:307–382.
24. Keeling PWN, Fielding JF: The irritable bowel syndrome. A review of 50 consecutive cases. *J Ir Coll Phys Surg* 1975; 4:91.
25. Fielding JF: The irritable bowel syndrome. *Clin Gastroenterol* 1977; 3:607–623.
26. Fielding JF: Surgery and the irritable bowel syndrome: The singer as well as the song. *Ir Med J* 1983; 1:33–34.
27. Preston DM, Lennard-Jones JE: Severe chronic constipation in young women: Idiopathic slow transit constipation. *Gut* 1986; 27:41–48.
28. Young SJ, Alpers DH, Norland CC, et al: Psychiatric illness and the irritable bowel syndrome. Practical implications for the primary physician. *Gastroenterology* 1976; 70:162–166.
29. Purtell JJ, Robins E, Cohen ME: Observations on clinical aspects of hysteria: A quantitative study of 50 hysteria patients and 156 control subjects. *JAMA* 1951; 146:902–909.
30. Woodruff RA, Goodwin DW, Guze SB: Hysteria (Briquet's syndrome), in *Psychiatric Diagnosis*. New York, Oxford University Press, 1974, pp 58–74.
31. Glick ME, Meshkinpour H, Haldeman S, et al: Colonic dysfunction in patients with thoracic spinal cord injury. *Gastroenterology* 1984; 86:287–294.
32. White JC, Verlot MG, Ehrentheil O: Neurogenic disturbances of the colon and their investigation by the colonmetrogram. *Ann Surg* 1940; 112:1042–1057.
33. Scott HW Jr, Cantrell JR: Colonmetrographic studies of the effects of section of the parasympathetic nerves of the colon. *Bull Johns Hopkins Hosp* 1949; 85:310–319.
34. Devroede G, Lamarche J: Functional importance of extrinsic parasympathetic innervation to the distal colon and rectum in man. *Gastroenterology* 1974; 66:273–280.
35. Devroede G, Arhan P, Duguay C, et al: Traumatic constipation. *Gastroenterology* 1979; 77:1258–1267.
36. Gunterberg B, Kewenter J, Petersen I, et al: Anorectal function after major resections of the sacrum with bilateral or unilateral sacrifice of sacral nerves. *Br J Surg* 1976; 63:546–554.
37. Schang JC, Devroede G, Hebert M, et al: Effects of rest, stress and food on myoelectric spiking activity of the left and sigmoid colon in man. *Dig Dis Sci*, 1988; 33(5):614–618.
38. Whorwell PJ, Prior A, Faragher EB: Controlled trial of hypnotherapy in the treatment of severe refractory irritable bowel syndrome. *Lancet* 1984; II:1232–1233.
39. Whorwell PJ, Prior A, Colgan SM: Hypnotherapy in severe irritable bowel syndrome: Further experience. *Gut* 1987; 28:423–425.
40. Groddeck G: Verstopfung als typus des Widerstands. *Die Arche* 1926; No. 8/9.
41. Goodwin JS, Goodwin JM: The tomato effect. Rejection of highly efficacious therapies. *JAMA* 1984; 251:2387–2390.
42. Pinkerton P: Psychogenic megacolon in children: The implications of bowel negativism. *Arch Dis Child* 1958; 33:371–380.
43. Tucker DM, Sandstead HH, Logan GM Jr, et al: Dietary fiber and personality factors as determinants of stool output. *Gastroenterology* 1981; 81:879–883.
44. Watkins GL, Oliver GA: Giant megacolon in the insane: Further observations on patients treated by subtotal colectomy. *Gastroenterology* 1965; 48:718–727.
45. Devroede G, Roy T, Bouchoucha M, et al: Constipation as a mirror of anxiety? Constipated women with colonic dysfunction have a distinct personality. *Dig Dis Sci*, submitted for publication.
46. Devroede G: The irritable bowel syndrome: Clinical and therapeutic aspects, in Poitras P (ed): *Proceedings of the First International Symposium on Small Intestinal and Colonic Motility*. Montreal, Canada, Centre de recherche cliniques, Hôpital Saint-Luc and Jouveinal Laboratories/Laboratoires, Inc., 1985, pp 129–139.
47. Devroede G: La constipation: du symptôme à la personne. *Psychologie Médicale* 1985; 17(10):1515–1524.
48. Likongo Y, Devroede G, Schang JC, et al: Hindgut dysgenesis as a cause of constipation with delayed colonic transit. *Dig Dis Sci* 1986; 31(9):993–1003.
49. Schang JC, Devroede G: Fasting and postprandial myoelectric spiking activity in the human sigmoid colon. *Gastroenterology* 1983; 85:1048–1053.
50. Schang JC: Colonic motility in subgroups of patients with the irritable bowel syndrome in Poitras P (ed): *Proceedings of the First International Symposium on Small Intestinal and Colonic Motility*. Montreal, Canada, Centre de recherche cliniques, Hôpital Saint-Luc and Jouveinal Laboratories/Laboratoires, Inc., 1985, pp 101–112.
51. Hinton JM, Lennard-Jones JE: Constipation: Definition and classification. *Postgrad Med* 1968; 44:720–723.
52. Asher R: Munchhausen's syndrome. *Lancet* 1951; 1:339–341.
53. Meadow R: Munchhausen syndrome by proxy. *Arch Dis Child* 1982; 57:92–98.

54. Arhan P, Devroede G, Jehannin B, et al: Segmental colonic transit time. *Dis Colon Rectum* 1981; 24:625–629.
55. Schang JC, Devroede G, Duguay C, et al: Constipation par inertie colique et obstruction distale: étude électromyographique. *Gastroenterol Clin Biol* 1985; 9:480–485.
56. Weber J, Ducrotte P, Touchais JY, et al: Biofeedback training for constipation in adults and children. *Dis Colon Rectum* 1987; 30:844–846.
57. Sandler RS, Drossman DA, Nathan HP, et al: Symptom complaints and health care seeking behaviour in subjects with bowel dysfunction. *Gastroenterology* 1984; 87:314–318.
58. Wald A: Colonic transit and anorectal manometry in chronic idiopathic constipation. *Arch Intern Med* 1986; 146:1713–1716.
59. Ducrotte P, Denis P, Galmiche JP, et al: Motricité anorectale dans la constipation idiopathique. Etude de 200 patients consécutifs. *Gastroenterol Clin Biol* 1985; 9:10–15.
60. Lanfranchi GA, Bazzoichi G, Brignola C, et al: Different patterns of intestinal transit time and anorectal motility in painful and painless chronic constipation. *Gut* 1984; 25:1352–1357.
61. Abrahamian FP, Lloyd-Still JD: Chronic constipation in childhood: A longitudinal study of 186 patients. *J Pediatr Gastroenterol Nutr* 1984; 3:460–467.
62. Bonfils S, Hachette JC, Danne O: *L'abord psychosomatique en gastro-entérologie*. Paris, Masson, 1982.
63. Pavlakis A, Wheeler JS Jr, Krane RJ, et al: Functional voiding disorders in females. *Neurourology and Urodynamics* 1986; 5:145.
64. Parks AG, Porter NH, Melzack J: Experimental study of the reflex mechanism controlling the muscles of the pelvic floor. *Dis Colon Rectum* 1962; 5:407–414.
65. Fry IK, Griffiths JD, Smart PJG: Some observations on the movement of the pelvic floor and rectum with special reference to rectal prolapse. *Br J Surg* 1966; 53:784–787.
66. Rutter KRP: Electromyographic changes in certain pelvic floor abnormalities. *Proc R Soc Med* 1974; 67:53–56.
67. Kerremans R: *Morphological and Physiological Aspects of Anal Continence and Defecation*. Bruxelles, Editions Arscia SA Bruxelles, Presses académiques européennes, 1969.
68. Wasserman IF: Puborectalis syndrome (rectal stenosis due to anorectal spasm). *Dis Colon Rectum* 1964; 7:87.
69. Preston DM, Lennard-Jones JE: Anismus in chronic constipation. *Dig Dis Sci* 1985; 30:413–418.
70. Womack NR, Williams NS, Holmfield JM, et al: New method for the dynamic assessment of anorectal function in constipation. *Br J Surg* 1985; 72:994–998.
71. Kuijpers HC, Bleijenberg G, De Morree H: The spastic pelvic floor syndrome. Large bowel outlet obstruction caused by pelvic floor dysfunction: A radiological study. *Int J Colorectal Dis* 1986; 1:44–48.
72. Jones PN, Lubowski DZ, Swash M, et al: Is paradoxical contraction of puborectalis muscle of functional importance? *Dis Colon Rectum* 1987; 30:667–670.
73. Turnbull GK, Lennard-Jones JE, Bartram CL: Failure of rectal expulsion as a cause of constipation: Why fibre and laxatives sometimes fail. *Lancet* 1986; 1:767–769.
74. Jennings PJ: Megarectum and megacolon in adolescents and young adults: Results of treatment at St. Mark's Hospital. *Proc R Soc Med* 1967; 60:805–806.
75. Percy JP, Swash M, Neill ME, et al: Electrophysiological study of motor nerve supply of pelvic floor. *Lancet* 1981; 1:16–17.
76. Hamel-Roy J, Devroede G, Arhan P, et al: Functional abnormalities of the anal sphincters in patients with myotonic dystrophy. *Gastroenterology* 1984; 86:1469–1474.
77. Reich W: *The Function of the Orgasm: Sex–Economic Problems of Biological Energy*. New York, Farrar, Straub and Giroux, 1943.
78. Lowen A: *Love and Orgasm*. New York, New American Library, 1967.
79. Bleijenberg G, Kuijpers HC: Treatment of the spastic pelvic floor syndrome with biofeedback. *Dis Colon Rectum*, 1987; 30:108–111.
80. Emery Y, Descos L, Meunier P, et al: Constipation terminale par asynchronisme abdomino-pelvien: analyse des données étiologiques, cliniques, manométriques, et des résultats thérapeutiques après rééducation par biofeedback. *Gastroenterol Clin Biol*, 1988; 12:6–11.
81. Hero M, Arhan P, Devroede G, et al: Measuring the anorectal angle. *J Biomed Eng* 1985; 7:321–325.
82. Kuijpers HC, Bleijenberg G: The spastic pelvic floor syndrome. A cause of constipation. *Dis Colon Rectum* 1985; 28:669–672.
83. Loening-Baucke VA, Cruikshank BM: Abnormal defecation dynamics in chronically constipated children with encopresis. *J Pediatr* 1986; 108(4):562–566.
84. Meunier P: Rectoanal dyssynergia in constipated children (abstract). *Dig Dis Sci* 1985; 30(8):784.
85. Meunier P, Louis D, Jaubert de Beaujeu M: Physiologic investigation of primary chronic constipation in children: Comparison with the barium enema study. *Gastroenterology* 1984; 87:1351–1357.
86. Wald A, Chandra R, Gabel S, et al: Anorectal manometry and continence studies in childhood encopresis (abstract). *Dig Dis Sci* 1984; 29(6):554.
87. Denis P, Cayron G, Galmiche JP: Biofeedback: The light at the end of the tunnel? Maybe for constipation. *Gastroenterology* 1981; 80:1089.
88. Ford MR: Interpersonal stress and style as predictors of biofeedback/relaxation training outcome: Preliminary findings. *Biofeedback Self Regul* 1985; 10:223–239.
89. Wallace WC, Madden WM: Experience with partial resection of the puborectal muscle. *Dis Colon Rectum* 1969; 12:196–200.
90. Barnes PRH, Hawley PR, Preston DM, et al: Experience of posterior division of the puborec-

talis muscle in the management of chronic constipation. *Br J Surg* 1985; 72:475–477.
91. Watier A, Devroede G, Duranceau A, et al: Constipation with colonic inertia. A manifestation of systemic disease? *Dig Dis Sci* 1983; 28(1):1025–1033.
92. Lane WA: The results of the operative treatment of chronic constipation. *Br Med J* 1908; Jan 18:126.
93. Tobon F, Schuster MM: Megacolon: Special diagnostic and therapeutic features. *Johns Hopkins Med J* 1974; 135:91–105.
94. Barnes PRH, Lennard-Jones JE, Hawley PR, et al: Hirschsprung's disease and idiopathic megacolon in adults and adolescents. *Gut* 1986; 27:534–541.
95. Preston JE, Lennard-Jones JE: Pelvic motility and response to intraluminal bisacodyl in slow-transit constipation. *Dig Dis Sci* 1985; 30:289–294.
96. Meunier P, Rochas A, Lambert R: Motor activity of the sigmoid colon in chronic constipation: Comparative study with normal subjects. *Gut* 1979; 20:1095–1101.
97. Dapoigny M, Tournut D, Trolese JF, et al: Activité myoélectrique colique à jeûn et en période post-prandiale chez le sujet sain et chez le colopathe. *Gastroenterol Clin Biol* 1985; 9:223–227.
98. Preston DM, Rees LH, Lennard-Jones JE: Gynaecological disorders and hyperprolactinaemia in chronic constipation. *Gut* 1983; 24:A480.
99. Krishnamurthy S, Schuffler MD, Rohrmann CA, et al: Severe idiopathic constipation is associated with a distinctive abnormality of the colonic myenteric plexus. *Gastroenterology* 1985; 88:26–34.
100. Henley FA: Pelvic colectomy for obstinate constipation. *Proc Roy Soc Med* 1967; 60:806–807.
101. Dyer NH, Dawson AM, Smith BF, et al: Obstruction of bowel due to lesion in the myenteric plexus. *Br Med J* 1969; 1:686–689.
102. Preston DM, Pfeffer JM, Lennard-Jones JE: Psychiatric assessment of patients with severe constipation. *Gut* 1984; 25:A582–A583.
103. Bard L: Le mégarectum, dilatation idiopathique d'origine congénitale. *La Semaine Médicale* 1910; 30(48):565.
104. Hillemand B: Mégarectum: Étiologie, pathogénie, clinique, traitement médical. *Arch des Maladies de l'Appareil Digestif et de la Nutrition (Paris)* 1965; 54:3–36.
105. Callaghan RP, Nixon HH: Megarectum: Physiological observations. *Arch Dis Child* 1964; 39:153–157.
106. Meunier P, Mollard P, Marechal JM: Physiopathology of megarectum: The association of megarectum with encopresis. *Gut* 1976; 17:224–227.
107. Arhan P, Devroede G, Persoz B, et al: Response of the anal canal to repeated distension of the rectum. *Clin Invest Med* 1979; 2:83–88.
108. Cummings JH, Wiggins HS: Transit through the gut measured by analysis of a single stool. *Gut* 1976; 17:219–223.
109. Hinton JM, Lennard-Jones JE, Young AC: A new method for studying gut transit times using radiopaque markers. *Gut* 1969; 10:842–847.
110. Eastwood HDH: Bowel transit studies in the elderly: Radiopaque markers in the investigation of constipation. *Gerontol Clin* 1972; 14:154–159.
111. Chaussade S, Roche H, Khyari A, et al: Mesure du temps de transit colique (TTC): Description et validation d'une nouvelle technique. *Gastroenterol Clin Biol* 1986; 10:385–389.
112. Metcalfe AM, Phillips SF, Zinsmeister AR, et al: Simplified assessment of segmental colonic transit. *Gastroenterology* 1987; 92:40–47.
113. Fleckenstein P: A probe for intraluminal recording of myoelectric activity from multiple sites in the human small intestine. *Scand J Gastroenterol* 1978; 13:767–770.
114. Fioramonti J, Bueno L, Frexinos J: Sonde endoluminale pour l'exploration électromyographique de la motricité colique chez l'homme. *Gastroenterol Clin Biol* 1980; 4:546–550.
115. Bueno L, Fioramonti J, Ruckebusch Y, et al: Evaluation of colonic myoelectrical activity in health and functional disorders. *Gut* 1980; 21:480–485.
116. Sarna S, Latimer P, Campbell D, et al: Electrical and contractile activities of the human rectosigmoid. *Gut* 1982; 23:698–705.
117. Schang JC, Hemond M, Hebert M, et al: Myoelectrical activity and intraluminal flow in human sigmoid colon. *Dig Dis Sci* 1986; 31:1331–1337.
118. Schuster MM, Hookman P, Hendrix TP, et al: Simultaneous manometric recording of internal and external sphincteric reflexes. *Bull Johns Hopkins Hosp* 1965; 116:79–88.
119. Devroede G, Vobecky S, Masse S, et al: Ischemic fecal incontinence and rectal angina. *Gastroenterology* 1982; 83(5):970–980.
120. Arhan P, Devroede G, Danis K, et al: Viscoelastic properties of the rectal wall in Hirschsprung's disease. *J Clin Invest* 1978; 62:82–88.
121. Farthing MJG, Lennard-Jones JE: Sensibility of the rectum to distension and the anorectal reflex in ulcerative colitis. *Gut* 1978; 19:64–69.
122. Denis P, Colin DR, Galmiche JP, et al: Elastic properties of the rectal wall in normal adults and patients with ulcerative colitis. *Gastroenterology* 1979; 77:45–48.
123. Barnes PRH, Lennard-Jones JE: Balloon expulsion from the rectum in constipation of different types. *Gut* 1985; 26:1049–1052.
124. Preston DM, Lennard-Jones JE, Thomas BM: The balloon proctogram. *Br J Surg* 1984; 71:29–32.
125. Lahr CJ, Rothenberger DA, Jensen LL, et al: Balloon topography. A simple method of evaluating anal function. *Dis Colon Rectum* 1986; 29:1–5.
126. Mahieu P, Pringot J, Bodart P: Defecography: I. Description of a new procedure and results in normal patients. *Gastrointestinal Radiology* 1984; 9:247–251.
127. Mahieu P, Pringot J, Bodart P: Defecography: II. Contribution to the diagnosis of defecation disorders. *Gastrointest Radiol* 1984; 9:253–261.

128. Sami-Ali: Corps réel, corps imaginaire. Dunod ed. Paris, 1984.
129. Sapir M: De soignant à soigné: le corps à corps. Mythe ou champ de recherche? *L'évolution psychiatrique* 1983; 48(4):989.
130. Almy TP, Hinkle LE Jr, Berle B, et al: Alterations in colonic function in man under stress. III. Experimental production of sigmoid spasm in patients with spastic constipation. *Gastroenterology* 1949; 12:437–449.
131. Nisard A, Jian R, Chevalier J, et al: Effet d'une cure thermale à Châtel-Guyon sur le temps de transit intestinal total de patients atteints de colopathie fonctionnelle. *Rev Fr de Gastroentérologie* 1982; 175:5.
132. Loening-Baucke VA: Abnormal rectoanal function in children recovered from chronic constipation and encopresis. *Gastroenterology* 1984; 87:1299–1304.
133. Hughes ESR, McDermott FT, Johnson WR, et al: Surgery for constipation. *Aust NZ J Surg* 1981; 51:144–148.

VIII
Endoscopic Therapy

43

Bleeding in the Upper Gastrointestinal Tract:

What is the rationale for endoscopic intervention?

STEVEN E. HAHN, M.D.
ROBERT I. GOLDBERG, M.D., F.A.C.P.

Does endoscopy alter the course of acute upper gastrointestinal (UGI) hemorrhage?

Despite developments in intensive care, sophisticated intravascular volume monitoring, and fiberoptic endoscopy, mortality from UGI bleeding has remained at approximately 10% for the past 40 years.[1] Many studies in the 1970s were performed to reassess the rationale of early UGI endoscopy in the patient with UGI bleeding. Some of these studies compared early endoscopy to UGI contrast radiography to determine if one or the other conferred an advantage or altered the course of bleeding. The conclusion of much of these data is that early endoscopy provides a more expeditious and accurate diagnosis than contrast radiography, but fails to alter the morbidity (transfusion requirements, need for emergency surgery, and duration of hospital stay) or mortality of the bleed.[2-9] It has become clear that as the vast majority of UGI bleeding ceases spontaneously, the value of diagnostic endoscopy is greatest in the select group that has continued bleeding throughout the resuscitative effort or recurrent bleeding during the hospital course.

The problem exists in how to identify this group of patients at the time of presentation. Morgan and co-workers studied a number of historic and clinical criteria as prognostic indicators in patients who continued bleeding or developed recurrent bleeding within 10 days of presentation.[10] He developed a series of patient "attributes" associated with a poor prognosis on presentation. These included age greater than 60 years; history of significant cardiac, respiratory, renal or hepatic disease; lack of alcohol or ulcerogenic medication usage; and congestive heart failure on presentation. Interestingly, binge drinking and salicylate use were associated with a more favorable prognosis. The risk of rebleeding or continued bleeding with two or more "poor patient attributes" was 30% and increased with the number of risk factors present. The mortality in the group with two or more risk factors also far surpassed the group with one or no risk factors.

Multiple studies have also confirmed the logical premise that the more significant the hemorrhage is hemodynamically, the more likely that bleeding will recur. Peterson and co-workers found that patients who rebled generally had lower hemoglobins (6.1 + 1.9 gm/L), greater time required for initial hemodynamic stabilization (3.0 + 1.7 hours), and higher initial transfusion requirements (3.9 units + 2.6).[9]

On the basis of these data it seems warranted to recommend urgent endoscopy in patients with associated severe illnesses, advanced age, and/or patients with hemodynamically significant hemorrhage on presentation. In the group of patients in whom bleeding ceases easily during the initial resuscitative effort, a case can be made to perform an elective diagnostic contrast study of the UGI tract to dictate further need for evaluation and therapy. This course of action, although undoubtedly less expensive and perhaps somewhat safer and better tolerated than endoscopy, can present serious diagnostic and therapeutic problems. Whereas contrast radiography can detect one or more significant mucosal lesions, endoscopic evaluation can detect stigmata of recent hemorrhage giving a more accurate assessment of the etiology of the bleed. A negative contrast study places the physician in the dilemma of not knowing whether the patient has bled from an ulcer with an adherent clot (which may obscure the accumulation of contrast material), a superficial mucosal lesion (e.g., Mallory-Weiss tear), "gastritis," or telangiectasias, or, in certain presentations, whether the patient had an upper tract bleed at all. An upper endoscopic evaluation can generally address all of the above doubts and in most cases can avoid the necessity for a subsequent lower tract evaluation. Finally, contrast material in the GI tract can create problems by obscuring the view of the endoscopist if rebleeding occurs without a definitive diagnosis, or by interfering with the interventional radiologist attempting to perform therapeutic angiography.

One of the strongest arguments in favor of an endoscopic role in UGI bleeding has been the advent of therapeutic endoscopic techniques to achieve hemostasis. The option of coupling endoscopic intervention to the initial diagnostic endoscopy may allow the endoscopist to alter the subsequent hospital course in a positive way, probably reducing transfusion requirements, need for emergency surgery, and perhaps mortality.

The remainder of the chapter will be a review of the different modalities currently available to the therapeutic endoscopist. We will not attempt to be overly comprehensive but rather will concentrate on those techniques that are generally available and in current use in the community. There is certainly no lack of imagination in the endoscopic community, and some ingenious ideas have met initial enthusiasm only to fall from favor. The purpose of the following is to provide some guidance to the internist, gastroenterologist, or endoscopic therapist based on the current literature and our own personal experiences.

THERMAL THERAPY

Thermal devices passed through the biopsy channel of an endoscope have received most of the attention in the recent literature and have been the most widely tested methods of endoscopic hemostasis both in the laboratory and in patient studies. All forms of heat therapy produce tissue edema, shrinkage and contraction of blood vessels, and coagulation of tissue proteins. Contact thermal devices contribute the additional dimension of "coaptive coagulation" or the ability to compress a bleeding site prior to the application of thermal energy. The advantage of this technique is to avoid the so-called heat sink effect or loss of thermal energy away from the bleeding site by flowing blood. Thermal cautery can be used either in the form of electrocoagulation, direct heat application, or laser.

Electrocoagulation—Monopolar Cautery

Electrocoagulation produces heat and eventual dessication of the tissue reducing the cauterized lesion into a necrotic mass. With monopolar cautery, the current flows from the electrode in contact with the tissue through the patient to a patient electrode or ground plate. Monopolar electrocoagulation was the first application of thermal therapy in gastrointestinal hemorrhage, having been transformed from its use in the operating room bovie to an endoscopic modality.

Papp has had the most extensive experience with the use of the monopolar cautery both in animal models and in humans. In an uncontrolled series of 86 patients with actively bleeding lesions (31 gastric ulcers, 6 marginal ulcers, 35 duodenal ulcers, 12 Mallory-Weiss tears, and 2 esophageal ulcers), effective hemostasis was achieved in 78 patients.[11, 12] Ten patients rebled and four underwent successful repeat therapy, leaving a successful therapeutic response in 83%.

In view of the high reported rate of rebleeding when a "visible vessel" is encountered in a mucosal lesion, Papp also evaluated the utility of monopolar cautery in reducing the rebleeding rate. Of 32 patients found to have visible vessels, 16 were randomized to cautery and 16 to a control of medical therapy with antacids and intravenous cimetidine.[11–14] Thirteen of 16 control patients rebled (81%), whereas only 1/16 (6%) of the cauterized group rebled, confirming both the high incidence of rebleeding with a visible vessel and the effectiveness of the monopolar cautery in the prevention of rebleeding. It should be noted that several recent studies have not confirmed the exceedingly high rebleeding rate reported in earlier studies with "visible vessels" or "sentinel clots." Whereas those endoscopic findings probably do portend a more aggressive course in many patients, the rebleeding rate seems to be closer to 50%.[15–17]

The technique as described by Papp consists of visualization of the bleeding or nonbleeding vessel, placement of the monopolar electrode within 2 to 3 mm of the vessel, and circumferential application of the cautery until bleeding ceases. The recommended setting is 5 on the electrocoagulation unit applied for 2 to 2.5 seconds in four to five circumferential applications. He stresses that the endoscopist should avoid direct application of the monopolar electrode to the visible vessel because this can result in destruction of the vessel and further bleeding.

Drawbacks in the use of monopolar cautery include the increased tendency to cause deeper penetration injury with the risk of perforation as well as "stickiness" of tissue to the electrode after coagulation which can result in increased bleeding. Piercy and co-workers, despite efforts to lower power and time of coagulation with monopolar cautery, reported excessively deep injury to the gastric wall.[18] Papp demonstrated that the size of the ulcer produced by monopolar cautery did not correlate with the depth of tissue injury when using higher amperage.[14]

Although universally available and undoubtedly an effective device for achieving hemostasis, the problem of the unpredictability of the depth of injury induced by monopolar cautery has hampered its widespread use for GI hemorrhage.

Bipolar or Multipolar Cautery (BICAP®)

Bipolar cautery and the newer and more widely used multipolar electrocoagulation device were developed as an offshoot of monopolar cautery to counteract the problem of excessive depth of injury. The multipolar cautery consists of an array of six equally spaced longitudinal electrodes along the side and over the rounded tip of a cylindrical probe. A central opening allows for water irrigation for improved visualization. The BICAP probe comes in diameters of 2.3 and 3.3 (7 and 10 Fr). Early power sources delivered a maximum of 25 watts, but new units now deliver 50 watts. Settings on the power source range from 1 to 10 for power and either 1 second, 2 seconds, or continuous for timed delivery. The water and coagulation modes are activated by a foot pedal.

Laine recently published an impressive endoscopic study evaluating the use of the BICAP in the treatment of UGI hemorrhage.[19] Patients with endoscopically documented active bleeding (defined as continuous flow of blood for at least 5 minutes of endoscopic observation) were randomized to either multipolar electrocautery or sham cautery to determine if the endoscopic therapy actually altered the course of the bleed. The results were heavily in favor of cautery; with 90% successful hemostasis (vs 13% in control group), 14% requiring surgery (vs 57% in control group), 2.4 unit mean transfusion requirement (vs 5.4 in control group), 4.4 day mean hospital stay (vs 7.2 days in control group), 0% mortality (vs 13% in control group), and $3,420 average hospital cost (vs $7,550 in control group). By including only endoscopically documented active bleeding for study, Laine has probably come closest to selecting a group of patients with a poor prognosis who might truly benefit from endoscopic intervention. Although the study population was quite small because active bleeding is not a common endoscopic finding, it seems clear that in this study, morbidity was reduced and surgery was in large part avoided secondary to endoscopic therapy. Many other small studies have demonstrated similar efficacy of the BICAP in achieving hemostasis and have shown it to compare favorably to other modalities.[19-24] Frequent rebleeding, however, remains a problem.

Advantages of the BICAP include[14]:
1. Low power at the tip of the probe, which allows direct placement on a vessel
2. Capability of immediately irrigating prior to electrocoagulation
3. End on, oblique, or lateral probe application
4. Limited depth of injury
5. The ability to compress an artery by the probe tip prior to cautery ("coaptive coagulation")

The BICAP is now widely accepted as an efficacious tool in achieving endoscopic hemostasis.

Heater Probe

The heater probe unit was developed in 1978 by Protell and co-workers for use in gastrointestinal bleeding.[25] The probe consists of a hollow aluminum cylinder with an inner heater coil and an outer coating of Teflon. A thermocouple element, contained within the probe tip, maintains the actual temperature at the desired level. A potent water jet provides excellent capacity for washing a lesion or breaking up a clot. The Olympus device comes in two diameters, 3.2 mm and 2.4 mm (approximately 10 Fr and 7 Fr, respectively). The probe tip delivers a preset quantity of energy (5 to 30 joules) when activated by a foot pedal.

Experience with the heater probe has generally been quite good. Of 16 patients treated by Shorvon and co-workers, initial hemostasis was achieved in 12.[26] Only 1 of 12 subsequently rebled and underwent successful repeat therapy.

Johnson and co-workers published a retrospective study of the use of the heater probe in major bleeding from peptic ulcers.[27] Selection criteria included either endoscopically observed arterial bleeding or a "sentinel clot" (raised visible vessel) in the setting of hemodynamically significant hemorrhage or recurrent bleeding. Of 20 patients in whom the heater probe was used, successful hemostasis was achieved in 19. Of six patients who rebled, five underwent successful repeat therapy for an overall success rate of 95%. No complications were noted during the study.

Storey treated 25 actively bleeding patients (15 gastric ulcers and 10 duodenal ulcers) already anesthetized for emergency surgery, who were elderly and/or compromised by associated illness.[28] Patients chosen for study had a 6.6 unit mean transfusion requirement. All but one of the gastric ulcer patients were able to avoid surgery initially due to successful endoscopic hemostasis. Two patients rebled with one requiring eventual surgery, for an overall efficacy rate of 87%. Less success was apparent with duodenal ulcers in which only two of ten were able to avoid surgery secondary to successful heater probe therapy. The author concludes that emergency surgery in compromised patients can often be avoided with the judicious use of the heater probe.

Several features of the heater probe make it particularly suitable for arterial hemostasis. It has a rounded tip for adequate compression or tamponade of a bleeding vessel. A Teflon coating reduces adherence to the lesion being treated. Proximal irrigation ports allow for excellent washing of the lesion even when it is forcefully applied to the site. The probe can be applied end on or tangentially, although the rigidity of the larger probe is desirable to permit effective tangential application.

Most authors recommend initial tamponade of the bleeding lesion by forceful compression of the probe tip to the lesion. Water irrigation at that point can clear blood or clot from the lesion. The heater probe is then applied either directly to the bleeding site or circumferentially with eventual application to the visible vessel. Some endoscopists, for fear of instigating further bleeding, prefer the latter approach. This allows a "cuff" of edema to facilitate hemostasis prior to direct application to the vessel. Johnston and co-workers showed in a canine model that the heater probe and BICAP could effectively coagulate and dessicate tissue without danger of tissue and vessel erosion.[29] In this study, tissue and vessel erosions were more problematic with monopolar cautery and laser, often interfering with effective arterial coagulation by disintegrating the vessel. These data support the safety of direct application of the heater probe and BICAP to the visible bleeding or nonbleeding vessel. In general, with lesions smaller than 0.5 cm, we feel comfortable with the initial application directly to the bleeding site (or visible vessel), whereas larger lesions are probably best treated circumferentially before direct application of heat energy.

BICAP vs Heater Probe—Any Difference?

Heater probe and BICAP have emerged as the favored and most widely used endoscopic devices for UGI bleeding. Despite definite similarities in manner of usage and efficacy, some differences exist and endoscopists have chosen sides.

BICAP delivers electric current between electrodes, and wattage and duration of pulsing can be set. The heater probe delivers a preset amount of energy (joules) as selected on the power generator and will not shut off until the desired amount of energy has been delivered. The area of current density is much smaller for the BICAP than for the heater probe.

The technique applied is essentially the same for both, with firm compression of the vessel followed by the application of cautery. With the 50-watt-BICAP at a setting of 7 for 1 second, 39 watts are delivered—usually three to five applications are necessary. With the heater probe, usually 25 to 30 joules are delivered for three to five applications. Because it takes 5 to 7 seconds for 30 joules to be delivered, the probe must be kept firmly in place; this is often difficult with the patient retching and with intestinal motility. For best hemostasis, repeat applications of the heater probe must be rapid without allowing the treatment area to cool.

Although earlier studies have demonstrated higher efficacy and less rebleeding with the heater probe, more recent work employing the newer 50-watt BICAP generator has not confirmed these differences. Jensen and co-workers, in a recent evaluation of BICAP and heater probe in severe ulcer bleeding, found essentially no differences in efficacy or safety.[30]

The heater probe and the BICAP are relatively inexpensive, induce predictable tissue damage, offer the advantage of coaptive coagulation, and are portable. Choice is generally made on the basis of availability and personal preference.

Laser

Interest and use of the laser for gastrointestinal hemorrhage has grown dramatically over the last 10 years. Laser beams are intense, easily focused, and monochromatic—all principles that make the device well-suited for endoscopic therapy. The light is absorbed by tissue and converted to heat which coagulates proteins, clots blood, and seals bleeding vessels.

The biologic effects of the laser depend on the physical properties of the beam. Both neodymium-yttrium-aluminum-garnet (Nd-YAG) and argon have been used with flexible waveguides adaptable for fiberoptic instruments. Argon laser radiation has a high coefficient of absorption such that the intensity of the light energy is quickly reduced as the beam enters deeper tissue (90% extinction at 1 mm).

The Nd-YAG laser has a greater depth of penetration (90% extinction at 4 mm). These properties, in part, determine which gastrointestinal lesions would be more amenable to therapy with each laser source (Table 43-1).

There was initial controversy as to whether argon or Nd-YAG laser was better suited for GI bleeding. Although argon penetrates less deeply and would theoretically be less likely to cause full thickness injury, its diminished potential to coagulate larger, deeper vessels hampers its utility in acute hemorrhage. The YAG laser is more versatile, being the preferred device for gastrointestinal tumor palliation. Clearly most centers can afford only one type of laser. At the present time, the argon laser has been relegated to endoscopic cauterization of angiodysplastic lesions, although even for this indication many authors prefer the Nd-YAG. As distinct from the thermal devices previously discussed, the laser is a noncontact device capable of achieving hemostasis by delivering energy at a distance from the lesion. This allows easier aiming that can be achieved by either the heater probe or BICAP which both require keeping the target site in alignment for several seconds. There is also no chance of inadvertently pulling off a clot or coagulum as is sometimes the case with the contact devices. It does not, however, offer the advantage of compression of the bleeding vessel (coaptive coagulation), and many investigators feel that tamponade of the lesion prior to coagulation is necessary to achieve lasting and effective hemostasis.

Flexible quartz fibers convey the beam from the laser to the target lesion. A plastic sheath generally encircles the 1-mm laser fiber with a space between for delivery of coaxial gas or water. The diameter of the entire sheathed fiber generally ranges from 2 to 2.4 mm, permitting it to be passed through the biopsy channel of a standard upper endoscope. Many endoscopists prefer to use a double channel scope, however, for simultaneous irrigation and suction.[31]

The recommended technique is to pass the laser fiber through the biopsy channel until it extends just into the field of view and 1 to 2 cm from the lesion. The scope is manipulated so that the lesion can be viewed en face. The efficacy of the coagulation is reduced, and the risk of induced bleeding is increased with tangential application of the laser. It has been recommended to use relatively high power settings (70 to 90 watts) and short pulse durations (0.3 to 0.5 seconds). Most investigators use either circumferential application around the ulcer or around the vessel if visualized, because the risk of vaporization and induced bleeding with direct application can be quite high (10% to 15%). Once a cuff of edema is observed, the endoscopist can proceed with relative safety in directly treating the vessel. Tissue edema and white coagulum around the vessel should be readily appreciated when adequate hemostasis has been achieved.

Efficacy of the Nd-YAG laser in the treatment of UGI hemorrhage has been examined in several studies. In one positive report, Rutgeerts and co-workers treated 152 patients with the Nd-YAG laser for UGI hemorrhage.[32] Peptic ulcers were responsible for over 90% of the bleeding, with the remaining lesions con-

TABLE 43-1.
Endoscopic Laser Treatment for Gastrointestinal Disease

Type of Laser	Wavelength (mm)	Coefficient of Absorption	Depth of Penetration	Visible to the Eye	Adaptable for Flex Scope
Nd-YAG	1.06	↓	↑ 90% penetration at 4 mm	No	Yes
Argon	.5	↑	↓ 90% extinction at 1 mm	Yes	Yes

sisting of Mallory-Weiss tears, gastric angiomas, and gastric carcinoma. All patients were endoscoped initially to determine if their lesions were amendable to the laser and only then were they included in the study. The authors felt that by eliminating all lesions that could not be treated with the laser due to poor location or technical factors, treatment failures encountered would not be failures of the endoscopist, but failures of the laser to achieve hemostasis. The patients were stratified into three groups: active arterial spurting lesions (phase I); active nonpulsatile bleeding (phase II); and nonbleeding lesions with significant stigmata of recent hemorrhage (phase III).

In phase I, of 23 patients with active arterial bleeding who underwent YAG therapy, hemostasis was achieved in 20 (87%). Eleven of 20 rebled (55%) and required surgery. Therefore, 14 of 23 patients (61%) required surgery, perhaps sparing the other 9 patients (39%) from otherwise necessary emergency surgery. However, the mortality rate was unaffected by laser therapy.

In phases II and III of the study, active nonpulsatile bleeding and nonbleeding lesions with stigmata of recent hemorrhage were compared with no therapy. In both phases, laser-treated groups fared better, with a statistically lower rate of rebleeding and need for urgent surgery. Mortality was again unaffected by laser therapy. The authors concluded that the YAG laser was both efficacious and safe (no free perforations out of 86 treated patients), but no significant effect on patient mortality could be demonstrated.

In a conflicting report, Krejs recently evaluated the use of the YAG laser in 174 ulcer patients with either active bleeding or stigmata of recent hemorrhage.[33] Although the laser was effective in achieving initial hemostasis in 88% of actively bleeding ulcers, no benefit could be demonstrated in reducing transfusion requirements, necessity for urgent surgery, length of hospital stay, or mortality rate. In addition, free perforation occurred in one patient and bleeding was precipitated in four patients, two of whom required surgery. Therefore, 3 of 85 patients (4%) had complications necessitating surgical intervention.

The laser is a large, expensive unit that for all practical purposes is not portable. As such, the patients must be brought to the laser, making it nearly impossible to couple therapy to the initial diagnostic endoscopy. As the lesion to be treated needs to be viewed en face, a large proportion of lesions are not endoscopically amenable to laser treatment. Being a noncontact device, larger energy applications are necessary to achieve hemostasis than with the contact probes. Finally, the use of laser photocoagulation carries a higher rate of perforation (1% to 2%) than the other thermal devices.[34]

New developments in laser technology may address some of these problems. Hashimoto and co-workers have developed a lateral prismatic tip to deliver the laser beam at a 60-degree to 90-degree angle which may make more lesions accessible to laser treatment, especially in the gastric fundus and duodenum.[35] Joffe has described his experience with the use of the endoscopic sapphire-tipped contact laser probe.[36] This can convert the laser to a contact device employing coaptive coagulation and probaby lessening the energy expenditure to achieve hemostasis.

Laser therapy has been reported to be of clinical benefit in patients with bleeding from angiodysplastic lesions and is clearly efficacious in the palliation of gastrointestinal obstructing tumors. For now, however, its therapeutic role in active UGI hemorrhage remains poorly defined.

SCLEROTHERAPY FOR NONVARICEAL LESIONS

In recent years interest has also turned to injection therapy of various sclerosant solutions for nonvariceal hemorrhage. Injection delivery systems are identical to those used for variceal sclerotherapy. Most of the initial investigations using this modality were performed in Japan and Europe, and few, if any, controlled studies have been performed in the United States.

In 1984, Hajiro reviewed the Japanese

experience, in the work of Asaki, who achieved initial hemostasis in 331 of 332 patients using *absolute alcohol* injection.[37] Only a 10% rebleeding rate was reported, although local ulceration was not uncommon, and perforation was noted in approximately 1% of patients.

Sugawa and co-workers reported on 48 patients with severe UGI hemorrhage treated with *98% ethanol*.[38] Eighty percent of those patients were actively bleeding at the time of endoscopy. No control group was included. The lesions included 17 gastric ulcers, 11 duodenal ulcers, 6 acute gastric mucosal lesions, 3 Mallory Weiss tears, 2 esophageal ulcers, 2 marginal ulcers, 1 gastric cancer, and 1 gastric leiomyoma. Initial hemostasis was achieved in 45 of 48 patients. Rebleeding occurred within 72 hours in only 3 of 45 patients. Five of the 48 patients died: 1 after emergency surgery, and 4 after seemingly successful hemostasis (3 of sepsis and 2 of pneumonia). The study included 20 patients with serious concomitant medical conditions at high surgical risk, and the authors speculate that mortality was reduced by successful hemostasis in many of these patients.

The tissue injury induced by ethyl alcohol, the most commonly used sclerosant, is mediated by dehydration resulting in vasoconstriction, vascular wall degeneration, and eventual thrombosis. The alcohol is generally injected through a 1-ml tuberculin syringe in amounts of 0.1 to 0.2 ml per injection at three or four sites surrounding the bleeding vessel. Experienced investigators emphasize the importance of injecting the ethanol slowly and of limiting the volume of injection to a total of 1 ml to prevent extension of the ulcer.

Other studies have investigated the efficacy of *1:10,000 epinephrine* injections in achieving hemostasis. Leung and co-workers reported on 37 patients with actively bleeding ulcers (10 gastric ulcers and 27 duodenal ulcers) who underwent injection therapy with epinephrine.[39] Volumes of 0.5 ml were injected into multiple sites around the vessel and eventually into the vessel itself. Total volumes ranged from 1.5 ml to 10 ml (mean 4.1 ml) with spurting vessels requiring larger total volumes of injection. All 27 patients had initial hemostasis, with a 17% rebleeding rate. No local or systemic complications were reported.

Hirao and co-workers described their techniques of injecting a solution of *hypertonic saline* and *1:10,000 epinephrine* into the base of a bleeding vessel, with permanent hemostasis achieved in 93.7% of 158 patients.[40] In their last 128 patients, the ulcer base was reinjected prophylactically 24 to 48 hours later and only 1 of these patients required emergency surgery.

Soehandra and co-workers, in an uncontrolled prospective study, reported on their experience with 50 pulsating and 64 oozing lesions treated with a combined injection method of *1:10,000 epinephrine* and *1% polidocanol*.[41] The lesions included 30 gastric ulcers, 30 duodenal-stomal ulcers, as well as angiodysplastic lesions, postpolypectomy and papillotomy hemorrhages. Five to 10 ml of epinephrine are injected submucosally into and around the bleeding vessel followed by injection of 5 ml of the sclerosant polidocanol. The epinephrine was thought to induce vasoconstriction and volume compression of the vessel with subsequent obliteration via the sclerosing effects of the polidocanol. Sixty-six percent of the patients with the pulsating type of bleeding attained permanent hemostasis in one sitting, with further sessions increasing the success rate to 84%. Ninety-two percent of the oozing type lesions were successfully treated. No comments were made regarding sclerosant-induced ulceration or possible untoward cardiovascular effects of the epinephrine, except to say that no serious complications were encountered.

Fuchs and co-workers, in an effort to avoid sclerosant-induced ulceration, reported on the prospective use of a *thrombin* solution to achieve hemostasis in actively bleeding lesions.[42] One hundred IUs of thrombin diluted in 3 ml of normal saline were injected into four quadrants surrounding the bleeding vessel. The injections were made adjacent to the vessel until bleeding ceased, usually requiring 10 to 15 ml of solution. Pulsatile bleeding was initially controlled in 10 patients, with three recurrences, for a success rate of 70%. Initial hemostasis was achieved in 12 of 13 oozing lesions, with recurrent bleeding in 2 patients, resulting in a success rate of 85%. Combining pulsatile and oozing lesions, 74% were controlled with thrombin injection, although some patients required multiple sessions. No systemic side effects of the injections nor injection-related ulceration was reported. The authors report that compared to their past experience, thrombin injection was more effective in achieving hemostasis in pulsatile bleeding, whereas polidocanol was more effective in oozing lesions.

Although much less expensive, universally available, and perhaps as effective as the thermal devices, injection therapy is not without associated side effects. Both alcohol and polidocanol have been demonstrated to induce ulceration and even cause perforations in a very small percentage of patients (up to 1%).[37, 41] Injections of thrombin have been used to avoid these complications, but there is a potential risk of transmitting hepatitis B virus.[42] Variceal sclerotherapy has been shown to cause bacteremia in a significant percentage of patients, and one can assume that a similar incidence can be expected with nonvariceal injections.

There is little doubt that nonvariceal injection therapy is an effective endoscopic modality to achieve hemostasis. As the majority of practicing endoscopists have experience with sclerotheray of esophageal varices, it would seem logical that many will expand this practice to include nonvariceal lesions. The combined solution of epinephrine and hypertonic saline described by Hirao may be the most logical choice of sclerosant because it appears to be both very safe and efficacious. Controlled studies comparing injection therapy to thermal devices and comparing different sclerosant solutions are needed to further guide the endoscopist. However, considering its low cost and availability, injection therapy holds exciting promise for the future.

CONCLUSIONS

The last 15 years have provided the technology to achieve endoscopic hemostasis and have forced the gastroenterologist (perhaps not so unwillingly) into the realm of interventional endoscopy. Today's endoscopist has to choose between many available modalities to stop bleeding, but more importantly, needs to decide when and when not to treat. It must be reiterated that 85% to 90% of UGI bleeding ceases without therapy. Endoscopic therapy should only be considered in the select group of patients who have significant initial bleeding, demonstrable recurrent bleeding, or concomitant medical conditions placing them at high risk for surgery or for tolerating another significant bleeding episode. This latter group of patients has been traditionally considered "too sick for endoscopy." In our opinion, early endoscopic evaluation and intervention have the greatest utility in these very patients.

The treatment of nonbleeding lesions with stigmata of recent hemorrhage is more controversial. Nonbleeding visible vessels or "sentinel clots" have been demonstrated in numerous studies to be associated with a substantial rate of rebleeding and need for emergency surgery. These lesions, if accessible endoscopically, should be treated to lessen the odds of rebleeding. However, we recommend that the endoscopist refrain from treating ulcers with clean white bases, small overlying black or red spots, or lesions with overlying clots (without underlying oozing). These lesions carry a low rebleeding rate (10%), and the small but definite risk of perforation or induced bleeding need not be taken.[1]

It is also important to realize the limitations of endoscopic therapy. Massive upper intestinal bleeding of nonvariceal origin resulting in shock is a surgical disease. If time permits, endoscopy should be performed for the express purpose of guiding the surgeon to the site of bleeding (preferably in the operating suite on an intubated patient).

In choosing the appropriate endoscopic

modality, one must be critical in evaluating the numerous studies presented in this chapter and elsewhere in the literature. Some of these studies are uncontrolled, retrospective rather than prospective, and many exclude hemodynamically unstable patients. More importantly, the investigators performing the endoscopic therapy in these studies are highly skilled, highly experienced endoscopists usually in centers with excellent surgical backup. It is naive to believe that their results can be reproduced by a less experienced endoscopist who only rarely treated actively bleeding patients.

We recommend that the endoscopist in practice become comfortable with one mode of therapy so that skill will increase as experience is accrued. The treatment modality chosen should be safe, effective, simple and easy to use with existing equipment, readily available in a community hospital, and of relatively low cost. In reviewing the data, the heater probe and BICAP seem to incorporate all of these features. Injection sclerotherapy of nonvariceal lesions may be shown to perform equally well when comparative studies are performed.

Endoscopic therapy of UGI hemorrhage is an extremely exciting area, bridging the gap between endoscopist and surgeon. Future technologic advances will no doubt further narrow this gap.

References

1. Silverstein FE, Gilbert DA, Tedesco FJ, et al: The National ASGE survey on upper gastrointestinal bleeding. *Gastrointest Endosc* 1981; 27(2):73–79.
2. Stevenson W, Cox RR, Roberts CJC: Prospective comparison of double-contrast barium meal examination and fiberoptic endoscopy in acute upper gastrointestinal haemorrhage. *Br Med J* 1976; 2:723–724.
3. Hoare AM: Comparative study between endoscopy and radiology in acute upper gastrointestinal haemorrhage. *Br Med J* 1975; 1:27–30.
4. Katon RM, Smith FW: Panendoscopy in the early diagnosis of acute upper gastrointestinal bleeding. *Gastroenterology* 1973; 65:728–734.
5. Morris DW, Levine GM, Soloway RD, et al: Prospective randomized study of diagnosis and outcome in upper gastrointestinal bleeding: Endoscopy versus conventional radiography. *Am J Dig Dis* 1975; 20:1103–1109.
6. Keller RT, Logan GM: Comparison of emergent endoscopy and upper gastrointestinal haemorrhage. *Gut* 1976; 17:180–184.
7. Thoeni RF, Cello JP: A critical look at the accuracy of endoscopy and double-contrast radiography of the upper gastrointestinal (UGI) tract in patients with substantial UGI haemorrhage. *Radiology* 1980; 135:305–308.
8. Cello JP, Thoeni RF: Gastrointestinal hemorrhage: Comparative values of double-contrast upper gastrointestinal radiology and endoscopy. *JAMA* 1980; 243:685–688.
9. Peterson WL, Barnett CC, Smith HJ, et al: Routine early endoscopy in upper gastrointestinal tract bleeding. A randomized controlled trial. *N Engl J Med* 1981; 304(16):925–929.
10. Morgan AG, McAdam WA, Walmsley GL, et al: Clinical findings, early endoscopy, and multivariate analysis in patients bleeding from the upper gastrointestinal tract. *Br Med J* 1977; 2:237–240.
11. Papp JP: Endoscopic electrocoagulation in the management of upper gastrointestinal tract bleeding. *Surg Clin North Am* 1982; 62(5):797–806.
12. Papp JP: Electrocoagulation in upper gastrointestinal bleeding. *Dig Dis Sci* 1981; 26(7):41–43.
13. Papp JP: Endoscopic electrocoagulation of the nonbleeding visible ulcer vessel. *Gastrointest Endosc* 1979; 25:45–46.
14. Papp JP: *Endoscopic Control of Gastrointestinal Hemorrhage.* CRC Press, 1981.
15. Storey DW, Bown SG, Swain CP, et al: Endoscopic prediction of recurrent bleeding in peptic ulcers. *N Engl J Med* 1981; 305:915–916.
16. Griffiths WJ, Neumann DA, Welsh JD: The visible vessel as an indicator of uncontrolled or recurrent gastrointestinal hemorrhage. *N Engl J Med* 1979; 300:1411–1413.
17. Wara P: Endoscopic prediction of major rebleeding. A prospective study of stigmata of hemorrhage in bleeding ulcer. *Gastroenterology* 1985; 88:1209–1214.
18. Piercey JRA, et al: Electrosurgical treatment of experimental bleeding gastric ulcers; Development and testing of a computer and a better electrode. *Gastroenterology* 1978; 74:527–534.
19. Laine L: Multipolar electrocoagulation in the treatment of active upper gastrointestinal tract hemorrhage. *N Engl J Med* 1987; 216(26):1613–1617.
20. Goff JS: Bipolar electrocoagulation versus Nd-YAG laser photocoagulation for upper gastrointestinal bleeding lesions. *Dig Dis Sci* 1986; 31(9):906–910.
21. Rutgeerts P, Vantrappen G, Van Hootegem P, et al: Neodymium-YAG laser photocoagulation versus multipolar electrocoagulation for the treatment of severely bleeding ulcers: A randomized comparison. *Gastrointest Endosc* 1987; 33(4):199–202.
22. Donahue PE, Mobarhan S, Layden TJ: Endoscopic control of upper gastrointestinal hemorrhage with a bipolar coagulation device. *Surg Gynecol Obstet* 1984; 159:114–118.
23. Morris DL, Brearley S, Thompson H: A compar-

ison of the efficacy and depth of gastric wall injury with 3.2 and 2.3 mm bipolar probes in canine arterial hemorrhage. *Gastrointest Endosc* 1985; 31(6):361–363.
24. Swain CP, Mills TN, Shemesh E, et al: Which electrode? A comparison of four endoscopic methods of electrocoagulation in experimental bleeding ulcers. *Gut* 1984; 35:1424–1431.
25. Protell RL, Rubin CE, Auth DC, et al: The heater probe: A new endoscopic method for stopping massive gastrointestinal bleeding. *Gastroenterology* 1978; 74:257–262.
26. Shorvon PJ, Leung JWC, Cotton PB: Preliminary clinical experience with the heat probe at endoscopy in acute upper gastrointestinal bleeding. *Gastrointest Endosc* 1985; 31(6):364–366.
27. Johnston JH, Sones JQ, Long BW, et al: Comparison of heater probe and YAG laser in endoscopic treatment of major bleeding from peptic ulcers. *Gastrointest Endosc* 1985; 31(3):175–180.
28. Storey DW: Endoscopic control of peptic ulcer haemorrhage using the "heater probe." *Gut* 1983; 24:A967–1012.
29. Johnston J, Jensen D, Auth D: Comparison of endoscopic lasers, electrosurgery and the heater probe in coagulation of canine arteries. *Gastrointest Endosc* 1984; 30:154.
30. Jensen DM, Machicado GA, Silpa M, et al: BICAP heater probe for hemostasis of severe ulcer bleeding. *Gastrointest Endosc* 1985; 31:175–180.
31. Fleischer D: Efficacy and safety of laser therapy for gastrointestinal bleeding. ASGE National Mid Year Course, January 1987. Washington, DC.
32. Rutgeerts P, Vantrappen G, Broeckaert L, et al: Controlled trial of YAG laser treatment of upper digestive hemorrhage. *Gastroenterology* 1982; 83(2):410–416.
33. Krejs GJ, Little KH, Westergaard H, et al: Laser photocoagulation for the treatment of acute peptic ulcer bleeding. *N Engl J Med* 1987; 316 (26):1618–1621.
34. Kiefhaber P, et al: Endoscopic control of massive gastrointestinal hemorrhage by irradiation with a high power neodymium YAG laser. *Prog Surg* 1977; 15:145–155.
35. Hashimoto D, Takami M, Idezuk Y, et al: Prismatic tip lateral radiation probe in YAG laser endoscopy. *Gastrointest Endosc* 1985; 31:153.
36. Joffe SN, Sankar MY, Salzer D, et al: Preliminary clinical applications of the contact surgical rod and endoscopic microbes with the Nd:YAG laser. *Gastrointest Endosc* 1985; 31:155.
37. Hajiro K: Japanese experience with local injection and hemoclips. Symposium on Endoscopy in Upper GI Bleeding. The XII International Gastrointestinal Endoscopy. The V European Gastrointestinal Endoscopy Congress. Lisbon, September 1984.
38. Sugawa C, Fujita Y, Ikeda T, et al: Endoscopic hemostasis of bleeding of the upper gastrointestinal tract by local injection of ninety-eight percent dehydrated ethanol. *Surg Gynecol Obstet* 1986; 162:159–163.
39. Leung JWC, Chung SCS: Endoscopic injection of adrenalin in bleeding peptic ulcers. *Gastrointest Endosc* 1987; 33:73–75.
40. Hirao M, et al: Endoscopic local injection of hypertonic saline-epinephrine solution to arrest hemorrhage from the upper gastrointestinal tract. *Gastrointest Endosc* 1985; 31:313–317.
41. Soehendra N, Grimm H, Stenzel M: Injection of nonvariceal bleeding lesion of the upper gastrointestinal tract. *Endoscopy* 1984; 16:115–117.
42. Fuchs KH, Wirtz HJ, Schaube H, et al: Initial experience with thrombin as injection agent for bleeding gastroduodenal lesions. *Endoscopy* 1986; 18:146–148.

44

Treatment of Bleeding Esophageal Varices

MICHAEL V. SIVAK, JR., M.D.
JOHN L. PETRINI, M.D.

Variceal hemorrhage, one of the more dramatic consequences of portal hypertension, is a difficult problem for the physician to manage. Although our knowledge of the anatomy of esophagogastric varices and the pathophysiology of portal hypertension has advanced, improvement in the prognosis for the gravely ill patient with variceal hemorrhage has been minimal.

The approach to variceal hemorrhage has changed radically in recent years. Confidence in portosystemic shunt surgery has waned, while enthusiasm for sclerotherapy and other noninvasive therapies has increased. In this chapter we present our approach to the management of variceal hemorrhage. As much as possible, this will be based on available data on the pathophysiology of portal hypertension and variceal bleeding as well as information on the technique and results of sclerotherapy.

There are many causes of portal hypertension and esophageal varices, and there are decided differences in outcome depending on the nature of the underlying disease. There are also marked differences in the approach to management. In this chapter we will be concerned exclusively with bleeding esophageal varices due to portal hypertension as a result of cirrhosis of the liver.

CLINICAL ASPECTS OF VARICEAL HEMORRHAGE

Proper management of any pathologic disorder is based on knowledge of its pathophysiology and natural course. Unfortunately, available information on the behavior of esophageal varices is imperfect and incomplete. Nevertheless, a concept of the mechanisms behind the formation of varices and the development of hemorrhage is of importance as each form of therapy is considered.

Prevalence, Morbidity, and Mortality

The results of studies of the prevalence of varices in patients with cirrhosis are inconsistent, presumably due to variability in methods of diagnosis and patient selection. Autopsy studies suggest that varices are present in approximately 60% of patients with cirrhosis.[1] In the past, antemortem studies relied on barium contrast radiography of the esophagus, but this method of diagnosis is less sensitive than endoscopy.[2] According to Galambos,[3] from 14% to 77% of patients with cirrhosis will have varices. Endoscopic series suggest that varices are present in from 33% to 98% of patients with cirrhosis.[2, 4]

Because the range of estimates for the prevalence of varices is so wide, it is difficult to arrive at an accurate estimate.

Information on the rate at which variceal bleeding develops in patients with cirrhosis is also inconsistent. In one series, 115 patients were followed for a mean of 3.3 years; variceal hemorrhage occurred in 28.6%.[5] In another study, 75 patients were observed for a maximum of 7 years, and variceal bleeding developed in 37%.[6] The autopsy study by Olsson found that 67% of patients with cirrhosis had bleeding prior to death, but the number with variceal hemorrhage could not be determined.[1] Resnick and co-workers[7] found that about 10% of patients with varices will develop hemorrhage per year of follow-up. Despite attempts to establish the risk of variceal bleeding in association with cirrhosis, the only valid conclusion is that varices confer a high probability of bleeding but not a certainty.

Mortality as a result of variceal hemorrhage ranges from about 15% to 90%. Bleeding ceases spontaneously in approximately 60% of cases, although bleeding recurs in about one-third.[8] If hemorrhage recurs during hospitalization for an episode of bleeding, the mortality is very high.[9] The mortality for variceal hemorrhage is highest during the first week after onset, with nearly 75% of the deaths occurring during this time.[8] In the survey of the American Society for Gastrointestinal Endoscopy (ASGE) on gastrointestinal bleeding, the mortality for variceal bleeding was over 30%.[10] Without some form of intervention, about two-thirds of patients who survive initial hospitalization will have recurrent bleeding.[11,12] At 6 weeks after the onset of bleeding, the mortality for patients with advanced cirrhosis is 42%.[8]

Pathophysiology of Variceal Bleeding

Shunting of blood from the portal venous system to the systemic circulation as a result of an increase in portal venous pressure is a prerequisite for variceal hemorrhage. Shunt channels include the azygous, gastroesophageal, umbilical, and hemorrhoidal venous systems. Hemorrhage may occur from any of these areas, but the gastroesophageal venous shunt is the most critical one in terms of risk to the patient. Occasionally, bleeding from hemorrhoidal vessels may be a serious problem.

Portal Venous Pressure

The gradient between wedged hepatic venous pressure and free hepatic venous pressure is known to closely reflect portal pressure.[13] Because clinical and biochemical data are unsatisfactory with respect to prediction of hemorrhage, many investigators have attempted to correlate this gradient with the occurrence of variceal bleeding. It is logical to expect that the level of portal hypertension should correlate with the propensity for variceal bleeding, although this does not appear to be the case.

There is a relation between portal venous pressure and the presence of varices in that a portohepatic gradient of about 10 to 12 mm Hg is required for the development of varices. Below this level it is less likely that varices will be present or that variceal bleeding will develop.[4,14] There is, therefore, a relation between portal pressure and the presence of varices in patients with early liver disease.[15] However, with established portal hypertension and varices there is no relation between the magnitude of the portal venous pressure and variceal bleeding.[16,17]

Variceal Size

Attempts have been made to correlate variceal size with the degree of portal hypertension. Some earlier studies suggested the existence of such a correlation.[18-20] However, as pointed out by Lebrec and co-workers,[4] these reports included patients with normal or only slightly increased portal pressure. If these patients are eliminated, and only those with frankly increased portal pressure are considered, the relation between variceal size and the level of portal hypertension is absent in these studies. Other investigations fail to demonstrate any relation between variceal size and degree of portal hypertension, and by consensus there appears to be no correlation between variceal size and the degree of portal hypertension.[4, 21-25]

Variceal size alone, without reference to portal pressure, has been studied in relation to the risk of hemorrhage. It must be noted that there is no standard classification of variceal diameter and linear extent. Although similar terms may be used in the endoscopic grading of varices in various studies, the definitions of these terms do not correspond.

Palmer and Brick[26] measured variceal diameter and linear extent in the esophagus in 201 patients with cirrhosis. A history of variceal bleeding was present in some but not all cases. At the time of hemorrhage, most patients had large-diameter varices that extended over a substantial length of the esophagus. Small varices tended to enlarge just before the onset of bleeding, and variceal size decreased during the interval between episodes of bleeding. Among 90 patients with cirrhosis and varices who underwent repeat endoscopy at intervals from 1 week to 1 year, spontaneous disappearance of the varices was observed in 14%, and varices developed in 10% of patients in whom the esophagus was previously normal. Because of the variable in variceal grade observed while following patients, Palmer and Brick[26] concluded that smallness alone offered no assurance that the chance for bleeding would be small.

Dagradi[6] reported a study of the natural history of esophageal varices in patients with alcoholic liver disease. The endoscopic classification of the varices was divided into five grades based on diameter. Grade 5 was equal to grade 4 except for the presence of "small varices on top of varices." The latter were bright red, small, telangiectatic vessels, also described as "cherry-red" spots. During follow-up, an increase in variceal diameter and linear extent occurred in 65% of patients who continued to drink alcohol. Varices usually increased in length to varying degrees before an increase in diameter to the next highest grade was noted. The mean time required for progression to the highest grades was 50 months. Varices never disappeared in patients who continued to consume alcohol, although a significant decrease in diameter and extent occurred in 80% of patients who stopped drinking. Dagradi[6] also concluded that high-grade varices would invariably rupture, especially those in excess of 5 cm in length.

Baker and co-workers[5] studied the natural history of varices in 115 cirrhotic patients without prior variceal bleeding. Variceal size was classified endoscopically according to diameter and extent. The incidence of bleeding was approximately the same in patients with varices in the lower grades, while it was twice as frequent among those with the largest vessels. However, the severity of bleeding was inversely proportional to grade. Only 28 patients had follow-up endoscopy, but varices were observed to disappear in 9 patients, decrease in grade in 7, remain unchanged in 6, and become more extensive in 6 patients. Baker and co-workers[5] concluded that variceal size fluctuates.

Lebrec and co-workers[4] reported a study of variceal size and the risk of bleeding in 100 patients. Of these patients, 47 were initially evaluated because of signs of liver disease and did not have bleeding. The other 53 patients had had bleeding that was due to gastric erosions in 27 patients and to varices in 26 patients. Barium swallow x-rays were performed in all patients within 2 weeks of entry, and the varices were classified according to size by two independent radiologists. Varices were graded as large or small depending on whether a varix was less or greater than 5 mm in diameter. There was agreement between the two radiologists in 94 patients. Radiographic and endoscopic grading of the varices were obtained in the 53 patients who had prior bleeding, and the authors stated that there was agreement between the radiologists and endoscopist in 52 cases. The prevalence of recent bleeding (i.e., prior to entry), whether due to varices or to acute gastritis, was significantly higher in those patients with large varices. Patients were followed for 1 year during which time bleeding reoccurred in 17 patients, 14 of these being in the group with prior bleeding, and 3 from the group that entered with only signs of liver disease. The incidence of gastrointestinal bleeding during follow-up was significantly greater in patients with large varices. Variceal size had been measured endoscopically in most patients with bleeding during follow-up, although in some cases the grading was done radiographically. Although all patients who bled during follow-up had large varices, in some cases the bleeding was due to acute gastritis.

There are several problems with the study of Lebrec and co-workers.[4] The radiographic diagnosis of esophageal varices is generally not as reliable as reported by these authors. Furthermore, the correlation in this study between endoscopic and radiographic assessment of varices is far better than reported by others.[27, 28] The authors found that the risk of variceal bleeding was significantly higher if the varices were large, but they also found that the risk of bleeding from gastric erosions was also significantly increased if the varices were large. The authors theorized that this is explained by the general increase in collateral circulation through gastric and esophageal veins which might favor bleeding from established gastric erosions.

Variceal Anatomy

Although an explanation of the exact events that initiate variceal bleeding remains elusive, a coherent concept of the pathologic venous anatomy of the gastroesophageal shunt is emerging. There appear to be three venous components within and associated with the esophagus[29, 30]; the extrinsic system (external to the esophageal muscle layer), the intrinsic system, and the perforating veins. Varices seen at endoscopy are part of the intrinsic system, this being a plexus of subepithelial and submucosal vessels. Perforating veins connect the extrinsic and intrinsic channels, and rudimentary valves within the perforating veins appear to direct flow from the intrinsic to the extrinsic system, or conversely to prevent flow from extrinsic to intrinsic veins.

The extrinsic veins are thought to constitute the main gastroesophageal-systemic shunt pathway in patients with portal hypertension. There are extensive anastomoses between the extrinsic system and other vessels including the left gastric vein and the azygous system. Although the intrinsic system also has abundant anastomoses in its proximal aspect, some anatomical studies suggest that interconnections between the intrinsic veins and gastric veins at the mucosal level are not as extensive as might be expected.[29] However, recent studies have demonstrated four distinct levels of veins in the region of the gastroesophageal junction.[30, 31]

Variceal Blood Flow

McCormack and co-workers[32] studied blood flow in esophageal varices by means of Doppler ultrasonography and injection of contrast medium into the submucosal veins. This investigation demonstrated that variceal blood flow may be directed either proximally or distally, that the direction of flow may reverse with respiration, and that the venous flow from the stomach is frequently not via the intrinsic variceal plexus.

The work of McCormack and co-workers[32] supports the concept that the extrinsic veins are the main portosystemic shunt pathway in the region of the stomach and esophagus. In this concept of variceal blood flow, the perforating veins have a central role in variceal bleeding. With increasing flow and pressure in the extrinsic shunt pathway, the valves of the perforating veins may become incompetent with a resultant increase in pressure in the intrinsic system and an increase in the prominence of these vessels.

"Red Color" Signs

At endoscopy, esophageal varices are raised structures that sometimes have a bluish tint. Larger vessels have a familiar undulating configuration, and they may also have certain curious surface features referred to collectively as "red color" signs. Dagradi[6] noted that large varices had certain distinguishing markings that he referred to as "varices on varices" or "cherry-red" spots.

The Japanese Research Society for Portal Hypertension has proposed a classification of esophageal varices based on size and appearance (Table 44–1).[33, 34] Using this scheme, Beppu and co-workers[33] carried out a restrospective analysis of 172 patients with varices to determine the relationship of the history of bleeding to the endoscopic classification of the varices. Only 9.1% of patients without red color signs had had bleeding, while 58.7% of those with red color signs had a history of variceal bleeding, a statistically significant difference. Similar conclusions have been reported by others.[34]

Although Beppu and co-workers[33] regarded red color signs as small dilated vessels or microtelangiectasias, the exact nature of these red spots is uncertain. Spence and co-workers[35] studied rings of esophageal tissue from 27 patients who underwent esophageal transection and reanastomosis for varices. These were compared with esophageal rings from patients with diseases other than varices. Dilated intraepithelial blood-filled channels were found in all of the rings from patients with varices. By electronmicrography these channels were seen to be lined by flattened cells that were not typical of endothelial cells. The authors suggested that these intraepithelial channels may correspond to the cherry-red spots seen endoscopically, and that these lesions may play a role in variceal hemorrhage.

THERAPY OF VARICEAL HEMORRHAGE

For patients with alcoholic liver disease, abstinence from alcohol is essential. Interventional forms of therapy for variceal hemorrhage include various pharmacologic agents, tamponade, sclerotherapy, and surgery. The efficacy of these forms of therapy, alone or in combination, is the subject of considerable investigative effort. However, an ideal approach to treatment of variceal hemorrhage has not been established, and management of the individual patient remains a matter of clinical judgment.

TABLE 44–1.
General Rules of the Japanese Research Society for Portal Hypertension for Recording Endoscopic Findings in Esophageal Varices

1. Red color signs (RCS)*
   (small dilated vessels or microtelangiectasia on varix surface)
   a. Red wale marking (RWM)
   b. Cherry-red spot (CRS)
   c. Hematocystic spot (HCS)
   d. Diffuse redness (DR)
2. Fundamental color
   a. White (Cw)
   b. Blue (Cb)
3. Form
   a. Small, straight varices (F1)
   b. Enlarged, tortuous, occupy less than ⅓ of lumen (F2)
   c. Largest coil-shaped, occupy more than ⅓ of lumen (F3)
4. Location (longitudinal extent)
   a. Lower ⅓ (Li)
   b. Mid ⅓ below tracheal bifurcation (Lm)
   c. Upper ⅓ above tracheal bifurcation (Ls)
5. Adjunctive finding
   a. Erosion (E+)

*The RWM and CRS are graded from 1+ to 3+ depending on number and extent.

General Measures

The initial measures for treatment of a patient with variceal hemorrhage are the same as those for gastrointestinal bleeding of any cause. The most immediate and critical concern is to stabilize the patient.

Hemodynamic resuscitation with intravenous fluids and blood products is essential to prevent the complications of prolonged hypotension. When there is any evidence of hemodynamic instability, at least two large-bore intravenous lines (18 gauge or larger) should be inserted. The desirability of central venous perfusion, as well as the necessity for other aggressive resuscitative measures, must be considered in relation to the circumstances of the individual case because such steps have attendant complications that represent a serious threat vis-á-vis the already compromised status of these patients.

There is a certain folklore regarding transfusion of patients with cirrhosis. It is a commonly held belief that transfusion should be restricted to the amount of blood necessary to maintain a hematocrit of 30% to 35% in order to avoid increasing portal pressure. The source of this notion is uncertain. However, most patients with cirrhosis tolerate this hematocrit level well, and reducing the amount of transfusion is always advisable.

Endotracheal intubation has been advocated to protect the airway from regurgitated blood but has not been evaluated critically.[36]

Although gastric lavage has been employed for decades as a method for control of gastrointestinal bleeding, there is no evidence of its efficacy and it cannot be advocated for any form of upper gastrointestinal hemorrhage. In the ASGE prospective survey of endoscopy in gastrointestinal bleeding, an active source of hemorrhage was found by endoscopy in 15.9% of patients with a clear gastric aspirate.[37]

Once vital signs are stable, a more detailed assessment of the patient should be undertaken. Clues to the cause of the bleeding should be sought in the history and physical examination. When there is evidence of portal hypertension and chronic liver disease, such as jaundice, ascites, spider angioma, and caput medusa, variceal hemorrhage must be included in the differential diagnosis with the recognition that there are many potential sources of bleeding in such patients. Particular attention should be given to the investigation for historic and/or physical evidence of other intercurrent illnesses, especially those that may be adversely affected by bleeding and hypotension, such as diabetes, heart disease, and hypertension. A thorough inquiry should be made concerning the use of medications, especially agents that have a deleterious effect in relation to gastrointestinal bleeding, such as aspirin and anticoagulants.

Endoscopy

There has been a considerable argument during the last three decades over the value of emergency endoscopy in patients with upper gastrointestinal bleeding. The merits of this debate are beyond the scope of this chapter, although it has become less relevant with the advent of various methods of endoscopic therapy.

Many reports of series of patients undergoing emergency endoscopy for upper gastrointestinal bleeding have emphasized that lesions other than varices are frequently responsible for bleeding in patients with portal hypertension including those with known varices.[9, 38–41] The reported percentage of patients with varices and a nonvariceal cause of bleeding ranges from 34%[9] to 72%.[40] More recent studies demonstrate that variceal hemorrhage is by far the most likely cause of bleeding in patients with known varices.[42–45] Nevertheless, variceal hemorrhage can never be assumed, even if the presence of varices is well established. Because certain therapeutic measures (vasopressin, tamponade, sclerotherapy) are specific for variceal hemorrhage, prompt endoscopy is required in every case in which there is any possibility of variceal bleeding. Variceal hemorrhage is by nature intermittent, and endoscopy should be prompt even if the patient's hemodynamic status is stable and bleeding appears to have stopped.

When endoscopy is performed in a patient with gastrointestinal bleeding and esophageal varices there are four possible results: active variceal bleeding, nonbleeding varices in the absence of any other potential source of bleeding, nonbleeding varices plus active bleeding from another source, and nonbleeding varices plus one or more other potential sources without active bleeding. In the first two instances, the varices may be accepted as the source of blood loss (although absolute certitude rests with the actual observation of blood flowing from a varix), and therapeutic measures may be introduced accordingly. In about 55% of patients with variceal bleeding there is no endoscopic evidence to implicate the varices as the source[37]; blood flowing or spurting from a varix will be noted at endoscopy in less than 10% of cases of variceal hemorrhage.[37] In the third possible result of endoscopy, variceal hemorrhage is eliminated from consideration by the endoscopic findings. However, the fourth situation, nonbleeding varices with another potential but nonbleeding source, can be especially complex. Sometimes careful endoscopic examination will provide a clue to the responsible lesion, for example, a visible vessel in an ulcer crater. If the source cannot be determined, lesions with an acid-peptic etiology can be treated accordingly, and endoscopy should be immediate if hemorrhage resumes, in order to pinpoint the source of bleeding.

Sometimes the passage of an endoscope through the esophagus will precipitate bleeding. However, this is a rare complication, encountered in 1.4% of patients in the ASGE survey,[37] and endoscopy should never be deferred for this reason.

Medical Therapy

Several types of medication for control of variceal hemorrhage have been evaluated in controlled trials. There are problems with the methodology of many of these studies including small numbers of patients.

Vasopressin

Vasopressin is the most extensively studied of the pharmacologic agents for control of variceal bleeding. It produces vasoconstriction in the skin, gut, skeletal muscle, and, to a lesser extent, heart, kidneys, and brain, and it has been administered systemically as well as by selective infusion to control variceal hemorrhage. Data from animal and human studies show that vasopressin decreases superior mesentery arterial flow, reduces portal flow and pressure, and increases mean aterial pressure at doses as low as 0.13 units/minute.[46] There seems to be little effect on the splanchnic flow at higher doses, although systemic effects are more pronounced. Nevertheless, administration of doses as high as 1.5 units/minute has been reported.[47]

In controlled trials, intra-arterial and intravenous infusions of vasopressin appear to be equally effective in controlling variceal hemorrhage, but this conclusion is based on data obtained in a very few patients. There have been five randomized, controlled trials of vasopressin versus placebo in the treatment of variceal hemorrhage. In one trial, no distinction was made between patients with variceal hemorrhage and those with peptic ulceration or mucosal bleeding.[48] Three of the other studies demonstrated numerical and sometimes statistically significant decreases in hemorrhage, although hospital mortality was not improved.[49-51] Efficacy ranges from 29% to 93% in these reports; the overall efficacy is 65% for combined data. One study showed no benefit for vasopressin.[52]

Vasopressin therapy has a complication rate as high as 71% with major side effects in 32% of cases.[53,54] A complication may occasionally be fatal. Myocardial ischemia can lead to congestive failure and ectopy. Stimulation of smooth muscle in the gastrointestinal tract and its blood supply can lead to diarrhea, cramping, and vascular thrombosis. Peripheral vasoconstriction often produces blanching of the skin, and necrosis has been reported.[55] Cerebrovascular effects can precipitate an ischemic stroke.

Vasopressin Analogues and Combination Therapy

There has been an effort to find vasopressin-like agents that have a selective gastrointestinal action but fewer side effects; glypressin (triglycyl vasopressin) is one possibility. Vosmik and co-workers[56] compared the outcome for 15 patients receiving glypressin with that of a control group of 13 patients. A numeric advantage in efficacy and mortality was noted in the glypressin-treated group, but cardiac effects (increase in blood pressure and pulse) were identical to those of vasopressin. Another study found a marked difference in efficacy between glypressin and vasopressin, but the rate of control of hemorrhage in the vasopressin-treated group was far lower than that of other reports. Side effects were less frequent in the glypressin group. Other studies have compared the hemodynamic effects of glypressin and vasopressin and found no difference in the two drugs.

Administration of a systemic vasodilator in combination vasopressin therapy has been used in an effort to control untoward cardiac side effects. Isoproterenol, nitroglycerin, and isosorbide dinitrate have been used. Recent data from Tsai and co-workers[57] and Gimson and co-workers[53] demonstrate that the combination of nitroglycerin and vasopressin resulted in similar or better control of bleeding, as well as statistical improvement in complication rate.

Somatostatin

Somatostatin is a 14-amino-acid peptide found in a wide variety of tissues, primarily the gastrointestinal tract and central nervous system. Of the several medications used to treat active variceal hemorrhage, only somatostatin has shown promise. It has a relatively specific vasoconstrictive effect on mesenteric smooth muscle which is rapid in onset, and due to an extremely short half-life (about 30 seconds), rapid in resolution. Two prospective randomized trials comparing somatostatin and vasopressin have been published[54, 58]; somatostatin was significantly more effective than vasopressin and had fewer side effects in one trial, while the other trial demonstrated that somatostatin was equal to vasopressin in controlling hemorrhage and had fewer side effects.

Propranolol

Lebrec and co-workers[59, 60] reported a trial of propranolol in good-risk patients which demonstrated a significant decrease in repeated episodes of hemorrhage compared to a control group. However, this therapy did not prove to be of value in another trial in patients with more severe liver disease.[61] Villeneuve and co-workers[62] studied the effect of propranolol on recurrent bleeding in unselected patients with recent variceal bleeding. There were no significant differences between propranolol-treated patients and controls with respect to the cumulative percentage of patients free of recurrent bleeding and survival. In a recently published prospective, randomized trial of propranolol in patients with varices but without prior bleeding, there was a significant reduction in the cumulative percentage chance of bleeding and mortality in those subjects who received the drug.[63]

It is difficult to explain the conflicting data from these various investigations. Propranolol does not reduce portal venous pressure uniformly in all patients, but this would not account for the varying results.

Tamponade

Compression of a bleeding point is a time-honored method for immediate control of bleeding and induction of hemostasis. This can be accomplished with bleeding esophageal varices by inflating balloons in the esophagus and stomach, a maneuver known as tamponade.

Three types of balloon tubes are currently in use. The Linton-Nachlas tube has three lumens (a large gastric balloon and gastric and esophageal suction ports) and relies on compression in the gastric cardia to reduce variceal flow. The Sengstaken-Blakemore tube (SB) has a gastric aspiration port, a gastric balloon, and an esophageal balloon. Direct pressure is exerted on the esophageal varices by inflating the esophageal balloon, which is held in position in the lower esophagus by the inflated gastric balloon. An additional tube must be placed in the esophagus above the esophageal balloon to prevent aspiration. The Minnesota modification of the SB tube incorporates an additional esophageal suction port and its gastric balloon accommodates a larger volume of air. The esophageal suction channel on the Minnesota tube is relatively small so that we often place an additional suction tube above the esophageal balloon.

The use of these inflatable devices to control variceal hemorrhage has been controversial. Several studies fail to demonstrate any significant control of hemorrhage, while others suggest that tamponade is effective.[64-66] There have been no randomized controlled trials of tamponade compared to supportive measures alone. The rate for reported complications averages 14% with a 3% fatality.[64] Some authors state that endotracheal intubation to protect the respiratory tract is necessary whenever balloon tamponade is used.[36]

Sclerotherapy

As will be discussed subsequently, endoscopic injection sclerotherapy is the fundamental component in our approach to the management of variceal hemorrhage. It will be considered in some detail.

Technique

A complete discussion of the technical aspects of sclerotherapy is beyond the scope of this chapter. Furthermore, most of the information on technique is empiric, there being relatively few published investigations of methodology. This is an unfortunate and conspicuous deficiency because it is possible that differences in technique influence outcome, favorably or adversely.

Variable factors in technique that might have a bearing on the results of sclerotherapy include the following: selection of sclerosing agent or agents, concentration of the agent(s), volume of sclerosant injected per puncture and per procedure, timing and schedule of procedures, the concomitant use of compression devices, paravariceal versus intravariceal injection or some combination of both, and the number and placement of injection sites. Some of these factors are interrelated. For example, there is probably an inverse relation between the concentration of the sclerosing agent and the volume injected (i.e., a lesser volume should probably be injected, perhaps with fewer injection sites, when an agent is used in high concentration).

The active sclerosing agent in our technique is sodium tetradecyl sulfate in a 0.75% solution. Injections are made intravariceally as much as possible. Each visible variceal column is injected as far distally as possible, and then injections are placed in each column at 2-cm intervals moving proximally in the esophagus up to about its midpoint. The volume injected depends on the size of the varix; up to 3 ml for a large vessel, 0.5 ml for a small one. The schedule of the sclerotherapy procedures is discussed in a later section.

Control of Variceal Hemorrhage

Acute Variceal Hemorrhage. Sclerotherapy is said to control acute variceal bleeding in at least 75% of episodes.[67-75] Alwmark and co-workers[76] reported cessation of bleeding for at least 24 hours in 95% of 72 acutely bleeding patients. Kjaergaard and co-workers[77] reported 94% hemostasis in 29 patients. Seventy-one patients with acute variceal hemorrhage were recently reported by Terblanche and co-workers.[78] Sclerotherapy combined with balloon tamponade was effective in controlling 95% of episodes.

In nearly all of these series, tamponade and/or intravenous vasopressin were used to stabilize patients prior to sclerotherapy.[67, 69, 70, 74, 76, 77, 79] However, in the series from Fleig and co-workers,[80] hemorrhage was controlled in 92% of patients unresponsive to balloon tamponade. Another report by Barsoum and co-workers[81] is of interest in this respect. Fifty patients were randomized to balloon tamponade, and 50 to sclerotherapy. Absence of hemorrhage for 1 month after treatment was considered a successful result. Sclerotherapy was successful in 74%, and tamponade alone was successful in 42% of patients.

Recurrent Variceal Hemorrhage After Sclerotherapy. It is difficult to assess the incidence of recurrent hemorrhage after sclerotherapy. Terblanche and co-workers[71] compared acute injection plus a long-term series of injections with acute sclerotherapy alone. There was a decrease in the number and severity of bleeding episodes in the former group. The reduction in rebleeding episodes and transfusion requirements in response to chronic sclerotherapy has also been emphasized by others,[82-84] although not by all groups.[85]

Controlled Trials. An important trial of sclerotherapy in 36 patients compared to medical management in 28 patients was reported in 1980 by Clark and co-workers.[70] In this investigation bleeding recurred in one-third of sclerotherapy patients versus two-thirds of control patients, and the difference between the two groups remained significant at various intervals of follow-up. This work was extended with a report by Macdougall and co-workers[86] in which recurrent bleeding was noted in 43% of injected patients versus 75% in the control group.

In the randomized trial of acute sclerotherapy versus conventional therapy (including tamponade when necessary) reported by Larson and co-workers,[87] 53% of patients receiving conventional therapy had recurrent bleeding compared to 23% of those undergoing sclerotherapy, a statistically significant difference. In this trial, patients were also stratified according to whether they had active bleeding at the time of randomization, and in this subgroup there was a significant difference in mean transfusion requirement in favor of the sclerotherapy-treated patients. Recurrent bleeding in patients with active hemorrhage at the point of randomization occurred in 55% (10 episodes) and 31% (4 episodes) of conventional therapy and sclerotherapy patients, respectively. There were two deaths from variceal hemorrhage in each group. Of the patients not actively bleeding at randomization, 27 received conventional therapy and 31 underwent sclerotherapy. Although there was no difference between the two groups with respect to the number of transfusions, there were significant differences in the number of patients with recurrent bleeding and number of episodes of bleeding in favor of the sclerotherapy group. There were no deaths among the sclerotherapy patients while four deaths occurred in the conventional therapy group, three of these being due to variceal hemorrhage.

In a study reported from Denmark,[88] 187 unselected patients were randomized to either medical treatment, including tamponade, or medical treatment plus sclerotherapy. Sclerotherapy appeared to have little effect on recurrent hemorrhage in the early follow-up period, although after 40 days there were significantly fewer patients with recurrent bleeding and significantly fewer episodes of recurrent bleeding in patients treated by sclerotherapy.

Soderlund and Ihre[89] reported a comparison of tamponade and/or vasopressin infusion ("conservative therapy") versus conservative therapy plus serial sclerotherapy. There were no differences between the two groups with respect to control of the initial bleeding episode and hospital mortality. Variceal eradication was possible in 83% of cases. During follow-up (minimum 1 year), the risk of bleeding was almost four times greater for control patients than for those undergoing sclerotherapy.

Korula and co-workers[90] reported a prospective randomized controlled trial in which there were 63 patients treated by sclerotherapy and 57 control patients. Mean follow-up was 12.5 months and 14.9 months for sclerotherapy and control patients, respectively. Significant differences were demonstrated with respect to mean bleeding risk factor, transfusion requirement, and the length of the bleeding-free interval.

Terblanche and co-workers[91] have reported a trial of long-term sclerotherapy in 37 patients versus medical management in 38 patients. Any patient in either group who developed recurrent bleeding during the trial was treated acutely by sclerotherapy. Varices were eradicated in nearly all patients in the sclerotherapy group, but there was a high rate of recurrence. The cumulative percentage chance to remain bleeding-free was slightly higher in the sclerotherapy patients from 6 months onward, but the difference was not statistically significant. However, bleeding in the sclerotherapy patients was usually mild while that in the control group was frequently life-threatening.

Variceal Obliteration

Obliteration of varices does not occur in a predicatable fashion after a fixed number of procedures. A long series of procedures may be required if varices are large at the outset.[92] It is possible to obliterate all variceal channels, but perhaps not in all patients. Thrombosed vessels may remain visible, and, after a series of injections, small interrupted, nodular-appearing vessels may still be present. With reference to variceal recurrence, there is relatively little information on long-term follow-up after obliteration.

Sarin and co-workers[93] followed 101 patients at monthly intervals (mean 17.9 months) after variceal obliteration. Varices recurred in 19 patients (18.8%), 12 of whom had underlying cirrhosis and 7 had noncirrhotic portal fibrosis. Recurrent varices were not observed in any patient with extrahepatic portal obstruction. Three patients (2.9%) bled from recurrent varices. Fifteen patients (14.9%) developed an esophageal stricture.

Westaby and Williams[94] followed 147 patients after variceal eradication (range 6 months to 6 years). New varices developed in 99 patients (67%), and in 28 (19%) there was also recurrent variceal bleeding. The majority of instances of recurrence as well as bleeding were noted within the first year after obliteration. Three patients died because of recurrent bleeding. Further sclerotherapy was effective in most patients, although varices recurred a second time in 20 patients, 8 of whom had further bleeding although there were no deaths.

Survival

An improvement in the survival of patients with variceal bleeding has been noted in several trials of sclerotherapy. Given the generally poor prognosis for variceal hemorrhage, any therapy that improves survival must be considered remarkable. Although there is skepticism over the validity of this conclusion, it seems clear that sclerotherapy has a beneficial effect with respect to severity and number of episodes of variceal hemorrhage, and it is therefore logical to expect that survival might be improved if deaths directly related to hemorrhage can be prevented. Nevertheless, there are not much data pertaining to survival, and these must be viewed with caution until more information becomes available.

In the study of Clark and co-workers[70] cited above, survival at 1 year was 46% in sclerotherapy-treated patients compared to 6% in the control population, although this difference was not significant. This series was extended with a report by Macdougall and co-workers[86] in which survival at 1 year was significantly better for sclerotherapy patients (75% versus 58%). The improvement in mortality was attributed to variceal obliteration. A third report from this group included 56 patients treated by sclerotherapy and 60 control patients.[95] The median follow-up was 37 months with a range of 19 to 68 months. For the sclerotherapy-treated patients, there were a significant reduction in mortality (18% versus 32%), fewer deaths (5% versus 25%), fewer episodes of hemorrhage, and an improvement in survival by cumulative life analysis. Other investigators have also found a favorable effect on survival.[76, 96–98]

Some reports do not demonstrate any

survival advantage for patients who undergo sclerotherapy.[98,99] In the randomized trial of Korula and co-workers,[90] 63 patients underwent sclerotherapy and there were 57 control patients (mean follow-up 12.5 and 14.9 months, respectively). Although sclerotherapy had a favorable effect on bleeding, there was no improvement in survival.

Thirty-seven patients undergoing sclerotherapy were compared to 38 patients who received medical therapy in the trial of Terblanche and co-workers,[91] and any patient in either group who developed recurrent bleeding during the trial was treated by acute sclerotherapy. There was no difference in survival between the two groups. The rate of recurrence of varices was high in this trial, which should be contrasted with the work of Macdougall and co-workers[86] who found an increase in survival that was attributed to an effort to obliterate varices. These contradictory results may relate to the fact that control patients in the trial by Terblanche and co-workers[91] received sclerotherapy for all acute episodes of bleeding.

Cello and co-workers[68] have reported a trial of sclerotherapy versus portacaval shunt in 52 patients with severe cirrhosis, each of whom had been transfused with at least six units of blood because of acute variceal hemorrhage. Twenty-eight patients were randomized to receive sclerotherapy and 24 to undergo operation. Survival at 30 days was about 40% in both groups and not significantly different. With respect to long-term outcome, univariate survival analysis (Kaplan-Meier) disclosed no significant difference between the two groups. Because a number of variables, such as the presence of ascites, shock, prolonged prothrombin time, and high serum bilirubin, may influence survival, Cello and co-workers[68] also carried out a multivariate analysis (Cox proportional-hazards model) and found that sclerotherapy significantly improved survival. However, the authors caution that the number of patients included in this statistical analysis was small and the number of variables was large. Furthermore, there were more inactive alcoholics in the sclerotherapy group, which the authors attribute to chance. However, this may have biased the results with respect to multivariate analysis.

In the study from Denmark[88] of 187 patients randomized to either medical treatment, including tamponade, or medical treatment plus sclerotherapy, overall survival in sclerotherapy-treated patients was not better than medical treatment alone. However, when other factors, such as the presence of ascites and/or encephalopathy, were taken into account, the overall mortality in the sclerotherapy group was significantly less than that in the group treated medically. Generally, the improvement in mortality for sclerotherapy-treated patients was attributed to better long-term survival. Although mortality was somewhat lower for sclerotherapy patients during the first 10 days, this was not statistically significant. Between 10 and 40 days' mortality was higher in the sclerotherapy group, but thereafter survival improved.

Sauerbruch and co-workers[100] found a highly significant difference in survival in relation to Child's classification in 96 patients undergoing sclerotherapy. Survival at 1 year for patients initially classified as Child's A was 100% versus only 38% of those in Child's class C.

Prophylactic Sclerotherapy

Several studies have shown sclerotherapy to be superior to conservative management in patients with esophageal varices but no prior variceal bleeding.[101,102]

Witzel and co-workers[102] reported a 25-month study of prophylactic sclerotherapy in which 56 patients underwent sclerotherapy and 53 patients served as controls. There were significant differences in favor of sclerotherapy-treated patients with respect to recurrent variceal bleeding (9% versus 57%), mortality (21% versus 55%), and death due to variceal hemorrhage (4% versus 18%).

Paquet and co-workers[103] have reported on several controlled trials of prophylactic sclerotherapy. Entry criteria included the presence of large varices with surface telangiectases (probably equivalent to red color signs) at endoscopy. In the first randomized series of patients reported by these authors the incidence of variceal bleeding in the control group was 66% and mortality was 42%.[103] The incidence of bleeding in patients treated by sclerotherapy was 6% with a mortality of 6%, a statistically significant difference.

In the trial of Koch and co-workers,[104] 30 patients were randomized to sclerotherapy and 30 to control status (mean follow-up 36 months). Bleeding reoccurred in 13.3% of patients who underwent sclerotherapy versus 30% of control patients. Mortality for patients classified as Child's A was 5.9% for sclerotherapy patients versus 25% for controls (statistically significant). However, for patients classified as Child's B and C the mortality for control patients was 40% and that for treated patients was 70%. Bleeding from esophageal varices was the most common cause of death among control patients, while liver failure was the most frequent cause in those undergoing sclerotherapy. The complication rate in the sclerotherapy group was 20%.

These favorable results of studies of prophylactic therapy from Europe must be considered in light of the preliminary report of the Veterans Administration cooperative study from the United States. In this study, the sclerotherapy-treated patients fared worse than control patients to the point that the study had to be halted.[105] The details of this multicenter trial have not been published yet.

Outpatient Sclerotherapy

The complication rate for elective sclerotherapy procedures appears to be relatively low, and there are several reports of sclerotherapy in nonhospitalized patients.[106, 107] These demonstrated no marked risk for stable patients undergoing outpatient sclerotherapy, although there is clear evidence of patient selection in most of the published work. In addition, outpatient procedures represent considerable savings in terms of cost. Whenever possible, we perform sclerotherapy on an outpatient basis. Although hospitalization is generally not necessary for most follow-up procedures, we seldom perform an initial procedure without hospitalizing the patient for at least 24 hours after the procedure.

Complications

Potential complications and complication rate have a direct bearing on the choice and outcome of therapy for bleeding varices. However, a comprehensive discussion of the untoward effects of sclerotherapy is beyond the scope of this chapter.

Because of the extensive collateral venous channels that develop in and around the esophagus in response to portal hypertension, as described above, any substance injected into a varix may reach virtually any part of the body. Sukigara and co-workers[108] demonstrated widespread systemic dissemination by combining technetium Tc 99m sodium pertechnetate with sclerosant. It is useful, therefore, to think of the complications of sclerotherapy as local esophageal effects and untoward results as a result of systemic dissemination.

Complication Rate. The complication rate for sclerotherapy ranges from 2% to 15% per patient.[68-70, 82, 109-111] Twenty-two major complications occurred in 18 of 66 patients (27%) in one series reported by Terblanche and co-workers.[78] A complication occurred in 21 of 107 patients undergoing 240 procedures in the series reported by Macdougall and co-workers.[86]

Minor Complications. Certain untoward results of sclerotherapy appear to have no lasting adverse effects. These may be considered side effects or minor complications, although their exact significance is uncertain. It is possible that in some cases they are a manifestation of a more serious underlying problem. Minor complications include chest pain, fever, altered esophageal physiology, and transient abnormalities on chest x-ray.

Chest pain that resolves occurs in from 25% to 50% of patients and is generally attributed to esophageal spasm.[112, 113] Odynophagia may also occur.[96]

Low-grade fever occurs after sclerotherapy in about 10% to 15% of patients, although Hughes and co-workers[82] reported temperature elevations in almost half of the patients treated. Fever resolves spontaneously and without apparent sequelae in almost all cases after a relatively slight rise which persists for 24 to 48 hours. It appears that temperature elevation postprocedure is not due to bacteremia, at least in the large majority of cases.[114]

Although no significant alterations in esophageal motility were found by some investigators,[115, 116] numerous other reports describe a wide variety of changes.[117-119] Defective clearance of acid from the esophagus has been found in some[120] but not all investigations.[121]

Chest x-rays obtained after sclerotherapy have revealed a variety of transient abnormalities including pleural effusions.[82] Saks and co-workers[122] discovered various radiographic abnormalities in 79% of cases, all of which resolved. Bacon and co-workers[123] found x-ray evidence of pleural effusions after 48% of sclerotherapy sessions.

Major Local Complications. Esophageal stricture occurs in about 3% of patients after sclerotherapy.[124] However, a much higher frequency of stricturing has been reported in some series in which paravariceal injections of a concentrated agent were performed.[77, 125] Although acid reflux has not been eliminated as an etiologic factor, stricture presumably results from the direct action of the sclerosant. Haynes and co-workers[126] compared the clinical course and management of 10 patients with sclerotherapy-related strictures and 14 patients without strictures after sclerotherapy. There were no significant differences between the two groups with respect to total volume of sclerosant, number of injections, number of sessions, volume of sclerosant, number of injections per session, number of esophageal ulcerations, and frequency of treatments.

Esophageal perforation occurs in about 1% to 2% of patients undergoing sclerotherapy. Several reports have emphasized the subtle nature and delay in the onset of symptoms of esophageal perforation.[127-129] Many perforations wall off and remain localized, and in time may heal.[130] Conservative management is usually indicated and should include broad-spectrum antibiotics and chest tube drainage in some cases.

Esophageal ulceration is common after sclerotherapy and probably is not a complication in most instances. Sanowski and co-workers[131] observed ulcers in 57% of patients. Exudate adherent to the varices was noted in one-third in this series, and erosions were noted in 14%. Sarin and co-workers[132] observed 48 patients undergoing sclerotherapy with absolute alcohol for the occurrence of esophageal ulcers. Ulcers were found in 94% of patients at 24 hours, 69% of patients at 1 week, and 12.5% of cases at 3 weeks.

Most ulcers heal, although a permanent, clinically insignificant defect in the esophageal wall may remain.[133] However, consequential ulceration and necrosis are possible, and serious bleeding may occur.[134] Ulceration, as with perforation, appears about 5 to 7 days after sclerotherapy.[135] Whether certain agents or techniques are ulcerogenic to a greater extent than others is problematic. In one animal study there was little difference in the local toxicity of various agents.[136] In the study of Sarin and co-workers,[132] there was a strong correlation between ulceration and the volume of sclerosant injected.

Variceal hemorrhage may be precipitated by sclerotherapy. However, in most cases this is controllable with additional injections.

Intramural hematomas have been reported; this led to bacteremia and death in one case, and perforation in another.[74, 137] Esophageal abscess with sepsis may occur.[138]

Major Systemic Complications. Bacteremia can occur with sclerotherapy, but the frequency is not established because of the conflicting results of the several available studies.[114, 139, 140] Low and co-workers[141] obtained blood cultures prior to sclerotherapy and at 5 and 10 minutes after 104 injection procedures in 38 patients. Pharyngeal cultures were obtained from each patient as well as cultures from the accessory channel of the endoscope. There was no significant difference in the rate of positive blood cultures before injection (1.9%) and after injection (4.3%). The same organism was isolated in the cultures obtained at 5 minutes and then at 10 minutes in only one patient. Organisms were cultured from the endoscope in 41% of the procedures, but none of these were subsequently found in positive blood cultures.

Acute respiratory failure after sclerotherapy has been reported in two patients who developed a clinical picture that in most respects resembled the adult respiratory distress syndrome.[142] However, Bailey-Newton and co-workers[143] found no clinically significant changes in pulmonary or systemic hemodynamics in eight patients who underwent intravariceal injections with sodium morrhuate. Also, Korula and co-workers[144] did not demonstrate any changes in lung function tests or gas exchange in 11 patients undergoing sclerotherapy.

Other, albeit rare, complications of sclerotherapy include spinal cord necrosis and paralysis,[145] bleeding from colorectal varices,[146, 147] portal vein thrombosis,[96, 148] and mesenteric venous thrombosis.[149] There is a recent report of three patients who developed pericarditis while undergoing sclerotherapy.[150] All of these patients had chest pain after sclerotherapy sessions.

Surgery

Portacaval Shunt

Randomized controlled trials of portacaval shunt surgery have demonstrated that this operation reduces bleeding from varices.[11, 151–154] However, there is no conclusive evidence in any trial that this type of operation improves survival. Conn[155] has suggested that the data taken collectively from the various reports indicate a reduction in mortality, while admitting that this is not valid statistically. Although the high incidence of postsurgical portal-systemic encephalopathy is thought to be the major drawback to shunt surgery, many patients in the control populations of the various trials developed encephalopathy, usually in response to bleeding. However, encephalopathy was more likely to be chronic in operated patients.

There are problems with the methodology of every trial of shunt surgery. This is not so much a criticism as a reflection of the difficulty this type of investigation represents. Diagnosis of gastrointestinal bleeding is one very obvious and common problem. Specifically, many of these trials were initiated at a time when endoscopy was not in widespread use, and some are based on less reliable means of establishing the existence of variceal hemorrhage, or indeed even the presence of varices. Another significant problem is that of patient selection. In addition, there was frequently a delay in randomization which in itself selects less seriously ill patients.

In actual practice, most portacaval shunts are performed on selected patients (i.e., those who have survived an episode of variceal hemorrhage with minimal or no encephalopathy and relatively good liver function). However, there are advocates for emergency portal decompressive surgery in all patients with variceal hemorrhage.[156–158] Although it is difficult to evaluate the outcome of this approach, there is a dramatic reduction in bleeding although the operative mortality is high, and it is not clear that this represents any improvement over the natural history of variceal bleeding. Although fewer patients die as a result of bleeding, this is balanced by the surgical mortality.

Shunt surgery has been performed in patients with varices that have not bled as a preventive measure. However, the results of this approach have been poor, and prophylactic shunt surgery cannot be recommended.[152, 159]

Selective Shunt Operations

The basic portacaval shunt operation has been modified technically in a number of ways in an effort to preserve hepatic portal flow and reduce the incidence of chronic postsurgical portal-systemic encephalopathy. The most promising and best-studied operation is the distal splenorenal shunt.[160–163] It remains difficult to decide the merits of this operation because many but by no means all studies demonstrate improvement vis-á-vis encephalopathy. In a long-term trial of portacaval shunt versus distal splenorenal shunt, Harley and co-workers[164] could find no significant difference between the two procedures with respect to portal-systemic encephalopathy or survival. In addition, there was an unusually high rate of recurrent variceal bleeding in the patients who underwent the selective shunt. Patients must be carefully chosen for the selective operation which is contraindicated if there is retrograde portal venous flow and should probably not be performed in patients with ascites.

Other Forms of Surgery

Other operations have been devised, such as devascularization and/or transection-reanastomosis of the esophagus using the stapling gun.[165–167] In general, these procedures have not been evaluated extensively in controlled trials.

Comparisons of Sclerotherapy and Surgery

Based on the information presented in this chapter thus far, it can be concluded that sclerotherapy and surgery are the two major forms of therapy for variceal hemorrhage. Fortunately, they are not mutually exclusive and can be used in the same patient. Depending on clinical circumstances, each type of therapy will have advantages and disadvantages. Therefore, certain important questions arise. Would a combination of the surgery and sclerotherapy improve outcome? If so, in what way should the two procedures be used? What circumstances favor one as opposed to the other?

Cello and co-workers'[68] trial of sclerotherapy versus portacaval shunt in patients with advanced cirrhosis and severe bleeding is described above. Twenty-eight patients received sclerotherapy, and 24 underwent operation. Significantly more patients had recurrent bleeding in the sclerotherapy group compared to those undergoing operation, although the total amount of blood transfused was greater in the shunted patients. Long-term, a significantly greater number of patients were rehospitalized for recurrent bleeding in the sclerotherapy group, and the total number of days spent in hospital for bleeding was also significantly greater. However, the total number of blood transfusions, number of patients rehospitalized for encephalopathy, total days in hospital for encephalopathy, and the resumption of alcohol abuse did not differ between the two groups.

Cello and co-workers[168] have recently reported the extended results of their investigation. With 32 patients randomized to each treatment group, the duration of initial hospitalization and total amount of blood transfused during hospitalization were significantly less in patients receiving sclerotherapy, but there was no difference in short-term survival. Mean follow-up was 530 days, and for those patients who survived the initial hospitalization, recurrent variceal bleeding and the amount of blood transfused was significantly greater in those who underwent sclerotherapy. Recurrent bleeding requiring shunt surgery developed in 40% of sclerotherapy-treated patients.

Sclerotherapy was superior to esophageal transection in a small number of poor-risk patients studied by Cello and co-workers.[169] Although there was no recurrent bleeding in the operated patients, the surgical mortality was 83%. Mortality in the sclerotherapy group was 67%, and about one-third of patients had further episodes of bleeding.

Huizinga and co-workers[170] reported a prospective randomized trial of sclerotherapy versus esophageal transection in which 39 patients underwent surgery and 37 patients underwent endoscopic therapy. Mortality at 30 days was significantly less in the transected patients versus those undergoing sclerotherapy. Early recurrence of bleeding was noted in 2.5% of operated patients versus 48.6% of those who received sclerotherapy, a highly significant difference.

The preliminary results of a prospective, randomized trial of sclerotherapy and distal splenorenal shunt have been reported recently by Warren and co-workers.[171] Thirty-six patients had sclerotherapy, and 35 underwent surgery. Nineteen of 36 (53%) of sclerotherapy-treated patients had recurrent bleeding versus 1 of 35 shunted patients (3%), a significant difference. Recurrent bleeding was controlled in all but 11 (31%) of the 36 sclerotherapy patients by repeated injection sessions. Those patients in whom sclerotherapy failed to control bleeding underwent surgery. Median follow-up was 26 months. At 2 years there was a significant improvement in survival in the sclerotherapy group (including patients who underwent sclerotherapy and surgery), which was 84%, versus survival in the shunted group, this being 59%.

Good-risk patients were randomized to either sclerotherapy (55 patients) or splenorenal shunt (57 patients) in a prospective controlled trial reported by Teres and co-workers.[172] Bleeding was recurrent in 37.5% of those undergoing sclerotherapy versus 14.3% of operated patients. However, portal-systemic encephalopathy developed in 24% of shunted patients versus 8% of those undergoing sclerotherapy. There was no significant difference in mortality between the two groups.

MANAGEMENT OF THE PATIENT WITH VARICEAL HEMORRHAGE

There is no entirely satisfactory solution to the problem of bleeding esophageal varices. All of the available data outlined above leave much to be desired. Virtually every trial is imperfect in some way. Nevertheless, the challenge of caring for the individual patient remains, and management decisions must be based on existing knowledge. In this respect, familiarity with the overall body of information pertaining to variceal hemorrhage is essential, and as a good general principle, a single report should never be taken at face value. Consideration of the clinical status of the individual patient is another important guideline because each form of therapy has good and bad points that may be more or less important in relation to specific clinical circumstances. Lastly, it is important to do what one does best. This does not mean rejection of promising methods of treatment, but the use of an unfamiliar therapy puts the individual patient at a disadvantage.

Any approach to the management of variceal hemorrhage is necessarily biased because of the imperfect nature of our knowledge. In this section, our approach, based insofar as possible on the foregoing discussion, will be presented. Our method is comprised of four basic elements: vasopressin, tamponade, sclerotherapy, and elective shunt surgery. In concept, pharmacologic therapy is attractive, but the data regarding propranolol are too confusing at present to advocate this treatment.

Patients with varices can be divided into three categories: those who have not bled; those with active bleeding; and those who have previously bled. Our approach to the management of each group is different.

Patients Who Have Not Bled

As noted, the results of prophylactic shunt surgery have been unsatisfactory, and this approach to management cannot be recommended.

Although studies from Europe suggest that certain patients selected according to variceal appearance at endoscopy may benefit from prophylactic sclerotherapy, this therapy must be considered with circumspection until the details of the cooperative trial of Gregory and co-workers[105] have been thoroughly evaluated.

Any beneficial outcome for prophylactic sclerotherapy must take into account the complications of sclerotherapy because patients are presumably clinically stable at the time treatment is initiated. It is not enough, therefore, to merely consider the prevention of bleeding. The European trials have also shown a survival benefit, but the trial in this country suggests an increase in mortality for patients undergoing prophylactic sclerotherapy. Because of the importance of this question, we prefer to remain skeptical on the value of prophylactic therapy until further data are available, and we do not recommend prophylactic sclerotherapy at this time.

The best management of the majority of

patients with cirrhosis (i.e., those with alcoholic cirrhosis) is to stop the offending agent. For those with biliary cirrhosis, primary sclerosing cholangitis, chronic active hepatitis, or other forms of cirrhosis, we prefer to follow the patient and treat only if variceal hemorrhage occurs.

Patients Who Are Actively Bleeding

The initial management of patients with acute/active gastrointestinal hemorrhage is resuscitation. The hemodynamic status of the patient can be stabilized in over 85% of cases with standard supportive measures. We use gastric lavage, but only to clear unclotted blood and assess the rapidity of hemorrhage.

Although variceal hemorrhage is the most likely cause of bleeding in patients with evidence of portal hypertension, endoscopy is the cornerstone of diagnosis of upper gastrointestinal bleeding. After resuscitation, certain specific therapies may be used if the bleeding is variceal in nature, and it is therefore necessary to know the cause of bleeding. Despite the likelihood of variceal bleeding, there is still a possibility that some other bleeding lesion may be found. In addition, diagnostic endoscopy may become therapeutic if variceal bleeding is confirmed and sclerotherapy is performed.

The details of our technique of sclerotherapy are outlined elsewhere.[173, 174] As with all types of therapy, the method of sclerotherapy must be individualized according to the status of the patient. It is usually possible to administer small amounts of sedation. We prefer intravenous meperidine because its effects can be promptly and readily reversed. However, it is advisable to place an endotracheal tube if the patient is obtunded and there is massive bleeding. The best endoscope, in our opinion, is one with two accessory channels because the ability to clear the endoscopic field of blood and debris enhances the success of the procedure. If a precise site of variceal bleeding can be located, injections should be made in this region. There are some differences in our placement of injections depending on whether an actual bleeding point is visualized.[173, 174]

If bleeding is massive and accurate visualization of the varices is impossible, an intravenous infusion of vasopressin is begun at a rate of 0.1 units/minute without any preceding intravenous bolus. The dosage can be advanced to a maximum of 0.8 units/minute if bleeding continues, but care must be taken to observe for complications. The concomitant use of nitroglycerin appears promising, but we feel that more data are required before this type of therapy can be advocated.

If bleeding is uncontrollable by the above measures, esophageal tamponade is instituted. We prefer the quadruple-lumen tube because its use reduces the risk of aspiration of esophageal blood or secretions, although we place a nasogastric tube above the esophageal balloon as an added precaution. Continuous esophageal and gastric suction must be established immediately upon insertion of the tamponade device.

The gastric balloon is inflated with 250 ml of air, and its position is verified by obtaining an x-ray film of the abdomen with the patient supine. After confirmation of correct positioning, the gastric balloon is inflated to its maximum volume of 700 ml. Its position is fixed in the cardia of the stomach by gentle traction. One of us prefers the football helmet method to anchor the tube externally. The other places a small sponge cube on the tube at the patient's nose. Gentle traction is made on the gastric balloon by withdrawing an additional 2-cm segment of the tube from the patient's nose. Then benzoin is applied to the sponge as well as the tube to prevent slippage and a length of ½-inch tape is wrapped around the sponge to hold it in place. A small piece of tape is wrapped around the tube next to the sponge as a marker for the correct position of the device.

If bleeding continues after maximum inflation of the gastric balloon, the esophageal balloon is inflated to a pressure of 35 to 40 mm Hg and clamped. The actual pressure in the esophageal balloon must be established accurately with a manometer. Some fluctuation in pressure will be noted with respiration.

The most important step in the use of balloon tamponade is the instruction of all nurses charged with the immediate care of the patient. They must be especially aware of the risk of asphyxiation if the device shifts in position. A pair of scissors should be kept at the bedside to be used to cut and remove the entire device in case the gastric balloon suddenly deflates and allows the esophageal balloon to migrate proximally and compromise respiration.

We generally release the pressure in the esophageal balloon every 4 to 6 hours for 10 to 15 minutes to prevent pressure necrosis of the esophagus and to check for cessation of bleeding.

One of the major limitations of tamponade is that it must not be used indefinitely. After 24 hours, the risk of pressure necrosis is great, and we therefore prefer to remove the device as soon as possible in all cases. If tamponade stops the hemorrhage, we leave the tube in place with the esophageal balloon deflated and the gastric balloon inflated for 8 to 10 hours. If no further bleeding occurs, the tube is removed.

When properly performed, esophageal tamponade controls variceal bleeding in all but the most severe cases. It can be used to buy time to properly stabilize the patient and to organize subsequent therapeutic steps. If sclerotherapy was not possible because of severe bleeding at the initial attempt at endoscopy, it is often advisable to perform endoscopy as the tamponade device is being removed because the endoscopic field should be clear enough to permit variceal injection.

If all of the above measures fail, surgery is the only remaining option. This can be an extremely difficult clinical decision. We do not advocate emergency portacaval shunt surgery except under the most extreme circumstances. Some patients may be salvaged by other surgical procedures, such as esophageal transection.

Patients in Whom Variceal Bleeding Has Stopped

Sclerotherapy is also the primary element in our approach to the long-term management of patients who have survived an episode of variceal hemorrhge. Although there is some argument over the value of long-term sclerotherapy, in most of the studies that demonstrate a benefit of sclerotherapy, efforts were made to eradicate all variceal channels. When sclerotherapy has been instrumental in controlling the initial episode of bleeding, we continue the procedures, usually with two subsequent sessions during the next 7 to 10 days. This schedule is often modified if a pronounced effect is noted in the esophagus as a result of any prior session. Sclerotherapy is then repeated at intervals of about 1 month until all varices have been eradicated. Patients are then evaluated at 6- to 12-month intervals for the development of new variceal channels.

Some patients will recover spontaneously from variceal bleeding, or they may have required minimal therapy without sclerotherapy. Provided the episode of variceal hemorrhage is well documented, we begin a course of sclerotherapy in these patients on a schedule similar to that described above.

If variceal hemorrhage resumes despite an optimal course of sclerotherapy, the patient is considered for shunt surgery. However, we may also elect to continue sclerotherapy if the course of treatment is thought to be suboptimal, because many patients with recurrent bleeding will respond to a more aggressive schedule of procedures.

References

1. Olsson R: The natural history of esophageal varices. *Digestion* 1972; 6:65–74.
2. Conn HO, Binder H, Brodoff M: Fiberoptic and conventional esophagoscopy in the diagnosis of esophageal varices. *Gastroenterology* 1967; 52:810–881.
3. Galambos JT: Esophageal variceal hemorrhage: Diagnosis and an overview of treatment. *Semin Liver Dis* 1982; 2:211–226.
4. Lebrec D, DeFleury P, Rueff B, et al: Portal hypertension, size of esophgeal varices, and risk of gastrointestinal bleeding in alcoholic cirrhosis. *Gastroenterology* 1980; 79:1139–1144.
5. Baker LA, Smith C, Lieberman G: The natural history of esophageal varices. A study of 115 cirrhotic patients in whom varices were diag-

nosed prior to bleeding. *Am J Med* 1959; 26:228–237.
6. Dagradi AE: The natural history of esophageal varices in patients with alcoholic liver cirrhosis: An endoscopic and clinical study. *Am J Gastroenterol* 1972; 57:520–540.
7. Resnick RH, Iber FL, Ishihara AM, et al: A controlled study of the therapeutic portacaval shunt. *Gastroenterology* 1974; 67:843–857.
8. Graham DY, Smith JL: The course of patients after variceal hemorrhage. *Gastroenterology* 1981; 80:800–809.
9. Novis BH, Duys P, Barbezat GO: Fiberoptic endoscopy and the use of the Sengstaken tube in acute gastrointestinal hemorrhage in patients with portal hypertension and varices. *Gut* 1976; 17:258–263.
10. Silverstein FE, Gilbert DA, Tedesco FJ, et al: The national ASGE survey on upper gastrointestinal bleeding. II. Clinical prognostic factors. *Gastrointest Endosc* 1981; 27:80–93.
11. Jackson FC, Perrin EB, Felix WR, et al: A clinical investigation of the portacaval shunt: V. Survival analysis of the therapeutic operation. *Ann Surg* 1971; 174:672–701.
12. Christensen E, Fauerholdt L, Schlichting P, et al: Aspects of the natural history of gastrointestinal bleeding in cirrhosis and the effect of prednisone. *Gastroenterology* 1981; 81:944–952.
13. Boyer TD, Triger DR, Horisawa M, et al: Direct transhepatic measurement of portal vein pressure using a thin needle. Comparison with wedged hepatic vein pressure. *Gastroenterology* 1977; 72:584–589.
14. Viallet A, Marleau D, Huet M, et al: Hemodynamic evaluation of patients with intrahepatic portal hypertension. Relationship between bleeding varices and the portohepatic gradient. *Gastroenterology* 1975; 68:1297–1300.
15. Reynolds TB: Interrelationships of portal pressure, variceal size, and upper gastrointestinal bleeding. *Gastroenterology* 1980; 79:1332–1333.
16. Reynolds TB, Ito S, Iwatsuki S: Measurement of portal pressure and its clinical application. *Am J Med* 1970; 49:649–657.
17. Garcia-tsao G, Groszmann RJ, Fisher R, et al: Portal pressure, presence of gastroesophageal varices and variceal bleeding. *Hepatology* 1985; 5:419–424.
18. Dagradi AE: Esophageal varices, splenic pulp pressure and "directional" flow patterns in alcoholic liver cirrhosis. A correlation study. *Am J Gastroenterol* 1973; 59:15–22.
19. Joly JG, Marleau D, Legare A, et al: Bleeding from esophageal varices in cirrhosis of the liver: Hemodynamic and radiological criteria for the selection of potential bleeders through hepatic and umbilicoportal catheterization studies. *Can Med Assoc J* 1971; 104:576–580.
20. Willoughby EO, David D, Smith CW, et al: The significance of small esophageal varices in portal cirrhosis. *Gastroenterology* 1964; 47:375–381.
21. Greene L, Weisberg H, Rosenthal WS, et al: Evaluation of esophageal varices in liver disease by splenic-pulp manometry, splenoportography, and esophagogastroscopy. Diagnostic discrepancies. *Am J Dig Dis* 1965; 10:284–292.
22. Westaby S, Wilkinson SP, Warren R, et al: Spleen size and portal hypertension in cirrhosis. *Digestion* 1978; 17:63–86.
23. Palmer ED: On correlations between portal venous pressure and the size and extent of esophageal varices in portal cirrhosis. *Ann Surg* 1953; 138:741–744.
24. Simert G, Lunderquist A, Tylen U, et al: Correlation between percutaneous transhepatic portography and clinical findings in 56 patients with portal hypertension. *Acta Chir Scand* 1978; 144:27–34.
25. Smith-Laing G, Camilo ME, Dick R, et al: Percutaneous transhepatic portography in the assessment of portal hypertension. Clinical correlations and comparison of radiographic techniques. *Gastroenterology* 1980; 78:197–205.
26. Palmer ED, Brick IB: Correlation between the severity of esophageal varices in portal cirrhosis and their propensity toward hemorrhage. *Gastroenterology* 1956; 30:85–90.
27. Conn HO: The varix volcano connection. *Gastroenterology* 1980; 79:1333–1336.
28. Conn HO, Mitchell JR, Brodoff MG: A comparison of the radiologic and esophagoscopic diagnosis of esophageal varices. *N Engl J Med* 1961; 265:160–164.
29. Butler H: The veins of the oesophagus. *Thorax* 1951; 6:276–296.
30. Kitano S, Terblanche J, Kahn D, et al: Venous anatomy of the lower oesophagus in portal hypertension: Practical implications. *Br J Surg* 1986; 73:525–531.
31. Vianna A, Hayes PC, Moscoso G, et al: Normal venous circulation of the gastroesophageal junction. A route to understanding varices. *Gastroenterology* 1987; 93:876–889.
32. McCormack TT, Rose JD, Smith PM, et al: Perforating veins and blood flow in esophageal varices. *Lancet* 1983; 2:1442–1444.
33. Beppu K, Inokuchi K, Koyanagi N, et al: Prediction of variceal hemorrhage by esophageal endoscopy. *Gastrointest Endosc* 1981; 27:213–218.
34. Fujita R: Endoscopic diagnosis and classification of esophageal varices in Japan, in Sivak MV Jr (ed): *Sclerotherapy of Esophageal Varices*. New York, Praeger, 1984, pp 35–42.
35. Spence RAJ, Sloan JM, Johnston GW, et al: Oesophageal mucosal changes in patients with varices. *Gut* 1983; 24:1024–1029.
36. Mandelstam P, Zeppa R: Endotracheal intubation should precede esophagogastric balloon tamponade for control of variceal bleeding. *J Clin Gastroenterol* 1983; 5:493–494.
37. Gilbert DA, Silverstein FE, Tedesco FJ, et al: The national ASGE survey on upper gastrointestinal bleeding. III. Endoscopy in upper gastrointestinal bleeding. *Gastrointest Endosc* 1981; 27:94–102.
38. Dagradi AE, Mehler R, Tan DTD, et al: Sources of upper gastrointestinal bleeding in patients with liver cirrhosis and large varices. *Am J Gastroenterol* 1970; 54:458–463.
39. Palmer ED: The vigorous diagnostic approach

to upper gastrointestinal tract hemorrhage. A 23-year prospective study of 14,000 patients. *JAMA* 1969; 207:1477–1480.
40. McCray RS, Martin F, Amir-Ahmadi H, et al: Erroneous diagnosis of hemorrhage from esophageal varices. *Am J Dig Dis* 1969; 14:755–760.
41. Waldram R, Davis M, Nunnerly H, et al: Emergency endoscopy after gastrointesintal hemorrhage in 50 patients with portal hypertension. *Br Med J* 1974; 4:94–96.
42. Dave P, Romeu J, Messer J: Upper gastrointestinal bleeding in patients with portal hypertension: A reappraisal. *J Clin Gastroenterol* 1983; 5:113–115.
43. Schoppe LE, Roark GD, Patterson M: Acute upper gastrointestinal bleeding in patients with portal hypertension: A correlation of endoscopic findings with etiology. *South Med J* 1983; 76:475–476.
44. Sutton FM: Upper gastrointestinal bleeding in patients with esophageal varices. What is the most common source? *Am J Med* 1987; 83:273–275.
45. Tabibian N, Graham DY: Source of upper gastrointestinal bleeding in patients with esophageal varices seen at endoscopy. *J Clin Gastroenterol* 1987; 9:279–282.
46. Blei AT, Groszmann RJ, Gusberg R, et al: Comparison of vasopressin and triglycyl-lysine vasopressin on splanchnic and systemic hemodynamics in dogs. *Dig Dis Sci* 1980; 25:688–694.
47. Chojkier M, Groszmann RJ, Atterbury CE, et al: A controlled comparison of continuous intraarterial and intravenous infusions of vasopressin hemorrhage from esophageal varices. *Gastroenterology* 1979; 77:540–546.
48. Mallory A, Schaefer J, Cohen JR, et al: Selective intraarterial vasopressin infusion for upper gastrointestinal tract hemorrhage. A controlled trial. *Arch Surg* 1980; 115:30–32.
49. Clanet J, Tournet R, Fourtanier G, et al: Treatment with pitressin for the hemorrhage from esophageal variceal rupture with cirrhosis. A controlled study. *Acta Gastroenterol Belg* 1978; 41:539–543.
50. Merigan TC, Poltkin GR, Davidson GS: Effect of intravenously administered posterior pituitary extract on hemorrhage from bleeding esophageal varices. *N Engl J Med* 1962; 266:134–135.
51. Conn HO, Ramsby GR, Storer EH, et al: Intraarterial vasopressin in the treatment of upper gastrointestinal hemorrhage. A prospective, controlled clinical trial. *Gastroenterology* 1975; 68:211–221.
52. Fogel MR, Knauer CM, Andres LL, et al: Continuous intravenous vasopressin in active upper gastrointestinal tract bleeding. *Ann Intern Med* 1982; 96:565–569.
53. Gimson AES, Westaby D, Hegarty J, et al: A randomized trial of vasopressin and vasopressin plus nitroglycerine in the control of acute variceal hemorrhage. *Hepatology* 1986; 6:410–413.
54. Jenkins SA, Baxter JN, Corbett W, et al: A prospective randomized controlled clinical trial comparing somatostatin and vasopressin in controlling acute variceal hemorrhage. *Br Med J* 1985; 290:275–278.
55. Korenberg RJ, Landau Price D, Penneys NS: Vasopressin-induced bullous disease and cutaneous necrosis. *J Am Acad Dermatol* 1986; 15:393–398.
56. Vosmik J, Jedlica K, Mulder JL, et al: Action of the triglycyl hormonogen of vasopressin (glypressin) in patients with liver cirrhosis and bleeding esophageal varices. *Gastroenterology* 1977; 72:605–609.
57. Tsai Y-E, Lay C-S, Kwok-Hung L, et al: Controlled trial of vasopressin plus nitroglycerine versus vasopressin alone in the treatment of bleeding esophageal varices. *Hepatology* 1986; 6:406–409.
58. Kravetz D, Bosch J, Teres J, et al: Comparison of intravenous somatostatin and vasopressin infusions in the treatment of acute variceal hemorrhage. *Hepatology* 198 4:442–446.
59. Lebrec D, Poynard T, Hillon P, et al: Propranolol for prevention of recurrent gastrointestinal bleeding in patients with cirrhosis, a controlled study. *N Engl J Med* 1981; 305:1371–1374.
60. Lebrec D, Poynard T, Bernuau J, et al: A randomized controlled study of propranolol for prevention of recurrent gastrointestinal bleeding in patients with cirrhosis: A final report. *Hepatology* 1984; 4:355–358.
61. Burroughs AK, Jenkins WJ, Sherlock S, et al: Controlled trial of propranolol for the prevention of recurrent variceal hemorrhage in patients with cirrhosis. *N Engl J Med* 1983; 309:1539–1542.
62. Villeneuve JP, Pomier-Layrargues G, Infante-Rivard C, et al: Propranolol for the prevention of recurrent variceal hemorrhage: A controlled trial. *Hepatology* 1986; 6:1239–1243.
63. Pascal JP, Cales P: Propranolol in the prevention of first upper gastrointestinal tract hemorrhage in patients with cirrhosis of the liver and esophageal varices. *N Engl J Med* 1987; 317:856–861.
64. Chojkier M, Conn HO: Esophageal tamponade in the treatment of bleeding varices. *Dig Dis Sci* 1980; 25:267–272.
65. Pitcher JL: Safety and effectiveness of the modified Sengstaken-Blakemore tube: A prospective study. *Gastroenterology* 1971; 61:291–298.
66. Hunt PS, Korman MG, Hansky J, et al: An 8-year prospective experience with balloon tamponade in emergency control of bleeding esophageal varices. *Dig Dis Sci* 1982; 27:413–416.
67. Terblanche J, Northover JMA, Bornman P, et al: A prospective evaluation of injection, sclerotherapy in treatment of acute bleeding from esophageal varices. *Surgery* 1979; 85:239–245.
68. Cello JP, Grendell JH, Crass RA, et al: Endoscopic sclerotherapy versus portacaval shunt in patients with severe cirrhosis and variceal hemorrhage. *N Engl J Med* 1984; 311:1589–1594.
69. Sivak MV Jr, Stout DJ, Skipper G: Endoscopic

injection sclerosis (EIS) of esophageal varices. *Gastrointest Endosc* 1981; 27:52–57.
70. Clark AW, Westaby D, Silk DBA, et al: Prospective controlled trial of injection sclerotherapy in patients with cirrhosis and recent variceal hemorrhage. *Lancet* 1980; II:552–554.
71. Terblanche J, Northover JMA, Bornman P, et al: A prospective controlled trial of sclerotherapy in the long term management of patients after esophageal variceal bleeding. *Surg Gynecol Obstet* 1979; 148:323–333.
72. von Ryll-Gryska P, Hedberg SE: Injection thrombosclerosis of esophageal varices. *Surg Gynecol Obstet* 1985; 161:438–444.
73. Spence RA, Anderson JR, Johnston GW: Twenty-five years of injection sclerotherapy for bleeding varices. *Br J Surg* 1985; 72:195–198.
74. Palani CK, Abuabara S, Kraft AR, et al: Endoscopic sclerotherapy in acute variceal hemorrhage. *Am J Surg* 1981; 141:164–168.
75. Lewis JW, Chung RS, Allison JG: Injection sclerotherapy for control of acute variceal hemorrhage. *Am J Surg* 1981; 142:592–595.
76. Alwmark A, Bengmark S, Borjesson B, et al: Emergency and long-term transesophageal sclerotherapy of bleeding esophageal varices. A prospective study of 50 consecutive cases. *Scand J Gastroenterol* 1982; 17:409–412.
77. Kjaergaard J, Fischer A, Miskowiak J, et al: Sclerotherapy of bleeding esophageal varices. Long-term results. *Scand J Gastroenterol* 1982; 17:363–367.
78. Terblanche J, Yakoob HI, Bornman PC, et al: Acute bleeding varices. A five-year prospective evaluation of tamponade and sclerotherapy. *Ann Surg* 1981; 194:521–530.
79. Stray N, Jacobsen CD, Rosseland A: Injection and sclerotherapy for bleeding oesophageal and gastric varices using a flexible endoscope. *Acta Med Scand* 1982; 211:125–129.
80. Fleig WE, Stange EF, Ruettenauer K: Emergency endoscopic sclerotherapy for bleeding esophageal varices: A prospective study in patients not responding to balloon tamponade. *Gastrointest Endosc* 1983; 29:8–14.
81. Barsoum MS, Bolous FI, El-Rooby AA, et al: Tamponade and injection sclerotherapy in the management of bleeding oesophageal varices. *Br J Surg* 1982; 69:76–78.
82. Hughes RW Jr, Larson DE, Viggiano TR, et al: Endoscopic variceal sclerosis: A one-year experience. *Gastrointest Endosc* 1982; 28:62–66.
83. Ayres SJ, Goff JS, Warren GH: Endoscopic sclerotherapy for bleeding esophageal varices: Effects and complications. *Ann Intern Med* 1983; 98:900–930.
84. Sivak MV Jr, Williams GW: Endoscopic injection sclerosis (EIS) of esophageal varices: Analysis of survival and transfusion requirement (abstract). *Gastrointest Endosc* 1981; 27:129.
85. Hennessy TPJ, Stephens RB, Keane FB: Acute and chronic management of esophageal varices by injection sclerotherapy. *Surg Gynecol Obstet* 1982; 154:375–377.
86. Macdougall BRD, Westaby D, Theodossi A, et al: Increased long-term survival in variceal haemorrhage using injection sclerotherapy. Results of a controlled trial. *Lancet* 1982; I:124–127.
87. Larson AW, Cohen H, Zweiban B, et al: Acute esophageal variceal sclerotherapy. Results in a prospective randomized controlled trial. *JAMA* 1986; 255:497–500.
88. Copenhagen Esophageal Varices Sclerotherapy Project: Sclerotherapy after first variceal hemorrhage in cirrhosis. *N Engl J Med* 1984; 311:1594–1600.
89. Soderlund C, Ihre T: Endoscopic sclerotherapy v. conservative management of bleeding oesophageal varices. A 5-year prospective controlled trial of emergency and long-term treatment. *Acta Chir Scand* 1985; 151:449–456.
90. Korula J, Balart LA, Radvan G, et al: A prospective randomized controlled trial of chronic esophageal variceal sclerotherapy. *Hepatology* 1985; 5:584–589.
91. Terblanche J, Bornman PC, Kahn D, et al: Failure of repeated injection sclerotherapy to improve long-term survival after oesophageal variceal bleeding. A five-year prospective controlled trial. *Lancet* 1983; II:1328–1332.
92. Rose JDR, Crane MD, Smith PM: Factors affecting successful endoscopic sclerotherapy for oesophageal varices. *Gut* 1983; 24:946–949.
93. Sarin SK, Sachdev G, Nada R: Follow-up of patients after variceal eradication. A comparison of patients with cirrhosis noncirrhotic portal fibrosis, and extrahepatic obstruction. *Ann Surg* 1986; 204:78–82.
94. Westaby D, Williams R: Elective sclerotherapy—technique and results. *Endoscopy* 1986; 18(Suppl 2):28–31.
95. Westaby D, Macdougall BR, Williams R: Improved survival following injection sclerotherapy for esophageal varices: Final analysis of a controlled trial. *Hepatology* 1985; 5:827–830.
96. Goodale RL, Silvis SE, O'Leary JF, et al: Early survival after sclerotherapy for bleeding esophageal varices. *Surg Gynecol Obstet* 1982; 155:523–538.
97. Hedberg SE, Fowler DL, Ryan RLR: Injection sclerotherapy of esophageal varices using ethanolamine oleate. A pilot study. *Am J Surg* 1982; 143:426–431.
98. Trudeau W, Prindiville T, Gibbert V, et al: Endoscopic injection sclerosis in Child's C patients with bleeding gastroesophageal varices (abstract). *Gastrointest Endosc* 1983; 29:168.
99. Trudeau W, Gibbert V, Young W, et al: Child's C patients receiving endoscopic injection sclerosis of bleeding esophageal varices fare no better than patients receiving conventional therapy (abstract). *Gastrointest Endosc* 1982; 28:148.
100. Sauerbruch T, Weinzierl M, Kopcke W, et al: Long term sclerotherapy of bleeding esophageal varices in patients with liver cirrhosis. An evaluation of mortality and rebleeding risk factors. *Scand J Gastroenterol* 1985; 20:51–58.
101. Paquet KJ: Prophylactic endoscopic sclerosing treatment of the esophageal wall in varices—a prospective controlled randomized trial. *Endoscopy* 1982; 14:4–5.
102. Witzel L, Wolbergs E, Merki H: Prophylactic

endoscopic sclerotherapy of oesophageal varices. A prospective controlled study. *Lancet* 1985; 1:773-775.
103. Paquet KJ, Koussouris P: Is there an indication for prophylactic endoscopic paravariceal injection sclerotherapy in patients with liver cirrhosis and portal hypertension? *Endoscopy* 1986; 18(Suppl 2):32-35.
104. Koch H, Henning H, Grimm H, et al: Prophylactic sclerosing of esophageal varices—results of a prospective controlled study. *Endoscopy* 1986; 18:40-43.
105. Gregory P, Hartigan P, Amodeo D, et al: Prophylactic sclerotherapy for esophageal varices in alcoholic liver disease: Results of a VA cooperative randomized trial (abstract). *Gastroenterology* 1987; 92:1414.
106. Drell E, Prindiville T, Trudeau W: Outpatient endoscopic injection sclerosis of esophageal varices. *Gastrointest Endosc* 1986; 32:4-6.
107. Korula J: Outpatient esophageal variceal sclerotherapy: Safe and cost-effective. A prospective study. *Gastrointest Endosc* 1986; 32:1-3.
108. Sukigara M, Omoto R, Miyamae T: Systemic dissemination of ethanolamine oleate after injection sclerotherapy for esophageal varices. *Arch Surg* 1985; 120:833-836.
109. Johnston GW, Rodgers HW: A review of 15 years' experience in the use of sclerotherapy in the control of acute haemorrhage for oesophageal varices. *Br J Surg* 1973; 60:797-800.
110. Moersch HJ: Further studies on the treatment of esophageal varices by injection of a sclerosing solution. *Ann Otol Rhinol Laryngol* 1941; 50:1233-1244.
111. Patterson CO, Rouse MO: The sclerosing therapy of esophageal varices. *Gastroenterology* 1947; 9:391-395.
112. Gebhard RL, Ansel HJ, Silvis SE: Origin of pain during variceal sclerotherapy (abstract). *Gastrointest Endosc* 1982; 28:131.
113. Shoenut JP, Micflikier AB: Retrosternal pain subsequent to sclerotherapy. *Gastrointest Endosc* 1986; 32:84-87.
114. Cohen LB, Korsten MA, Scherl EJ, et al: Bacteremia after endoscopic injection sclerosis. *Gastrointest Endosc* 1983; 29:198-200.
115. Larson GM: Esophageal motility after injection sclerotherapy (abstract). *Gastrointest Endosc* 1983; 29:164.
116. Simon C, Cohen L, Scherl E, et al: Esophageal motility and symptoms after endoscopic injection sclerotherapy (abstract). *Gastrointest Endosc* 1983; 29:192.
117. Ogle SJ, Kirk CJC, Bailey RJ, et al: Oesophageal function in patients undergoing injection sclerotherapy for oesophageal varices. *Digestion* 1978; 18:178-185.
118. Reilly JJ Jr, Schade RR, Van Thiel DS: Esophageal function after injection sclerotherapy: Pathogenesis of esophageal stricture. *Am J Surg* 1984; 147:85-88.
119. Soderlund C, Thor K, Wiechel KL: Oesophageal motility after sclerotherapy for bleeding varices. *Acta Chir Scand* 1985; 151:249-253.
120. Snady H, Korsten MA: Esophageal acid-clearance and motility after endoscopic sclerotherapy of esophageal varices. *Am J Gastroenterol* 1986; 81:419-422.
121. Sauerbruch T, Wirsching R, Holl J, et al: Effects of repeated injection sclerotherapy on acid gastroesophageal reflux. *Gastrointest Endosc* 1986; 32:81-83.
122. Saks BJ, Kilby AE, Dietrich PA, et al: Pleural and mediastinal changes following endoscopic injection sclerotherapy of esophageal varices. *Radiology* 1983; 149:639-642.
123. Bacon BR, Bailey-Newton RS, Connors AF Jr: Pleural effusions after endoscopic variceal sclerotherapy. *Gastroenterology* 1985; 88:1910-1914.
124. Sivak MV Jr: Endoscopic injection sclerosis of esophageal varices: ASGE survey (letter). *Gastrointest Endosc* 1982; 28:41.
125. Sorensen T, Burcharth F, Pedersen ML, et al: Oesophageal stricture and dysphagia after endoscopic sclerotherapy for bleeding varices. *Gut* 1984; 25:473-477.
126. Haynes WC, Sanowski RA, Foutch PG, et al: Esophageal strictures following endoscopic variceal sclerotherapy: Clinical course and response to dilation therapy. *Gastrointest Endosc* 1986; 32:202-205.
127. Huizinga WKJ, Keenan JP, Marszalek A: Sclerotherapy for bleeding oesophageal varices—a fatal complication. A case report. *S Afr Med J* 1984; 65:436-438.
128. Soderlund C, Wiechel K-L: Oesophageal perforation after sclerotherapy for variceal haemorrhage. *Acta Chir Scand* 1983; 149:491-495.
129. Carr-Locke DL, Sidky K: Broncho-oesophageal fistula: A late complication of endoscopic variceal sclerotherapy. *Gut* 1982; 23:1005-1007.
130. Shemesh E, Bat L: Esophageal perforation after fiberoptic endoscopic injection sclerotherapy for esophageal varices. *Arch Surg* 1986; 121:243-245.
131. Sanowski RA, Kozarek RA, Brayko C, et al: Esophageal variceal sclerotherapy (EVS): Course and complications (abstract). *Gastrointest Endosc* 1983; 29:193.
132. Sarin SK, Nanda R, Vij JC, et al: Oesophageal ulceration after sclerotherapy—a complication or an accompaniment? *Endoscopy* 1986; 18:44-45.
133. Scherl EJ, Fabry TL: Pseudodiverticula secondary to injection sclerotherapy. *J Clin Gastroenterol* 1983; 5:401-403.
134. Subramanyam K, Patterson M: Chronic esophageal ulceration after endoscopic sclerotherapy. *J Clin Gastroenterol* 1986; 8:58-60.
135. Novis B, Bat L, Pomerantz I, et al: Endoscopic sclerotherapy of esophageal varices. *Isr J Med Sci* 1983; 19:40-44.
136. Shepherd MM, Lee RG, Bowers JH: Local toxicity of sclerosing agents used in canine esophagus (abstract). *Gastrointest Endosc* 1983; 29:188.
137. Harris OD, Dickey JD, Stephenson PM: Simple endoscopic injection sclerotherapy of oesophageal varices. *Aust NZ J Med* 1982; 12:131-135.
138. Barthel JS, Sprouse RF, Dix JD, et al: Fatal *Candida* esophageal abscess and sepsis complicat-

ing endoscopic variceal sclerosis. *Gastrointest Endosc* 1987; 33:107–110.
139. Camara DS, Gruber M, Barde CJ, et al: Transient bacteremia following endoscopic injection sclerotherapy of esophageal varices. *Arch Intern Med* 1983; 143:1350–1352.
140. Brayko CM, Kozarek RA, Sanowski RA: Bacteremia during esophageal variceal sclerotherapy: Its cause and prevention (abstract). *Gastrointest Endosc* 1983; 29:159–160.
141. Low DE, Shoenut JP, Kennedy JK, et al: Infectious complications of endoscopic injection sclerotherapy. *Arch Intern Med* 1986; 146:569–571.
142. Monroe P, Morrow CF Jr, Millen JE, et al: Acute respiratory failure after sodium morrhuate esophageal sclerotherapy. *Gastroenterology* 1983; 85:693–699.
143. Bailey-Newton RS, Connors AF Jr, Bacon BR: Effect of endoscopic variceal sclerotherapy on gas exchange and hemodynamics in humans. *Gastroenterology* 1985; 89:368–373.
144. Korula J, Baydur A, Sassoon C, et al: Effect of esophageal variceal sclerotherapy (EVS) on lung function. *Arch Intern Med* 1986; 146:1517–1520.
145. Seidman E, Weber AM, Morin CL, et al: Spinal cord paralysis following sclerotherapy for esophageal varices. *Hepatology* 1984; 4:950–954.
146. Foutch PG, Sivak MV Jr: Colonic variceal hemorrhage after endoscopic injection sclerosis of esophageal varices: A report of three cases. *Am J Gastroenterol* 1984; 79:756–760.
147. Keane RM, Britton DC: Massive bleeding from rectal varices following repeated injection sclerotherapy of oesophageal varices. *Br J Surg* 1986; 73:120.
148. Barsoum MS, Mooro HAW, Bolous FI, et al: The complications of injection sclerotherapy of bleeding oesophageal varices. *Br J Surg* 1982; 69:79–81.
149. Thatcher BS, Sivak MV Jr, Ferguson DR, et al: Mesenteric venous thrombosis as a possible complication of endoscopic sclerotherapy: A report of two cases. *Am J Gastroenterol* 1986; 81:126–129.
150. Knauer CM, Fogel MR: Pericarditis: Complication of esophageal sclerotherapy: A report of three cases. *Gastroenterology* 1987; 93:287–290.
151. Jackson FC, Perrin EB, Dagradi AE, et al: Clinical investigation of the portacaval shunt. I. Study design and preliminary survival analysis. *Arch Surg* 1965; 91:43–54.
152. Resnick RH, Chalmer TC, Ishihara AM, et al: A controlled study of the prophylactic portacaval shunt. A final report. *Ann Intern Med* 1969; 70:675–688.
153. Reuff B, Degos F, Degos JD, et al: A controlled study of therapeutic portacaval shunt in alcoholic cirrhosis. *Lancet* 1976; I:655–659.
154. Reynolds TB, Donovan AJ, Mikkelsen WP, et al: Results of a 12-year randomized trial or portacaval shunt in patients with alcoholic liver disease and bleeding varices. *Gastroenterology* 1981; 80:1005–1011.
155. Conn HO: Ideal treatment of portal hypertension in 1985. *Clin Gastroenterol* 1985; 14:259–288.
156. Orloff MJ, Bell RH Jr, Hyde PV, et al: Long-term results of emergency portacaval shunt for bleeding esophageal varices in unselected patients with alcoholic cirrhosis. *Ann Surg* 1980; 192:325–340.
157. Villeneuve JP, Pomier-Layrargues G, Duguay L, et al: Emergency portacaval shunt for variceal hemorrhage. A prospective study. *Ann Surg* 1987; 206:48–52.
158. Orloff MJ, Bell RH Jr: Long-term survival after emergency portacaval shunting for bleeding varices in patients with alcoholic cirrhosis. *Am J Surg* 1986; 151:176–183.
159. Conn HO, Lindenmuth WW, May CJ, et al: Prophylactic portacaval anastomosis. A tale of two studies. *Medicine* 1972; 51:27–40.
160. Fischer JE, Bouer RS, Atamian S, et al: Comparison of distal and proximal splenorenal shunts: A randomized prospective trial. *Ann Surg* 1981; 194:531–544.
161. Langer B, Rotstein LE, Stone RM, et al: A prospective trial of the selective distal splenorenal shunt. *Surg Gynecol Obstet* 1980; 150:45–48.
162. Reichle FA, Fahmyu WF, Golsorkhi M: Prospective comparative clinical trials with distal splenorenal and mesocaval shunts. *Am J Surg* 1979; 137:13–21.
163. Rikkers LF, Rudman D, Galambos JT, et al: A randomized controlled trial of the distal splenorenal shunt. *Ann Surg* 1978; 188:271–282.
164. Harley HA, Morgan T, Redeker AG, et al: Results of a randomized trial of end-to-side portacaval shunt and distal splenorenal shunt in alcoholic liver disease and variceal bleeding. *Gastroenterology* 1986; 91:802–809.
165. Hassab MA: Nonshunt operations in portal hypertension without cirrhosis. *Surg Gynecol Obstet* 1970; 131:648–654.
166. Sugiura M, Futagawa S: Further evaluation of the Sugiura procedure in the treatment of esophageal varices. *Arch Surg* 1977; 112:1317–1321.
167. Johnston GW: Six years' experience of oesophageal transection for oesophageal varices, using a circular stapling gun. *Gut* 1982; 23:770–773.
168. Cello JP, Grendell JH, Crass RA, et al: Endoscopic sclerotherapy versus portacaval shunt in patient with severe cirrhosis and acute variceal hemorrhage. Long-term follow-up. *N Engl J Med* 1987; 316:11–15.
169. Cello JP, Crass R, Trunkey DD, et al: Endoscopic sclerotherapy versus esophageal transection in Child's class C patients with variceal hemorrhage. Comparison with results of portacaval shunt. Preliminary report. *Surgery* 1982; 91:333–338.
170. Huizinga WK, Angorn IB, Baker LW: Esophageal transection versus injection sclerotherapy in the management of bleeding esophageal varices in patients at high risk. *Surg Gynecol Obstet* 1985; 160:539–546.
171. Warren WD, Henderson JM, Millikan WJ, et al: Distal splenorenal shunt versus endoscopic sclerotherapy for long-term management of

variceal bleeding. Preliminary report of a prospective, randomized trial. *Ann Surg* 1986; 203:454–462.
172. Teres J, Bordas JM, Bravo D, et al: Sclerotherapy vs. distal splenorenal shunt in the elective treatment of variceal hemorrhage: A randomized controlled trial. *Hepatology* 1987; 7:430–436.
173. Sivak MV Jr: Sclerotherapy for esophageal varices, in Silvis SE (ed): *Therapeutic Gastrointestinal Endoscopy*. New York, Igaku Shoin, 1985, pp 31–66.
174. Sivak MV Jr: Sclerotherapy of esophageal varices, in Bayless TM (ed): *Current Therapy in Gastroenterology and Liver disease—2*. Toronto, B. C. Decker Inc., 1986, pp 48–54.

45

Gastric Bubble Insertion:
Is this a rational approach to managing obesity?

STANLEY B. BENJAMIN, M.D., F.A.C.P.

Like many ideas and techniques, the concept of placing an iatrogenic bezoar in the stomach to facilitate weight loss is not a new one. It is the general availability of specific commercial devices for this purpose that has kindled both interest and controversy regarding this concept. It would certainly be logical to assume that such a device would be important in promoting weight loss because one of the major complications of naturally occurring or postgastric surgery bezoars is weight loss. It can be assumed then that the first attempts at placing such a device derive from this observation. Similarly, as we will see, the complications of these devices could have been predicted from these same clinical observations.

The intent of this presentation is to review the available data on this group of devices designed to treat obesity, to offer my opinions regarding their use, and, perhaps most importantly, to discuss the future of this area of therapeutics.

DEFINITIONS AND DESCRIPTIONS

As always, understanding of terminology is crucial to further discussion. As defined in a standard dictionary, a *balloon* is a large airtight bag and a *bubble* is a film or liquid enveloping air or gas.[1] For purposes of this discussion and clarity of communication in general, all iatrogenic bezoars used as adjuncts to diet and behavioral modification should be referred to as balloons, with specific devices referred to by their proprietary names when they differ (e.g., Garren-Edwards Gastric Bubble).

At the time of this writing, seven such devices are commercially available in parts of the world, under development, or undergoing preclinical evaluation (Table 45–1).

HISTORIC PERSPECTIVES

Bezoars have a colorful and unique history. Having been recognized since antiquity, they have more often been perceived as materials with special healing powers than a medical or surgical problem. This is especially true of the trichobezoar which was a valued possession to many, one even being present with the British crown jewels!

As a medical problem, it was observed that weight loss was an important part of the clinical syndrome seen in individuals with this condition. Based on these observations, attempts were made to place an iatrogenic bezoar in the stomachs of obese individuals. Silicone breast implants and toy balloons represent some of the early attempts at artificially producing reduced caloric intake and early satiety.[2,3]

In the last 15 years, several commercial

523

TABLE 45-1.
Commercially Available Balloons, 1987*

Ballobes Balloon—Free floating or air-filled polyurethane
Garren-Edwards Gastric Bubble—Free floating, air-filled polyurethane
Percival Balloon—Attached, fluid-filled silicone
Gau Balloon—Free floating, fluid-filled, silicone
Riepe/Bard Balloon—Free floating, fluid-filled, latex
Taylor Balloon—Free floating, fluid-filled, silicone
Wilson-Cook Intragastric Balloon—Attached, air-filled polyurethane

*These are the iatrogenic bezoars, either free floating or attached by a small-caliber nasogastric tube, available or under evaluation at this time.

devices that would provide these benefits were marketed. The individual dynamics of these separate devices are testimony to a group of committed, innovative individuals, often performing their initial work without the support of the medical technologies industry.

The skyrocketing of this concept in the United States came with Food and Drug Administration approval of the Garren-Edwards Gastric Bubble in September 1985. The frustrations of obesity treatment, the huge population of patients, and, presumably, economic considerations led to what has been referred to as "bubble mania." The rapid spread of the use of this device in the absence of conclusive data showing efficacy produced a backlash of opinion, especially as complications typical to bezoars began to surface. Initially lost in this sea of emotion were both the genuine concerns of the developers to address these issues and the data being collected on the other devices. A review of these data will hopefully provide an intelligent answer to the question of whether balloons should be used.

BALLOONS—WHAT DO WE REALLY KNOW?

Perhaps the greatest disappointment and one of the major concerns is the lack of controlled observation from which to make decisions related to any of these devices. If the scanty preliminary data available related to these devices are compiled (Table 45-2), it can be seen that similar degrees of weight loss, generally in the range of 1 to 2 lb per week, can be expected.[3-10] On the surface, this would appear to be a positive response, in fact representing the kind of weight loss considered "healthy." A major concern, however, has been raised by the several sham-controlled studies which have been performed with the Garren-Edwards Gastric Bubble.[7-11] In these studies there was no difference between sham patients and bubble patients. Of note, however, was the fact that all groups lost weight during these studies. Given the Food and Drug Administration requirement that this device be used as an adjunct to diet and behavioral modification, all these studies entered patients in such a program. The conclusion from these observations is that the Garren-Edwards Gastric Bubble is no better than diet and behavioral modification in producing weight loss except that these devices add cost and the risk of significant morbidity. On review, however, several questions still remain. The natural history of obesity is not weight loss; however, in these studies—both sham-controlled and initial efficacy trials—it would appear that these devices serve as a "hook" to get patients into an effective method of weight loss (i.e., diet and behavioral modification).

The unanswered questions relate to subgroups in the syndrome of obesity for whom bubble therapy may be effective, the potential entry biases of trials performed to date, and the potential that other balloons for which no controlled data are available may, in fact, be effective when compared to diet and behavioral modification alone.

COMPLICATIONS

As previously stated, bezoars naturally occurring have a similar and predictable constellation of complications: gastric ulceration, bleeding, and bowel obstruction.[11-17] It is not surprising that iatrogenic bezoars carry along with them the same risks. The only question, actually,

TABLE 45–2.
Balloons: Is there a difference?

	Weight Loss Data		
Balloon	Per week (mean) (lb/week)	12 weeks (total) (lb)	38 weeks (lb)
Ballobes[2]	1.22	14.7*	
Garren-Edwards			
Garren & Garren[5, 6]	2.5	30.0	
Hogan et al[7]†	1.56	18.7	
Bejamin et al[8]†	1.51‡	18.0	
Percival[3]	1.7		
Ripe/Bard[20]			
Single blinded	1.9	22.8	
Open trial	1.4	16.8	
Taylor[4]	1.37	16.5	
Wilson-Cook[19]	1.5		57.2

*Represents median weight loss.
†Controlled, blinded trial, no difference to sham.
‡Represents all patients with bubbles, first 3 months.

should have been the relative incidence of these predictable complications.

With the notable exception of overt, clinically significant bleeding, all these complications have been reported from these devices. Ulcers are reported with considerable frequency in association with the Garren-Edwards Gastric Bubble. An initial incidence of 6% was reported in the original Garren data submitted to the Food and Drug Administration. This was followed by a decrease in the inflation volume from 250 cc to 200 cc and a reduction in ulcer incidence to 2%. In a variety of subsequent studies, the rates have varied from 10% to 15%.[7–10] One gastric perforation has been reported to the manufacturer due to penetration of a gastric ulcer.

In preliminary data from other balloon studies, reflecting a much smaller user experience, gastric ulcers have been reported, and it should be anticipated that ulceration will be a complication for some percentage of all balloon use.[18] Whether or not concomitant use of medication such as H_2-receptor blockers will, as preliminarily reported, decrease this incidence is unknown.

The major complication of balloon use is spontaneous deflation and passage into the small bowel with small bowel obstruction and the need for surgical removal (Fig 45–1). Representing the major morbidity of naturally occurring bezoars, this complication led to a dampening of interest in the Garren-Edwards Gastric Bubble.[19] This complication has been seen with other anti-obesity balloons, but the relative risks of other devices is not yet established.[20] The nature of the material used in the production of these devices, their shape, and design of deflation or fluid loss will all play important roles in defining the relative risk of such an event.

The major lesson should be, however, that these devices are foreign bodies and, in a large enough population exposure, small bowel obstruction is to be anticipated. When this occurs these devices *must be* managed as blunt foreign bodies with the risk of small bowel necrosis, peritonitis, and even death! Should anti-obesity balloons become generally accepted, one of the major issues will relate to the frequency with which they pass into the small bowel and produce obstruction.

BALLOONS, BUBBLES, OR NOTHING?

I think that the answer to this question is easy for the short term and unknown for the future. At a recent multidiscipli-

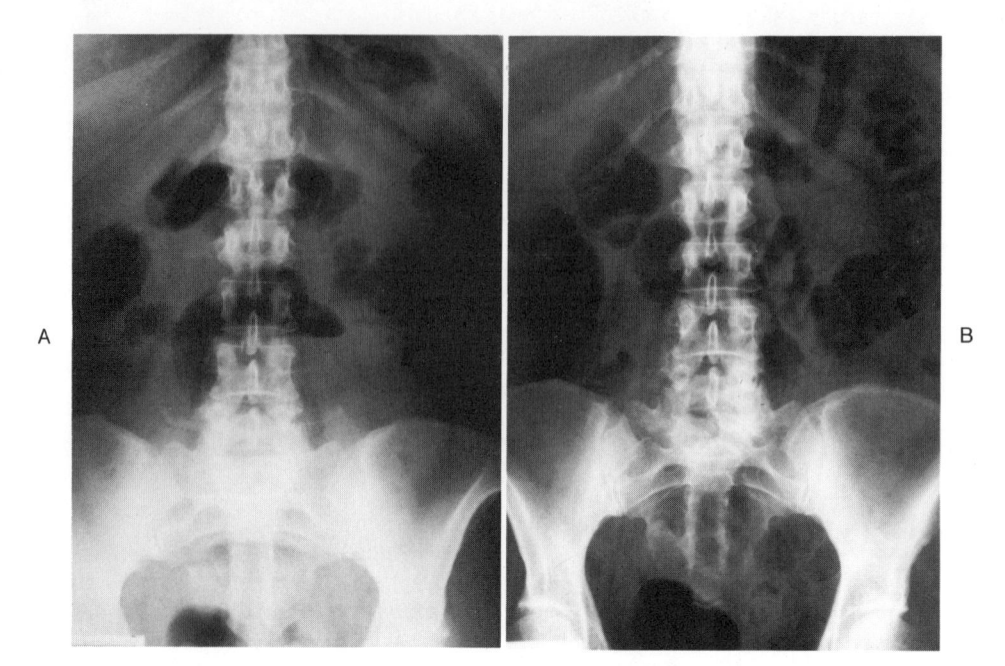

FIG 45–1.
A, patient with Garren-Edwards Gastric Bubble lodged in small bowel, presenting with small bowel obstruction. **B,** after medical treatment bubble is now visible in colon.

nary conference on balloons, the consensus of experts, including bariatric surgeons, diet and behavioral modification specialists, and gastroenterologists, was that insufficient data exist to warrant the general use of these devices outside of controlled clinical trials.[21]

However, given the magnitude of the problem of obesity, its significant co-morbidity and frustrating treatment, the concept of balloon therapy should not be too quickly abandoned. Insufficient data have been generated to answer definitively the questions that have been raised. How these questions are answered will require close cooperation among the disciplines involved in obesity management.

Appropriate protocol design, comparative studies between devices, large carefully documented user experiences, and comparisons of trials of these devices with no diet or behavioral modification are all necessary to place the concept of balloon therapy in its proper niche.

At the present time, then, balloons or bubbles should not be used outside of well-designed, carefully monitored clinical trials. Whether or not the medical device industry will bear the financial burden associated with answering these questions remains to be seen. We as a group have learned a great deal about these concepts, exposed some human foibles, and will hopefully approach the next era of balloon therapy in a much more organized and less impatient fashion.

References

1. *Webster's New World Dictionary,* College Edition. Cleveland and New York, The World Publishing Co., 1962.
2. Nieben OG, Harboe H: Intragastric balloon as an artificial bezoar for treatment of obesity. *Lancet* 1983; 1:198–199.
3. Percival WL: The balloon diet: A non-invasive treatment for morbid obesity: Preliminary report on 108 patients. *Can J Surg* 1984; 27:135–136.
4. Taylor TV, Pullan BR: Initial experience with a free floating intragastric balloon in the treatment of morbid obesity (abstract). *Gut* 1983; 24:979.
5. Garren LR, Garren M: The Garren gastric bubble. An endoscopic aid to treatment of morbid obesity (abstract). *Gastrointest Endosc* 1984; 30:153A.
6. Garren L, Garren M, Giordano F, et al: Further experience with the Garren-Edwards gastric

bubble as an adjunctive therapy in obesity (abstract). *Gastrointest Endosc* 1986; 32:170–171.
7. Hogan RB, Johnson JH, Long BW, et al: The gastric bubble vs. sham endoscopy: A prospective, randomized, controlled, double-blinded comparison as adjunct to a standard weight loss program. *Gastrointest Endosc* 1987; 33:172A.
8. Benjamin SB, Maher K, Ciarleglio C, et al: A double-blind crossover study of the Garren-Edwards anti-obesity bubble. *Gastrointest Endosc* 1987; 33:168A.
9. Meshkinpour H, Hso D, Farivar S: The effect of gastric bubble as a weight reduction device: A controlled crossover study. *Gastroenterology* 1987; 92:A1532.
10. Levine GM, Goldstein M, Lowe M, et al: The gastric bubble, fad or fantastic? *Gastroenterology* 1987; 92:A1505.
11. Buchholz PR, Harston AS: Phytobezoars following gastric surgery for duodenal ulcer. *Surg Clin North Am* 1972; 52:341–352.
12. Goldstein HM, Cohen LE, Hagen RO, et al: Gastric bezoars, a frequent complication in the postoperative ulcer patient. *Radiology* 1973; 107:341–344.
13. Mir AM, Mir MA: Phytobezoar after vagotomy with drainage or resection. *Br J Surg* 1973; 60:846–848.
14. Moriel EZ, Avalon A, Eid A, et al: An unusually high incidence of gastrointestinal obstruction by persimmon bezoars in Israeli patients after ulcer surgery. *Gastroenterology* 1983; 84:752–754.
15. Rigler RA, Grininger DR: Phytobezoar after partial gastrectomy. *Surg Clin North Am* 1970; 50:380–386.
16. Krausz MM, Moriel EZ, Avalon A, et al: Surgical aspects of gastrointestinal persimmon phytobezoar treatment. *Am J Surg* 1986; 152:526–530.
17. Goldstein SS, Lewis JH, Rothstein R: Intestinal obstruction due to bezoars. *Am J Gastroenterol* 1984; 79:313–318.
18. Mathus-Vliegen EMH: Intragastric balloons for morbid obesity results, patient tolerance and balloon life-span. Presented at a scientific workshop on intragastric balloons for obesity. Tarpon Springs, FL, March 1987.
19. Benjamin SB: Small bowel obstruction and the Garren-Edwards bubble: Lessons to be learned. *Gastrointest Endosc* 1987; 33:183A.
20. Riepe S: Antiobesity gastric balloon. Presented at a scientific workshop on intragastric balloons for obesity. Tarpon Springs, FL, March 1987.
21. Holland S, Bach D, Duff J: Balloon therapy for obesity—when the balloon bursts. *J Can Assoc Radiol* 1985; 36:347–348.
22. Schapiro M, Benjamin SB, Blackburn G, et al: The intragastric balloon for obesity treatment—Summary of a scientific workshop. *Gastrointest Endosc* 1987; 33:323–328.

46

Colonoscopic Polypectomy of Polyps with Adenocarcinoma:
When is it curative?

LAWRENCE B. COHEN, M.D.
JEROME D. WAYE, M.D.

It is now widely accepted that most colon and rectal cancers result from malignant transformation of benign colon adenomas.[1] This adenoma–cancer sequence evolves through several stages, from the benign adenomatous polyp to in situ cancer to invasive cancer as the malignant cells invade the submucosa. In this sequence, the adenomatous elements are progressively replaced by cancer cells, ultimately producing a polypoid cancer, a lesion in which no benign adenomatous tissue is present. As the cancerous cells extend deeper into the polyp stroma, and the proportion of malignant cells within the adenoma increases, so too does the risk of cancer penetration into the wall of the colon and the possibility of distant metastases via the lymphatic and vascular channels.

The adenomatous polyp is a true neoplasm, which develops as a result of unrestricted cell proliferation and incomplete cellular maturation.[2] The histologic architecture of an adenoma is composed of closely packed glandular elements in a "picket-fence" configuration, arranged in a tubular or villous pattern, or a combination of the two. An adenoma is characterized by cellular atypia, or dysplasia, which can range from mild to severe. The small adenoma is usually composed of tubular elements with a mild degree of dysplasia, but with increasing size of the polyp both the proportion of villous features and the degree of cellular atypia increase.[3,4] Severe dysplasia, also termed carcinoma-in-situ or mucosal cancer, has no risk of metastasis because the lymphatic plexus within the colon does not extend above the muscularis mucosae into the mucosa.[5] It is the presence of a dense lymphatic network within the submucosa of a colonic adenoma that enables invasive cancer cells to metastasize.

A malignant polyp is defined as an adenoma in which cancer cells have broken through the muscularis mucosae to invade the submucosal stroma. At times, the pathologist may have difficulty in distinguishing invasive cancer extending through the muscularis from islands of trapped benign adenomatous tissue within the submucosa, called "pseudocarcinomatous invasion."[6]

The incidence of cancer within a polyp is related to its size and histology. For a polyp less than 0.6 cm in diameter, the cancer risk is extremely low, on the order of 0.1%. About 1% of polyps 1 cm in diameter will contain carcinoma, while the rate may be as high as 40% in large polyps greater than 3 cm.[7] An increase in the proportion of villous features is similarly associated with a higher incidence of cancer in adenomas, from 5% for the tubular adenoma, to more than 40% in the villous polyp.[8] Overall, about 4% to 5% of all adenomatous polyps will contain invasive cancer.[9] In this chapter, we will review the endoscopic and histopathologic features of the malignant colon polyp and set out guidelines for a rational approach to the management of this controversial problem.

THE ENDOSCOPIC ASSESSMENT

More than 90% of all colonoscopically resected malignant polyps are found distal to the splenic flexure.[10–12] In part, this reflects the tendency of left colon lesions to produce detectable blood loss, leading to their discovery at an earlier time when they may still be amenable to endoscopic removal. Right-sided colon tumors are often clinically quiescent and usually become symptomatic only after the tumor becomes quite large and cancer cells have extended through the wall of the colon. At this stage of the disease, surgical resection of the tumor is required. Case selection may also contribute to the predominance of malignant polyps within the left colon because the endoscopist is more willing to resect large sessile lesions in the rectum and sigmoid, while the same size lesion in the cecum would often be referred directly to the surgeon, bypassing inclusion in an endoscopic series.

There are several factors to be considered as the endoscopist visually engages a colon polyp. The operator should first decide if endoscopic resection of the tumor is necessary. Any lesion that has the appearance of a large bowel carcinoma rather than an adenoma should be biopsied, and the polypectomy decision should be deferred. A large broad-based bulky exophytic lesion that appears to extend into the wall of the colon rather than merely sitting on its surface, an annular lesion that involves more than half the circumference of the bowel wall, or a flat, sessile ulcerated villous adenoma is best left for the surgeon. Ulceration of a polyp or an area of firmness detected by instrument palpation is a strong indication of cancerous invasion of the polyp. When an irregular-shaped polyp and the underlying wall move together when the lesion is probed, it is likely that cancer cells have invaded the submucosa of the colon, and polypectomy should not be attempted.

Upon encountering a cancer that requires surgical resection, the endoscopist need not remove other polyps that will be included in the resected segment of bowel. However, the remainder of the colon should be examined whenever possible to exclude a concurrent cancer or polyp, which occur in 2% and 35% of cases, respectively.[13] All polyps discovered outside the anticipated margins of surgical resection should be removed endoscopically.

The size and attachment of a colonic polyp are additional factors in the polypectomy decision. A pedunculated adenoma, regardless of the size of the polyp head, can always be safely removed endoscopically, provided that it has a true pedicle and that adequate electrocoagulation is given prior to stalk transection.[7] Some sessile adenomas have a pseudopedicle created by pulling out the underlying mucosa. This is often an indication that cancer cells have invaded the bowel wall, and caution should be exercised when resecting such a lesion.[14] The gross endoscopic appearance of a polyp and its location are important factors because a large sessile polyp in the rectum may be endoscopically removed without difficulty, whereas a similar lesion in the right colon may require surgical resection. There is little role for endoscopic biopsy of the adenomatous polyp in which there is a suspicion of invasive cancer, because superficial pinch biopsies will often not reflect the pathologic nature of the entire lesion.[15]

Several observations should be made during endoscopic polypectomy. First, the ease of polyp transection should be noted. Was transection readily accomplished without the need for either extended electrocoagulation time or excessive tension on the snare wire, or was excessive resistance encountered? Malignant invasion of the resected tissue should be suspected if the length of time required to produce separation is longer than expected for the size of the polyp. The endoscopist should also evaluate the adequacy of polypectomy. When the polyp is pedunculated, transection through the stalk will resect all adenomatous tissue, because the pedicle is composed of normal colonic mucosa. However, when a large sessile lesion is resected in a piecemeal fashion, it is possible for some residual adenomatous tissue to remain on the colon wall. At times it may be difficult to determine the adequacy of polypectomy. In such cases, reexamination should be performed in 4 to 6 weeks, after the coagulum has sloughed and reepithelialization has taken place. In some instances, it may be desirable to mark the site of a resected polypoid lesion. By injecting India ink into the submucosa of the bowel wall at the site of polypectomy, the precise area of concern is permanently marked, allowing it to be easily recognized either during subsequent endoscopic examinations or by the surgeon at the time of bowel resection.[16]

It is the responsibility of the endoscopist to prepare the specimen for pathologic evaluation. Whenever possible, the lesion should be preserved in one piece rather than in several fragments. A pin should be used to mark the base or stalk of the polyp, and the tissue should be delivered immediately to the laboratory for processing. The specimen should be accompanied by a written description of the lesion, including its size, location, type of attachment, and an assessment of the adequacy of the resection.

THE HISTOPATHOLOGIC EVALUATION

The histopathologic evaluation requires that the entire polyp be submitted and processed, and the polyp must be sectioned to demonstrate the normal anatomical relationship of the head and stalk. The pathologist should be requested to provide the following information:[10]
1. The histologic elements of the adenoma; tubular, villous, or tubulovillous
2. The precise extent of cancerous invasion within the polyp. Are cancer cells present deep to the muscularis mucosae, or is the process limited to the mucosa? Is the cancer mucosal or invasive?
3. The histologic grade of the cancer cells; well-differentiated, moderately differentiated, or poorly differentiated
4. The proportion of adenomatous tissue replaced by cancer
5. The presence or absence of cancer cell invasion into lymphatic or vascular channels
6. The depth of cancer extension into the polyp
7. The presence of cancer cells at or close to the margin of resection

It is the responsibility of the pathologist to clearly communicate the microscopic findings to the clinician.[17] Of foremost importance is the question of cancerous invasion. Severe dysplasia, carcinoma in situ, mucosal cancer, and intraepithelial carcinoma are synonyms to describe a biologically benign lesion without tumor invasion beyond the muscularis mucosae, and endoscopic resection of such a polyp is curative. If cancer does invade the stroma of a polyp, the ratio of benign to malignant tissue within the polyp should be stated. As the volume of cancerous cells increases relative to the amount of remaining adenoma, the risk of metastasis becomes greater.[2] The depth of cancer invasion with respect to the line of resection is an important measurement, and this distance should be reported in millimeters. As cancer spreads into the deeper layers of the polyp, the likelihood of tumor penetration of the colon wall increases. Upon careful review of the histologic findings, the clinician and the pathologist together can then judge the adequacy of endoscopic polypectomy.

THE MALIGNANT POLYP: A CLINICIAN'S DILEMMA

There is tremendous controversy over the proper management of the malignant polyp. There are those who advise secondary bowel resection for all polyps found to contain invasive cancer,[18] while others advocate a more conservative approach, claiming that endoscopic resection is adequate treatment for the great majority of cancerous polyps.[10, 19] In an attempt to resolve these divergent viewpoints, two basic questions must be addressed:

1. *What is the risk of residual or metastatic cancer when a malignant polyp has been endoscopically resected?* Are the various features of the cancer, such as the degree of cellular differentiation, level of invasion, or involvement of the lymphatic or vascular channels of prognostic significance? Do differences in the attachment of a polyp affect this risk? Are there high-risk patients in whom the probability of residual disease after polypectomy justifies the need for further treatment?
2. *Does surgical intervention improve the survival of patients with residual disease after endoscopic resection?* What are the circumstances that would impact on the decision for subsequent surgery? Does the potential benefit of early surgery outweigh the risks and disadvantages to those patients not known to have residual disease?

The pertinent studies that deal with these two critical issues will be reviewed in order to develop a strategy for the management of the malignant polyp.

The Risk of Residual Disease

A number of well-designed studies have evaluated the risk of residual disease after endoscopic removal of a malignant polyp. However, their results are difficult to compare due to a lack of consistency with respect to case selection, terminology, pathologic assessment, and methods used to evaluate the outcome of treatment. Some series are based solely on endoscopic polypectomy,[10, 12] while others mix colonoscopic and surgical data.[11, 20–23] Although the morphologic features of a polyp should not pose a problem, they are not all classified as sessile or pedunculated, but may be reported in terms of long stalks, short stalks, pseudopedicles, or the type of attachment may not be differentiated at all. Because of these differences between published studies, the findings are not easily interpreted, and a single unified concept does not emerge.

After colonoscopic polypectomy of an adenoma that contains invasive cancer, the risk of subsequently developing recurrent or metastatic cancer depends on the presence of any remaining cells. The residual disease may be either grossly evident or microscopic and can occur within the bowel wall, regional lymph nodes, or in distant organs. Knowledge of the probability of residual disease is necessary in order to accurately determine the need for further therapy following removal of a malignant polyp.

There are two methods to determine the presence of residual cancer. The most direct is exploratory surgery with resection of involved segments of colon along with the regional lymph nodes. The other approach requires surveillance for the development of further disease. Because of the relatively long latency period before metastatic colon cancer becomes clinically apparent, follow-up must be maintained for up to 10 years before a patient can be declared free of disease. Most studies have used a combination of these two methods for identifying residual cancer, but in some, the mean duration of follow-up has been too short for an accurate assessment of the results.

The reported risk of residual disease ranges widely, from 0% to 40%, with the variation related to differences in study design. In their thorough review of the literature, Wilcox and co-workers[24] reported a 10.4% incidence of recurrence from studies reported before endoscopy, and a 10.1% cumulative risk following colonoscopic polypectomy. An overall 14% cumulative risk of residual or recurrent disease has been compiled from six well-documented studies reported between 1978 and 1986 (Table 46–1).

In 1975, Wolff and Shinya[25] proposed guidelines for separating malignant polyps into two histologic categories, favorable and unfavorable, based on the histologic grade of the malignancy, the presence or absence of cancer at the resec-

TABLE 46-1.
Malignant Colon Polyp: Correlation of Histologic Features with Risk of Residual Disease

	No. of cases	Cancer at/near* Resection Margin No.	Cancer at/near* Resection Margin Residual Disease	Poorly Differentiated Cancer No.	Poorly Differentiated Cancer Residual Disease	Lymph/Vascular Invasion No.	Lymph/Vascular Invasion Residual Disease	Residual Disease No.	Residual Disease %
Colacchio et al[18]	24	0	0	2	1	4	2	6	25
Cooper[20]	56	24	7	3	2	6	1	8	14
Lipper et al[21]	22	2	1	0	0	1	0	2	9
Haggitt et al[11]	64	28†	7	2	1	2	1	8	12
Morson et al[10]	60	9	0	3	0	NA	NA	3	5
Cranley et al[12]	38	22	10	4	3	4	1	10	26
Total	264	85	25	14	7	17	5	37	14
Positive predictive value (%)			29.4		50		29.4		

*Cancer within 3 mm of resection margin.
†Level 4 invasion.

tion margin, and cancer cell invasion of the lymphatic or vascular channels. Since that time, numerous studies have examined these and other histologic criteria in an attempt to identify risk factors for residual disease.

The presence of cancer extending to the margin of resection is the most important factor in predicting the risk of residual disease. In early studies, Lockart-Mummery,[26] Scarborough,[27] and Carden and Morson[28] proposed the importance of tumor at the resection margin as a risk factor for recurrence and recommended further treatment for such cases. More recently, Coutsoftides found a 50% incidence of residual disease in six patients who had cancer remaining at the cautery margin.[29] In a series of 56 endoscopically resected malignant polyps, Cooper found a 28% incidence of either residual or recurrent disease in 24 cases in which cancer was at or near the resection margin.[20] Morson evaluated 60 endoscopically resected malignant polyps, including 9 polyps with tumor extending to the diathery margin.[10] There was no residual disease in the one patient who subsequently underwent exploration, and no evidence of recurrent disease was found in the remaining eight patients with a follow-up of more than 5 years. Morson concluded that a positive polypectomy margin does not necessarily require surgical resection because "diathermy coagulation would destroy any residual malignant tissue at the site of polypectomy" and that surgery was indicated only when endoscopic resection of the polyp was judged to be incomplete by endoscopic and pathologic criteria, or when the specimen contained poorly differentiated cancer. Haggitt reported on 64 malignant polyps that were resected either endoscopically (39 polyps) or by colectomy (25 polyps).[11] He introduced yet another grading system for depth of cancer invasion, ranging from noninvasive, superficial cancer limited to the mucosa (level 0) to infiltration into the submucosa of the bowel wall (level 4). In his study, 25% of cases with level 4 invasion had residual or recurrent disease, but the admixing of data derived from both surgical resection and colonoscopic polypectomy causes problems with identification of bowel wall invasion which is difficult to determine endoscopically. Cranley found that the presence of cancer at or near (within 3 mm of) the resection margin was the most accurate predictor of residual disease, with a sensitivity of 100% and a positive predictive value of 45% (10 of 22 cases with cancer at or near the resection margin).[12]

The histologic grade of the cancer may be the next most important predictive feature of the malignant polyp. Although the risk of residual cancer approaches 50% in the poorly differentiated malignant polyp, it is a less useful prognostic tool because this histologic feature is found in less than 10% of all cancerous polyps. Further, it may not be an independent risk factor for recurrent disease because most often, the presence of poorly differentiated cells is accompanied by positive resection margins.[11, 12] Similarly, the presence of lymphatic or vascular invasion has a relatively high positive predictive value, but the low frequency of its occurrence as the only unfavorable finding and the pathologist's difficulty with its recognition make this factor a less valuable prognostic feature. The proportion of an adenoma occupied by malignant cells is not an independent risk factor for residual disease, and even the polypoid cancer is not an absolute indication for secondary bowel resection.[10-12, 20]

Whether a malignant polyp is pedunculated or sessile, the most important risk factor for cancer recurrence is the distance between tumor cells and the margin of resection. Although it is relatively simple to be certain that polypectomy of an adenoma with a stalk has been complete, the adequacy of resection of a sessile polyp may be more difficult to determine. To this extent, the management of the pedunculated polyp containing invasive cancer is less complicated. However, the risk factors for residual cancer are independent of polyp morphology, and cancer at the cautery margin remains the most important criteria for residual disease according to the published literature.[10-12, 20]

In summary, the overall risk of residual disease following resection of a malignant polyp is in the range of 10% to 14%. However, if one eliminates from consideration those malignant polyps that have one or more poor prognostic indicators, the likelihood of residual cancer falls to 2% to 3%.[30] The most important prognostic factor is cancer cells at or within 2 or 3 mm of the margin of resection, which, if present, increase the probability of residual cancer to 25% to 30%. Cancer that is poorly differentiated and infiltration of the vascular or lymphatic channels are other unfavorable histologic findings, although the relative infrequency of these two features make them of lesser importance. While complete excision of the sessile polyp is at times technically more difficult than resection of a pedunculated adenoma, the presence or absence of a pedicle does not influence the risk of residual disease apart from the endoscopist's assessment of the completeness of polypectomy and the histologic findings described above.

The Risks and Benefits of Surgical Resection

There is insufficient information in the literature to permit a precise analysis of the benefits of secondary surgical resection for a patient discovered to have a polyp that contains invasive cancer. As the likelihood of residual cancer increases, so does the probability that surgical intervention will improve the outcome. Residual disease may be found in the wall of the colon, in the lymph nodes outside of the bowel, or in distant organs. Surgery will clearly benefit those patients in the first category, will probably help the second group, and will most likely be of little or no value when cancer is widely metastatic.

In a review of the cumulative findings in five studies of patients with cancerous polyps who underwent secondary surgical resection, Wilcox and Beck reported an 18% incidence of residual disease among 98 patients, with cancer limited to the lymph nodes in 61% and distant spread in the remaining 39% of patients.[31] The authors concluded that the operative efficacy, that is, the fraction of patients having residual disease who are curable by resection, is 61%. However, it remains to be determined whether the majority of these "potentially curable" patients have benefited from surgery and will subsequently live longer. There are no comparable figures from nonoperative series with which to compare these data, and long-term follow-up of large numbers of patients who are managed with only endoscopic polypectomy is needed.

The overall operative mortality for segmental resection of the colon is approximately 2%.[32] In healthy individuals below the age of 50, mortality rates as low as 0% have been reported, while the rate may be 15% to 20% in patients over the age of 70 with complicating medical problems.[33] In one series of 61 patients over the age of 80, the operative mortality for colon surgery was 2.2%.[34] Most studies agree that the surgical risk is correlated with the presence of associated medical diseases rather than the age of the patient.

Wilcox and Beck[31] have developed a mathematical model for decision tree analysis of the malignant polyp. Based on their calculations of the probability of residual disease, the potential efficacy of surgery, and the operative mortality, they concluded that for patients with a low operative risk (no complicating medical problems, age less than 70), "resection would yield the best outcome in terms of life expectancy" as long as the probability of residual disease was in excess of 0.5%. Although some of the premises and assumptions in this paper may not be entirely accurate, we do agree that surgery is indicated for those patients with a malignant polyp characterized by one or more of the following features: (1) cancer at the resection margin, (2) poorly differentiated cancer, or (3) invasion of lymphatic or vascular channels by cancer cells. In patients who are elderly (older than age 70) or who have complicating medical illness, the need for secondary bowel resection must be made more cautiously.

CONCLUSION

On the basis of these findings, the following conclusions and recommendations are made about the malignant colon polyp:
1. An adenomatous polyp should be considered "malignant" only when cancer cells extend beyond the muscularis mucosae into the submucosal stroma of the lesion.
2. The malignant polyp is uncommon, comprising only 4% to 5% of all colonic adenomas. The great majority of malignant polyps are located distal to the splenic flexure.
3. The endoscopic features that suggest the presence of invasive cancer within a polyp include: ulceration, areas of firmness, fixation of the lesion to the underlying bowel wall, or a pseudopedicle. Further, the endoscopist must assess the adequacy of polypectomy, particularly in sessile polyps.
4. The histopathologic evaluation requires that the specimen be entirely submitted, that the polyp sectioned to demonstrate proper orientation of the head and stalk, and that the important pathologic features of the malignant polyp carefully assessed.
5. Three histologic features have predictive value in assessing the risk of residual disease: (a) cancer at the margin of resection, (b) poorly differentiated cancer, and (c) cancer cells in the lymphatic or vascular channel.
6. The indications for secondary surgical resection of a malignant polyp include the following:
   - An endoscopic assessment that polypectomy was incomplete
   - Cancer at the resection margin of the excised polyp
   - Poorly differentiated cancer cells
   - Cancer cell infiltration into the lymphatic or vascular space

These criteria for recommending surgery should be modified for the patient who is older than 70 years of age or who has complicating medical problems.

References

1. Morson BC: Evolution of cancer of the colon and rectum. *Cancer* 1974; 34:845–849.
2. Fenoglio CM, Pascal RR: Colorectal adenomas and cancer. Pathologic relationships. *Cancer* 1982; 50:2601–2608.
3. Shinya H, Wolff WI: Morphologic, anatomic distribution and cancer potential of colonic polyps. An analysis of 7000 polyps endoscopically removed. *Ann Surg* 1979; 190:679–683.
4. Morson BC, Konishi F: Contribution of the pa-

thologist to the radiology and management of colorectal polyps. *Gastrointest Radiol* 1982; 7:275–281.
5. Fenoglio CM, Kaye GI, Lane N: Distribution of human colonic lymphatics in normal, hyperplastic and adenomatous tissue. *Gastroenterology* 1973; 64:51–66.
6. Muto T, Bussey HJ, Morson BC: Pseudo-carcinomatous invasion in adenomatous polyps of the colon and rectum. *J Clin Pathol* 1973; 26:25–31.
7. Cohen LB, Waye JD: Treatment of colonic polyps: Practical considerations, in Classen M (ed): *Clinics in Gastroenterology*. London, WB Saunders, 1986, pp 359–376.
8. Morson BC: Genesis of colorectal cancer, in Sherlock P, Zamcheck N (eds): *Clinics in Gastroenterology*. London, WB Saunders, 1976, pp 505–525.
9. Gillespie PE, Chambers TJ, Chan KW, et al: Colonic adenomas—a colonoscopic survey. *Gut* 1979; 20:240–245.
10. Morson BC, Whiteway JE, Jones EA, et al: Histopathology and prognosis of malignant colorectal polyps treated by endoscopic polypectomy. *Gut* 1984; 25:437–444.
11. Haggitt RC, Glotzbach RE, Soffer EE, et al: Prognostic factors in colorectal carcinomas arising in adenomas: Implications for lesions removed by endoscopic polypectomy. *Gastroenterology* 1985; 89:328–336.
12. Cranley JP, Petras RE, Carey WD, et al: When is endoscopic polypectomy adequate therapy for colonic polyps containing invasive cancer? *Gastroenterology* 1986; 91:419–427.
13. Morson BC, Dawson IMP: *Gastrointestinal Pathology*, ed 2. Oxford, Blackwell Scientific Publications, 1979.
14. Waye JD, Shapiro R, Scher L, et al: An endoscopic determinant of the need for subsequent surgery in the malignant polyp (abstract). *Gastrointest Endosc* 1985; 31:150.
15. Livstone EM, Troncale FJ, Sheahan DG: Value of a single forceps biopsy of colonic polyps. *Gastroenterology* 1977; 73:1296–1298.
16. Ponsky J, King J: Endoscopic marking of colonic lesions. *Gastrointest Endosc* 1975; 22:42–43.
17. Riddell RH: Hands off cancerous large bowel polyps. *Gastroenterology* 1985; 89:432–435.
18. Colacchio TA, Forde KA, Scantlebury VP: Endoscopic polypectomy. Inadequate treatment for invasive colorectal carcinoma. *Ann Surg* 1981; 194:704–707.
19. Macrae FA, Whiteway J, Jones E, et al: Malignant polyps: Five year follow up confirms colonoscopic polypectomy as adequate treatment for selected patients (abstract). *Gastrointest Endosc* 1983; 29:179.
20. Cooper HS: Surgical pathology of endoscopically removed malignant polyps of the colon and rectum. *Am J Surg Pathol* 1983; 7:613–623.
21. Lipper S, Kahn LB, Ackerman LV: The significance of microscopic invasive cancer in endoscopically removed polyps of the large bowel. A clinicopathologic study of 51 cases. *Cancer* 1983; 52:1691–1699.
22. Frei JV: Endoscopic large bowel polypectomy. Adequate treatment of some completely removed, minimally invasive lesions. *Am J Surg Pathol* 1985; 9:355–359.
23. Fried GM, Hreno A, Duguid WP, et al: Rational management of malignant colon polyps based on long-term follow-up. *Surgery* 1984; 96:815–821.
24. Wilcox GM, Anderson PB, Colacchio TA: Early invasive carcinoma in colonic polyps. A review of the literature with emphasis on the assessment of the risk of metastasis. *Cancer* 1986; 57:160–171.
25. Wolff WI, Shinya H: Definitive treatment of malignant polyps of the colon. *Ann Surg* 1975; 182:516–525.
26. Lockart-Mummery HE, Dukes CE: The surgical treatment of malignant rectal polyps. *Lancet* 1952; 2:751–755.
27. Scarborough RA: The relationship between polyps and carcinoma of the colon and rectum. *Dis Colon Rectum* 1960; 3:336–342.
28. Carden ABG, Morson BC: Recurrence after local excision of malignant polyps of the rectum. *Proc R Soc Med* 1964; 57:559–561.
29. Coutsoftides T, Sivak MV, Benjamin SP, et al: Colonoscopy and the management of polyps containing invasive cancer. *Ann Surg* 1978; 188:638–641.
30. Rossini FP, Ferrari A, Spandrte M, et al: Closcopic polypectomy in diagnosis and management of cancerous adenomas: An individual and multicentric experience. *Endoscopy* 1982; 14:124–127.
31. Wilcox GM, Beck JR: Early invasive cancer in adenomatous colonic polyps (malignant polyps). Evaluation of the therapeutic options by decision analysis. *Gastroenterology* 1987; 92:1159–1168.
32. Welch CE, Malt RA: Abdominal surgery. *N Engl J Med* 1979; 300:705–712.
33. Boyd JB, Bradford B, Watne AL: Operative risk factors of colon resection in the elderly. *Ann Surg* 1980; 192:743–746.
34. Hobler KE: Colon surgery for cancer in the very elderly. Cost and 3-year survival. *Ann Surg* 1986; 203:129–131.

47

Nontoxic Megacolon:
Is endoscopic therapy appropriate?

JAMIE S. BARKIN, M.D., F.A.C.P., F.A.C.G.
IRA AGATSTEIN, M.D.

Colonic pseudo-obstruction (CPO), or Ogilvie's syndrome, is a form of colonic ileus. It is characterized by an adynamic, dilated, unobstructed colon. The key to the successful treatment of this condition is early recognition and exclusion of mechanical obstruction.

ETIOLOGY

The mechanism has remained elusive since Ogilvie's original description of malignant invasion of the prevertebral ganglia causing CPO. Many underlying illnesses have been associated with colonic pseudo-obstruction; Table 47–1 lists the possible associations.[1] An alteration of the autonomic innervation of the colon may be the common pathway by which these entities cause CPO. This hypothesis is supported by the fact that both clonidine and epidural anesthesia, which can result in CPO, are sympatholytic. Another contributing factor may be the presence of a large populace of anaerobic intestinal microflora. The presence of anaerobes is believed to be the etiology of the CPO occurring as a late complication of jejunoileal bypass.[2] In a random sequence, double-blind crossover study of patients with CPO after jejunoileal bypass, it was reported that antibiotics that decreased the anaerobic flora resulted in clinical improvement.[3]

PHYSICAL FINDINGS

Abdominal distention is present in virtually all patients. This may occur gradually over a few days, although in some patients there may be rapid distention within a 24-hour period. Bowel sounds are usually normal, but may be high-pitched. However, the presence of high-pitched tinkles should suggest mechanical obstruction.

Abdominal tenderness is usually absent; however, mild tenderness may be felt in the right lower quadrant. Peritoneal signs suggests cecal perforation.

The sudden development of fever or tachycardia must alert one to possible intestinal necrosis.

X-RAY FINDING

A gas-filled colon without fluid levels, often with an abrupt cut-off of distention in the gas pattern at the hepatic, splenic, or sigmoid flexures, is highly suggestive of CPO. A barium enema that does not demonstrate an obstruction has been used in the past to confirm this entity. Once barium reaches the dilated colon without evidence of distal mechanical obstruction, the examination should be terminated.[4] However, in the appropriate clinical setting with abdominal x-rays that are highly suggestive of CPO, a barium enema may

TABLE 47–1.
Underlying Illnesses in Patients with Colonic Pseudo-obstruction*

1. *Cardiovascular*
   Myocardial infarction
   Congestive heart failure
   Retroperitoneal hemorrhage
   Mesenteric thrombosis or insufficiency
2. *Drug/Toxic*
   Analgesics
   Phenothiazines
   Clonidine
   Anti-parkinsonian drugs
   Lead poisoning
   Anticholinergics
   Monoamine oxidase inhibitors
3. *Infectious/Inflammatory*
   Appendicitis
   Cholecystitis
   Gastritis
   Pancreatitis
   Pelvic abscess
   Peptic ulcer disease
   Pneumonia
   Sepsis
   Burns
4. *Malignant*
   Leukemia (chemotherapy?)
   Retroperitoneal metastases
5. *Metabolic*
   Alcoholism
   Electrolyte abnormalities esp. hypokalemia
   Thermal injury
	6. *Neurologic*
	   Epidural anesthesia
	   Post myelogram
	   Multiple sclerosis
	   Parkinson's disease
	   Spinal cord injury
	   Cerebrovascular disease
	7. *Obstetric/Gynecologic*
	   Cesarean section
	   Gynecologic surgery
	   Vaginal delivery
	   Intracavitary radiation
	8. *Surgical*
	   Intra-abdominal surgery
	9. *Urinary Tract*
	   Renal failure
	   Urinary calculus
	10. *Orthopedic*
	   Fractures—pelvic, hip
	   Hip surgery including pinning
	11. *Idiopathic*

*Modified from Romeo D, Solomon GD, Hover AR: Acute colonic pseudo-obstruction: A possible role for the colocolonic reflex. *J Clin Gastroenterol* 1985; 7(3):256.

not be desirable, because it will only serve to inhibit endoscopic visualization and delay endoscopic therapy. If, however, the area of dilatation is not reached by the endoscopist, a barium study should be done to rule out mechanical obstruction.

We need to direct our attention to the cecum when looking at abdominal radiographs in patients with suspected CPO, because it is the most likely site of colonic perforation. This is because of its large diameter, and, as shown by Kozarek and Sanowski, the cecum requires the least amount of pressure to cause perforation.[5] The exact diameter at which cecal perforation will occur is unknown. However, the usual cecal diameter is below 7.5 cm, and when the diameter exceeds 12 cm, there is a significant risk of complications.[6] Unfortunately, using only cecal diameter as an indicator of impending perforation is fraught with uncertainty, and other authors have advocated using cecal diameters of between 14 and 16.5 cm as the critical point at which operative decompression is warranted.[7] Patients with considerable small-intestine distention, in addition to that of large bowel, seem to tolerate the distention better than those without small-intestine distention.[8] This may be due to partial decompression of the colon by an incompetent ileocecal valve, thus avoiding a "closed-loop" situation. However, the small bowel distention may just be a reflection of aerophagia. Abdominal flat and upright x-rays should be obtained at 12-hour intervals when the patient is initially seen and at

24-hour intervals when the patient is stable and the cecal diameter is decreasing or following therapy. This is mandatory because it is the only method that allows us to assess progression prior to perforation.

PROGNOSIS

In most patients, recovery is the rule if complications of CPO are avoided and the underlying illness is reversed.[1] The serious consequences that occur if it is not recognized early and vigorous therapy is not instituted are related to progressive dilation of the cecum. As dilation increases, serosal splitting of the tenial coli ensues, followed by the development of mucosal ischemia, leading to areas of gangrene and infarction which may progress to perforation. The point at which cecal distention culminates in perforation depends on a number of factors including the rapidity of dilation, systemic circulatory support, and oxygenation of tissue.[9] A mortality of 25% to 40% is usually associated with cecal perforation.[10]

THERAPY

The therapeutic approach to the patient with CPO is best described in three levels of care.[11] Level I is general supportive measures to eliminate, when possible, the underlying etiology. Level II is colonoscopic and radiologic guided decompression. Level III is surgical intervention. The overlying theme is effective colonic decompression to prevent colonic perforation with its attendant high morbidity and mortality.

Level I

Proper fluid and electrolyte balance should be achieved, and the patient should be kept npo with nasogastric suction. Contributing drugs (i.e., narcotics, clonidine, thorazine, and anticholinergic agents) should be discontinued, and, theoretically, neostigmine should be given,[12] although this is not proven. In addition, there should be recognition and correction of hyponatremia and hypokalemia. Hypomagnesemia was found in 60% of patients as reported by Nano.[13] Proctosigmoidoscopy should be performed to rule out mechanical causes of obstruction. Preparation for this procedure should include enemas to eliminate the formed stool in the rectum and distal colon (see section entitled "Preparation for Colonoscopy").

The role of antibiotic therapy is controversial; it seems prudent, however, to initiate early antibiotic coverage with an anerobic spectrum. This belief is supported by studies in patients with CPO following jejunoileal bypass.[2,3]

Hubbard has found mobilization and, particularly, frequent turning of the patient to be helpful.[14] This concept has been used for management of the patient with toxic megacolon.

Level II

Therapy at this stage consists primarily of endoscopic decompression. There is an obvious advantage to colonoscopic decompression versus laparotomy, because it avoids opening the bowel with the risk of contamination by bacteria into the peritoneum. It is unclear exactly when endoscopic therapy should be instituted, but it would seem reasonable that if level I therapy is unsuccessful after 12 hours, endoscopic therapy should begin, because these techniques can prove effective only before mucosal ischemia and necrosis occur. This conclusion is supported by the observation that decompression of the colon has been shown to facilitate blood circulation to the colon and possibly also initiate colonic peristalsis to prevent recurrence of this condition.[15] If the initial evaluation of the patient reveals that cecal dilatation is greater than 12 cm, it is reasonable to initially use both supportive level I and endoscopic level II therapy.[16] Colonoscopy is contraindicated if bowel perforation or necrosis has occurred. While the former can be found on x-ray, clinical diagnosis of the latter is very difficult, because the markedly distended cecum may be very tender to palpation.

Preparation for Colonoscopy

Most authors recommend no specific bowel preparation prior to attempted colonoscopic decompression, because the colon is dilated and the fecal material beyond the sigmoid colon is usually liquid. The colonoscope can be advanced above the fecal–air interface. Preparation with tap-water enemas allows the evacuation of solid material in the rectosigmoid as well as making the remaining stool in the distal part of colon liquid and therefore easier to aspirate.[16]

Technique of Colonoscopy

The scope is passed above the fecal–air interface keeping the lumen in view, and the smallest amount of air possible is inserted to visualize the lumen. Most air insertion will take place when the colonoscope is in the left colon, and because there is colonic dilatation in the transverse colon, very small amounts of air will be needed in this area. Colonoscopic visualization of mucosal necrosis or ulceration is a sign of impending cecal perforation.[17] If any ischemic or gangrenous mucosa is found during the procedure, the procedure should be terminated and surgery should be planned.[16]

When the ascending colon is reached, an attempt should be made to visualize the entire cecal mucosa to look for ulceration and/or gangrene.[18] The area in the cecum that must be visualized is the antimesenteric aspect of the anterior colonic wall, because this is the site at which cecal perforation will most likely occur.[17] Thereafter, slowly withdraw the colonoscope while keeping the lumen in view and using suction to remove both air and fluid contents. Frequent irrigation is usually necessary to maintain good visibility.

It has been suggested that it is advisable to use CO_2 for insufflation instead of air. The rationale is that as air is replaced by the CO_2 further decompression of the colon occurs when the CO_2 is absorbed from the lumen of the bowel.[18] Further studies will be needed to confirm this.

How Far Do We Proceed at Colonoscopy?

It seems prudent to proceed as proximal as possible toward the cecum. This allows visualization of the cecum to determine if colonic ulcerations (ischemic areas) are present and to definitely exclude mechanical causes of obstruction. Cecal decompression may at times be accomplished by suction through the colonoscope or by tube placement with suction in the transverse colon.[20] Unfortunately, this has not been successful in other patients.[7] Fausel found that gross decompression of abdominal distention could not be achieved until the colonoscope was passed beyond the hepatic flexure.[11]

Comparison of Treatment Modalities

Fausel and Goff compared the levels of treatment needed in 35 episodes of CPO.[11] Twelve episodes responded to level I treatment; however, three recurred. One of these three occurrences responded again to level I therapy. In summary, 10 of 12 episodes required only level I care.

Twelve patients underwent colonoscopic decompression; nine were successfully treated. Symptoms recurred in three. One patient had resolution with a second colonoscopy; one had a technically unsuccessful repeat colonoscopy; the third patient was successfully decompressed a second time, but symptoms recurred and surgery was necessary.

What is the Initial Effectiveness of Colonoscopic Depression?

Overall, when reported series are combined, colonoscopic decompression is initially successful in 80% of patients with

CPO.[21, 22] The reasons for failure are exemplified in the series of patients reported by Nivatvongs. Of three unsuccessful colonoscopic decompressions, two were because of technical reasons that precluded successful colonoscopy (i.e., presence of stool and a fixed colon secondary to metastasis), and the third was because of the presence of colonic gangrene.[20]

Should Repeat Colonoscopy Be Performed for Recurrence?

Initial colonoscopy may not successfully decompress the cecum, and repeat colonoscopy may be necessary.[7] When reported studies are combined, 17% of patients had an unsuccessful initial decompression. In this combined series, 18 patients had recurrences of CPO which was successfully treated, however 9 of the 18 had a second or additional colonoscopy. Colonoscopic decompression of CPO appears to be associated with a significant recurrence rate after initial successful colonoscopic decompression.[7] Therefore, even when obstruction is relieved, the patient must be followed carefully by serial abdominal x-rays and continued medical management to be sure the obstruction does not recur.

In this combined series definitive treatment by colonoscopic decompression was obtained in approximately 75% of patients.[21]

Is Colonoscopy in the Distended Colon Dangerous?

Overall, in the combined series, which totalled 105 patients, there was a 2% complication rate. This is in the range of the perforation rate of 0.2% to 2% that occurs during diagnostic colonoscopy.

Colonoscopic damage may not result in frank perforation, and although the true incidence of this damage is unknown in three patients who had previously undergone unsuccessful colonoscopic decompression and who underwent laparotomy, no colonoscopic complications were seen.[23]

Should Endoscopic Catheter or Tube Placement Be Used for Continued Drainage?

Although colonoscopy has provided us with an effective means of treating patients with CPO, approximately 20% of initial treatments are unsuccessful and 18% of patients have recurrence of disease. This has led to additions to colonoscopy with the aim of increasing its initial effectiveness and preventing recurrences. The initial modification was catheter or tube placement for continued decompression. Bernton and co-workers modified a 16 Baker jejunostomy tube with an inflatable balloon at its tip by sewing four 1-inch loops of 1.0 silk suture along the distal 12 inches of the tube at 3-inch intervals.[24] In addition more drainage points were cut in the tube. The distal silk loop is grasped with a colonoscopic biopsy forceps which is withdrawn into the endoscope, and the tube and colonoscope are passed together. Upon entry to the ascending colon the tube is pushed ahead of the colonoscope, the balloon is inflated, and the colonoscope alone is withdrawn. This can be fluoroscopically confirmed. The tube is connected to gravity drainage with a gas vent. Positioning a long Baker tube in the cecum allows for continuous decompression and time for causative illness to resolve. Depending on the nature of the contents evacuated, frequent irrigation may be required to maintain patency. Groff has used a salem sump instead of a Baker tube and a double-channel colonoscope so that suction continues while one channel is blocked by the biopsy forceps.[25] Kozarek has used this type of tube with continued success (personal communication). If only a single-channel colonoscope is available, tube placement can be via a Seldinger technique. Once the colonoscope has reached the desired location, a 0.052 flexible-tip guidewire is placed through the biopsy channel and the colonoscope is withdrawn (using fluoroscopic guidance to assure that the wire remains in situ), a nasogastric tube is passed over the wire with fluoroscopic guidance (H. Parker, personal communication) or a commercially available cecal decompression tube. The wire is withdrawn, and the tube is taped to the buttocks to maintain its location. We are uncertain, however, whether tube placement subsequent to colonoscopic decompression is advantageous, because Nano found no difference between recurrent rates in those patients who underwent colonoscopic decompression solely versus those who underwent colonoscopic decompression with tube placement.[13] The failure of tube placement to make a difference may be due to technical factors such as tube obstruction or displacement.

Ponsky and co-workers obtained effective decompression in two patients by applying the principles of percutaneous gastrostomy to the colon, performing a percutaneous, endoscopically guided cecostomy.[26] This technique provides a large-caliber tube cecostomy, which is effective in providing and maintaining colonic decompression.

Radiologic Methods for Decompression

Nonoperative percutaneous needle decompression of the colon in a patient with CPO has been reported by Crass.[27] This technique offers an alternative therapeutic approach for the patient in whom colonoscopy is technically unsuccessful. CT-guided needle aspiration was successfully performed, using a posterior (retroperitoneal) approach to avoid spillage of colonic contents into the peritoneal cavity.

Level III

Level III consists of surgical cecostomy or resection. The former will probably be used less frequently as endoscopic and possibly radiologic methods are applied more liberally. Surgical exploration is indicated in the presence of peritoneal signs or x-ray evidence of perforation, including free intra-abdominal air or air in the colon wall. Surgical mortality in these compromised patients ranges from 24% to 46%.[23]

CONCLUSIONS

1. Initial colonoscopic decompression can be accomplished in 80% of patients with CPO, with only moderate difficulty.
2. Definitive treatment can be provided by colonoscopy in 75% of patients.
3. Colonoscopic decompression is not associated with significant morbidity or mortality.
4. Colonoscopic decompression may avoid laparotomy in severely ill patients.
5. Colonoscopy can identify those patients with impending perforation.

References

1. Romeo PR, Solomon GD, Hover AR: Acute colonic pseudo-obstruction: A possible role for the colocolonic reflex. *J Clin Gastroenterol* 1985; 7(3):256–260.
2. Barry RE, Benfield P, Nicell P, et al: Colonic pseudo-obstruction: A new complication of jejunoileal bypass. *Gut* 1975; 16:903–908.
3. Barry RE, Chow AW, Billesdon J, et al: Colonic pseudo-obstruction complicating jejuno-ileal bypass: The role of intestinal flora. *Gut* 1975; 16(10):825.
4. Fletcher JP, Little JM: Intestinal pseudo-obstruction. *Med J Aust* 1979; 2:339–341.
5. Kozarek RA, Sanowski RA: Use of pressure release valve to prevent colonic injury during colonoscopy. *Gastrointest Endosc* 1980; 26(4):139–142.
6. Terhune DW, Petrochko N Jr, Jordan GH, et al: Ogilvie's syndrome developing after ethanol ablation of renal cell carcinoma. *J Urol* 1985; 133:838–839.
7. Geelhoed GW: Colonic pseudo-obstruction in surgical patients. *Am J Surg* 1985; 149:258–265.
8. Lescher TJ, Teegarden DK, Pruitt BA Jr: Acute pseudo-obstruction of the colon in thermally injured patients. *Dis Colon Rectum* 21(8):618–622.
9. Spira IA, Wolff WI: Colonic pseudo-obstruction following termination of pregnancy and uterine operation. *Am J Obstet Gynecol* 1976; 126(1):7–12.
10. Nanni C, Garbini A, Luchetti P, et al: Ogilvie's syndrome (acute colonic pseudo-obstruction): Review of the literature (October 1948 to March 1980) and report of four additional cases. *Dis Colon Rectum* 1982; 25(1):157–166.
11. Fausel CS, Goff JS: Nonoperative management of acute idiopathic colonic pseudo-obstruction (Ogilvie's syndrome). *West J Med* 1985; 143:50–54.
12. Bardsley D: Pseudo-obstruction of the large bowel. *Br J Surg* 1974; 61:963–969.

13. Nano D, Prindiville T, Pauly M, et al: Colonoscopic therapy of acute pseudoobstruction of the colon. Am J Gastroenterol 1987; 82(2):145–148.
14. Hubbard CN: Correspondence. J Bone Joint Surg 1983; 65A(6):872.
15. Clayman RV, Reddy P, Nivatvongs S: Acute pseudo-obstruction of the colon: A serious consequence of urologic surgery. J Urol 1981; 126:415–417.
16. Nakhgevany KB: Colonoscopic decompression of the colon in patients with Ogilvie's syndrome. Am J Surg 1984; 148:317–320.
17. Strodel WE, Nostrant TT, Eckhauser FE, et al: Therapeutic and diagnostic colonoscopy in nonobstructive colonic dilatation. Ann Surg 1983; 4:416–421.
18. Spira IA, Wolff WI: Gangrene and spontaneous perforation of the cecum as a complication of pseudo-obstruction of the colon: Report of three cases and speculation as to etiology. Dis Colon Rectum 1976; 19(6):557–562.
19. Goedkoop KP, Verhagen PF: Acute pseudoobstruction of the colon (letter). Neth J Surg 1986; 38(6):192.
20. Nivatvongs S, Vermeulen FD, Fang DT: Colonoscopic decompression of acute pseudo-obstruction of the colon. Ann Surg 1982; 196(5):598–600.
21. Bode WE, Beart RW Jr, Spencer RJ, et al: Colonoscopic decompression for acute pseudo-obstruction of the colon (Ogilvie's syndrome). Report of 22 cases and review of the literature. Am J Surg 1984; 147:243–245.
22. Starling JR, Weese JL: Letter to the editor. Dis Colon Rectum 1984; 27(2):147.
23. Strodel WE, Dent TL, Nostrant TT, et al: Treatment alternatives in renal failure and renal transplantation patients with non-obstructive colonic dilatation. Transplantation 1983; 36:37–40.
24. Bernton E, Myers R, Reyna T: Pseudo-obstruction of the colon: Case report including a new endoscopic treatment. Gastrointest Endosc 1982; 28(2):90–92.
25. Groff W: Colonoscopic decompression and intubation of the cecum for Ogilvie's syndrome. Dis Colon Rectum 1983; 26(4):503–506.
26. Ponsky JL, Aszodi A, Perse D: Percutaneous endoscopic cecostomy: A new approach to nonobstructive colonic dilatation. Submitted for publication.
27. Crass JR, Simmons RL, Frick MP, et al: Percutaneous decompression of the colon using CT guidance in Ogilvie syndrome. AJR 1985; 144:475–476.

48

Sigmoid Volvulus:
Is it a difficult twist to manage?

KEVIN P. MORRISSEY, M.D.

For the first half of the 20th century, acute sigmoid volvulus was a surgical emergency. Early surgery in excellent hands saved the lives of 85% of patients with a viable colon, whereas patients with a gangrenous colon as a consequence of delay in diagnosis or surgery faced up to a 50% operative mortality.

In 1947 Bruusgaard reported his experience with nonoperative decompression of the colon by proctoscopy in 91 patients with sigmoid volvulus.[1] This report of a 90% success rate with a dramatic drop in mortality figures to 2.9%, established the role of endoscopic decompression for the vast majority of cases of acute sigmoid volvulus. Many subsequent reports confirmed Bruusgaard's experience and provided valuable data on the natural history of nonoperatively treated patients, as well as of those subsequently operated upon electively.[2-7]

The development of flexible colonoscopy from 1970 to the present and the popularization of the flexible sigmoidoscope over the past 8 years might be expected to further modify the endoscopic approach to volvulus. Currently, the initial, emergent treatment modality for acute sigmoid volvulus continues to be an attempt at endoscopic decompression of the twisted obstructed sigmoid loop. If this fails, emergency exploratory laparotomy is necessary. The real problem in the management of acute sigmoid volvulus is not the "difficult twist" requiring special expertise in endoscopic manipulation, but rather the conceptual approach to the overall management of this life-threatening condition, which so often strikes the elderly, debilitated, high-risk patient.

This problem has been heightened in recent years by the passage of many gastrointestinal emergencies, formerly triaged to surgery, into the hands of gastroenterologists and the inpatient medical service. Although internists have long cooperated with surgeons in the emergent care of patients with such GI emergencies as bleeding peptic ulcer, obstructive jaundice, and toxic megacolon, they have had little experience in the total care of intestinal volvulus, particularly the decision for surgery. Until gastroenterologists familiarize themselves with the natural history of volvulus, best found in the surgical literature, careful consideration of surgery may be neglected, and definitive surgical correction of volvulus may not often enough follow upon its emergent decompression.

The management of sigmoid volvulus can be divided into three stages: diagnosis, initial endoscopic management, and definitive treatment. This chapter will focus on the technique and short-term results of endoscopic decompression, in the context of the total management of the patient.

DIAGNOSIS

There are major variations in the incidence, pathogenesis, and clinical patterns of volvulus around the world. These have been collectively reviewed in a series of reports by Ballantyne and co-workers.[3, 8–10] In most Western countries, acute sigmoid volvulus commonly presents as diffuse abdominal distention, often in elderly, chronically ill patients confined to bed or in nursing homes. It may also strike generally healthy individuals within a broad age range (30 to 80 years) who have only a long history of constipation and laxative use or require constipating medication for neuropsychiatric conditions such as Parkinson's disease and depression.

Some patients may be able to give a clearly interpretable history of antecedent attacks of volvulus, and one should always ask for it because nonsurgically treated volvulus carries a greater than 60% recurrence rate. Other patients, without realizing it, may have been spontaneously decompressing less severe attacks of partial volvulus in the past. These latter patients usually admit to a long history of constipation, occasionally punctuated by episodic, explosive bowel movements with relief of the obstipation and distention; or they may give a history of diarrhea, denoting partial large bowel obstruction and possibly colonic bacterial overgrowth, in the weeks preceding an attack of complete obstruction from volvulus.

The major and frequently only sign of early volvulus may be moderate to massive abdominal distention with obstipation. Abdominal pain may not occur at all or may not be very remarkable in the elderly, chronically constipated person. In the younger individual with stronger peristaltic activity or a tight sigmoid twist of 360 degrees or more, there may be significant pain accompanied by nausea, vomiting, and, before long, signs of dehydration and third-spacing of extracellular fluid volume. Rarely is the degree of abdominal distention so great that diaphragmatic elevation compromises respiration with production of a respiratory acidosis; if there is accompanying dehydration, one may see hypotension and metabolic acidosis as well. We have witnessed this dramatic sequence unfold in a woman who appeared agonal, but whose condition was immediately reversed by bedside endoscopic decompression (Fig 48–1).

The history and physical exam are usually sufficient to distinguish between mechanical small-bowel obstruction and conditions producing large-bowel distention. However, one may not as easily distinguish volvulus from other processes involving the large bowel, such as diffuse colonic ileus or an obstructing rectosigmoid carcinoma. The plain abdominal film alone is diagnostic in 40% to 60% of patients with sigmoid volvulus.[6] Rigid sigmoidoscopy can also be expected to confirm a diagnosis of volvulus in approximately 60% to 70% of affected patients. However, if volvulus or a rectosigmoid neoplasm is not the cause of the distention, the procedure is not diagnostic; when the volvulus occurs higher in the sigmoid (an estimated 24% of cases[11]), sigmoidoscopy yields a dangerous false-negative result with the risk of delayed diagnosis, bowel gangrene, and a significantly higher patient mortality.

Some states of colonic ileus so closely mimic sigmoid volvulus, often including some degree of torsion of the hugely distended colon, that it may not be possible to tell endoscopically whether one has bypassed a true obstructing twist of the bowel, or just rounded an area of angulation in a colonic ileus. Although satisfactory temporary decompression may be achieved by endoscopy alone in either ileus or volvulus, a clear diagnosis may not have been made, and an inappropriate definitive treatment may have been advised. The difficulties in making the correct diagnosis of mechanical large-bowel obstruction versus ileus without use of contrast radiography are clearly documented in a paper by Stewart.[12]

Whenever the clinical situation permits, we favor confirming the suspected diagnosis of sigmoid volvulus by a water-soluble contrast (Gastrograffin) enema. It takes but a few minutes to perform the x-ray. Even without any preparatory enemas, the gross demonstration of a point of sigmoid or rectosigmoid obstruction is usually enough to distinguish volvulus from a carcinoma, while the demonstration of unobstructed flow of contrast media higher into the colon rules out sigmoid volvulus and points toward a nonmechanical form of colonic inertia.

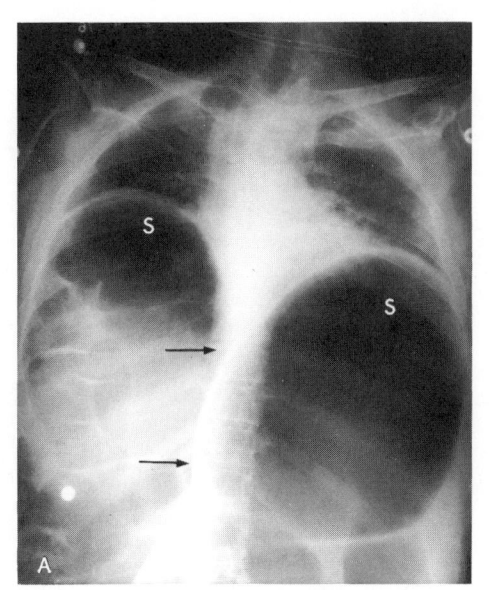

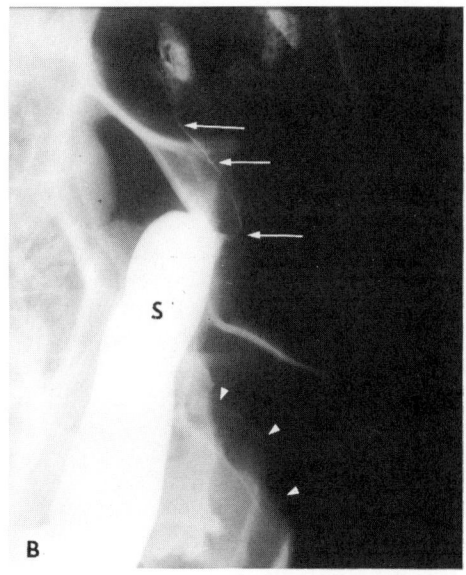

FIG 48–1.
A, massive colonic dilatation pushing up the diaphragm in a 64-year-old female with a history of prior volvulus operatively detorted, presented again with volvulus, respiratory acidosis and shock. Bedside colonoscopy immediately relieved the crisis. **B,** same patient's barium enema days later, demonstrating persistent twisted, partially obstructed segment *(arrows).* Repeat colonoscopic decompression was necessary. Elective sigmoid resection 2 weeks later was without complication or recurrence of volvulus. S = sigmoid distal to the obstructed segment pointed to by the arrows. The arrowheads outline the iliac crest. S = sigmoid colon abutting diaphragm; arrows outline the interface between the two limbs of sigmoid loop.

Rarely have our radiologists needed to instill barium instead of water-soluble contrast media in order to make a working diagnosis. Barium hinders subsequent colonoscopic decompression, either for sigmoid volvulus or a colonic ileus, whereas Gastrograffin does not. Gastrograffin is also a good stimulus to distal bowel evacuation prior to colonoscopy, and, as in one of our patients, occasionally may bring about partial decompression of the twisted segment of bowel.

There are situations in which diagnostic maneuvers such as contrast x-ray and endoscopy may not be indicated or will only dangerously delay appropriate treatment. The clinical progression of symptomatic volvulus may be insidious and far advanced, particularly in a patient in a nursing home or a bedridden elderly patient living alone. In these instances, when bowel viability is often already compromised, overall mortality is greatly increased at the time of suspected diagnosis.[13] The initial management should bypass usual diagnostic maneuvers and center on cardiorespiratory and fluid resuscitation of the patient, followed immediately by either an emergency room or bedside attempt at endoscopic decompression and/or exploratory laparotomy. In patients in whom gangrenous obstruction may have set in, endoscopic decompression may be impossible, or, even if successful, may be ultimately fruitless because of the finding of significant mucosal ischemia. Even in the unlikely event that such a bowel could be decompressed, emergency laparotomy, sigmoid resection, and colostomy are still indicated, because the risk of subsequent sepsis and death is high.

INITIAL ENDOSCOPIC MANAGEMENT

Once the suspected diagnosis of volvulus is confirmed by plain film or contrast x-ray, in the more usual setting in which the distended patient is not toxic or in danger of cardiovascular collapse, an attempt at endoscopic decompression of the twisted loop should be carried out promptly. A number of classic studies have clearly demonstrated that endoscopic decompression with the rigid sigmoidoscope is successful in 85% of cases and carries less than a 3% mortality rate.[1, 2, 4] This is in contrast to a 40% mortality rate following emergency surgery of any sort without prior endoscopic decompression and time for mechanical bowel preparation.

Results of Colonoscopic Decompression

Currently there are only sparse data regarding decompression of sigmoid volvulus with flexible endoscopes. There are scattered case reports[14-17] and a few larger series.[11, 17-19] Starling has reported successful decompression in eight out of eight patients.[18] Brothers and co-workers recently reported success in five of eight attempts.[11] Arigbabu has accumulated a series of 92 cases in Nigeria where sigmoid volvulus is the most common cause of large bowel obstruction. Colonoscopic decompression was successful in all but nine cases in which ischemic changes of strangulation were found and colonoscopy was abandoned for emergency surgery.[19]

Our experience at New York Hospital-Cornell Medical Center from 1976 to 1987 is summarized in Table 48–1. In 12 of the 14 patients (86%), colonoscopy was successful 19 out of 22 times for primary or recurrent volvulus. There were no major complications or deaths. The three patient failures were by insufficiently experienced endoscopists; one of these patients had been successfully decompressed previously by another endoscopist. By chance, none of the patients in our series had evidence of irreversible ischemic change, although mild changes—edema, erythema, hyperemia, congestion, and focal erosions—were noted in 7 of the 14 patients. During the same time period at our institution, at least two cases of unsuccessful rigid sigmoidoscopy not in this series were found at surgery to have strangulating obstruction. Another patient presenting with volvulus was so toxic that endoscopic decompression was not even attempted. Gangrenous bowel was also found at operation.

Further analysis of our series of colonoscopic decompression for sigmoid volvulus revealed (Table 48–1) that rigid sigmoidoscopy had initially been attempted ten times in nine patients but failed in seven of them. A subsequent attempt at colonoscopic decompression was success-

TABLE 48–1
Endoscopic Decompression in 14 Patients with Sigmoid Volvulus

	Success		Failure		Recurrence	
	Patients	%	Patients	%	Patients	%
Rigid Sigmoidoscopy (RS)						
9 Primary procedures	2	22	7	78	2	100
1 Secondary procedure			1	100		
Flexible colonoscopy (FC)						
5 Primary procedures	5	100			2	40
17 Secondary procedures	8	73	3	27	7	88
2 After successful RS	2	100			2	50
7 After failed RS	5	71	2	29	5*	100
8 After successful FC	6	86	1	14	6*	100
Total of 14 patients	12	86	2	14	8	67
Total of 22 colonoscopies	(19/22)	86	(3/22)	14	(9/19)	47

*One patient's volvulus could not be decompressed by rigid sigmoidoscopy and recurred twice following colonoscopic decompression. A rectal tube had not been passed.

ful in five of the seven failures (71%). Some of these successes were undoubtedly due to the longer length of the colonoscope and its ability to reach a point of torsion beyond the length of the rigid instrument. However, our success rate of 28.5% with the rigid instrument is misleadingly low. This is only partly due to house officer inexperience in rigid sigmoidoscopy. The majority of patients presenting with volvulus during this time period are not contained in this series, and of the cases available for review, 14 out of 22 were successfully decompressed by the proctoscope. Starling in his series also noted that five of his eight patients successfully decompressed with the colonoscope had failed rigid sigmoidoscopy,[18] while Brothers and co-workers noted similar failure with the rigid instrument in 9 of 21 attempts.[11]

There was a very high recurrent rate of volvulus averaging 67% regardless of whether rigid or flexible endoscopy was successful in decompressing the colon. This is consistent with data reported by others for recurrence during the same hospitalization[5,6] and underscores two important points stressed by Aufses (in his invited commentary on Welch and Anderson's paper[6] and Boley[13]: (1) endoscopic decompression is only a temporizing maneuver, whose effectiveness can be prolonged by passage of a long rectal tube at the completion of the endoscopic procedure, and (2) the long-term recurrence rates of simply decompressed sigmoid volvulus are probably much higher than 60%.

Technique of Endoscopic Decompression

In my experience, decompression of sigmoid volvulus with flexible instruments has been technically easy and uniformly successful when carried out by an experienced endoscopist. The preliminary gastrograffin enema usually provides adequate distal bowel preparation for visualization of the volvulized segment. Sedation is generally not necessary. Gentle pressure against the point of extrinsic compression, as well as insufflation of small amounts of air and water to maintain visibility are usually all that are necessary to pass through the twisted segment, using direct advancement of the colonoscope shaft rather than a torqueing motion or sharply angulating the tip of the instrument with the tip controls. One may appreciate edema, hyperemia, and congestion in this narrowed segment, and immediately above it in the obstructed dilated sigmoid, a dark vast chamber with copious air and liquid stool puddling on one side of the lumen. The gas and liquid feces can be rapidly aspirated with immediate relief of the patient's symptoms of distention, abdominal tightness, and any respiratory difficulty.

Once the endoscope has been advanced into the distal twisted segment of sigmoid and symptoms are relieved, it is very tempting to try to pass further up the colon, beyond the proximal point of torsion (Fig 48–2, A) and then to attempt to detort or untwist the entire loop of volvulized sigmoid. This is a waste of time, needlessly risky and uncomfortable for the unsedated patient, and unnecessary, if not generally hard to do. We have tried to detort the entire segment in two patients and were unable to do so after over 30 minutes maneuvering in both instances. It is clear from reviewing the published reports of colonoscopic decompression of sigmoid volvulus that in most instances the sudden relief of symptoms was due to the decompression or release of gas and stool, and not to a change in the rotation of the colon. Moreover, none of the published accounts actually have documented by contrast x-ray a change in the pre- and postendoscopic configuration of the sigmoid.

It should be no surprise that one cannot reasonably hope to obtain or maintain a true detorsion of a sigmoid volvulus. Our operative series, as well as others', contains patients presenting with recurrent sigmoid volvulus in whom operative detorsion alone had been carried out years previously. At elective operation for volvulus, one often finds a shortened, scarred, and fixed sigmoid mesentery which rests easily in a partially twisted

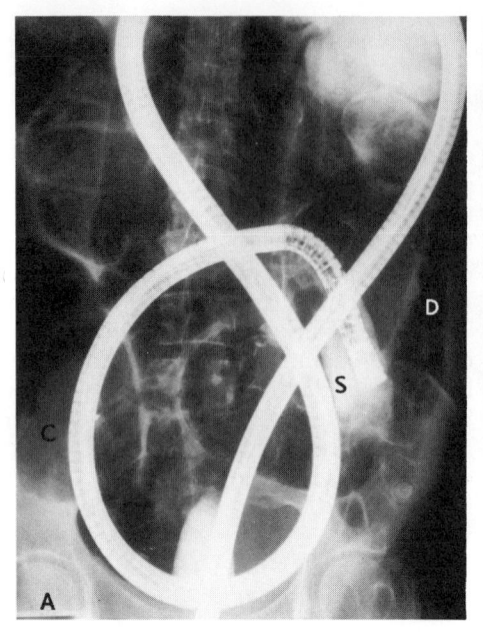

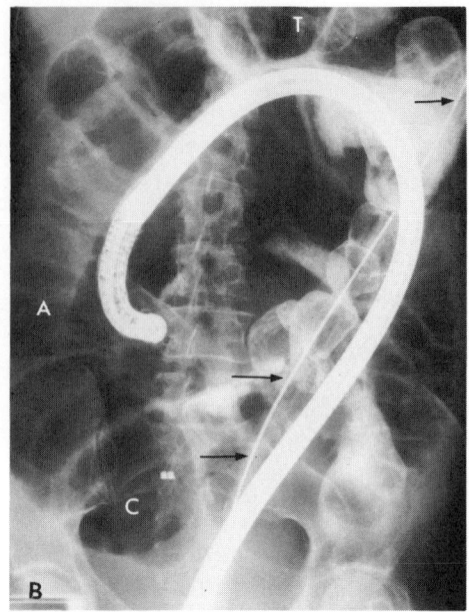

FIG 48–2.
A, sixty-year-old female colonoscoped after only partial decompression by rigid sigmoidoscopy. The colonoscope is swallowed up in the massive rigid sigmoidoscopy. The colonoscope is swallowed up in the massive sigmoid loop during an abortive attempt to pass beyond it into the descending colon and "detort" the twisted loop. **B,** same patient with colonoscope at adequate level of intubation to satisfactorily *decompress* the obstructed loop. A rectal tube has been advanced alongside the colonoscope into the distal sigmoid to maintain decompression, pending surgical resection. S = sigmoid; D = descending colon; T = transverse colon; A = ascending colon; C = cecum; arrows point to rectal tube.

state in the opened peritoneal cavity. The long loop of acutely distended bowel, filled with air and semisolid feces and crowded by other viscera, is quite immobile and resists the weak force moment of torque generated by the colonoscope in an attempt to rotate the giant sigmoid loop over a great arc and surface area within the closed peritoneal space. Even if one is lucky enough to partially or completely untwist the segment, the inevitable return of constipation with accumulation of air and stool again will generate a force moment strong enough to twist the bowel on its axis once more.

I believe that one can as easily accomplish a well-defined goal of sigmoid loop decompression by simply using a 60-cm flexible sigmoidoscope to decompress the distal segment. This instrument, in my hands, is far easier to handle and has a larger more useful suction channel than the colonoscope. There is no comparison in its ease of use over the rigid sigmoidoscope, with additional comfort to both the patient and the endoscopist, and far less chance of being hit in the face by an explosion of feces and flatus.

Passage of a rectal tube up into the decompressed segment of bowel is a particularly helpful maneuver. Review of our data shows that in several cases in which this was not done, repeat endoscopic decompression was necessary from 2 to 8 days after the initial procedure. The reported series of decompression with the rigid sigmoidoscope also note the value of placing a large caliber rectal tube at the conclusion of the procedure and leaving it as long as possible for the brief hospital interval between emergent decompression and elective surgery. In order to pass a rectal tube at the conclusion of colonoscopic decompression, one passes a guide wire down the endoscope channel, withdraws the instrument, and then passes a soft 26 to 30 F chest or rectal tube over the guide wire. The tube should be firmly taped to the perianal region or it will migrate distally and become ineffective. A plain film at the conclusion of the entire procedure, which takes about 15 to 30 minutes, will confirm the correct position of the tube (Fig 48–2, B).

Failure to immediately decompress the colon by endoscopy is an indication for emergency surgery. As noted above, we have not, in this series, encountered a situation in which significant vascular compromise was present. Such a state will not always permit endoscopic decompression or the opportunity to document the corresponding mucosal changes. If significant changes are noted suggestive of irreversible gangrene (e.g., bloody colonic contents, blue or black colonic mucosa), then immediate operation is advised, even if the sigmoid colon has been decompressed. In questionable cases, the patient must be observed very carefully over the next 12 to 24 hours, and repeat endoscopic visualization of the affected segment should be done to determine the progression or regression of ischemic changes in the sigmoid mucosa. Irreversible vascular compromise has been missed by surgeons at the time of operative detorsion of the sigmoid, without resection. Unless the condition is recognized and the patient is reoperated upon early, the patient's chances of dying increase manyfold.

It should be reiterated that some patients with sigmoid volvulus present with such an acute abdomen that the likelihood of strangulation is high. Constant and colicky abdominal pain, abdominal tenderness, and a palpable bowel loop are particularly suspicious symptoms and signs for infarction. Endoscopic decompression should not be done. Surgical consultation is indicated immediately.

DEFINITIVE TREATMENT

There appears to be less controversy now about the definitive treatment of sigmoid volvulus than 15 years ago when Arnold and Nance published their large series advocating elective resection only for good-risk patients.[2] The current recommendations are clear-cut in the younger or good-risk patient: initial endoscopic decompression, if possible, followed by elective bowel resection and anastomosis preferably within the same hospitalization. It is in the elderly, very high-risk patients that one has to individualize recommendations and more carefully weigh nonsurgical and various surgical options. The ease of nonoperative treatment by endoscopic decompression, and the overall high-risk population involved, with limited outlook on life, naturally led many physicians in the past to a policy of watchful waiting without definitive surgery. However, the high incidence rates of recurrent volvulus from 50% to over 80%, with corresponding mortality figures as high as 20%,[5,13] have induced most knowledgeable physicians to recommend elective sigmoid resection in most instances, as soon as the decompressed sigmoid colon and the patient's general condition can be optimally prepared for surgery.

Current mortality data for elective resection are as low as 5.6% to 8.5%.[3,7,13] Ballantyne has analyzed the results of all types of surgical therapy for sigmoid volvulus throughout the world and found that the major determinant of patient mortality is the viability of the colon. When the colon is viable, the mortality is 12.4%, whereas when the colon is gangrenous, the mortality is 52.8%, referred to as "the mortality of delay."[13]

In assessing the risks of surgery in the elderly, it is well to recall the tremendous evolution in intensive care unit management, and more accurate risk assessment, particularly of the elderly patient. One of our patients with severe ASCVD, CHF, and COPD as the setting for her acute volvulus was initially judged by her internist to be too high a risk for surgery. She sustained three recurrences of volvulus while awaiting transfer to a convalescent home but was fortunate enough to be successfully decompressed each time. She went on to survive a subtotal colectomy for her volvulus and three incidentally encountered colonic cancers from cecum to splenic flexure; and then survived a reoperation for small bowel obstruction from adhesions, finally going on to live another year in reasonable comfort before succumbing to metastatic colon cancer.

In our series of 14 patients endoscopically decompressed, the average age was 64 years, and 7 of the patients were 75 to 89 years of age. Thirteen patients were operated upon, 12 within the same hospitalization, and one 2 months later in England. One patient, an 84-year-old man, died at home of a massive myocardial infarction 1 month following sigmoid resection. There were no subsequent recurrences of volvulus or other major morbidity of surgical treatment except for two instances of small bowel obstruction requiring reoperation. Bak and Boley's recently reported experience with the treatment of sigmoid volvulus in elderly patients is the best analysis to date of the long-term consequences of nonoperative treatment—a 70% recurrence rate and a 21% mortality versus operative treatment with a 6.7% mortality and an acceptable 26% morbidity rate, the predominant complication being seven instances of mechanical bowel obstruction, four of which required reoperation.

For some aged, high-risk patients, or those with severely impaired mental function and no reasonable prospect of improved quality of life, more difficult decisions regarding definitive treatment or disposition will have to be made. Certainly, for some bedridden patients, a resection with end-sigmoid colostomy may well be preferable to anastomosis, and may actually facilitate daily nursing care in a home or institution. Some other patients should clearly not be subjected to surgery electively and a program of regular enemas or passage of a flatus tube at home or in an institution may be more humane management of an insoluble situation.

In summary, endoscopy is still the best mode of initial management of acute sigmoid volvulus. Recent data suggest that flexible limited colonoscopy is as efficacious and safe as rigid sigmoidoscopy in decompressing the obstructed sigmoid loop. As the practice of rigid endoscopy wanes, one may expect that flexible sigmoidoscopy will supplant its emergent role in volvulus. However, it remains a temporizing maneuver which should be followed by definitive surgical resection in the vast majority of cases.

References

1. Bruusgaard C: Volvulus of the sigmoid colon and its treatment. *Surgery* 1947; 22:466–478.
2. Arnold GJ, Nance FC: Volvulus of the sigmoid colon. *Ann Surg* 1973; 177:527–537.
3. Ballantyne GH: Review of sigmoid volvulus: History and results of therapy. *Dis Colon Rectum* 1982; 25:494–501.
4. Drapanas T, Stewart JD: Acute sigmoid volvulus: Concepts in surgical treatment. *Am J Surg* 1961; 101:70–77.
5. Hines JR, Geurkink RE, Bass RT: Recurrence and mortality rate in sigmoid volvulus. *Surg Gynecol Obstet* 1967; 124:567–570.
6. Welch GH, Anderson JR: Acute volvulus of the sigmoid colon. *World J Surg* 1987; 11:258–262.
7. Wertkin MG, Aufses AH: Management of volvulus of the colon. *Dis Colon Rectum* 1978; 21:40–45.
8. Ballantyne GH, Brandner MD, Beart RW, et al: Volvulus of the colon: Incidence and mortality. *Ann Surg* 1985; 202:83–92.
9. Ballantyne GH: Review of sigmoid volvulus. *Clinical Patterns and Pathogenesis* 1982; 25:823–830.
10. Ballantyne GH: Sigmoid volvulus: High mortality in county hospital patients. *Dis Colon Rectum* 1981; 24:515–520.
11. Brothers TF, Strodel WE, Eckhauser FE: Endoscopy in colonic volvulus. *Ann Surg* 1987; 206:1–4.
12. Stewart PJ, et al: Does a water soluble contrast enema assist in the management of acute large bowel obstruction: A prospective study of 117 cases. *Br J Surg* 1984; 71:799–804.
13. Bak MP, Boley SJ: Sigmoid volvulus in elderly patients. *Am J Surg* 1986; 151:71–75.
14. Ghazi A, Shinya H, Wolff WI: Treatment of volvulus of the colon by colonoscopy. *Ann Surg* 1976; 183:236–265.
15. Biery DL, Hoffman SM: Colonoscopic reduction of sigmoid volvulus. *JAOA* 1977; 77:543–545.
16. Sanner CJ, Saltzman DA: Detorsion of sigmoid volvulus by colonoscopy. *Gastrointest Endosc* 1977; 23:212–213.
17. Starling JR: Initial treatment of sigmoid volvulus by colonoscopy. *Ann Surg* 1979; 190:36–39.
18. Starling JR: Treatment of the non-toxic megacolon by colonoscopy. *Surgery* 1983; 94:677–682.
19. Arigbabu AO, Badejo OA, Akinola DO: Colonoscopy in the emergency treatment of colonic volvulus in Nigeria. *Dis Colon Rectum* 1985; 11:795–798.

49

Endoscopic Sphincterotomy: When is it appropriate?

JEROME H. SIEGEL, M.D., F.A.C.P., F.A.C.G.

At the introduction of endoscopic sphincterotomy, controversy surrounded its use in the management of retained common bile duct stones and papillary stenosis.[1-6] In spite of the success of endoscopic sphincterotomy and the acceptable morbidity and mortality rates of this endoscopic procedure in the elderly or high-risk groups,[4-6] its use in younger patients with gallstone pancreatitis and in patients with intact gallbladders continues to stimulate discussion.[7,8] However, for those of us with large series and extensive experience, sphincterotomy performed in any of these patient groups has proven to be safe and effective with few long-term complications or recurrent disease.[9,10] After 15 years' experience with endoscopic sphincterotomy and nearly 60,000 procedures performed worldwide, cumulative data support the earlier impression that sphincterotomy is safer and more cost-effective than surgical exploration of the common bile duct. And enough evidence is available to show that endoscopic sphincterotomy is as therapeutically effective as surgery.[7-10] Therefore, sphincterotomy should no longer be a controversial issue in treating patients with retained common bile duct stones regardless of the age of the subject. My assignment then will be to discuss its use in patients with cholecystitis, cholangitis, and pancreatitis.

CHOLECYSTITIS

For the most part, patients presenting with cholecystitis are managed very effectively either conservatively (medically) or more aggressively (surgically). In most cases, the acute phase is safely managed with intravenous fluids and antibiotics with or without nasogastric suction. Surgical consultation should be obtained early in the course of presentation in the event of progression of the disease and imminent danger of perforation or hydrops. In most cases the initial evaluation of such an index patient includes routine blood work, ultrasonography, and cholescintigraphy (i.e., HIDA or Desida).[11-14] Endoscopic retrograde cholangiopancreatography (ERCP), in general, is infrequently employed in patients with cholecystitis unless the patient presents with cholestatic liver function tests and/or jaundice. When a patient presents with concomitant cholangitis, urgent performance of ERCP and sphincterotomy may be necessary. At ERCP, choledocholithiasis and, possibly, cholelithiasis may be confirmed. Whether cholelithiasis *will be* confirmed by ERCP depends on the patency of the cystic duct and whether or not contrast material can be forced into the cystic duct in a retrograde fashion to opacify that structure and the gallbladder.

In performing an ERCP in a patient

with an occluded cystic duct proven by scintigraphy, the endoscopist may attempt to dislodge the obstructing stone either by: (1) selectively cannulating the cystic duct and physically pushing the stone back into the gallbladder or (2) forcefully injecting contrast material into the cystic duct. Neither of these procedures can be relied on to successfully achieve its goal because selective cannulation of the cystic duct is arbitrary.

INTACT GALLBLADDER

Sphincterotomy for the treatment of common bile duct stones and coexisting cholelithiasis is gaining acceptance in this country as it has in Europe and Japan.[15-20] However, to my knowledge, few people, if any, are performing sphincterotomy for cholelithiasis alone. Satisfactory results of sphincterotomy for the treatment of choledocholithiasis and cholelithiasis have convinced most skeptics that an intact gallbladder after sphincterotomy is not a liability. In fact, in our own large combined series, Safrany and I reported long-term results that showed that sphincterotomy in patients with choledocholithiasis and cholelithiasis significantly reduces the annual incidence of cholecystitis.[21] These results certainly do not justify the performance of sphincterotomy for cholelithiasis alone, and its performance in such patients should be restricted to a rigid controlled trial under a strict investigational protocol conducted in a prospective, randomized fashion. Only then can an assessment of results be made and recommendations followed.

Even though I have stated that sphincterotomy is not indicated in patients with cholecystitis or cholelithiasis alone, ours and other data concerning sphincterotomy in patients with intact gallbladders may help to formulate a controlled trial of sphincterotomy in patients with cholelithiasis. Some patients in our series[22] had acalculous gallbladders and underwent sphincterotomy for the treatment of sphincter of Oddi dysfunction. These patients have been followed a minimum of 5 years without evidence of cholecystitis.

Published and unpublished data from Vennes' group may support a controlled trial of sphincterotomy for cholecystitis and/or cholelithiasis. In their published reports,[23, 24] Vennes and co-workers demonstrated that sphincterotomy actually prevented the formation of stones in prairie dogs fed a lithogenic diet. In that study only one animal in the sphincterotomized group formed stones while all but one animal in the sham sphincterotomy group formed stones. This study and the follow-up study in similar animals which were randomized for sphincterotomy and sphincterotomy with atropine support the hypothesis that loss of sphincter of Oddi function prevents gallstone formation. Vennes has also performed further studies in sphincterotomized prairie dogs in which glass beads were implanted in their gallbladders to determine the mechanism of disappearance of stones as well as the tolerance of the cystic duct. At last account, beads as large as 6 mm passed out of the animals' gallbladders supporting the hypothesis that sphincterotomy promotes emptying of the gallbladder.[25]

Even though data are available to support the hypothesis that sphincterotomy of the sphincter of Oddi may prove effective for gallbladder disease, the leaders in the field of ERCP and sphincterotomy should not advocate its performance before data from controlled trials can be evaluated. This proposed study will give us the opportunity of proving a hypothesis through established protocols rather than relying on retrospective data.

SPHINCTEROTOMY IN THE TREATMENT OF ACUTE, SUPPURATIVE CHOLANGITIS

For many years endoscopists have performed sphincterotomy in patients with cholangitis.[26-27] In most clinical situations, cholangitis, which is usually secondary to choledocholithiasis, responds to hydration, vasopressors, and antibiotics before ERCP is performed. However, before performing ERCP, one should attempt to stabilize the patient hemodynamically and to reduce the fever. Sphincterotomy and insertion of prostheses have been performed in emergency situations to provide immediate decompression of the biliary tree. My analogy to this clinical scenario is incision and drainage of an abscess. And, at ERCP, purulent effluent is usually seen on the papilla, and, after sphincterotomy, the duct spontaneously drains this purulent material. Following sphincterotomy and drainage, the clinical condition improves immediately.

Prior to the introduction of sphincterotomy, the only interventional therapy available for the treatment of cholangitis was surgery. Because of the tenuous clinical condition of many patients who underwent surgery, the morbidity and mortality rates were very high especially when patients were elderly with intercurrent medical problems.[28] The advent of percutaneous drainage techniques[29-32] did improve some of the complications associated with surgery, however, complications with the radiologic techniques also remain high in emergency situations.

Surprisingly, the morbidity and mortality of endoscopic techniques for the management of acute cholangitis have remained acceptably low. In a previous report in which we included all patients with cholangitis, acute-unstable, acute-stable, and subacute or resolving cholangitis, we successfully treated more than 900 patients who underwent ERCP, sphincterotomy, and/or placement of either a prosthesis or nasobiliary tube without a death or the need for emergency surgery.[27] The majority of these patients were stable (Fig 49-1), while 28% were considered to be acutely ill. As shown in the illustration, this latter group of patients was further subdivided into groups which were hemodynamically stable with fever and those who were unstable requiring vasopressors and antibiotics.

My approach to the treatment of patients with cholangitis who are acutely ill and unstable has been to attempt decompression using any acceptable endoscopic method (i.e., sphincterotomy with/or without prosthesis, insertion of a prosthesis and/or nasobiliary tube) (Fig 49-2). If patients are unstable and poor operative risks, I prefer to decompress the obstructed duct as expeditiously as possible. In addition, my philosophy is to be as conservative as determined by the patient's clinical condition. In other words, if the patient is too sick to undergo surgery, I prefer the conservative approach (prosthesis) to sphincterotomy to avoid

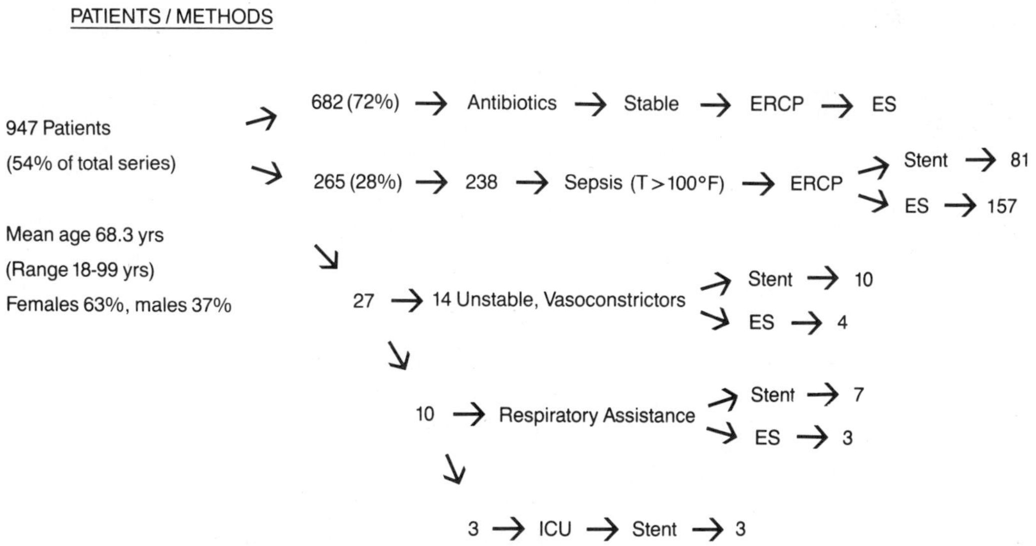

PATIENTS / METHODS

947 Patients
(54% of total series)

Mean age 68.3 yrs
(Range 18-99 yrs)
Females 63%, males 37%

→ 682 (72%) → Antibiotics → Stable → ERCP → ES

→ 265 (28%) → 238 → Sepsis (T > 100°F) → ERCP → Stent → 81
                                                    → ES → 157

↓
27 → 14 Unstable, Vasoconstrictors → Stent → 10
                                    → ES → 4
↓
10 → Respiratory Assistance → Stent → 7
                              → ES → 3
↓
3 → ICU → Stent → 3

FIG 49-1.
Distribution of 947 patients presenting with cholangitis, and methods of endoscopic treatment. (From Siegel, JH: *Endoscopic Retrograde Cholangiopancreatography: Technique, Diagnosis and Therapy.* New York, Raven Press, in press. Used by permission.)

complications, such as bleeding, which may require emergency surgery. If the intention of performing a less invasive procedure is to avoid prolonged, more complicated surgical intervention, then I recommend inserting a prosthesis, which should provide adequate decompression and subsequent clinical improvement. After the patient has improved in several days or weeks, a definitive endoscopic sphincterotomy can be performed on an elective basis when the patient is stable. This approach has enabled us to enjoy near total success with little morbidity, no emergency surgery, and no deaths.

Of the total number of patients we treated with cholangitis, 13 were so unstable that they were in the intensive care unit and all were on respirators. Ten of these patients were endoscoped in the radiology department under fluoroscopic control as is usually the procedure for routine ERCP. However, the patients were maintained on respiratory assistance during the performance of ERCP. Because of the presence of a respirator and endotracheal tube, most patients were left in a supine position or slightly obliqued for performance of ERCP. Decompression was successful in all subjects without complication. The remaining three patients were too unstable to be moved from intensive care. Therefore, the procedure was brought to the bedside and performed without fluoroscopic control. In the latter group of patients, a catheter and guide wire were advanced blindly into the bile duct and a prosthesis was inserted. Positioning of the prosthesis in the bile duct is confirmed visually when bile is seen flowing into the duodenum after separation of the guide wire and pusher tube. Immediate clinical improvement and stabilization occurred in these patients after drainage was established, which was indeed gratifying.

Now that endoscopic sphincterotomy has become established in providing definitive therapy for cholangitis in both routine and emergency clinical situations, surgical intervention with its attendant complications should be considered less desirable, and, more than likely, surgery will acquiesce to the endoscopic methods.

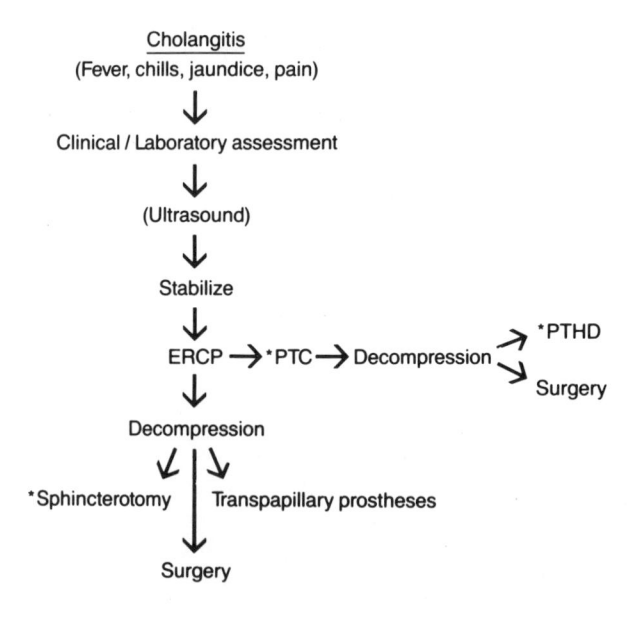

```
              Cholangitis
    (Fever, chills, jaundice, pain)
                  ↓
    Clinical / Laboratory assessment
                  ↓
              (Ultrasound)
                  ↓
               Stabilize
                  ↓                              → *PTHD
           ERCP → *PTC → Decompression
                  ↓                              ↘ Surgery
            Decompression
            ↙        ↘
  *Sphincterotomy │ Transpapillary prostheses
                  ↓
                Surgery
```

*Normal coagulation

FIG 49–2.
Flow chart (algorithm) for managing patients with cholangitis. (From Siegel JH: *Endoscopic Retrograde Cholangiopancreatography: Technique Diagnosis and Therapy.* New York, Raven Press, in press. Used by permission.)

Informing primary care physicians and noninterventional gastroenterologists of this progress has enabled us to continue making giant leaps forward in this critical area of patient management. Parenthetically, the latter group of physicians has been slow to accept any forms of therapy other than surgery regardless of our success in reducing morbidity and mortality.

ENDOSCOPIC SPHINCTEROTOMY IN ACUTE PANCREATITIS

First, we need to clarify the subject of this subchapter. As you recall from the earlier literature, acute pancreatitis had previously been considered a contraindication to the performance of ERCP.[4, 5] However, these earlier tenets of gastroenterology have changed with progress and time. If the etiology of pancreatitis is thought to be due to gallstones, which is referred to as gallstone pancreatitis, ERCP and the performance of sphincterotomy are clearly indicated. Therefore, the historic presentation of pancreatitis needs clarification. The primary care physician and gastroenterologist must pursue the cause of pancreatitis and be fully aware of all possible etiologies in order to provide sufficient and adequate care (i.e., rule out alcohol, drugs, infection, medication, and trauma).

When a patient presents with abdominal pain and symptoms compatible with pancreatitis, a sonogram is usually performed as the test of first choice to rule out biliary tract disease (i.e., cholelithiasis and a dilated biliary tree). When all biochemical, radiologic, and clinical parameters are assessed and gallstone pancreatitis is confirmed, ERCP may become a consideration, but, in my experience, consideration of its performance is totally dependent on the clinical picture.[2, 8] If the patient shows evidence of clinical improvement, I prefer to wait until the ileus resolves, and the patient is tolerating diet and, in general, returns to near normal function before scheduling the ERCP. However, if the patient's clinical condition deteriorates, and he or she becomes hemodynamically unstable, a decision must be made to intervene.

In earlier reported series,[33, 34] emergency sphincterotomy was performed in patients who were seriously compromised and moribund with excellent results. Despite the extremely unstable condition of these patients, no complications or deaths occurred. These results contradict those reported when only medical therapy was instituted or when emergency surgery was performed.[35-38] Still, despite the acceptable results of sphincterotomy in this patient group, I prefer the conservative approach especially when the patient shows signs of improvement. It is my philosophy to avoid intervention, because the procedure may cause harm, and to postpone it until the patient's tolerance has improved.

The natural history of gallstone pancreatitis has been studied previously, and the cause/effect relationship is attributed to the passage of a stone into the ampulla occluding both the bile duct and pancreatic duct. This situation usually develops when the anatomical arrangement of these ducts forms a common channel. In most cases, the inciting stone passes through the papilla, and, as a result of meticulous work reported independently by Acosta and Kelly,[39-41] the stone was retrieved in the stool of affected patients. This latter finding led to the concept that pancreatitis was a one-time event, because by careful analysis of histories and other parameters, Acosta and Kelly concluded that most patients never experienced a second episode.

However, the recommendation that cholecystectomy be performed subsequent to the index episode of pancreatitis to prevent recurrent and possibly fatal attacks has become an accepted principle of management. I recommend that before the patient undergoes cholecystectomy, he or she should have an index ERCP performed to rule out common bile duct stones. Although most stones may pass spontaneously, we have found that the stone remains in the bile duct freely floating and should be removed endoscopically before cholecystectomy. Again, the philosophy of this approach is to clear the bile duct endoscopically and minimize the surgical exploration.

Controversy has not only surrounded the performance of endoscopic sphincterotomy but the performance of surgical sphincterotomy for acute gallstone pancreatitis.[42, 43] Many surgeons disagree with the advocate for surgical sphincterotomy, Stone, whose experience, initially dismal, did improve. This experience was reflected by good results with less morbidity and mortality than earlier reported. He firmly believes that sphincterotomy performed emergently will reduce the morbidity associated with pancreatitis (i.e., pseudocyst and abscess). Because of Stone's work and his improved results, endoscopic sphincterotomy has become a more acceptable alternative to surgery.

One other consideration should be made in this chapter concerning the performance of sphincterotomy in patients with a history of cholelithiasis and pancreatitis. In our series of 61 patients treated for pancreatitis, 11 underwent sphincterotomy prophylactically (Fig 49–3). This subgroup of patients had experienced as many as three episodes of pancreatitis with serious, life-threatening presentations. There were seven men and four women, mean age 59 years, range 43 to 83 years. The common denominator in these cases was intercurrent medical problems such as severe chronic obstructive pulmonary disease (three patients) or severe arteriosclerotic heart disease with unstable angina, post myocardial infarction, and coronary bypass (eight patients). Each patient had an intact gallbladder and cholelithiasis. Because the next attack of pancreatitis could be potentially fatal, each patient was referred for sphincterotomy which was performed uneventfully.

Anatomically, if the bile duct sphincter is transected, this creates a new biliary-digestive fistula separating the bile duct effluent from the ampulla and the pancreatic duct. Thus a sphincterotomy will permit the passage of stones through it into the duodenum avoiding impaction in the ampulla and subsequent pancreatitis. Although the indications for performing sphincterotomy in these patients are not "hard," none of these patients has expe-

Males	7
Females	4
Mean Age	59
Age Range	43-83 yrs
COPD	3
ASHD	8
Complications	0
Surgery	0
Deaths	0

FIG 49–3.
Prophylactic sphincterotomy in 11 patients with gallstone pancreatitis. (From Siegel JH: *Endoscopic Retrograde Cholangiopancreatography: Technique, Diagnosis and Therapy.* New York, Raven Press, in press. Used by permission.)

rienced a recurrent episode of pancreatitis subsequent to sphincterotomy. Therefore, one can conclude that "prophylactic" sphincterotomy in patients with cholelithiasis and a previous episode of pancreatitis who are poor risks for cholecystectomy should be considered candidates for endoscopic sphincterotomy.

In conclusion, I have been given several controversial topics to discuss, all dealing with tentative indications for the performance of endoscopic sphincterotomy. I have attempted to discuss the advantage of sphincterotomy over surgery in certain clinical situations and have advised caution and a conservative approach in others. Because endoscopists are on the threshold of making inroads into the management of pancreaticobiliary disorders, we should continue to proceed with caution and support our approach with hard data obtained, when possible, through the successful completion of randomized controlled trials.

References

1. Kawai K, Akasaka Y, Murakami K, et al: Endoscopic sphincterotomy of the ampulla of Vater. *Gastrointest Endosc* 1974; 20:148–151.
2. Classen M, Safrany L: Endoscopic papillotomy and removal of gall stones. *Br Med J* 1975; 4:371–374.
3. Classen M, Ossenberg FW: Progress report: Nonsurgical removal of common bile duct stones. *Gut* 1977; 18:760–769.
4. Safrany L: Duodenoscopic sphincterotomy and

gall stone removal. *Gastroenterology* 1977; 72:338–343.
5. Siegel JH: Endoscopic management of choledocholithiasis and papillary stenosis. *Surg Gynecol Obstet* 1979; 148:747.
6. Siegel JH: Endoscopy and papillotomy in diseases of the biliary tract and pancreas. *J Clin Gastroenterol* 1980; 2:337–347.
7. Siegel JH: Endoscopic papillotomy in the management of patients with intact gallbladders and coexisting choledocholithiasis and cholelithiasis. *Gastrointest Endosc* 1979; 25.
8. Safrany L, Neuhaus B, Krause S, et al: Endoskopishe papillotomie bei akuter, biliar bedinster pancreatitis. *Dtsch Med Worchenschr* 1980; 105:115–1190.
9. Siegel JH: Endoscopic papillotomy in the treatment of biliary tract disease: 258 procedures and results. *Dig Dis Sci* 1981; 26:1057–1064.
10. Classen M, Burmeister W, Hagenmuller F, et al: Longterm examinations after endoscopic papillotomy. Scientific Program, American Society of Gastrointestinal Endoscopy, New Orleans, LA, May 1979.
11. Taylor, KJW, Rosenfield AT: Part III: Ultrasound scanning. *Clin Gastroenterol* 1979; 7(2):488–516.
12. Lapie JL, Orlando RC, Mittelstaedt CA, et al: Ultrasonography in the diagnosis of obstructive jaundice. *Ann Intern Med* 1978; 89:61–63.
13. Weissmann MS, Frank M, Rosenblatt R, et al: Cholescintigraphy, ultrasonography and computed tomography in the evaluation of biliary tract disorders. *Semin Nucl Med* 1979; 9:22–35.
14. Koch H, Rosch W, Schappner O, et al: Endoscopic papillotomy. Gastroenterology 1977; 73:1393–1396.
15. Seifert E: Endoscopic papillotomy and removal of gallstones. *Am J Gastroenterol* 1978; 69:154–159.
16. Demling L: Recent advances in gastrointestinal endoscopy. *Am J Gastroenterol* 1978; 69:533–543.
17. Cotton PB: Non-operative removal of bile duct stones by duodenoscopic sphincterotomy. *Br J Surg* 1980; 67:1–5.
18. Siegel JH: The intact gallbladder and duodenoscopic sphincterotomy: Safety in numbers (abstract). *Gastrointest Endosc* 1985; 31:144.
19. Cotton PB: 2–9 year followup after sphincterotomy for stone in patients with gallbladders (abstract). *Gastrointest Endosc* 1986; 32:157–158.
20. Siegel JH, Safrany L, Pullano WE, et al: The significance of duodenoscopic sphincterotomy in patients with gallbladders in situ: 11 year followup of 1272 patients (abstract). *Gastrointest Endosc* 33:159.
21. Siegel JH, Safrany L, Pullano WE, et al: Does endoscopic sphincterotomy reduce the annual incidence of cholecystitis in patients with intact gallbladders? Analysis of longterm results in 1555 patients (abstract). *Gastrointest Endosc* in press.
22. Siegel JH, Safrany L, Pullano WE, et al: The significance of duodenoscopic sphincterotomy in patients with gallbladders in situ; 11 year followup in 1272 patients. *Am J Gastroenterol* in press.
23. Hutton SW, Sievert CE Jr, Vennes JA, et al: The effect of sphincterotomy on gallstone formation in the prairie dog. *Gastroenterology* 1981; 81:663–667.
24. Hutton SW, Sievert CE Jr, Vennes JA, et al: Intribition of gallstone formation by sphincterotomy in the prairie dog: Reversal by atropine. *Gastroenterology* 1982; 82:1308–1313.
25. Vennes JA: Personal communication.
26. Siegel JH: Endoscopic papillotomy: A definitive treatment for cholangitis (abstract). *Gastroenterology* 1980; 78:1259.
27. Siegel JH, Ramsey WH, Pullano W: Endoscopic management of 947 patients with cholangitis. Proven safety and efficacy (abstract). *Gastrointest Endosc* 1986; 32:154–155.
28. Gogel WK, Runyon BA, Volpicelli NA, et al: Acute suppurative obstructive cholangitis due to stones: Treatment by urgent endoscopic sphincterotomy. *Gastrointest Endosc* 1987; 33:210–213.
29. Gold RP, Casavella WJ, Stern G, et al: Transhepatic cholangiography: The radiological method of choice in suspected obstructive jaundice. *Radiology* 1979; 133:39–44.
30. Nakayama T, Ikeda A, Okuda K: Percutaneous transhepatic drainage of the biliary tract: Technique and results in 104 cases. *Gastroenterology* 1978; 74:554.
31. Perieras RV Jr, Rheingold OJ, Hutson D, et al: Relief of malignant obstructive jaundice by percutaneous insertion of a permanent prosthesis in the biliary tree. *Ann Intern Med* 1978; 89:589.
32. Ring EJ, Oleaga JA, Feinman DB, et al: Therapeutic application of catheter cholangiography. *Radiology* 1978; 128:333.
33. van der Spuy S: Endoscopic sphincterotomy in the management of gallstone pancreatitis. *Endoscopy* 1981; 13:25–26.
34. Safrany L, Cotton PB: A preliminary report, urgent duodenoscopic sphincterotomy for acute gallstone pancreatitis. *Surgery* 1981; 89:424–428.
35. McSherry CK, Glenn F: The incidence and causes of death following surgery for non-malignant biliary tract disease. *Ann Surg* 1980; 191:271–275.
36. Rosseland AR, Solhang JH: Early or delayed endoscopic papillotomy (EPT) in gallstone pancreatitis. *Ann Surg* 1984; 199:165-7.
37. Ranson JHC: The timing of biliary surgery in acute pancreatitis. *Ann Surg* 1979; 189:654–662.
38. Kelly TR: Gallstone pancreatitis, the timing of surgery. *Surgery* 1980; 88:345–349.
39. Acosta JM, Ledesma CL: Gallstone migration as a cause of acute pancreatitis. *N Engl J Med* 1974; 290:484–487.
40. Kelly TR: Gallstone pancreatitis. *Arch Surg* 1974; 109:294.
41. Acosta JM, Rossi R, Ledesma CL: The usefulness of stool screening for diagnosing cholelithiasis in acute pancreatitis. *Dig Dis Sci* 1977; 22:168–172.
42. Stone HH, Fabian TC, Dunlope WE: Gallstone pancreatitis biliary tract pathology in relation to time of operation. *Ann Surg* 1981; 194:305–310.
43. Strow PR, Stone HH: A technique for transduodenal sphincteroplasty. *Surgery* 1980; 92:546–550.

Index

A

Abdominal angina, 365–366
Abdominal distention, 544; *see also* Distention
Abdominal pain
  angina and, 365–366
  chronic, 433–446
    diagnosis and, 439–441
    etiology and pathogenesis and, 436–439
    management of, 441–443
    prevalence of, 433
    syndromes and, 434–436
  pancreatic pain and, 192–197
Abdominal surgery preceding liver transplant, 228
Abscess
  Bartholin's gland, 390
  liver, 162
  metronidazole and, 384
  pancreatic, 145, 147, 181–191
    anatomic definition of, 186
    percutaneous drainage and, 190
    treatment and, 156–157
Abuse, laxative, 311
Acetaminophen, 78
Achalasia
  clinical data and, 29–33
  etiology and pathogenesis of, 28–29
  manometric criteria for, 6
  manometry and, 7
  pseudo-, 33–34
  treatment of, 34–42
Achlorhydria, 80
Acid-peptic autodigestion, 75
Acid perfusion test, 8, 24
Acid reflux test, 23
Acid secretion
  esophageal motility disorder and, 14
  gastritis and, 75–76
  heartburn and, 4
  short bowel syndrome and, 333
Acquired immune deficiency syndrome, 329, 448, 453–454
ACTH, 382
Adaptation, intestinal, 336–337
Adenocarcinoma
  Barrett's esophagus and, 22, 46–53
  gastroesophageal junction and, 33–34
  polyp and, 412, 528–535
ADH; *see* Antidiuretic hormone
Adhesion, 436
Adjuvant therapy
  colon cancer and, 413–415
  gastric cancer and, 124–125, 126
  failure and, 127
Adrenal gland, 55
Adrenergic agent, 35
Adult respiratory syndrome, 138
Aerophagia, 437
Age
  cholecystectomy and, 175–176
  ulcerative proctitis and, 369
Alacrima, 29
Alcohol-induced disease
  common bile duct stone and, 161
  esophageal varices and; *see* Esophageal varices
  liver transplantation and, 232
Aldosterone, 218
Algorithm, 11
Alimentary diarrhea, 310
Alkaline phosphatase
  common bile duct stone and, 162
  liver transplantation and, 238
Alkaloid, vinca, 59
Allergic proctitis, 375
Allograft rejection, 236
Alpha$_1$-antitrypsin deficiency, 232
Alpha$_2$-macroglobulin, 151
ALT as hepatitis marker, 275–276
Ambulatory 24–hour pH monitoring, 10–11, 13, 23
Amebiasis, 372
Amino acid solution, 333
5–Aminosalicylic acid
  toxic megacolon and, 398–399
  ulcerative proctitis and, 376
Amoxicillin, 100
Amylase
  common bile duct stone and, 162
  pancreatitis and, 135, 148–149
Amyl nitrate, 34
Analgesic, 193
Anal sphincter
  continence and, 349–350

559

Anal sphincter (cont.)
  electromyography, 478
  ileal pouch-anal anastomosis and, 405
Anastomosis
  Billroth, 166
  esophageal, 122
  ileal pouch and, 402–406
Anemia
  iron deficiency, 114
  pernicious, 80
Anesthesia, 292
ANF; see Atrial natriuretic factor
Angina, abdominal, 365–366
Angiodysplasia, 430–431
Angiography
  diarrhea and, 316
  intestinal ischemia and, 262–263
  massive rectal bleeding and, 428
Angiotensinogen, 218
Angle, anorectal
  anatomy and, 350
  ileal pouch-anal anastomosis and, 405
Anismus, 469–473
Antireflux surgery, 52
Anorectal anatomy, 349–351
Anorectal angle
  anatomy and, 350
  ileal pouch-anal anastomosis and, 405
Anorectal pressure studies, 478
Antacid
  duodenal ulcer and, 96
  gastric ulcer and, 91
  stress-related gastritis and, 76–77
Antibiotic
  colonic pseudo-obstruction and, 538
  Crohn's disease and, 384
  flatus and, 344–345
  pancreatitis and, 153, 154–155
  sclerosing cholangitis and, 300
  toxic megacolon and, 398–399
  ulcerative proctitis and, 372
Antibody, 80
Anticholinergic agent
  achalasia and, 35
  duodenal ulcer and, 96
  esophageal motility disorder and, 14
  hypertrophic gastropathy and, 83
Anticoagulant, 363
Antidepressant
  chronic pain and, 442
  duodenal ulcer and, 96
Antidiarrheal agent
  Crohn's disease and, 385
  toxic megacolon and, 396
Antidiuretic hormone, 219
Antifibrinogenic agent, 310
Antigen, Australia, 268–269, 271–272
Antihistamine; see H_2-receptor antagonist
Anti-inflammatory drug, nonsteroidal, 77–79
Antilymphocyte globulin, 235
Antimuscarinic anticholinergic drug, 96
Antireflux surgery
  achalasia and, 41
  Barrett's esophagus, 50–52
  esophageal motility disorder and, 14
  gastric volvulus and, 114–115

Antisecretory drug
  duodenal ulcer and, 96
  hypertrophic gastropathy and, 83
Antithymocyte globulin, 235
Antiulcer drug, 79
Antrum
  aberrant pacemaker and, 68
  biopsy and, 100
  gastroparesis and, 65
Anus
  ileal pouch and, 402–406
  imperforate, 357
Anxiety, constipation and, 464
Aperistalsis, 28
Appendicitis, 436
Applied impedance tomography, 69
Arginine vasopressin, 219
Arterial thrombosis, 237–238
Arteriography, 425
Ascites
  gastric cancer and, 121
  hepatorenal syndrome and, 254
  liver transplantation and, 223
Aspiration, pancreas and, 186–188, 210–211
Aspirin
  gastric ulcer and, 93
  gastritis and, 77, 78
Atherosclerosis, 365–366
Atresia, biliary, 232
Atrial natriuretic factor, 219
Atrophic gastritis, 80–82
Atropine, 9
Atypia, gastric cancer and, 119
Australia antigen, 268–269, 271–272
Autodigestion, acid/peptic, 75
Autoimmune disease
  atrophic gastritis and, 80–81
  hepatitis and, 246, 248, 250–251
    liver transplantation and, 230–231
AVP; see Arginine vasopressin
Azathioprine
  liver transplantation and, 235–236
  sclerosing cholangitis and, 310
Azotemia, 253–261

B

Bacille Calmette-Guérin, 414
Bacteremia
  esophageal sclerotherapy and, 511–512
  sclerosing cholangitis and, 300
Bacteria
  malabsorption and, 312
  pancreatic abscess and, 186
Baker jejunostomy tube, 540–541
Balloon
  common bile duct and, 438
    stone extraction and, 169–170
  esophagus and, 12
    varices and, 505–506, 515–516
  gallbladder pain and, 319
  obesity and, 523–527
Band, congenital obstructive, 110–111
Barium studies
  Barrett's esophagus and, 46

diarrhea and, 314
enema and
  colonic pseudo-obstruction and, 536–537
  colon ischemia and, 364–365
  massive rectal bleeding and, 428
  occult blood and, 423
  sigmoid volvulus and, 545
  toxic megacolon and, 396
  ulcerative proctitis and, 373
endoscopy and, 425
gastric volvulus and, 113
gastroesophageal reflux and, 23, 24
gastroparesis and, 68
Barrett's esophagus, 45–55
  antireflux surgery and, 50–52
  background of, 45–46
  barium swallow and, 24
  cancer risk and, 46–48
  endoscopic surveillance and, 48–50
  gastric cancer and, 119
  management of, 52–53
  mucosa and, 22
Bartholin's gland abscess, 390
Basal cell hyperplasia, 21
Belching, 341–342
Belsy-Mark IV procedure, 25
Bernstein test, 8, 24
Beta-adrenergic agonist, 35
Bethanechol
  gastroesophageal reflux and, 25
  gastroparesis and, 71–72
Betiromide test, 316
Bezoar, iatrogenic, 523–527
BICAP; see Bipolar cautery
Bile acid, 287
Bile duct
  chronic pain and, 438
  common; see Common bile duct stone
  liver transplantation and, 232
Bile reflux, 81
Bile salt catharsis, 309
Biliary bypass, 212
Biliary disorder, 281–304
  atresia and, 232
  cirrhosis and
    bile duct obstruction and, 162
    liver transplantation and, 229–230
  colic and, 161
  dyskinesia and, 434
  gallstones and, 283–297; see also Gallstone
  pain and, 440
  postoperative pain and, 317–325
  sclerosing cholangitis and, 298–304
Bilirubin
  common bile duct stone and, 162
  gallstone and, 284
Billroth anastomosis, 166
Biofeedback
  anismus and, 472–474
  fecal incontinence and, 354
    spina bifida and, 357
Biopsy
  adenomatous polyp and, 413
  antral, 100
  Barrett's esophagus and, 46
  Crohn's disease and, 381

hepatitis and, 247
liver, 299
small intestine and, 326–331
ulcerative proctitis and, 372, 373
  child and, 375
Bipolar cautery
  heater probe versus, 491
  upper gastrointestinal tract bleeding and, 489–490
Bismuth
  Campylobacter pylori and, 100
  duodenal ulcer and, 96, 101
Bleeding
  colonic ischemia and, 364
  Crohn's disease and, 389–393
  duodenal ulcer and, 102
  endoscopic retrograde sphincterotomy and, 173
  erosive gastritis and, 74–79
  esophageal varices and; see Esophageal varices
  gastric ulcer and, 89
  massive rectal, 427–432
  occult, 420–426
  ulcerative proctitis and, 374
  upper gastrointestinal tract and, 487–497
Bleomycin, 59
Bloating, 342–344
  chronic pain and, 437
Blood count
  common bile duct stone and, 162
  pancreatic cancer and, 208
Blood flow, variceal, 501
Blood gases, 155
Blood test, stool
  colon cancer and, 411
  diarrhea and, 314
  positive, 420–426
Bochdalek's hernia, 108, 114–115
Bone disease, 334
Bovine pancreatic protease, 193
Bowel; see Large intestine
Breast disease, 460
Brooke ileostomy, 406
Brown-McHardy dilator, 37–38
Bruit, 435
Bubble, gastric, 523–527
Budd-Chiari syndrome, 231
Buffered aspirin, 78
Bulimia, 307–308
Burn patient, 74–75
Bypass, biliary, 212

C

Calcium, 155
Calcium channel blocker
  achalasia and, 35–36
  esophageal motility disorder and, 14
Calculus
  common bile duct; see Common bile duct stone
  gallstone; see Gallstone
  uric acid, 335
Campylobacter
  duodenal ulcer and, 99–100, 101
  gastritis and, 81–82
  infectious colitis and, 449
  traveler's diarrhea and, 452

Campylobacter (cont.)
  ulcerative proctitis and, 370
Canal, anal, 405
Cancer
  Barrett's esophagus and, 46–53
  colon, 410–419
    bloating and, 342
    diarrhea and, 309
  esophagus and
    prognostic variables and, 56–57
    staging and, 55–56
    therapy and, 57–61
  gastric glandular, 117–130; *see also* Gastric carcinoma
  gastric ulcer and, 89–90
  obstipation and, 460
  pancreatic, 207–213
  polypectomy and, 528–535
  pseudoachalasia and, 31
Candida, 93
Cannulation
  common bile duct and, 167–168
  pancreas divisum and, 198–201, 203
Capmul; *see* Monooctanoin
Carbohydrate, 344
Carbon dioxide in barium studies, 364
Carbuterol, 35
Carcinoid tumor, 80–81
Carcinoma
  achalasia and, 34
  Crohn's disease and, 381–382, 386
  gastric
    glandular, 117–130; *see also* Gastric carcinoma
    partial gastrectomy and, 81
Cardiac chest pain, 3, 4, 5, 6
Cardioplasty, 41
Catharsis, bile salt, 309
Catheter
  colonic pseudo-obstruction and, 540–541
  pancreas and
    pancreatitis and, 156
    pigtail, 188
    pseudocyst and, 157, 181–191
Cautery, 488–490
CCK; *see* Cholecystokinin
CDCA; *see* Chenodeoxycholic acid
Cecum, 537
Celiac artery syndrome, 435
Celiac plexus block, 195
Celiac sprue, 330
Central nervous system; *see* Neurologic disorder
Central venous pressure, 256
Cephalosporin, 82
Cephalothin, 403
Chagas' disease, 28
Chalasia, 20
Charcoal, 344–345
Charcot's triad, 161
Chemotherapy
  colon cancer and, 415–416
  esophageal cancer and, 59–61
  pancreatic cancer and, 212
Chenodeoxycholic acid, 285–289
Chest pain
  achalasia and, 29–30
  ambulatory 24-hour pH monitoring and, 10–11
  cause of, 4–5
  gastric volvulus and, 112
  initial evaluation and, 5
  irritable bowel syndrome and, 13
  new tests for, 12–13
  origin of, in esophageal disease, 3–4
  sclerotherapy and, 510
  testing and, 5, 7–9
  therapy and, 13–15
Child
  fecal incontinence and, 352–353
    treatment of, 357
  icteric hepatitis and, 266
  liver transplantation and, 232–233
  ulcerative proctitis and, 374–375
Chlamydia trachomatis
  infectious colitis and, 450
  traveler's diarrhea and, 452
  ulcerative proctitis and, 371
Cholangiocarcinoma, 300
Cholangiogram
  percutaneous transhepatic, 163, 169
  T-tube, 164, 175
Cholangitis, 161
  endoscopic sphincterotomy and, 552–555
  sclerosing, 230
Cholangiopancreatography; *see* Endoscopic retrograde cholangiopancreatography
Cholecystectomy
  diarrhea and, 309
  necrotizing pancreatitis and, 150
  postoperative pain and, 317–325
Cholecystitis
  endoscopic sphincterotomy and, 551–552
  intact gallbladder and, 175
Cholecystokinin, 193, 195–196
Choledocholithiasis, 160–180; *see also* Common bile duct stone
Cholelitholytic therapy, 286–287
Cholesterol gallstones, 283–285
Cholinesterase inhibitor, 8–9
Cholinomimetic agent, 71–72
Chronic abdomen, 433–446
Chylous ascites, 221
Chymex test, 316
Chymotrypsin, 193
Cimetidine
  duodenal ulcer and, 98
    relapse and, 99, 102
  gastritis and, 76, 77
  gastroesophageal reflux and, 25
Cirrhosis
  ascites and, 217
  esophageal varices and, 498–522; *see also* Esophageal varices
  liver transplantation and, 229–231
Cisapride
  gastroesophageal reflux and, 25
  gastroparesis and, 72
Cisplatin
  esophageal cancer and, 59
  gastric cancer and, 128
Clostridium difficile
  elderly patient and, 454–455
  infectious colitis and, 449–450

traveler's diarrhea and, 452
ulcerative proctitis and, 371
Coagulation
  endoscopic retrograde sphincterotomy and, 165–166
  gastritis and, 77
Colchicine, 310
Colic
  biliary, 161
  intestinal, 162
  postcholecystectomy syndrome and, 318
Colitis
  diarrhea and, 307
  diversion, 371
  infectious, 447–457
  toxic megacolon and, 394
  ulcerative
    sclerosing cholangitis and, 298
    surgery outcomes and, 409
Colitis cystica profunda, 371–372
Colloidal bismuth, 96
Colon; see Colonoscopy; Large intestine
Colonic pseudo-obstruction, 536–542
Colonoscopy
  colonic pseudo-obstruction and, 538–540
  diarrhea and, 314
  massive rectal bleeding and, 429–430
  occult blood and, 423–424
  polypectomy and, 528–535
  sigmoid volvulus and, 546
  ulcerative proctitis and, 373
Colorectal cancer, 422; see also Cancer
Colostomy, 371
Columnar epithelium, 45
Coma, hepatic, 258–259
Common bile duct; see Common bile duct stone
  manometry and, 321
  pain and, 318–319
Common bile duct stone, 160–180
  clinical manifestations and, 160–162
  diagnosis and, 162–163
  endoscopic retrograde sphincterotomy and, 165–169
    complications and, 172–174
    intact gallbladder and, 175–176
  gallstones and, 174–176
  laboratory findings and, 162
  large, 169–172
  treatment of, 163–165
Compression of varices, 505–506; see also Decompression
Computerized tomography
  esophageal cancer and, 55, 56
  liver transplantation and, 237
  pancreas and
    abscess and, 156–157
    cancer and, 210–211
    necrosis and, 151
    pancreatitis and, 137–138, 149, 154, 155, 181, 188
Conditioning, operant, 354
Congenital obstructive band, 110–111
Congestive heart failure
  biliary disease, 162–163
  intestinal ischemia and, 362
Constipation
  incontinence and, 352

obstipation and, 458–484; see also Obstipation
treatment and, 356–357
Continence; see Incontinence, fecal
Continent ileostomy, 406–408
Contraction
  achalasia and, 29
  esophagus and, 5
  external anal sphincter and, 355
Contrast radiography; see Barium studies
Coronary artery disease, 3, 4
Corticosteroid
  Crohn's disease and, 382
  liver transplantation and, 235
  toxic megacolon and, 398
Cortisol, 312
Crater, ulcer, 97
C-reactive protein, 151
Creatinine, 254
Crigler–Najjar syndrome, 226
Crohn's disease, 380–388
  perineal fistula and, 389–393
  small intestine biopsy and, 330
  ulcerative proctitis and, 369, 371
Cryptosporidium, 454
Cullen's sign, 135
Culture
  pancreatic abscess and, 186
  stool, 449
Cupruretic agents, 310
Curling's ulcer, 74
Cushing's ulcer, 74
Cyclophosphamide, 235–236
Cyclosporine
  hepatotoxicity and, 238
  liver transplantation and, 235–236
  sclerosing cholangitis and, 310
Cystgastrostomy, danger of, 157–158
Cytomegalovirus, 238

D

Davol catheter, 156
Decompression
  colonic pseudo-obstruction and, 538–540
  gastric volvulus and, 114
  gastroparesis and, 69
  pancreas divisum and, 203
  pancreatic pseudocyst and, 157
  sigmoid volvulus and, 546–549
  toxic megacolon and, 398–399
Defecation; see also Incontinence, fecal
  denial of, 466–468
  dynamic evaluation of, 478
Dehydration, 450
Delta hepatitis, 250, 269
Demeclocycline, 255
Denol; see Tripotassium dicitratobismuthate
Depression, 442
Dermatomyositis, 67
Derotation, 114
Desyrel; see Trazodone
Diabetes mellitus
  diarrhea and, 311–312
  fecal incontinence and, 351
  treatment and, 355–356

Diabetes mellitus *(cont.)*
    gastropathy and, 68
Dialysis
    hepatic coma and, 258–259
    hepatorenal syndrome and, 257
Diarrhea
    colon ischemia and, 364
    fecal incontinence and, 356
    history and examination and, 297–309, 311–312
    homosexual male and, 452–454
    incontinence and, 352
    infectious colitis and, 448
    small intestine biopsy and, 329, 330
    work-up for, 312–314, 316
Dicyclomine, 14
Diet; *see* Nutrition
Diffuse esophageal spasm, 6
Digitalis, 362
Dilatation
    achalasia and, 37–40, 41
    esophageal motility disorder and, 14
Diltiazem
    achalasia and, 35
    esophageal motility disorder and, 24–25
Diphenoxylate, 356
Discharge, mucous, 389–393
Dissecting microscopy of jejunal biopsy, 330–331
Distal antral pacemaker, 68
Distention balloon
    chronic pain and, 437
    intestinal, 342–344
        ischemia and, 361–262
    nontoxic megacolon and, 537–538
Diuretic
    ascites and, 221
    hypertrophic gastropathy and, 83
Diversion colitis, 371
Diversion proctitis, 372
Diverticula
    chronic pain and, 436
    diarrhea and, 311
    rectal bleeding and, 430
DNA
    gastric cancer and, 122
    hepatitis B virus and, 268
Domperidone, 25
Dopamine antagonist, 71–72
Doxorubicin, 128
Drainage
    common bile duct and, 176, 321
    pancreas divisum and, 202
    pancreatic pseudocyst and abscess and, 157, 181–191
Dressing, 156
Drug-induced disease
    diarrhea and, 311
    gastritis and, 77–79
    hepatitis and, 246, 251
    pancreatitis and, 134
Duct
    common bile; *see* Common bile duct stone
    pancreas divisum and, 198
Dumping syndrome, 66–68
Duodenal ulcer, 95–107
    Campylobacter pylori and, 99–100
    dyspepsia and, 97–98
    initial therapy and, 96–97
    maintenance therapy, 98–99
    management and, 101–105
    natural history of, 95–96
    recurrence and, 100–101
    symptom-ulcer crater disparity, 97
D-xylose test, 366
Dyskinesia
    biliary, 434
    gastroduodenopyloric, 67
Dyspepsia
    gastric ulcer and, 89
    nonulcer, 97–98
        chronic pain and, 434, 440
Dysphagia
    achalasia and, 29
    manometry and, 7
Dysplasia
    Barrett's esophagus and, 49, 53, 119
        antireflux surgery and, 51–52
    obstipation and, 460
Dyssynergia, rectosphincteric, 469–473

E

EAS; *see* External anal sphincter
Ecchymosis, 135
Ectasia, vascular, 430–431
Edema
    hypertrophic gastropathy and, 82–83
    pancreatitis and, 154
Edrophonium test, 8–9, 29
Elastase, 193
Elderly patient, 454–455
Electrical stimulation, 319
Electrocoagulation, 488–490
Electrohydraulic lithotripsy, 171, 172
Electrolyte abnormality
    infectious colitis and, 450–451
    short bowel syndrome and, 333
Electromyography
    anal sphincter and, 478
    colon and, 477–478
Embolus, mesenteric artery, 359–363
Embryology, 198
Encopresis, 352
Endocrine neoplasm, 309
Endoscopic retrograde cholangiopancreatography
    cancer and, 210–211
    cholecystitis and, 551–552
    common bile duct stone and, 163
    diarrhea and, 316
    pain and, 192
    pancreas divisum and, 198–201
    pancreatitis and, 134, 134
    postcholecystectomy syndrome and, 318, 320–322
Endoscopy
    achalasia and, 31
    Barrett's esophagus, 48–50, 53
    bleeding and
        esophageal varices and, 498–522
        upper gastrointestinal tract and, 487–497
    cholangiopancreatography and; *See* Endoscopic retrograde cholangiopancreatography

diarrhea and, 314, 316
duodenal ulcer and, 95
erosive gastritis and, 77
esophageal cancer and, 56–57
gastric bubble insertion and, 523–527
gastric cancer and, 119
gastric ulcer and, 89–90
gastric volvulus and, 113, 114
gastroparesis and, 68
infectious colitis and, 450
internal cystgastrostomy, danger of, 157–158
nontoxic megacolon and, 536–542
pancreas divisum and, 203
polypectomy and, 528–535
pseudoachalasia and, 34
retrograde cholangiopancreatography and; See Endoscopic retrograde cholangiopancreatography
retrograde sphincterotomy and
    Cimetidine, 163, 164–169
    gallstone pancreatitis and, 174
    prophylactic, 176
sigmoid volvulus and, 543–550
small intestine biopsy and, 326–327
sphincterotomy and, 551–557
Enema
    barium
        colonic pseudo-obstruction and, 536–537
        colon ischemia and, 364–365
        massive rectal bleeding and, 428
        occult blood and, 423
        sigmoid volvulus and, 545
        toxic megacolon and, 396
        ulcerative proctitis and, 373
    encopresis and, 357
    Gastrograffin, 544–545
    hydrocortisone, 375–376
Entameoba histolytica, 452
Enteral feeding, 336–338
Enteric-coated aspirin, 78–79
Enteritis, 307
Enterogastrone, 333
Enuresis, 460
Enzyme, 193
Eosinophilia, 314
Epinephrine, 494
Epithelium
    Barrett's esophagus and, 45, 50–51
    gastritis and, 78
    obstipation and, 460
Epstein-Barr virus, 238
ERCP; see Endoscopic retrograde cholangiopancreatography
Erosive gastritis, 74–79
ERS; see Endoscopy, retrograde sphincterotomy and
Eructation, 341–342, 343
Erythromycin
    Campylobacter pylori, 82
    ileal pouch-anal anastomosis and, 403
Escherichia coli, 454
Esophageal varices, 498–522
    clinical aspects and, 498–502
    patient management and, 514–516
    therapy of, 502–514
Esophagogastric junction, 113
Esophagomyotomy, 40–42

Esophagoscopy, 46
Esophagus, 2–61
    achalasia and, 28–45; see also Achalasia
    anastomosis and, 122
    Barrett's; see Barrett's esophagus
    cancer and, 55–64
        prognostic variables and, 56–57
        staging and, 55–56
        therapy and, 57–61
    chest pain and, 3–17; see also Chest pain
    esophagitis and, 40–41
    gastrectomy and, 123
    heartburn and, 18–27; see also Heartburn
    motility disease; see Motility disease, esophageal
    pH monitoring and, 10–11
    sphincter and; see Sphincter, lower esophageal
    varices and; see Esophageal varices
Esophagus ligament, 110
Estrogen, 20
Ethanol sclerotherapy, 494
Ether, methyl tertiary butyl
    bile duct stone and, 172
    gallstones and, 291–292
Etoposide, 128
Eventration, 108, 110
Exocrine pancreatic cancer, 207–208
External anal sphincter
    biofeedback and, 355
    continence and, 349–350
Extracellular fluid, 260–261
Extracorporeal focused electrohydraulic lithotripsy, 171
Extracorporeal therapy, 257–258
Extract, pancreatic, 193–194
Extrapancreatic fluid, 186
    percutaneous drainage and, 190

F

Factitious pain, 439
Famotidine
    duodenal ulcer and, 96, 98
    gastritis and, 76
    gastroesophageal reflux and, 25
Fat, 338
Fatigue, 243, 246
Fat sequestra, 148, 157–158
Fecal blood test, positive, 420–426
Fecal impaction, 312
Fecal incontinence, 349–358
    obstipation and, 460
Fertility, Crohn's disease and, 382
Fever
    cholangitis and, 161
    pancreatitis and, 188
    sclerotherapy and, 510
Fiber, vasoactive intestinal polypeptide, 29
Fiberoptic endoscopy, 373
Fistula
    Crohn's disease and, 387, 389–393
    metronidazole and, 384
Fistulotomy instrument, 168
Flatus, 344–345, 437
Floxuridine, 417

Fluid
  ascites and, 219, 220–221
    gastric cancer and, 121
    hepatorenal syndrome and, 254
    liver transplantation and, 223
  extrapancreatic, 190
  hepatorenal syndrome and, 256, 260–261
  pancreatic necrosis and, 154–155
  pancreatic pseudocyst and, 184
  pancreatitis and, 151–152, 182
  peripancreatic, 157
  short bowel syndrome and, 333
5–Fluorouracil
  colon cancer and, 414, 415–416
  esophageal cancer and, 59
  gastric cancer and, 126, 128
    failure of, 127
Fulminant hepatic failure, 231
Fulminant pancreatitis, 155
Fundoplication
  gastric volvulus and, 114–115
  gastroesophageal reflux and, 25
Furazolidone, 100

G

Gallbladder, 281–304
  common bile duct stone and, 160–180; see also Common bile duct stone
  gallstones and, 283–297; see also Gallstone
  sclerosing cholangitis and, 298–304
  upper-quadrant pain and, 317–325
Gallstone, 283–297
  background on, 283–286
  dissolution therapy and, 286–292
  endoscopic sphincterotomy and, 175–176, 552
  pancreatitis and, 138, 150, 174–175
  short bowel syndrome and, 335
Gamma flutamyl transpeptidase, 238
Ganglion cells, 28
Garren-Edwards Gastric Bubble, 523–527
Gas
  chronic pain and, 434, 437
  intestinal, 341–345
Gastrectomy
  hypertrophic gastropathy and, 83
  operative risk and, 122–124
  partial, 81
Gastric artery, 122
Gastric balloon
  esophageal varices and, 515–516
  obesity and, 523–527
Gastric carcinoma, 117–130
  adjuvant therapy and, 124–125
    failure of, 127
  advanced, 127–128
  Barrett's esophagus and, 119–120
  early diagnosis and, 118–119
  failure patterns and, 126
  incurable, 125–126
  spleen and, 124
  staging and, 120–122
  surgery and, 112–124
Gastric emptying, 65–73

Gastric fundus-type epithelium, 45
Gastric hypersecretion, 333
Gastric lavage, 503
Gastric outlet obstruction, 67
Gastric pullup, 58
Gastric ulcer, 88–94
  antral and acid-bearing mucosa and, 120
  cancer and, 118–119
Gastric volvulus, 108–110
Gastrin, 314
Gastrinoma, 309
Gastritis
  erosive, 74–79
  hypertrophic and, 82–83
  nonerosive, 79–82
Gastrocolic ligament, 110
Gastroduodenopyloric dyskinesia, 67
Gastroesophageal junction, 33–34
Gastroesophageal reflux
  chest pain and, 3–17; see also Chest pain
  gastric cancer and, 120
  heartburn and, 18–27
  measurement of, 22–23
Gastrograffin enema, 544–545
Gastrohepatic ligament, 110
Gastrointestinal series; see Upper gastrointestinal series
Gastrokinetic agent, 71–72
Gastroparesis, 65–73
  diagnosis and treatment of, 68–72
  physiology and, 65–66
  symptoms and etiology of, 66–68
Gastropathy, diabetic, 68
Gastropexy, 114, 115
Gastrophrenic ligament, 110
Gastrostomy, 115
Giant gastric ulcer, 92–93
Gland, Bartholin's, 390
Glandular carcinoma, gastric, 117–130; see also Gastric carcinoma
Globulin
  antilymphocyte, 235
  hepatitis, 265–268, 274–275
Glomerular filtration rate, 257
Glucocorticoid
  achalasia and, 29
  liver transplantation and, 235
Glypressin, 505
Graft rejection, 236
Grey Turner's sign, 135
Guaiac test, false-negative, 420–421

H

H_2-receptor antagonist
  duodenal ulcer and, 96, 100
  gastric ulcer and, 91
  gastritis and
    anti-inflammatory drug and, 79
    stress-related, 76
  gastroparesis and, 71
  short bowel syndrome and, 333
HAV; see Hepatitis
HbsAg; see Hepatitis

Head of pancreas, 208–209
Heartburn, 18–27
  clinical sequelae of, 21–22
  diagnosis of, 22–24
  gastroesophageal reflux and, 4–5
  management of, 24–26
  pathogenesis of, 18–21
Heart failure
  biliary disease, 162–163
  intestinal ischemia and, 362
Heater probe, 490–491
Heller myotomy, modified, 40–41
Hematology, 246
Hematoma, 511
Heme-positive stool, 420–426
Hemodialysis, 257
Hemoperfusion, 258
Hemorrhage; see Bleeding
Hemorrhoid, external, 390
Hepatic artery, 237–238
Hepatic disorder; see Hepatitis; Liver
Hepatic vein thrombosis, 231
Hepatitis
  clinical profile and, 243, 246
  definition of, 243
  immunization and, 264–280; see also Immunization, hepatitis
  laboratory findings and, 246–247
  liver biopsy and, 247–248
  liver transplantation and, 230–231, 252
  pregnancy and, 251
  presentation and, 243
  treatment and, 248–251
Hepatitis B immune globulin, 275
Hepatorenal syndrome, 253–263
  clinical features of, 253–254
  diagnosis and, 254–255
  functional renal failure and, 217
  pathogenesis and, 255
  treatment and, 255–261
Hernia
  hiatal
    Barrett's esophagus, 119
    gastric volvulus and, 113, 114
  paraesophageal, 108
Herpes simplex
  liver transplantation and, 238
  ulcerative proctitis and, 371
Hiatal hernia
  Barrett's esophagus, 119
  gastric volvulus and, 113, 114
Hill procedure, 25
Histamine antagonist; see H_2-receptor antagonist
Homosexual male
  diarrhea and, 452–454
  infectious colitis and, 447–457
Hormone, antidiuretic, 219
Hydralazine
  esophageal motility disorder and, 14
  intestinal ischemia and, 362
Hydrocortisone enema, 375–376
Hyperadrenalism, 311–312
Hyperaldosteronism, 218–219
Hyperalimentation, 222–223
Hyperamylasemia, 148

Hypercalciuria, 334
Hypergammaglobulinemia, 329
Hyperlipemia, 134
Hyperlipoproteinemia, 226
Hyperparathyroidism, 334
Hyperplasia, basal cell, 21
Hypersecretion, acid; see Acid secretion
Hypertension
  liver transplantation and, 237
  lower esophageal sphincter and, 6
Hyperthyroidism, 311–312
Hypertonic saline, 494
Hypertrophy
  achalasia and, 28
  gastropathy and, 82–83
Hypochondria, 442
Hyponatremia
  ascites and, 220–221
  paracentesis and, 221–222
Hypoproteinemia, 82–83
Hysteria, 442

I

IAS; see Internal anal sphincter
IBS; see Irritable bowel syndrome
Icteric hepatitis, 266
IF; see Intrinsic factor
Ileal pouch-anal anastomosis, 402–406
Ileorectostomy, 408–409
Ileostomy
  continent, 406–408
  Crohn's disease and, 385
Immune globulin, hepatitis and, 265–268, 274–275
Immunization, hepatitis, 264–280
  A, 264–268
  B, 268–269, 271–272
  non-A, non-B, 272–273
  transfusion-associated, 273–276
Immunosuppression
  Crohn's disease and, 383–384
  liver transplantation and, 234–236
  sclerosing cholangitis and, 310
  small intestine symptoms and, 329
Impaction, fecal
  diarrhea and, 312
  prevention of, 357
Impedance tomography, 69
Imperforate anus, 353, 357
Implant, 128
Incarcerated hernia, 108
Incontinence, fecal
  adults and, 351–352
  child and, 352–353
    treatment of, 357
  diagnosis of, 353–354
  diarrhea and, 309
  mechanisms of, 349–351
  obstipation and, 460
  treatment of, 354–357
Infant, chalasia and, 20
Infarction
  colon and, 365
  intestinal ischemia and, 362

Infarction (cont.)
  myocardial, 162
Infection
  Campylobacter pylori, 81–82
  colitis and, 447–457
  common bile duct stone and, 161
  Crohn's disease and, 381
  diarrhea and, 308
  ileal pouch-anal anastomosis and, 404–405
  liver transplantation and, 237, 238
  pancreatic
    abscess and, 181–191
    catheter and, 157
    pancreatitis and, 136–137, 145, 146–147
    percutaneous drainage and, 188–190
    pseudocyst and, 189–190
    treatment and, 155–156
  total parenteral nutrition and, 334
  toxic megacolon and, 395–396
  ulcerative proctitis and, 370–371
Inflammation
  Crohn's disease and, 380–388
  diarrhea and, 308–309
  infectious colitis and, 448
  rectal mucosa and, 368–370
Infusion
  esophagus and, 4
  liver, 416–418
Interferon, 248
Interlobular bile duct, 232
Intermittent gastric volvulus, 112
Intermittent therapy for duodenal ulcer, 104–105
  relapse and, 102
Internal anal sphincter, 349–350
Internal cystgastrostomy, endoscopic, 157–158
Interstitial pancreatitis, 144
  anatomic definition of, 181–182
  natural history of, 144, 145
  treatment and, 154
Intestinal angina, 365–366
Intestinal colic, 162
Intestinal peptide, vasoactive
  achalasia and, 29
  diarrhea and, 309, 314
Intestinal pseudo-obstruction, 68
Intestine; see Large intestine; Small intestine
Intraluminal manometry, 23–24
Intraperitoneal drug delivery, 128
Intravenous fluid
  ascites and, 221
  toxic megacolon and, 398
Intrinsic factor, 80
Iron deficiency anemia, 114
Irritable bowel syndrome
  balloon distention and, 319
  bloating and, 342
  chronic pain and, 434
  diagnosis and, 440
  diarrhea and, 309–311
  esophagus and, 13
  postcholecystectomy syndrome and, 319
  psychotherapy and, 443
Ischemia, 359–367
  colon and, 363–365
  hepatorenal syndrome and, 256–257

  mesenteric
    acute, 359–363
    chronic, 365–366
  proctitis and, 371
Isoamylase, 149
Isopropamide, 96
Isosorbide dinitrate, 35–36

J

Jaundice
  common bile duct stone and, 161, 163
  hepatorenal syndrome and, 254
  myocardial infarction and, 162
  pancreatic cancer and, 209
Jejunal biopsy, 330–331
Jejunostomy tube, 540–541
Junctional-type epithelium, 45

K

Kidney; see Renal disorder
Kock ileostomy, 406–408
  Crohn's disease and, 385

L

Lacrimal probe, 203
Lacrimation, 29
d-Lactic acidosis, 335
Lactose tolerance test, 311, 314, 316
Lactulose, 357
Laparotomy
  gastric volvulus and, 114
  intestinal ischemia and, 363
  pancreatic cancer and, 210–211
  pseudoachalasia and, 34
Large intestine, 347–484
  cancer and, 410–419
  colonoscopy; see Colonoscopy
  Crohn's disease and, 380–388
    perineal fistula and, 389–393
  fecal incontinence and, 349–358
  heme-positive stool and, 420–426
  infectious colitis and, 447–457
  inflammation and, 308–309
  irritable bowel syndrome and; see Irritable bowel syndrome
  ischemic bowel and, 359–367
  obstipation and, 458–484; see also Obstipation
  pouch versus stoma and, 402–409
  toxic megacolon and, 394
  ulcerative proctitis, 368–379
Laser, 491–493
Lavage
  esophageal varices and, 503
  necrotizing pancreatitis and, 155
  peritoneal, 138
Laxative, 311
Legionella, 238
Leukocytosis
  infectious colitis and, 449

intestinal ischemia and, 362
Licorice, 96
Ligament, gastric volvulus and, 110–111
Lipase, 148–149
Lipid, 148, 157–158, 333
Lithotripsy, 170–171, 172, 292–294
Liver, 215–280
　abscess and, 162
　ascites and, 217–224
　esophageal cancer and, 55
　esophageal varicies and, 498–522
　hepatic coma and, 258–259
　hepatitis and, 243–253; see also Hepatitis
　hepatorenal syndrome and, 253–263; see also Hepatorenal syndrome
　infusion, and, 416–418
　metastasis and, 121, 126
　pancreatic cancer and, 208–210
　sclerosing cholangitis and, 299
　transplantation and, 225–242
　　candidates for, 225–229
　　graft rejection and, 236
　　hepatorenal syndrome and, 260
　　immunosuppression and, 234–236
　　indications for, 229–233
　　infection and, 238
　　late liver dysfunction and, 238
　　postoperative period and, 233–234, 236–238
　　quality of life and, 238–239
　　retransplantation and, 236
Loperamide, 356
Low compliance infusion system, 4
Lower esophageal sphincter; see Sphincter, lower esophageal
Lower gastrointestinal tract bleeding, 427–432
Lymph node
　gastrectomy and, 123
　gastric cancer and, 121–122, 126
Lymphoma, 384

M

Macroglobulin, alpha$_2$, 151
Magnetic resonance imaging, 56
Maintenance therapy for duodenal ulcer, 102, 103–104
Malabsorption
　diarrhea and, 312
　Schilling test and, 315
Malignancy; see Cancer
Malingering, 439
Malnutrition, 222
Manometry
　achalasia and, 32
　esophageal, 6, 7
　fecal incontinence and, 354
　lower esophageal sphincter and, 23–24
　papilla and, 202
　sphincter of Oddi and, 318, 320–322
Massive rectal bleeding, 427–432
Meadow's syndrome, 466
Mechanical lithotriptor, 170–171
Mechanical obstruction
　gastroparesis and, 66–68

stomach and, 67
Mechanical stapling, 58
Medication; see Drug-induced disease
Megacolon
　nontoxic, 536–542
　prevention of, 357
　toxic, 394–401
　　Crohn's disease and, 386
Megarectum, 476–477
　prevention of, 357
Meningomyelocele, 352–353
Mentrier's disease, 82
6–Mercaptopurine, 383, 392
Mesenteric ischemia, 359–363
　chronic, 365–366
Mesenteroaxial volvulus, 109
　complications and, 112
Metabolic disease
　diarrhea and, 311–312
　liver transplantation and, 226, 227
　total parenteral nutrition and, 334
Metaclopramide, 343
Metaplastic esophageal mucosa, 119–120
Metastasis, 55, 59–60
　esophageal cancer and, 55, 59–60
　liver, 121
　　colon cancer and, 417
　　gastric cancer and, 126
　lymph node, 121–122
Methocholine, 29
Methotrexate, 310
Methyl-CCNU
　colon cancer and, 414
　gastric cancer and, 126
　failure of, 127
Methyl tertiary butyl ether
　bile duct stone and, 172
　gallstones and, 291–292
Metoclopramide, 71–72
Metronidazole, 384, 391–392
Microscopy of jejunal biopsy, 330–331
Mineral oil, 357
Mitocycin C
　esophageal cancer and, 59
　gastric cancer and, 127, 128
Mixed connective-tissue disease, 21
Monitoring, esophageal, 10–11
Monooctanoin
　bile duct stone and, 172
　gallstones and, 298–290
Monopolar cautery, 488–489
Morphine, 138
Motility disorder
　chronic pain and, 437
　esophageal
　　chest pain and, 4–5
　　lower esophageal sphincter and, 18
　　manometric criteria for, 6, 6
　　Raynaud's disease and, 21
　gastroparesis and, 65–73
Mucosa
　Barrett's esophagus and, 45
　gastric ulcer and, 88–94
　gastroesophageal reflux and, 21
　pyloric, 81–82

Mucosa (cont.)
  stress-related gastritis and, 74–79
  ulcerative proctitis and, 368–379
Mucous discharge, 389–393
Multipolar cautery, 489–490
Munchausen's syndrome
  chronic pain and, 434
  constipation and, 465–466
Muramyl tripeptide, 128
Muscle
  hypertrophy and, 28
  puborectalis, 350, 351
Muscle relaxant, 24–25
Musculoskeletal syndrome, 5
Mycobacterium avium-intracellulare, 454
Myocardial infarction, 162
Myoelectric activity, 437
Myotomy
  esophageal motility disorder and, 14
  modified Heller, 40–41

N

Nasogastric tube decompression, 114
Natriuretic factor, atrial, 219
Nd-YAG laser, 491–493
Necrosis, pancreatic, 136
  anatomic definition of, 182
  cholecystectomy and, 150
  pancreatitis and, 138, 145, 146–147
  percutaneous drainage and, 188–189
  treatment and, 154–156
Needle aspiration, 186–188
Neisseria gonorrhoeae, 452
Neodymium-yttrium-aluminum-garnet laser, 491–493
Neomycin, 403
Neoplasm; *see* Cancer
Nephrolithiasis, 335
Nerve block, 195
Nervous system, parasympathic, 462
Neurohumoral agents, 19
Neurologic disorder
  liver transplantation and, 237
  incontinence and, 351–352
    treatment and, 356
Neuromuscular disease, 68
Nifedipine
  achalasia and, 35–36
  esophageal motility disorder and, 24–25
Nissen fundoplication, 25
Nitrate, 14
Nitroglycerin
  achalasia and, 35
  esophageal motility disorder and, 14
  intestinal ischemia and, 362
Nitroprusside, 362
Nocturnal acid reflux, 23
Non-A, non-B hepatitis, 248
  immunization and, 272–273
Nonadherant dressing, 156
Noncardiac chest pain, 3–17; *see also* Chest pain
Nonerosive gastritis, 79–82
Non-narcotic analgesic, 193

Nonsteroidal anti-inflammatory drug
  drug-induced gastritis and, 77–79
  duodenal ulcer and, 104
  erosive gastritis and, 77–79, 79
  gastric ulcer and, 93
  hepatorenal syndrome and, 255
Nontoxic megacolon, 536–542
Nonulcer dyspepsia, 97–98
  chronic pain and, 434, 440
Norepinephrine, 218
5–Nucleotidase, 162
Nursing home patient, 454–455
Nutcracker esophagus
  irritable bowel syndrome and, 13
  manometry and, 6, 7
Nutrition
  bloating and, 343
  diarrhea and, 307
  gastroparesis and, 70
  pancreatic pain and, 193
  pancreatitis and, 153
  parenteral
    Crohn's disease and, 385
    short bowel syndrome and, 334–338
    toxic megacolon and, 398

O

Obesity, 523–527
Obliteration of varices, 508
Obstipation
  definition of, 458–460
  etiology and, 462–463
  evaluation of, 477–479
  mechanisms of, 466–477
  psychologic factors and, 463–466
  risks of, 460–462
  sigmoid volvulus and, 544
  treatment of, 479–480
Obstruction
  gastric volvulus and, 110–111
  gastroparesis and, 65–73
  ileal pouch-anal anastomosis and, 404–405
  pseudo, 536–542
Occult blood, 420–426
Oddi's sphincter; *see* Sphincter, of Oddi
Omeprazole, 97
Operant conditioning, 354
Organoaxial volvulus, 109
  complications and, 112
Osmotic diarrhea, 310

P

Pacemaker, aberrant distal antral, 68
Packing, pancreatitis and, 156
Pain
  abdominal angina and, 365–366
  chest, 3–17; *see also* Chest pain
  cholangitis and, 161
  chronic abdominal, 433–446
  pancreas divisum and, 202
  pancreatitis and, 134
  upper-quadrant, 317–325

Pancreas, 131–213
  cancer and, 207–213
  common bile duct stone and, 160–180; see also
      Common bile duct stone
  diarrhea and, 316
  necrosis and, 154–156
  pain and, 192–197
  pancreas divisum and, 198–206
  pancreatitis; see Pancreatitis
  pseudocyst and abscess and, 181–191
Pancreatectomy, 195
Pancreatic extract therapy, 193–194
  bloating and, 343
Pancreatitis
  alcohol abuse and, 133
    common bile duct stone and, 161
  anatomic definitions of, 181–182, 184, 186
  clinical course and, 135–136
  complications and, 136–137
  diagnosis and, 134, 148–151
  endoscopic sphincterotomy and, 555–556
  gallstones and, 174–175
  imaging and, 137–138
  laboratory tests and, 135
  management and, 153–158
  natural history of, 144, 146–148
  physical examination and, 134–135
  treatment and, 138–140, 151, 153
Papilla
  cannulation and, 198–201, 203
  endoscopic retrograde cholangiopancreatography
      and, 321
  endoscopic retrograde sphincterotomy and, 166
  manometry, 202
Papillotomy, 168
Paracentesis
  ascites and, 221
  hepatorenal syndrome and, 256–257
Paraesophageal hernia, 108, 110, 114–115
Parasite, 449
Parasympathetic innervation, 462
Parenteral nutrition; see Nutrition, parenteral
Partial thromboplastin time, 247
Pelvic floor muscle, 351
Pelvic pain, 434
Penicillamine, 251
Penicillin, 82
Peptic stricture, 21–22
Peptic ulcer
  Barrett's esophagus and, 45
  radiology and, 425
Peptide, vasoactive intestinal, 309, 314
Pepto-bismol; see Bismuth
Percutaneous aspiration cytology, 210–211
Percutaneous drainage, 181–191
Percutaneous transhepatic cholangiography
  common bile duct stone and, 163
  papillotome and, 169
Percutaneous transhepatic ultrasonic lithotripsy,
    171–172
Perforation
  duodenal ulcer and, 102
  endoscopic retrograde sphincterotomy and, 173
  esophageal dilation and, 39
  esophageal sclerotherapy and, 511
Perianastomotic sepsis, 404–405

Peripancreatic fat sequestra, 157–158
Peripancreatic necrosis, 148
Peritoneum
  dialysis and, 257
  gastric cancer and, 121, 126
  pancreatitis and, 138
  venous shunt and, 222
Peritoneovenous shunt, 259–260
Pernicious anemia, 80
pH
  achalasia and, 32
  esophagus and, 5, 7–9
Phenophthalein, 311
Phenothiazine, 71
Phlegmon, 181
pH monitoring, esophageal, 10–11, 13, 23
Phosphate enema, 357
Phospholipase A, 149
Pigment gallstone, 283–285
Pigtail catheter drainage, 188
Pirenzepine, 96
Placebo, 343
Plasma, paracentesis, 221
Platelet, 247
Pneumatic dilatation
  achalasia and, 41
  esophageal motility disorder and, 14
Pneumocystic carinii, 238
Polidocanol, 494
Polyacrylonitrile hemodialysis, 258
Polyp, 409
  adenomatous, 412
  colonoscopy and, 528–535
  gastric cancer and, 119
Polypeptide fiber, vasoactive intestinal, 29, 309, 314
Polyposis coli, 409
Portacaval shunt
  esophageal varices and, 512
  hepatorenal syndrome and, 260
  liver transplantation and, 228–229
Portal venous pressure, 499
Postcholecystectomy syndrome
  chronic pain and, 436
  upper-quadrant pain and, 317–325
Postexposure immunization for hepatitis, 266–267,
    272
Potassium, 218
Pouch, Kock, 406–408
Prazosin, 362
Prednisolone
  ascites and, 222
  hepatitis and, 250
Pre-exposure immunization for hepatitis, and, 267,
    269, 271–272
Pregnancy
  Crohn's disease and, 382
  heartburn and, 20
  hepatitis and, 251–252
Pressure
  esophageal, 13
  portal venous, 499
Probe, heater, 490–491
Prochlorperazine, 71
Proctitis, ulcerative, 368–379
Proctocolectomy
  Crohn's disease and, 389

Proctocolectomy *(cont.)*
    sclerosing cholangitis and, 310
Proctosigmoiditis, 368–379
Progesterone, 20
Prokinetic agent, 71–72
Propantheline bromide, 83
Prophylaxis
    duodenal ulcer and, 102
    esophageal varices and, 509–510
    stress-related gastritis and, 76–77
Propoxyphene, 193
Propranolol, 505
Prostaglandin
    ascites and, 219
    duodenal ulcer and, 96
    gastritis and, 76, 79
Protein, 333
Prothrombin time
    common bile duct stone and, 162
    hepatitis and, 247
Provocative testing
    esophagus and, 7–9
    gastroesophageal reflux and, 24
    postcholecystectomy syndrome and, 323
Pseudoachalasia, 33–34
    cancer and, 31
Pseudocyst
    pancreatic, 141, 145
        pancreatitis and, 147, 157–158, 181–186
        percutaneous drainage and, 189–190
        radiography and, 186–188
Pseudomembranous colitis, 454–455
Pseudo-obstruction
    colonic, 473–476, 536–542
    neuromuscular disorder and, 68
Pseudosyndrome, abdominal, 435–436
Pseudotumor, 364–365
Psychologic factors
    chronic pain and, 438–439
    obstipation and, 463–466
Psychotropic drug, 14, 15
PTT; *see* Partial thromboplastin time
Puborectalis muscle
    continence and, 350
    fecal incontinence and, 351
Pullup, gastric, 58
Pulmonary disorder; *see* Respiratory disorder
Pyloroduodenal dysmotility, 437–438
Pylorus
    atrophic gastritis and, 80, 81–82
    gastroparesis and, 65, 67

R

Radiation
    esophageal cancer and, 58–61
    pancreatic cancer and, 212
    proctitis and, 371, 372
Radiography
    achalasia and, 30
    barium contrast, 23
    Barrett's esophagus, 46
    colonic pseudo-obstruction and, 536–537
        decompression and, 541
    intestinal ischemia and, 362
    needle aspiration of pancreas and, 186–188
    pancreatitis and, 149
    toxic megacolon and, 395
Radionuclide imaging
    achalasia and, 30–31
    gastroparesis and, 69
    massive rectal bleeding and, 428
    scintigraphy and, 23
    upper gastrointestinal series and, 425
Ranitidine
    duodenal ulcer and, 96, 98
    gastritis and, 76
    gastroesophageal reflux and, 25
    side effects of, 102
Raynaud's disease and, 21
Realimentation, 70–71
Rectal disorder
    cancer and, 528–535
        Crohn's disease and, 386
        obstipation and, 460
    fecal incontinence and, 351–352
        treatment and, 356
    massive bleeding and, 427–432
    occult blood loss and, 422–424
    reservoir capacity and, 350–351
    stricture and, 387
    ulcerative proctitis and, 368–379
Rectal tube, 548–549
Rectosphincteric dyssenergia, 469–473
Rectovaginal fistula, 390
Recurrence
    duodenal ulcer and, 98–99
    gastric ulcer and, 92
    ulcerative proctitis and, 374
Red color signs, 501–502
Red scarring, 92
Reflex, anorectal, 478
Reflux
    esophageal motility disorder and, 14
    gastroesophageal, 18–27
    postoperative esophagitis and, 40–41
    test of, 23
    vesicoureteral, 460
Regional enteritis, 307
Regurgitation, 29
Renal disorder
    ascites and, 217
    common bile duct stone and, 162
    hepatorenal syndrome and, 253
    pancreatitis and, 136, 138
    paracentesis and, 222
Renin-angiotensin system, 218
Respiratory disorder
    esophageal sclerotherapy and, 512
    liver transplantation and, 237
    pancreatitis and, 138
    toxicty of chemotherapy agents and, 60
Restitution, epithelial, 78
Retransplantation, liver, 236
Retrograde cholangiopancreatography; *see* Endoscopic retrograde cholangiopancreatography
Rotation, gastric volvulus and, 108–116
Roux-en-Y reconstruction, 81

S

Salicylate
  gastritis and, 77
  toxic megacolon and, 398–399
  ulcerative colitis and, 376
Saline sclerotherapy, 494
Salivary amylase, 135
Salmonella
  colitis and, 454
  ulcerative proctitis and, 370
Schilling test, 315
Scintigraphy
  gastroesophageal reflux and, 23
  gastroparesis and, 69
Scleroderma
  esophagus and, 20–21
  gastroparesis and, 67
Sclerosing cholangitis, 298–304
  liver transplantation and, 230
Sclerotherapy
  esophageal varices and, 506–512
    surgery and, 513–514
  nonvariceal lesions and, 493–495
Secretin-cholecystokinin-PZ test, 316
Secretin-stimulated dorsal pancreatic juice, 202–203
Secretin ultrasound test, 202
Secretion, acid; see Acid secretion
Secretory diarrhea, 309, 310
Sedation, 292
Sengstaken-Blakemore tube, 506
Sepsis; see Infection
Sequestra, fat, 148, 157–158
Serine protease, 193
Serum alkaline phosphatase, 162
Serum amylase
  common bile duct stone and, 162
  pancreatitis and, 135, 148–149
Serum lipase, 148–149
Sexually transmitted disease, 450
SGOT, 162
SGPT, 275–276
Shigella
  elderly patient and, 454
  traveler's diarrhea and, 452
  ulcerative proctitis and, 370
Shock
  intestinal ischemia and, 362
  pancreatitis and, 136
Short bowel syndrome, 332–340
Shunt
  esophageal varices and, 512–513
  peritoneal venous, 222, 259–260
  portacaval
    hepatorenal syndrome and, 260
    liver transplantation and, 228–229
Sigmoid esophagus, 30
Sigmoidoscopy
  colon ischemia and, 364
  infectious colitis and, 450
  massive rectal bleeding and, 428
  occult blood and, 423
Sigmoid volvulus, 543–550
Simethicone, 343

Small intestine, 304–345
  biopsy and, 326–331
  diarrhea and, 307–316; see also Diarrhea
  gas and, 341–345
  nontoxic megacolon and, 537–538
  short bowel syndrome and, 332–340
  upper-quadrant pain and, 317–325
Smoking, 97, 105
Smooth muscle relaxant, 24–25
SO; see Sphincter, of Oddi
Sodium
  ascites and, 217, 220
  hepatorenal syndrome and, 256
  paracentesis and, 222
Solid test meal, 69
Solitary rectal ulcer syndrome, 371–372
Somatostatin, 505
Sorbitol, 307
Spasm, esophageal, 4–6
Spastic pelvic floor syndrome, 469–473
Sphincter; see also Sphincterotomy
  anal
    continence and, 349–350
    electromyography and, 478
    ileal pouch-anal anastomosis and, 405
  lower esophageal
    achalasia and, 28
    assessment of, 23–24
    gastric cancer and, 119
    gastroesophageal reflux and, 18
    incompetence of, 19–20
  of Oddi
    dysfunction and, 322–323
    gallstone pancreatitis and, 174
    manometry and, 320–322, 318
Sphincteric disobedience syndrome, 469–473
Sphincterotomy, 551–557
  chronic pain and, 442
  common bile duct stone and, 176
  endoscopic retrograde
    cimetidine and, 163, 164–169
    gallstone pancreatitis and, 174
    prophylactic and, 176
    intact gallbladder and, 175–176
  papilla, 203–204
Spina bifida, 352–353, 357
Splanchnic vessels, 365–366
Spleen, gastrectomy and, 124
Splenectomy
  hepatitis and, 246
  pancreatic necrosis and, 155–156
Splenic flexure syndrome, 435
Squamous mucosa, 45
Stapling, 58
Static dilatation, 14
Steatorrhea
  pancreatic enzyme and, 193
  short bowel syndrome and, 338
Stent
  common bile duct stone and, 176
  pancreas divisum and, 202, 203
Sterile pancreatic necrosis, 188–189
Sterile pseudocyst, 189
Steroid, 398
Stimulation, electrical, 319

Stomach, 65–130; see also Gastric entries
  gastric ulcers and, 88–94
  gastric volvulus and, 108–110
  gastritis and, 74–87
  gastroparesis and, 65–73
  glandular carcinoma and, 117–130; see also Gastric carcinoma
Stone
  common bile duct; see Common bile duct stone
  gallstone and; see Gallstone
  uric acid, 335
Stool
  blood test and
    colon cancer and, 411
    positive, 420–426
  examination of, 312–314
  infectious colitis and, 449
Stress-related gastric erosion, 74–77
Stress ulcer, 153
Stricture
  Crohn's disease and, 387
  esophageal sclerotherapy and, 511
  gastroesophageal reflux and, 21–22
Substernal burning, 4–5
Sucralfate
  anti-inflammatory drug and, 79
  duodenal ulcer and, 96
  gastric ulcer and, 91
  stress-related gastritis and, 76
Sulfalazine, 376
Sulfasalazine, 383
Supperative cholangitis, 552–555
Surgery
  abdominal, liver transplantation and, 228
  achalasia and, 40–41
  anal sphincter and, 351
  antireflux, 50–52
  ascites and, 222
  common bile duct stone and, 163–164
  Crohn's disease and, 385
    perineal, 392–393
  esophageal cancer and, 57–58
    chemotherapy and, 60–61
  esophageal motility disorder and, 14
  esophageal varices and, 512–514
  gastric ulcer and, 92
  gastric volvulus and, 114
  pancreas divisum and, 204
  pancreatic cancer and, 211–212
  pancreatic pain and, 195
  rectal, 549–550
  sclerosing cholangitis and, 301
  toxic megacolon and, 400
Surrogate market, 275–276
Swallow, barium
  Barrett's esophagus and, 46
  gastroesophageal reflux and, 24
Syphilis, 453

T

Tachygastria, 68
Tamponade, esophageal varices and, 505–506
Technetium-99m, 428
Tensilon test, 8–9

Tetracycline, 82
Thermal therapy, 488–493
Thiethylperazine, 71
Thromboplastin time, partial, 247
Thrombosis
  hepatic artery, 237–238
  hepatic vein, 231
Tinidazole, 100
Tomography
  applied impedance, 69
  computerized; see Computerized tomography
Tonic contraction, 29
Tonometry, 366
Torsion, 108–110
Total parenteral nutrition
  short bowel syndrome and, 333, 334–338
  toxic megacolon and, 398
Toxicity, cyclosporine, 238
Toxic megacolon, 394–401
  Crohn's disease and, 386
Trace mineral deficiency, 334–335
Tracheal-bronchial tree, 59–60
Tracheal invasion of esophageal cancer, 55, 59–60
Transfusion, 503
  hepatitis and, 273–276
Transhepatic percutaneous cholangiography, 163
Transit time, obstipation and, 477–479
Transplantation, liver; see Liver, transplantation and
Trauma
  anal sphincter and, 351
  gastric volvulus and, 111
Traveler's diarrhea, 451–452
Trazodone, 14, 15
Triazinate, 128
Tricyclic antidepressant
  chronic pain and, 442
  duodenal ulcer and, 96
Triglycyl vasopressin, 505
Tripotassium dicitratobismuthate, 100–101
Trypanosoma cruzi, 28
Trypsinogen, 149
T-tube cholangiogram, 164, 175
Tube
  colonic pseudo-obstruction and, 540–541
  nasogastric, 114
  rectal, 548–549
Tube feeding, 336
Tumor, carcinoid, 80–81; see also Cancer
Tyrosinemia, 232

U

UDCA-CDCA, 292–294
Ulcer
  duodenal, 95–107
  endoscopic therapy and, 487–497
  erosive gastritis and, 74–79
  esophagus and, 21
    sclerotherapy and, 511
  gastric, 88–94
    antral and acid-bearing mucosa and, 120
    cancer and, 118–119
  gastric bubble and, 525
  peptic, 425
    Barrett's esophagus and, 45

stress, 153
Ulcerative colitis
  diarrhea and, 307
  sclerosing cholangitis and, 298
  surgery outcomes and, 409
Ulcerative proctitis, 368–379
Ultrafiltration, 257
Ultrasound
  common bile duct stone and, 164
    lithotripsy and, 171–172
  liver transplantation and, 237
  pancreas divisum and, 202
  pancreatic abscess and, 156–157
  pancreatitis and, 137–138, 149
Upper gastrointestinal series
  bleeding and, 424–426
  esophageal pain and, 11
  gastric ulcer and, 89
  gastric volvulus and, 113
  gastroparesis and, 68
Upper gastrointestinal tract bleeding, 487–497
Upper-quadrant pain, 317–325
Uric acid stone, 335
Urinary tract infection, 460
Urine, 254–255
Urodeoxycholic acid, 285–289

V

Vagotomy, 309
Varices, esophageal; see Esophageal varices
Vascular disease
  bleeding and, 430–431
  short bowel syndrome and, 333
Vasoactive intestinal peptide, 309, 314
  achalasia and, 29
Vasopressin
  ascites and, 219
  esophageal varices and, 504–505
Vasopressor, 362
Vein, hepatic, 231
Venous pressure, portal, 499
Venous shunt, peritoneal, 222
Verapamil, 35
Vesicoureteral reflux, 460
Villous lesion, 328, 329

Vinblastine, 59
Vinca alkaloid, 59
Violaceous discoloration, 390
VIP; see Vasoactive intestinal polypeptide
Virus
  hepatitis and; see Hepatitis
  liver transplantation and, 237, 238
Vitamin B_{12}, 80, 81
Volume expander, 256
Volvulus
  gastric, 108–110
  short bowel syndrome and, 333
  sigmoid, 543–550
VP-16, 128

W

Water; see Fluid
Weight loss
  esophageal cancer and, 57
  gastric bubble and, 523–527
White scarring, 92
Wilson's disease
  liver transplantation and, 231–232
  treatment of, 251

X

d-Xylose test, 316
  abdominal angina and, 366

Y

Yersinia
  infectious colitis and, 450
  traveler's diarrhea and, 452
  ulcerative proctitis and, 370

Z

Zollinger-Ellison syndrome, 314, 316

THE OTTO C. BRANTIGAN, M.D.
MEDICAL LIBRARY
SAINT JOSEPH HOSPITAL
7620 YORK ROAD
TOWSON, MD. 21204